PERIODONTOLOGY AND PERIODONTICS:
Modern Theory and Practice

NOTICE

Dentistry is an ever-changing science. As new research and clinical experience broaden our knowledge, changes in treatment are required. The authors and the publisher of this work have made every effort to ensure that the procedures herein are accurate and in accord with the standards accepted at the time of publication.

PERIODONTOLOGY AND PERIODONTICS: Modern Theory and Practice

Sigurd P. Ramfjord, L.D.S., M.S., Ph.D.
Professor of Dentistry, Emeritus
Department of Periodontology

Major M. Ash, Jr., B.S., D.D.S., M.S.
Marcus L. Ward Professor of Dentistry
Department of Periodontology

University of Michigan
School of Dentistry
Ann Arbor, Michigan

Ishiyaku EuroAmerica, Inc.
St. Louis • Tokyo

Book Editor: Gregory Hacke, D.C.
Index Editor: Stephen Graef, M.M.
Graphic Design: Ray Mangin

Ishiyaku EuroAmerica, Inc.
716 Hanley Industrial Court, St. Louis, Missouri 63144

Library of Congress Catalogue Card Number 89-83509

ISBN 0-912791-40-3

Ishiyaku EuroAmerica, Inc.
St. Louis • Tokyo

Composition by Graphic World, Inc.
St. Louis, Missouri
Printed in Japan

PREFACE

The main objective of the present book is to provide a compiled source of scientific knowledge on periodontics for anyone concerned with periodontal health and disease—from patients, students, hygienists, and general dentists, to periodontists and insurance carriers. In order to reach this goal within a book of manageable length, much of the style is compact with abundant selected references to be used if the reader wants to evaluate and go into greater depth.

Much progress has been made both in the science and in the art of periodontics in the last decade, which means that outmoded concepts and procedures have to be left behind. These advances may mean a radical change in philosophy and clinical practice for many. If surgical pocket elimination, soft tissue curettage, and bone surgery have been proved to be misguided efforts, why carry these procedures along in practice and insurance coverage?

The responsibility of teachers to patients and the dental profession has directed us always to avoid the teaching of experimental procedures until they have been proven safe and valuable by long-term, well-controlled clinical trials. This approach goes for chemical treatments and for a number of existing "regenerative procedures." As long as well-established, safe and successful procedures are available, they should be given preference.

Interest in maintaining natural dentition for psychological and functional reasons is increasing rapidly, and the information presented in this book should be of significant help in reaching that goal.

We wish to acknowledge the assistance of Professor William Brudon for rendering our sketches into meaningful illustrations; the library reference assistance given by librarians Sue Seger and Ruth Cressman; the considerable help of Marian Brockie and Joanne Kazluaskas in typing the manuscript; and the editorial assistance of Dr. Greg Hacke.

Sigurd P. Ramfjord
Major M. Ash, Jr.

CONTENTS

PERIODONTAL STRUCTURES

Periodontium literally means "around the tooth." Several variations of this word were used by G.V. Black (1887) to designate the "periodontal membrane" and "periosteum of the tooth."[3] The word was commonly used when the American Academy of Periodontology was founded in 1914, but the modern concept of the periodontium as a functional system originated with Weski in 1921.[11] This functional system, which receives the impact of mechanical function of the teeth, includes the gingiva (both attached and free gingiva, including the epithelial attachment), the periodontal membrane, the cementum, and the alveolar bone.

Pathological processes originating in and affecting the function of the periodontium are called *periodontal diseases*. Conventionally, neoplastic, dermatologic, and metabolic diseases affecting the periodontium are not designated as periodontal diseases.

The science that deals with the structures and behavior of the periodontium in health and in disease is called *periodontology*, and the branch of denistry concerned with prevention and treatment of periodontal disease is termed *periodontics* or *periodontia*.

PERIODONTAL STRUCTURES

Gingiva

The *gingiva* refers to the fibrous connective tissue and mucosa surrounding the teeth and covering the coronal portion of the alveolar process. The marginal part of the gingiva that can be deflected from the tooth surface is called the *free gingiva* or *marginal gingiva*, and the coronal border of the free gingiva is called the *free gingival margin* or the *gingival crest* (Fig. 1-1). The free gingiva is attached at the tooth surface as junctional epithelium, which forms the base of the

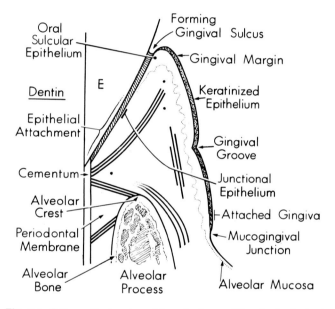

Fig. 1-1. Schematic drawing of the gingiva and the dentogingival junction.

gingival sulcus. In probing with a thin probe (Fig. 1-2) or deflecting the free gingiva from the tooth, the tendency is for the probing or the separation to extend close to the fiber attachment to the tooth at the base of the junctional epithelium. The depth of this gingival crevice when assessed with a thin probe is 1 to 2 millimeters (mm) buccally and lingually and 2 to 3 mm interproximally.[7] There may be no well-defined anatomical boundary of the oral surface of the free gingiva in an apical direction.[8] However, a slight linear depression in the mucosa (parallel to the free gingival margin) called the *free gingival groove*[9] may be present in about 33% of persons with normal gingivae.[1] This gingival groove, when present, is located about 1.0 to 1.5 mm from the free gingival margin[1,9] and corresponds

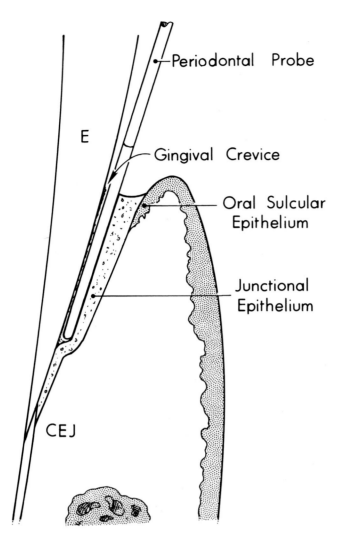

E

Periodontal Probe

Gingival Crevice

Oral Sulcular Epithelium

Junctional Epithelium

CEJ

Fig. 1-2. Schematic representation of periodontal probe and crevice.

roughly to the clinically measurable bottom of the gingival crevice.

The interproximal gingival tissues are called *gingival* or *interproximal papillae* and may be considered as part of the free gingiva. With teeth making interproximal contacts, the interdental tissues extend almost to the contact areas of the teeth, and with convex interproximal tooth surfaces on posterior teeth there often appear to be a buccal and a lingual papilla with a slight depression, a saddle or "col"[5] area between the papillae (Fig. 1-3).

Attached gingiva. The firm part of the gingiva that extends apically to the free gingiva is called *attached gingiva* because it is attached firmly to the buccal and lingual alveolar processes and to the neck of the teeth. The apical border of the attached gingiva is demarcated by the mucogingival junction or line, indicating the coronal extent of the soft, movable alveolar mucosa, which is not part of the periodontium.

The width of the attached gingiva varies widely among different teeth and jaws.[1,4] The widest zone of attached gingiva is found in the anterior regions and decreases from the cuspids distally. The narrowest zone of attached gingiva is on the buccal aspect of the mandibular first bicuspids,[4] while the widest zone is in the maxillary anterior region. On the lingual aspect in the mandible it is 3 to 4 mm wide, while in the palate there is no distinguishing anatomical feature between the attached gingiva and the palatal mucosa. The width of the attached gingiva tends to increase with age if there is no gingival recession.[2] It appears that the position of the mucogingival line relative to the lower border of the mandible is constant with time, so that the attached gingiva increases in width with compensatory eruption of the teeth.[2] A band of keratinized attached gingiva does not appear to be essential for the maintenance of a disease-free periodontium.[6]

Periodontal membrane

The fibrous attachment system of the teeth to the bone is called the *periodontal membrane* or *periodontal ligament*. This structure has both a membranous and a ligamentous function. Anatomically, it has a rich vascularity that is not found in true ligaments, and its function is in part hydrodynamic. Therefore, we prefer the term *periodontal membrane* to *periodontal ligament*. Like the tissues between the tooth and the bone, the various gingival fiber structures also help attach the tooth to the bone.

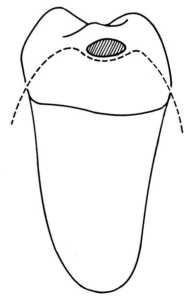

Fig. 1-3. Schematic drawing with the interproximal dip in the broken line indicating the "col" between the buccal and lingual papillae.

Alveolar bone

The wall of the bone housing of the tooth is called *alveolar bone* or *cribriform plate* because it is penetrated by numerous holes for vascular supply to the periodontal membrane. The rest of the bone that makes up the alveolar process is called *supporting bone,* or simply *alveolar process.* This bone is not considered to be part of the periodontium. The coronal margin of the alveolar bone is called the alveolar crest; it normally is located 1 mm from the cementoenamel junction of the teeth. The periodontal fibers are anchored to the alveolar bone by partially calcified Sharpey's fibers entering the bone in relatively heavy bundles, while the attachment to the cementum, also by Sharpey's fibers, is mediated by a large number of smaller fiber bundles surrounded and partially penetrated by apatite crystals, which are mainly arranged parallel to the long axis of the fibers.

REFERENCES

1. Ainamo, J., and Löe, H.: Anatomical characteristics of gingiva. A clinical and microscopic study of the free and attached gingiva, J. Periodont. 37:5, 1966.
2. Ainamo, J., and Talari, A.: The increase with age of the width of attached gingiva, J. Periodont, Res. 11:182, 1976.
3. Black, G.V.: A Study of the Histological Characters of the Periosteum and Periodontal Membrane, Chicago: W.T. Kenner, 1887.
4. Bowers, G.M.: A study of the width of attached gingiva, J. Periodont. 34:201, 1963.
5. Cohen, B.: Morphological factors in the pathogenesis of periodontal disease, Br. Dent. J. 107:31, 1959.
6. Dorfman, S., et al: Longitudinal evaluation of free autogenous gingival grafts. A four year report, J. Periodontol. 53:349, 1982.
7. Fuder, E.J., and Jamison, H. C.: Depth of gingival sulcus surrounding young permanent teeth, J. Periodont. 34:457, 1963.
8. Lang, N.P., and Löe, H.: The relationship between the width of keratinized gingiva and gingival health, J. Periodont. 43:623, 1972.
9. Orban, B.: Clinical and histologic study of surface characteristics of the gingivae, Oral Surg. 1:827, 1948.
10. Wenneström, J., et al: The role of keratinized gingiva in plaque associated gingivitis in dogs, J. Clin. Periodontol. 9:75, 1982.
11. Weski, O.: Rontgenologisch - Anatomische Studien aus dem Gebiete der Kieferpatholoogie. II. Die chronischen marginalen Entzundungen des Alveolarfortsatzes mit besonderer Beruchsichtung der Alveolar-Pyorrhoe, Viertel. J. Schr. f. Zahnheilk. 37:1, 1921.

The *periodontal epithelium* consists of the keratinized surface epithelium, the sulcular and junctional epithelium, and Malassez's epithelial rests. The keratinized gingival epithelium, the oral sulcular epithelium, and the junctional epithelium provide a barrier to the entrance of bacteria into the underlying connective tissues. The epithelium and the intracellular attachment mechanisms, as well as their attachment to the tooth structure, are important to the defense against bacteria and their antigenic and toxic products, which continually challenge the dento-gingival junction.

GINGIVAL SURFACE EPITHELIUM

The outer or oral surface of the gingiva, termed the *masticatory gingiva*, is covered by squamous epithelium with varying degrees of keratinization. The surface has a pitted appearance or texture, called "stippling."[14] This stippling is more prominent on the labial than on the lingual surfaces, and in adults more than in children, but it may disappear in old age. It usually stops slightly short of the free gingival margin, but, in persons who vigorously practice oral hygiene, the stippling may extend to the free gingival margin and the tip of the interdental papillae (Fig. 2-1).

In the stippled area, the bottoms of the pits correspond to deep ridges or projections of epithelium into lamina propria of the connective tissue (Fig. 2-2). The protruding parts of the stippling correspond to thinner epithelium over ridges or projections of the connective tissue. In histological sections, the epithelial projections resemble pegs and have been called *rete pegs*. The biological significance of stippling is not known, but the ridge-and-peg arrangements between the epithelium and the connective tissues provide excellent mechanical stability between the two tissue

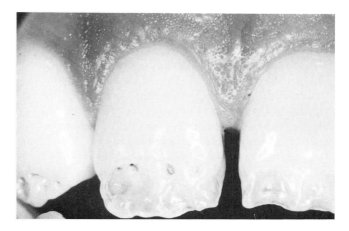

Fig. 2-1. Picture of gingival stippling extending to the free gingival margin. Vigorous toothbrushing with hard toothbrush in young women.

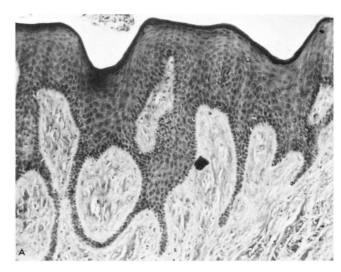

Fig. 2-2. Histological section of heavily keratinized and stippled attached gingiva. Note that dips in the surface correspond to epithelial projections ("rete pegs") within the connective tissue.

components, as well as a large contact interphase for metabolic interchange.

Histologically, the surface epithelium of the gingiva exhibits the common structural arrangement of keratinized, stratified squamous mucosa: (1) stratum basale or basal cell layer; (2) stratum spinosum or spinocellular layer; (3) stratum granulosum or granular layer; and (4) stratum corneum, which has various degrees of keratinization.

Epithelial cell ultrastructure

The cell has a nucleus composed of nucleoplasm (karyoplasm) surrounded by protoplasm (cytoplasm) and is confined within a cell membrane (plasmalemma). Every living cell is enclosed by a plasma membrane that selectively regulates the flow of nutrients and ions between the interior of the cell and its external environment. Most of the metabolic processes take place at the surfaces and interfaces of these membranes. Within the nucleus and cytoplasm are a number of structures called *organelles*, including those involved in cell division, formation of proteins, production of energy, and production of enzymes.

Lysosomes are the cytoplasmic organelle complex that has received most attention in periodontology. A large number of acid hydrolases have been identified from lysosomal fractions. Lysosomes retain their hydrolytic enzymes inside a single membrane until some membrane-active agent, such as testosterone, irradiation, or endotoxins, injures the membrane. As the enzymes are released, lytic activity is initiated. These enzymes play an active role in the breakdown of injured cells and the intracellular lysis of phagocytized bacteria or other foreign matters.

Basement lamina. Through the light microscope it appears that the basal epithelial cells rest on a PAS positive (periodic acid-Schiff), 1 to 2 micrometers (μm) thick, basement membrane, which was assumed to act as a gluing ground substance interphase between the epithelium and the connective tissue. However, studies using the electron microscope have revealed that the basement lamina has at least two or more components, and this junctional region as seen by electron microscopy does not entirely correspond to the basement membrane seen by light microscopy.[5] The boundary membrane observed in electron microscopy has an outer dense zone towards the connective tissue, called *lamina densa*, and an inner electronlucent zone close to the epithelium, called *lamina lucida*. Both these zones together are called *basement lamina* (Fig. 2-3). The lamina densa is about 30 to 60 nanometers (nm) thick, and is composed of a dense granular stroma and a system of fine filaments that extend from the connective tissue through the lamina lucida to the cell membrane of the basal cells. Lamina lucida is a less dense homogenous zone (30 to 50 nm

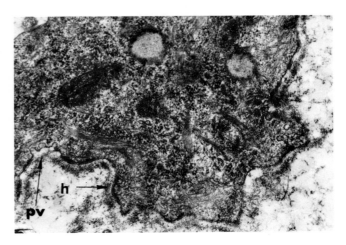

Fig. 2-3. Basal surface of basal cell and electron microscopic basement lamina. Pinocytotic vesicles (*pv*) and hemidesmosomes (*h*) are distributed irregularly along the basement lamina. Human gingiva. Original magnification, ×34,000.

wide) between the lamina densa and the cell wall of the basal cells.[4]

The basement membrane is not penetrated by blood or lymph vessels. All metabolic interchanges must therefore be mediated through this membranous structure, which may be altered greatly by inflammation.

Cell junctions. Electron microscope studies have established that epithelial cells are not held together by cell bridges with cytoplasmic continuity; rather, opposing extensions of cell membranes are held together by *desmosomes* (connecting bodies) (Fig. 2-4). The desmosomes[7] are bipartite lamellated structures on opposing cell membranes. They appear as thickening of the surface of the cell membrane, surrounded by a layer of fine filaments that are embedded in a condensation of the cytoplasmic matrix, and with surface attachment plaques. The distance between the two opposing attachment plaques is 35 to 39 nm. These types of junctions also have been called "spot" desmosomes because they hold the cells together in the fashion of spot welds.[33]

Half- or hemidesmosomes attach the basal epithelial cells to the basement membrane and the connective tissue. The hemidesmosome has only 1 attachment plaque, about 20 nm thick. This plaque is in contact with the inner leaflet of the cell membrane and a peripheral density in the lamina lucida close to the plaque.[34] The anchorage of the hemidesmosomes to the lamina lucida appears to be relatively strong, and persists even with inflammation. The nature of this attachment is assumed to be similar to that of the attachment between regular desmosomes.

A second type of cell junction is called a *tight junc-*

tion. In the region of a tight junction, the plasma membranes of two adjacent epithelial cells appear to fuse, providing an area of intimate contact that completely encircles each cell.[7] The two plasma membranes are not actually cemented together but fused at a series of points.[33]

A third type of junction is the *gap junction.* The intercellular spaces in gap junctions are narrowed to about 3 nm instead of the normal width of 25 nm. The gap junctions have intercellular pipes or channels that apparently bridge both the adjacent membranes and the intercellular space.[2] Gap junctions apparently are also the major pathways for direct intercellular communication.

Cell types

About 90% of the gingival epithelial cells are keratin-forming cells (keratinocytes). The remainder of the cells, which lack desmosomes and other junctional complexes, are referred to as *nonkeratinocytes* or *clear cells.* In the stratum spinosum, the nuclei have more

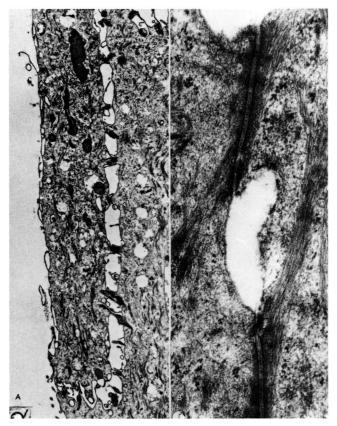

Fig. 2-4. *A,* Superficial crevicular cells with marked intracellular degeneration but with persistence of desmosomes. Original magnification, × 8400. *B,* Intercellular area from superficial crevicular epithelium. Typical desmosomes with tonofilaments inserting into the inner leaflets of the attachment plaques. Original magnification, × 57,000.

indentations than in the basal cells. There is a smaller nucleus-to-cytoplasm ratio, possibly due to a shrinkage in size of the nuclei. The intercellular spaces are wider and the cell junctions more frequent than in the basal cell layer. In the stratum granulosum, the nuclei are elongated and often pyknotic. Desmosomes, tight junctions, and intermediate or gap junctions are numerous, but the interproximal spaces are more narrow than in the stratum spinosum.

In highly keratinized epithelium, as in the palate, the intercellular spaces are more narrow. The desmosomes may be modified so that attachment plaques cannot be identified. Tight junctions and the modified desmosomes appear close to the surface.[34]

The nonkeratinocytes of the gingival epithelium are (1) melanocytes, (2) Langerhans' cells, and (3) nonspecific cells. All three types are dendritic in appearance, with branched cytoplasmic processes.

The melanocytes are characterized by melanin granules (melanosomes), which sometimes may also be observed in keratinocytes, but which presumably are formed in melanocytes. Melanocytes may be classified as active or inactive, depending on presence or absence of mature melanosomes. They are found in both light- and dark-skinned individuals. Both melanin-producing and melanin-containing cells may be present without any clinical evidence of gingival pigmentation.

The Langerhans' cells are identifiable by their rod-shaped bodies and gold-chloride-positive granules. Langerhans cells are immunologically competent keratinocytes that appear to react with T helper cells (lymphocytes) and perhaps with Granstein cells (another type of dendritic antigen-presenting cell). Granstein cells react similarly with suppressor T cells to maintain a positive balance in the immune response of lymphocytes to potentially harmful invaders. Their presence in keratinized gingiva may relate to the protective/destructive effects of immune responses in periodontal disease. The nonspecific third type of dendritic cells has basic morphological features similar to those of melanocytes and the Langerhans' cells, but lacks the specific identifying characteristics of those cells. These clear cells, or dendritic nonkeratinocytes, are found in the basal and spinocellular layers, but have not been observed in the granular and keratinized layers of the gingiva.

Metabolism of keratinocytes. The four cell layers of keratinizing gingiva (basal, spinous, granular, and corneal) represent stages of histogenesis in a system of histodifferentiation starting at the basal cell layer. The keratinocytes go through a migration and transformation cycle from basal cells until they are desquamated as keratin "ghost cells" without visible nuclei, or as parakeratotic cells with pyknotic nuclei and a keratinized cytoplasm.

The role of genetic programming versus environmental factors in cell migration and cytodifferentiation to keratin is not fully known. However, cell mitosis and renewal migration rate can be altered by environmental factors. According to tritiated thymidine studies, the average renewal time for gingival surface epithelium in mammals such as marmoset monkeys is about 10 days.[32] The time is assumed to be similar for humans. Mechanical stimulation, mild irritation and inflammation, and hormones such as estrogen and testosterone will increase mitotic rate, while hypoglycemia, cortisone, and nutritional disturbances may decrease mitotic rate and cell turnover.

It is not known what determines the degree of keratinization locally, nor why some cells complete their life cycle with parakeratosis while other cells go through complete keratinization. Clinically, it appears that parakeratosis is associated with gingival inflammation, while keratosis indicates a noninflammatory state. It has been shown that keratinization of the gingiva can be increased by mechanical surface stimulation,[12] but no biochemical explanation has been established for this phenomenon.

DENTO-GINGIVAL JUNCTION

The dento-gingival junction is an anatomical and functional interface between the gingiva and tooth structure. Of particular interest is the development of the gingival sulcus and the presence of junctional epithelum. Together, these provide for the attachment of the gingiva to the enamel surface via hemidesmosomes.

When the crown of an unerupted tooth is completely formed, it is covered by reduced enamel epithelium. The cells joining the enamel surface still have the columnar shape of ameloblasts arranged perpendicular to the surface, but they appear to be inactive with regard to cell division, as are the rest of the cells making up the reduced enamel epithelium. Only very rarely will a single cell of the outer layer of this epithelium (where it contacts the connective tissue) take up tritiated thymidine, providing an indication of initiated cell division.

Development

Just before the reduced enamel epithelium comes in contact with the oral epithelium during tooth eruption, the mitotic activity in the basal cells of the oral epithelium at the cusp tips of the erupting teeth decreases. At the same time, the approaching reduced enamel epithelium in the basal cell layer close to the cusp tip starts to display high mitotic activity.

After the erupting cusp tip has become exposed in the oral cavity, it is surrounded by a shallow sulcus ending in the still attached reduced enamel epithelium and bordered orally by the free gingival margin.

This margin is covered by parakeratotic oral epithelium. As the tooth erupts, one can clearly distinguish 2 epithelial structures facing the tooth. One is a sulcular nonkeratinized squamous epithelium, and the other is a residual reduced enamel epithelium still attached to the tooth (Fig. 2-5). It appears that, as the tooth erupts, the reduced enamel epithelium is gradually replaced through proliferation of its basal cells as these cells become stimulated following partial exposure of the tooth in the oral cavity.[18,32]

As the reduced enamel epithelium is replaced through cell proliferation, the new epithelium joining the tooth surface is called *junctional epithelium*.[30] The attachment of this epithelium to the tooth surface is called the *epithelial attachment*.

Ultimately, under controlled conditions in which plaque irritants do not cause inflammation (e.g., in germ-free animals), the junctional epithelium extends from the cementoenamel junction to the free gingival margin. Thus, under ideal conditions, the gingival sulcus approaches a depth of zero. The base of the gingival sulcus is the junctional epithelium.

In one study, the change from reduced enamel epithelium to junctional epithelium was reported to be complete when the teeth reached functional occlusion,[5] while in other studies reduced enamel epithelium has been observed as long as 1 to 2 years following

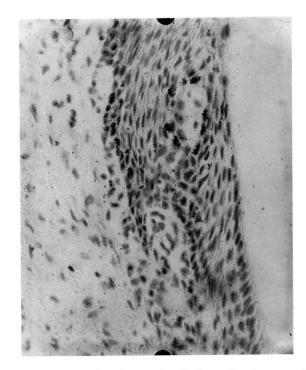

Fig. 2-5. *Bottom,* reduced enamel epithelium with columnar cells (residual ameloblasts) at bottom half of picture. *Top,* squamous epithelial cells from proliferating basal cells have replaced the reduced ameloblasts (monkey).

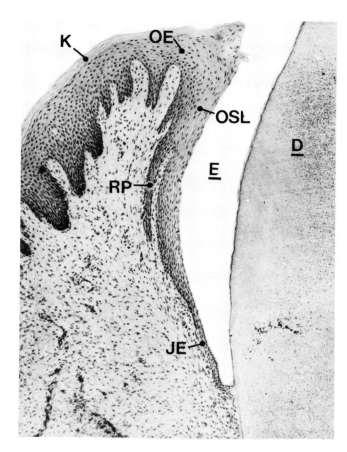

Fig. 2-6. Healthy gingiva of a monkey. Minimal inflammation. Rete peg (*RP*) projection from sulcus epithelium. *D* is dentin; *JE* is junctional epithelium; *K* is keratinized surface of gingiva; *OE* is oral epithelium; *E* is enamel space; and *OSE* is oral sulcular epithelium.

the eruption of the teeth.[30] The rate at which this conversion takes place may depend on stimulation from inflammation and function as well as on anatomical variations in the surrounding structures and their relation to the teeth.

It has been stated that the reduced enamel epithelium will persist for several years in the interdental col area,[4] and that this persistence would cause inferior resistance to surface irritants. This assumption is unlikely for several reasons: (1) it has not been shown that the reduced enamel epithelium persists longer for the interproximal than for the other tooth surfaces, (2) the mature sulcular epithelium may originate from the junctional epithelium without being structurally inferior, and (3) the morphological epithelial peculiarities in the col area credited to persistent reduced enamel epithelium have also been observed following gingivectomy, when all junctional and sulcular epithelium has been removed.[30]

Following complete excision of both the free gingiva and these epithelia, the morphological and ultrastructural appearance of the regenerated sulcus and junc-

tional epithelium is indistinguishable from the normal initial structures,[6] regardless of whether the epithelium contacts enamel, dentin, or cementum.[9,21,22]

The oral sulcular epithelium is fairly thick and made up entirely of basal and prickle cells of polyhedral shape, whereas the junctional epithelium is thin, containing only a few cell layers, with the cells appearing flattened, as if pressed against the tooth surface. The junction between the sulcular and junctional epithelium (Fig. 2-6) may usually be identified histologically by one or more irregular projections of epithelial pegs or ridges that arise from the apical border of the sulcular epithelium.

Histology of sulcular epithelium

The oral sulcular epithelium is made up of basal cells and stratum spinosum or prickle cells (Fig. 2-7). These cells are basically keratinocytic, but they do not go through the complete process of keratinization. The border to the connective tissue is often irregular, with epithelial projections, but there is no regular rete peg arrangement as in the gingival surface epithelium. Studies of specific enzyme activity within the oral sulcular epithelium have to be accepted with caution because of the common presence of inflammation and inflammatory cells in this region. In general, except for the lack of keratinization, the metabolic activities seem to be similar to those described for the surface gingival epithelium. Some recent studies indicate that the lack of keratinization in the sulcular epithelium is related to local environmental factors rather than to genetic factors. This conclusion would be expected, because the oral sulcular epithelium may derive from the keratinizing surface epithelium. Physiological defense mechanisms of the sulcus and the junctional epithelium are discussed in chapter 5.

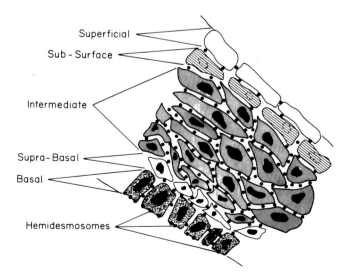

Fig. 2-7. Schematic drawing of oral sulcular epithelium.

JUNCTIONAL EPITHELIUM, DENTAL CUTICLES, AND PELLICLES

The excellent monograph by Schroeder and List-garten is recommended for comprehensive study of the junctional epithelium and associated structures.[30]

Histology of junctional epithelium

The junctional epithelium is composed of basal and prickle cells (Fig. 2-8). It is normally a thin band of epithelium, of 12 to 28 cell layers, with a total thickness of 30 to 100 μm.[29] It contains a higher number of intercellular spaces and a lower desmosome density than does the surface gingival epithelium. There are only a few tight junctions and minimal cytoplasmic filaments. All these features may explain why the junctional epithelium is easily penetrated and separated mechanically.

The junctional epithelium-tooth interface (internal basement lamina) and the epithelium-connective tissue interface (outer basement lamina) are structurally similar when studied by electron microscopy. In both instances, the attachment is by hemidesmosomes and a basement lamina.[19,29,30] The hemidesmosomes are closer together along the tooth surface than along the epithelial connective tissue junction.

Since there is a higher-than-normal density of hemidesmosomes on the cell surfaces contacting the tooth, it appears that at least some of these hemidesmosomes have been formed at the contact interface rather than being previously disconnected desmosomes. How these hemidesmosomes move along the tooth surface during cell renewal migration is not known, but the process may be similar to epithelial cell migration over the connective tissue on a wound surface. Similar hemidesmosomal attachment has also been described between junctional epithelium and cementum. The attachment seems to be to laminar or cuticular structures on the tooth surface rather than to the calcified surfaces themselves.

Cuticular structures and epithelial attachment

At least thirty different names and concepts have been applied to the highly controversial cuticular structures encountered on the surfaces of the teeth.[1] Cuticles have been classified as preeruptive and posteruptive or acquired structures,[37] or as primary and secondary cuticles.[13] More recent names are *integuments*[36] and *pellicles*.[1]

Nasmyth (1839) described an organic coating over the enamel of unerupted and newly erupted teeth.[26] This coating, which could be floated off after placing the teeth in acid for a short time, was called Nasmyth's membrane. Much later came Gottlieb's well-known theories of a primary calcified enamel cuticle formed as an end product of the function of the ameloblasts, and of a keratinized secondary enamel cuticle that formed during the transformation of the ameloblasts into reduced squamous enamel epithelium.[13] Gottlieb postulated that these two cuticulae were intimately and organically connected, and with the epithelial cells attached to the secondary cuticle they were thus also attached to the enamel (Fig. 2-9). Various modifications of this theory prevailed for several decades, but have now been discarded.

On the basis of light and phase microscopy, there was general agreement for over 100 years that an organic Nasmyth's membrane covered unerupted teeth following completion of the amelogenesis. It appeared to be 0.5 to 1.0 μm thick[22] and attached to the reduced ameloblast. It was assumed to be partially calcified.

With the advent of electron microscopy, several of these past concepts have been refuted. Ussing observed a membrane at the distal end of the ameloblasts of unerupted teeth,[38] but it was only 20 to 50 nm thick, while the cuticular structure seen with the light microscope was 1 μm thick (equal to 1000 μm). These structures could therefore not be identical. Later, Listgarten failed to find any enamel cuticle in electron microscopic studies of unerupted teeth. He suggested that the cuticle seen with light or phase microscopy is the result of an optical phenomenon.[22] He described in detail a cellular attachment of the reduced ameloblast to the enamel surface. The most frequent mode of attachment of the ameloblast to adjacent enamel, he reported, was by hemidesmosomes on the enamel

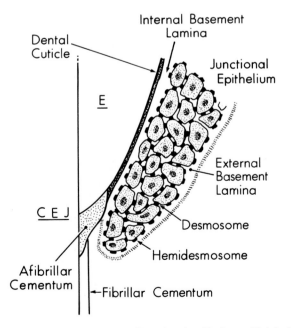

Fig. 2-8. Schematic drawing of junctional epithelium with labeling of the various structures. *E,* Enamel; *CEJ,* cementoenamel junction.

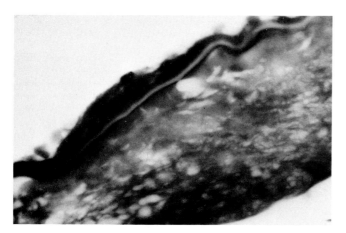

Fig. 2-9. Primary and secondary enamel cuticle. Decalcified enamel is seen at bottom of picture. Junctional epithelial cells occur on the surface of the cuticle.

side of the cell membrane. These hemidesmosomes corresponded in size and structure to those of other epithelial membrane-connective tissue junctions and to the hemidesmosomes observed at the gingivo-dental junction of erupted teeth.

Another mode of attachment Listgarten found involved a cuticle-like granular layer covering the enamel close to the cementoenamel junction (Listgarten cuticle A or primary cuticle). It extended coronally from the cementoenamel junction for only 50 μm or less. In erupted teeth, the layer may be slightly thicker and extend a little farther coronally. The cuticle was often covered by cementum near to the cementoenamel junction, and it appeared to be mineralized.

On the basis of this[22] and other, more recent, reports,[19,29] it appears that the reduced enamel epithelium is attached to the enamel surface or to cuticle A by a basement lamina and hemidesmosomes rather than through a Nasmyth's membrane or a secondary enamel cuticle.

Erupted functional teeth also have the electron-dense cuticle A or primary cuticle on the enamel close to the cementoenamel junction. However, a second type of cuticle (Listgarten cuticle B), the dental cuticle[30], was observed to cover the primary cuticle or the enamel surface directly where no primary cuticle was present. It was less granular than the primary cuticle, had a mottled appearance, and was connected to the junctional epithelium by basement lamina and hemidesmosomes.

The thickness of the dental cuticle as seen with the light microscope may be as much as 50 μm, while in electron microscopic study it appears to be much thinner (0.04 to 0.7 μm). The thickness is greatest at the most coronal part of the junctional epithelium and thinner toward the cementoenamel junction.[30]

The true origin of the dental cuticle is still unknown, but it has been linked theoretically to a continuous secretion of basement lamina material from the junctional epithelium.[29] It may instead be a secretion product from the connective tissues, forming as a seepage along the tooth surface;[8,20] alternatively, it has been suggested but not proven that the cuticle originates from degenerated erythrocytes.[17,18] It may be that what is seen in light microscopy as a dental cuticle is an amorphous layer of coagulated tissue fluid adherent to the tooth surface.[20] The main unsolved problem concerning the epithelial attachment is the origin and nature of the secondary dental cuticle, which mitigates almost all epithelial contact with the tooth.

Dental pellicles

Soon after a tooth has been cleaned and polished, the exposed surfaces of the teeth in vivo are covered by a thin (1-3 μm) organic structure called the *dental pellicle*. When less than 1 μm in thickness, it is sometimes called a cuticle. It cannot be removed by regular toothbrushing, not even following scrubbing with a hard bristle brush and soap or detergents in tap water,[36,37] but requires polishing with an abrasive to be removed. It can be separated from the tooth by immersion in a decalcifying solution for 10 minutes, after which it can be teased off or lifted away.

The pellicle consists of specific salivary proteins, some of which promote specific colonization and maintenance of indigenous oral flora, while others function as antimicrobial factors. The composition of the pellicle is variable but includes proteins, glycoproteins (mucins), and a substantial amount of lipids as well.

Although in vitro studies have shown that bacteria will adhere to hydroxyapatite, the adherence is enhanced by salivary pellicle, and the colonization of plaque on the tooth surface involves interaction between the surface of the bacteria and the absorbed pellicle.[16] In electron micrographs of dental pellicle, the surface often has a honeycomb appearance from adherent bacteria, and bacterial plaque is apparent on the surface of the pellicle.

MALASSEZ'S EPITHELIAL RESTS

Rests and strands of epithelial cells are found in the periodontal membrane (Fig. 2-10). These cells have been considered to be remnants of the Hertwig root sheath,[15] and were first described by Malassez in 1885.[24] Epithelial rests may be seen throughout the periodontal membrane, but they are usually located close to the cementum. They are most numerous in the apical[27] and cervical areas[40] of the teeth, and seem to become reduced in number by age. The cells have the ultramicroscopic appearance of basal cells attached to a well-defined basement lamina. Based on ultrastructural morphology and histochemical evidence,

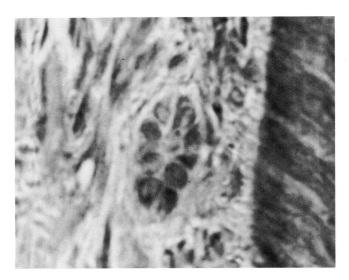

Fig. 2-10. *Center,* Malassez epithelial rests with glandlike appearance. Human specimen.

Valderhaug and Nylen characterized these cells as "resting epithelial cells."[39] Only occasional[3] thymidine labeling has been observed in cell rests located in noninflamed periodontal tissues.[11,35] However, when stimulated in an area of inflammation, in tissue culture, or by orthodontic tooth movement, they may undergo frequent mitosis. It is assumed that they may provide the epithelial components of radicular and lateral root cysts.

In cross-sections, the epithelial rests often have a rosette, glandlike appearance,[35] but no secreting function has been demonstrated.[39] Speculations with regard to the role of these rests in the formation of cementum or periodontal pockets have not been substantiated, and such functions appear to be unlikely.

REFERENCES

1. Armstrong, W.G.: Origin and nature of the acquired pellicle. P. Roy, S. Med. 61:923, 1968.
2. Barnett, M.L., and Szabo, G.: Gap junctions in human gingival keratinized epithelium. J. Periodont. Res. 8:117, 1973.
3. Caffesse, R.G., Karring, T., and Nasjleti, C.: Keratinizing potential of sulcular epithelium, J. Periodont. 48:140, 1977.
4. Cohen, B.: A study of the periodontal epithelium, Br. Dent. J. 112:55, 1962.
5. Engler, W.O., Ramfjord, S.P., and Hiniker, J.J.: Development of epithelial attachment and gingival sulcus in rhesus monkeys, J. Periodont. 36:44, 1965.
6. Engler, W.O., Ramfjord, S.P., and Hiniker, J.J.: Healing following simple gingivectomy. A tritiated thymidine radioautographic study. I. Epithelialization, J. Periodont. 37:298, 1966.
7. Farquhar, M.G., and Palade, G.E.: Junctional complexes in various epithelia, J. Cell Biol. 17:375, 1963.
8. Frank, R.M., and Cimasoni, G.: Ultrastructure de l'epithelium cliniquement normal du sillon et de la junction gingivodentaires, Z. Zellforsch. 109:356, 1970.
9. Frank, R.M., et al.: Ultrastructural study of epithelial and connective gingival reattachment in man, J. Periodont. 45:626, 1974.
10. Gibbons, R.J.: Adherent interactions which may affect microbial ecology in the mouth, J. Dent. Res. 63:378, 1984.
11. Gilhuus-Moe, O., and Kvam, E.: Behaviour of the epithelial remnants of Malassez following experimental movement of rat molars. Acta Odont. Scand. 30:139, 1972.
12. Glickman, J., Petralis, R., and Marks, R.M.: The effect of powered toothbrushing and interdental stimulation upon microscopic inflammation and surface keratinization of the interdental gingiva. J. Periodont. 38:105, 1965.
13. Gottlieb, B.: Der Epithelansatz am Zähne. Dtsch. Monatschr. Zahnheilk. 39:142, 1921.
14. Greene, A.H.: Study of the characteristic of stippling and its relation of gingival health, J. Periodont. 33:176, 1962.
15. Hertwig, W.: Archiv für Mikr. Anat. Bd. XI, Suppl. VII, 1874.
16. Hillman, J.D., van Houte, J., and Gibbons, R.J.: Sorption of bacteria to human enamel powder, Arch. Oral Biol. 15:899, 1970.
17. Hodson, J.J.: The distribution, structure, origin and nature of the dental cuticle of Gottlieb, Part I. Periodontics. 5:237, 1967.
18. Hodson, J.J.: The distribution, structure, origin and nature of the dental cuticle of Gottlieb, Part II. Periodontics. 5:295, 1967.
19. Kobayashi, K., Rose, G. G., and Mahan, G. J.: Ultrastructure of the dento-epithelial junction, J. Periodont. Res. 11:313, 1976.
20. Lie, T., and Selvig, K.A.: Formation of an experimental dental cuticle, Scand. J. Dent. Res. 83:145, 1975.
21. Listgarten, M.A.: The ultrastructure of human gingival epithelium. Am. J. Anat. 114:49, 1964.
22. Listgarten, M.A.: Phase-contrast and electron microscopic study of the junction between reduced enamel epithelium and enamel in unerupted human teeth, Arch. Oral Biol. 11:999, 1966.
23. Listgarten, M.A.: Ultrastructure of the dentogingival junction after gingivectomy, J. Periodont. Res. 7:151, 1972.
24. Malassez, L.: On the existence of masses of epithelium round the roots of adult teeth in a normal state. J. Brit. Dent. Assoc. 6:370, 1885.
25. Melcher, A.H.: The nature of the "basement membrane" in human gingiva, Arch. Oral Biol. 10:783, 1965.
26. Nasmyth, A.: On the structure, physiology, and pathology of the persistent capsular investments and pulp of the teeth. Microchir. Trans. Chir. Soc. London. 22:310, 1839.
27. Reeve, C.M., and Wentz, F.J.: The prevalence, morphology and distribution of epithelial rests in the human periodontal ligament. Oral Surg. 15:785, 1962.
28. Schroeder, H.E.: Melanin containing organelles in cells of the human gingiva. II. Keratinocytes, J. Periodont. Res. 4:235, 1969.
29. Schroeder, H.E.: Ultrastructure of the junctional human gingiva, Helv. Odont. Acta. 13:65, 1969.
30. Schroeder, H.E., and Listgarten, M.A.: Fine structure of the developing epithelial attachment of human teeth. S. Karger, 1971.
31. Schroeder, H.E.: Histopathology of the gingival sulcus. In The Borderline Between Caries and Periodontal Disease, ed. T. Lehner. London: Academic Press, 1977.
32. Skougaard, M.R., and Beagrie, G.S.: The renewal of gingival epithelium in marmosets (Calithrix jacchus) as determined through autoradiography with thymidine-H3, Acta Odont. Scand. 20:467, 1962.
33. Staehelin, L.A., and Hull, B.E.: Junctions between living cells. Sci. Am. 238:141, 1978.

34. Thilander, H., and Bloom, G.D.: Cell contacts in oral epithelia, J. Periodont. Res. 3:96, 1968.
35. Trowbridge, H.O., and Shibata, F.: Mitotic activity in epithelial rests of Malassez, Periodontics, 5:109, 1967.
36. Turner, E.P.: The integument of the enamel surface of the human tooth. I. The developmental integument, Dent. Pract. 8:341, 1958.
37. Turner, E.P.: The integument of the enamel surface of the human tooth. II. The acquired enamel cuticle, Dent. Pract. 8:373, 1958.
38. Ussing, M.J.: the development of the epithelial attachment, Acta Odont. Scand. 13:123, 1955.
39. Valderhaug, J.P., and Nylen, M.U.: Function of epithelial rests as suggested by their ultrastructure, J. Periodont. Res. 1:69, 1966.
40. Valderhaug, J.P., and Zander, H.: Relationship of "epithelial rests of Malassez" to other periodontal structures, Periodontics. 5:254, 1967.

3

CONNECTIVE TISSUES

GINGIVAL CONNECTIVE TISSUES

The gingival connective tissues are dense fibrous connective tissues with a complex functional orientation that is developed gradually during tooth eruption and is later modified by functional demands. The structural orientation of these tissues is well suited to meet the physical stresses of mastication and swallowing.

Structural orientation

The fibers have an interwoven pattern, and numerous gingival fibers are not even attached to the surface of the tooth. The function of the fibers is to stabilize the attached gingiva to the alveolar process and to the tooth, and, to a lesser extent, to stabilize the tooth to the bone. A circumferential arrangement of the fibers (ligamentum circulare) holds the functional epithelium in close contact with the tooth and helps to maintain the epithelial seal to the tooth, while interdental fibers add to the stability of the teeth.

Fibers can be observed (fig. 3-1) to occur in the following directions: (1) from the cementum to the free gingiva (the free gingival fibers); (2) from the cementum to the tip of the interproximal papillae (free gingival or papillary fibers); (3) interproximally from tooth to tooth (the transseptal fibers); (4) surrounding the tooth completely or partially in a ringlike fashion (the circular of semicircular fibers);[13] (5) from the cementum to the alveolar crest (the alveolar crest fibers); (6) from the free gingiva to the alveolar crest (gingival crest fibers); (7) from the basement lamina of the attached and free gingival mucosa to the alveolar process (alveolar process fibers); (8) more or less parallel to the aveolar process without any apparent functional orientation; (9) radially arranged dentogingival fibers described as traversing the buccal attached gingiva and terminating the muscle fibers of facial muscles.[21]

Cellular components

Exclusive of vascular and nerve tissues, more than half of all cells in the gingiva are fibroblasts, which produce the connective tissue substances that determine the morphological and physical characteristics of the gingiva. Mast cells are present in great numbers in normal human gingiva.[25] Macrophages are numerous in healthy gingival tissues, with a dense zone of macrophages just under the junctional epithelium. These cells have small oval or indented nuclei and abundant cytoplasm. Under electron microscopy, they display scattered lamellae of rough endoplasmic reticulum, lysosomes, and microfilaments. Macrophages may produce hydrolytic enzymes and act as scavenger and detoxification cells in normal gingiva. They may also contain phagocytized melanin, which appears to be degraded in the macrophages.[17]

Connective tissue fibers

Classically, connective tissue fibers have been divided into three different types: collagen, reticular fibers, and elastic fibers. Lately, a fourth group of fibers, called oxytalan fibers, has been described. Collagen fibers make up more than 50% of the volume of the human gingiva. The main function of these fibers is to provide tensile strength and mechanical support for the periodontal tissues. In the gingiva, there is a high proportion of acid-soluble collagen. This has been taken to mean that there is a high rate of new collagen formation and thus a high collagen turnover.

Reticular fibers are present in the gingiva,[11] as well as elastic fibers, which give the tissues their suppleness and ability to spring back to their normal position after stretching. There are only a few elastic fibers in the gingiva, mainly in vessel walls.

Oxytalan fibers were initially described by Fullmer.[5]

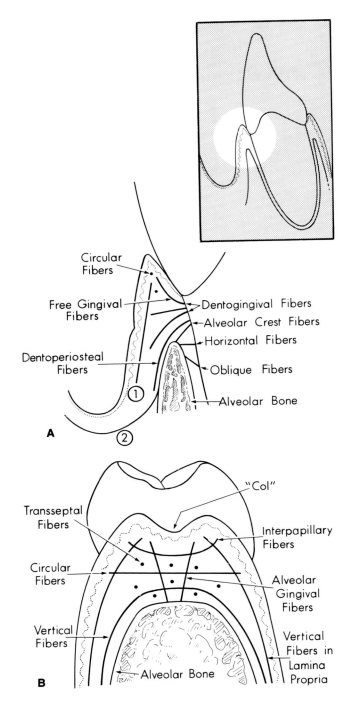

Fig. 3-1. *A*, Schematic drawing of buccal or lingual gingival fibers. *B*, Schematic drawing of interproximal gingival fibers. *1*, Subepithelial fibers. *2*, Fibers to facial muscles.

The chemical composition of the oxytalan fiber is essentially unknown, and no specific function has been established. It may be that oxytalan fibers represent a modified type of elastic fiber, since a chemical as well as functional relationship to elastic fibers has been suggested.[6]

Ground substance

The cells, fibers, nerves, and vessels of the gingiva are embedded in a viscous, gel-like ground substance. This ground substance is made up mainly of a large variety of proteoglycans and hyaluronic acid, but chondroitin sulfates and other polysaccharides are also important components.[24] The term *proteoglycans* includes molecules that were previously classified as mucopolysaccharides.

One of the most important properties of the ground substance is its very high viscosity in aqueous solutions. It is assumed that this property acts as a barrier to the spread of bacteria. Some of the most invasive bacteria produce the enzyme hyaluronidase, which depolymerizes hyaluronic acid in the ground substance, and thus permits the spread of bacteria and their toxins.

Gingival vasculature

The superior and inferior dental arteries extend branches into the gingiva, interproximally as well as buccally and lingually. Branches of these vessels also anastomose with arteries supplying the adjacent oral mucosa, as stated in the classic paper by Hayashi (1932) concerning the arterial blood supply of the periodontium.[7] His findings have been reconfirmed by several authors using various methods of investigation.

The gingival tissues have a double blood supply: an internal one from bone and periodontal membrane, and an external one through the periosteum.[9] An extensive system of anastomoses assures ample circulatory interchange from the gingival tissues, even if some intervening obstruction should block a considerable number of vessels.[4] Experimental occlusion of gingival arterioles by microspheres has indicated that the blood supply to the dentogingival junction is primarily from the periodontal membrane,[8] but it can also be reestablished from the periosteal side of the aveolar process. The main blood supply to the attached gingiva is through periosteal vessels.[4]

The lymphatic drainage of the gingiva extends from the connective tissue papillae and progresses into a collecting network on the surface of the periosteum on the alveolar process,[16,20] then into the regional lymphatics. Lymphatics beneath the junctional epithelium extend into the periodontal membrane[16] and open into collecting vessels associated with veins.

Innervation

The gingivae are innervated by the maxillary and mandibular branches of the trigeminal nerve. The nerve trunks generally follow the paths of the blood vessels. The palatal gingiva of the maxillary incisors and cuspids is supplied by the nasopalatine nerve, and the palatal gingiva of the molars and bicuspids is innervated by branches of the anterior (greater) palatal nerve. The labial gingiva of the maxillary incisors and cuspids is supplied by the labial branch of the infraorbital nerve, and the buccal gingiva of the posterior maxillary teeth by the superior alveolar nerve.

The lingual gingiva of all mandibular teeth is supplied by the lingual nerve, and the labial gingiva of the mandibular anterior teeth (incisors, cuspids, and sometimes bicuspids) by the mental nerve. The buccal gingiva of the mandibular molars, and often of the bicuspids, is supplied by the long buccal nerve. The interdental tissues are mostly innervated by intraosseous branches of the dental and alveolar nerves.

The attached gingiva, with its numerous connective tissue papillae, has the most nerve endings in the gingival tissues, while nerve endings are less frequent in the free gingiva.[15] A large variety of "free nerve endings" have been described in the gingiva. Numerous free-ending nerve fibers apparently enter the subepithelial papillae from a subepithelial nerve plexus. Many of these fibers do not lose their myelin sheath until they approach close to the epithelium, where they divide into two or more terminal branches.

Organized terminations of nerves resembling Meissner's corpuscles have been described in the connective tissue papillae and close to the epithelium.[15] End bulbs of the Krause type have been observed both in the papillae and in the underlying lamina propria. A third type of small encapsulated end bulb has also been observed in the gingiva. These bulbs may be coiled[3] or knoblike structures.[15] The correlation between individual types of nerve endings and function is controversial, since the physiological behavior of the various nerve endings has not been determined with certainty.

Autonomic nerves have been identified histologically in the gingiva[14] and it is assumed that these nerves contribute to autonomic regulatory mechanisms such as vascular flow.

PERIODONTAL MEMBRANE

The periodontal membrane may be considered to be an extension of the gingival connective tissues into a space between the root of the tooth and the alveolar bone. This membrane is attached to the cementum, acting as a pericemental covering, and to the alveolar bone, acting as a periosteum, but its main function is to provide support for the teeth and proprioceptive impulses for occlusal function.

Structural arrangement

A large part of the periodontal membrane in functioning teeth is made up of collagenous fiber bundles connecting the tooth and the bone. The fibers have a functional orientation and have been divided into the following groups: alveolar crest fibers, horizontal fi-

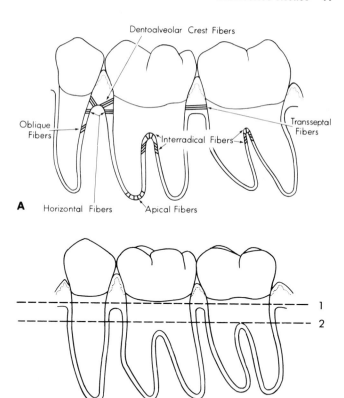

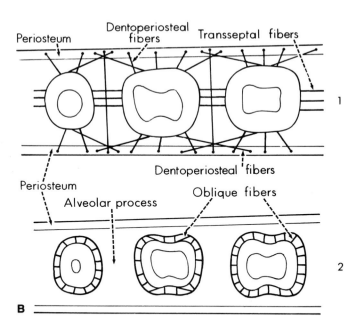

Fig. 3-2. *A,* Schematic drawing of periodontal membrane fibers showing functional orientation so that occlusal forces in various directions can be transmitted as pull to the alveolar bone. *B,* Schematic drawing of supracrestal horizontal cross-section through the teeth (*1*) and subcrestal cross-section through the alveolar process and the roots of the teeth (*2*). Note the complex functional fiber orientation.

bers, oblique fibers, apical fibers, and interradicular fibers (fig. 3-2).[12] This division, however, is a great oversimplification, based on axial sections through teeth and periodontium with heavy function. In human periodontium with average function, the main part of the periodontal membrane is made up of connective tissues without such obvious functional arrangement except at the alveolar crest. If horizontal sections (cross cut of the teeth) are studied, fiber bundles appear to run from the tooth to the bone in many directions, giving stability to torque as well as to intrusive forces. With decrease in functional demand, there is a gradual decrease in functional fiber orientation.

The width of the periodontal space (distance from tooth to alveolar bone) or thickness of the periodontal membrane varies with age and function from 0.15 to 0.38 mm.[2] It is narrowest at the middle of the root and wider at the alveolar crest and at the apex, but these small physiological variations of 0.05 to 0.10 mm cannot be observed in a roentgenogram. With increased tooth mobility, the variations may be much greater and thus observable in roentgenograms.

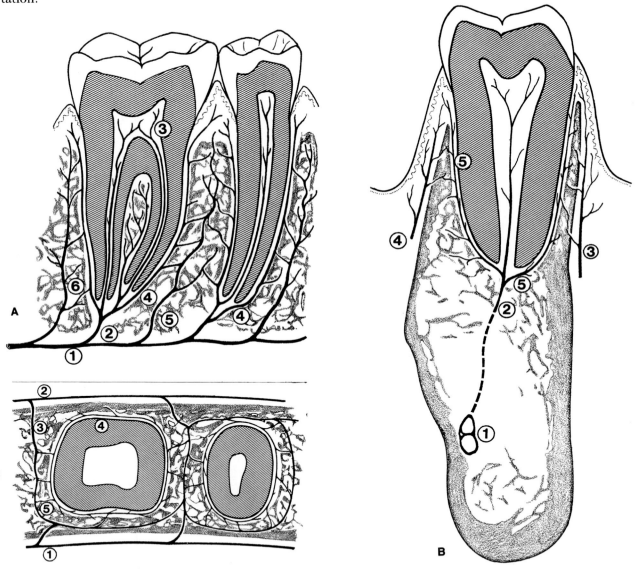

Fig. 3-3. *A,* Schematic drawing of longitudinal vertical section through teeth and alveolar process showing distribution names. *1,* Inferior alveolar artery; *2,* dental arteriole; *3,* pulpal branches; *4,* periodontal ligament arteriole; *5,* intermediate (interalveolar) arteriole; *6,* perforating branch. *B,* Schematic drawing of vertical cross-section through the mandible and a mandibular molar showing the vascular distribution to the periodontium. *1,* Inferior alveolar artery; *2,* dental arteriole; *3,* facial periosteal arterioles; *4,* lingual periosteal arterioles; *5,* periodontal membrane arterioles. *C,* Schematic drawing of horizontal subcrestal cross-section through the roots of a mandibular molar and a bicuspid with the surrounding alveolar bone and alveolar process. The pattern of the vascular supply is indicated and labeled. *1, 2, 3,* Lingual, facial, and interalveolar arterioles; *4,* periodontal ligament arteriole; *5,* perforating branches of interalveolar arteriole.

Tissue components

The cellular components, the fibers, and the ground substance are similar to the corresponding structures in the gingiva, with some quantitative differences. The rate of collagen synthesis is very high in the periodontium, and alveolar fibers show a higher activity than cemental fibers.[23] The next highest activity is in the middle of the periodontal membrane.

Vascularity

The inferior dental artery goes through the mandibular canal and is accompanied by a number of inferior dental veins. The main artery gives off a series of dental branches (fig. 3-3) consisting of eight to twelve main channels and some fine branches, which supply the mandibular teeth and their surrounding bone. The veins that drain the venous network of the alveoli and interalveolar septa follow a course different from the arteries and terminate in a number of inferior dental veins accompanying the main artery. The venous drainage from the mandible goes upward to the pterygoid plexus, and then downward to the facial and external jugular veins.

The Spalteholtz injecting and clearing technique[22] has been used in several studies of the intrabony and intraperiodontal course of blood vessels, and recent studies have reconfirmed the classic descriptions by Hayashi (1932) of the dental artery giving off branches to the pulp, to the apical part of the periodontal membrane, and of interalveolar branches with numerous small arteries penetrating through holes in the alveolar bone and through the interdental septa.[7] The veins within the alveolar bone, especially those coming from the periodontal membrane, join one another and also join the veins in the interalveolar septa. Within the periodontal membrane, the vessels branch in various directions and form a plexiform pattern, which is closer to the alveolar bone than to the cementum,[4] but which includes small vessels extending close to the cementum.[24]

The lymphatic system of the periodontal membrane has not received much attention in periodontal research. It has been reported that, in marmosets, lymph capillaries in the periodontal ligament originate as blind-ending diverticula that later open into collecting vessels associated with veins, and that lymphatics follow the pathways of the veins and drain into the regional lymph nodes.[19]

Innervation

The inferior dental nerve and the anterior, middle, and posterior superior dental nerves follow the paths of the inferior, anterior, middle, and posterior arteries and penetrate the bone into the periodontal membrane in company with these arteries. Nerve fibers enter the periodontal membrane both at the apex and through openings in the alveolar wall. The small terminal nerve fibers, however, do not follow the paths of the blood vessels.[15] The richest nerve supply is in the apical portion of the periodontal membrane, and in this region the nerve bundles are thicker and have more nerve endings than in the cervical portion. Both thick and thin nerve fibers are found in the periodontal membrane. The thicker fibers are myelinated and the thinner fibers have free endings relating to pain.[10]

REFERENCES

1. Cohen, L.: The venous drainage of the mandible. Oral Surg. 12:1447, 1959.
2. Coolidge, E.D.: The thickness of the human periodontal membrane. J.A.D.A. 24:1260, 1937.
3. Dixon, A.D.: Sensory nerve terminations in the oral mucosa. Arch. Oral Biol. 5:105, 1961.
4. Folke, L.E.A., and Stallard, R.E.: Periodontal microcirculation as revealed by plastic microspheres, J. Periodont. Res. 2:53, 1967.
5. Fullmer, H.M. Differential staining of connective tissue fibers in areas of stress, Science 127:1240, 1958.
6. Fullmer, H.M., Sheetz, J.H., and Narkates, A.J.: Oxytalan connective tissue fibers. A review, J. Oral Pathol. 3:291,1974.
7. Hayashi, S.: Untersuchungen über die arterille Blutversorgung des Periodontiums, Dtsch. Monatsschr. F. Zahnheilkd. 50:145, 1932.
8. Kennedy, J.: Experimental ischemia in monkeys, II. Vascular response, J. Dent. Res. 48:888, 1969.
9. Kindlova, M.: The blood supply of the marginal periodontium in Macacus rhesus, Arch. Oral Biol. 10:869, 1965.
10. Kizor, J.E. Cuozzo, J.W., and Broman, D.C.: Functional and histologic assessment of the sensory innervation of the periodontal ligament of the cat, J. Dent. Res. 47:59, 1968.
11. Melcher, A.M.: Histologic recognition of gingival reticulum, Arch. Oral Biol. 11:219, 1966.
12. Orban, B.: Dental Histology and Embryology. Philadelphia: P. Blakiston and Son, 1929.
13. Page, R.C., et al.: Collagen fibre bundles of the normal marginal gingivae in the marmoset, Arch. Oral Biol. 19:1039, 1974.
14. Raab, H.: Die Klinische Bedeutung des Nachweises von adrenergen, autonomen Nerven im menschlichen Zahnfleisch, Oesterr. Z. Stomatol. 67:381, 1970.
15. Rapp, R., Kristine, W.D., and Avery, J.K.: Study of neural endings in the human gingiva and periodontal membrane, J. Can. Dent. Ass. 23:637, 1957.
16. Ruben, M.P., et al.: Visualization of lymphatic microcirculation of oral tissues. II. Vital retrograde lymphography, J. Periodont. 42:774, 1971.
17. Schroeder, H.E.: Melanin containing organelles in cells of the human gingiva. III. Connective tissue cells, Helv. Odont. Acta. 13:46, 1969.
18. Schroeder, H.E., Munzel-Pedrazzoli, S., and Page, R.: Correlated morphometric and biochemical analysis of gingival tissue in early chronic gingivitis in man, Arch. Oral Biol. 18:899, 1973.
19. Schweitzer, G.: Die Lymphgefasse des Zahnfleisches und der Zahne, Arch. f. mikr. Anat. 69:807, 1907.
20. Shapiro, L., and Ruben, M.P.: Visualization of lymphatic microcirculation of oral tissues. I. Development, structure and physiology of the lymphatic complex, J. Periodont. 42:334, 1971.

21. Smukler, J., and Dreyer, C.J.: Principal fibers of the periodontium, J. Periodont. Res. 4:19, 1969.
22. Spalteholtz, W.: Die Arterien der Herzwand. Leipzig: S. Hirzel, 1924.
23. Stallard, R.E.: The utilization of H³-proline by the connective tissue elements of the periodontium, Periodontics 1:185, 1963.
24. World Workshop in Periodontics. Ed. S.P. Ramfjord, D.A. Kerr, and M.M. Ash. Ann Arbor, Michigan: The University of Michigan, 1966.
25. Zachrisson, W.B.: Mast cells of the human gingiva. II. Metachromatic cells at low pH in healthy and inflamed tissue, J. Periodont. Res. 2:87, 1967.

4

CEMENTUM AND ALVEOLAR BONE

This chapter describes the cementum and alveolar bone as they relate to clinical practice. More specifically, those features of cementum and bone that are of interest in periodontics are discussed here.

CEMENTUM

Cementum is a calcified bonelike substance that covers the roots of the teeth and provides attachment for the periodontal fibers. It is not quite as hard as dentin, but has the same mineral and crystal patterns as dentin and bone.[15] The main difference is the lack of blood vessels and nerves in cementum.

Cementogenesis

Cementogenesis follows dentinogenesis during root development.[18] As residual cells from the Hertwig's root sheath are separated from the newly formed dentin, a fibrillar cementoid matrix is deposited around cells that look like fibroblasts positioned close to the dentinal surface. These cells take on the common shape of cementoblasts, and calcification of the cementoid material is initiated. The initial layer of cementum is usually acellular, but during rapid cementogenesis, cementoblasts may become entrapped in the newly formed cementum. The cementoblasts appear to be specialized fibroblasts extending cytoplasmic processes among the collagen fibrils into the cementoid or precementum layer. Cementoblasts that become incorporated into cementum are called *cementocytes.*

Cementum usually covers the entire root of human teeth, including the apical opening to the pulp, and often extends for a short distance over the enamel at the cementoenamel junction.[10] However, in some instances, the cementum does not join up with the enamel, and residual remains of Hertwig's root sheath, instead of cementum, may cover the root surface. Enamel extensions and enamel pearls may also cover small areas of the root surface that are devoid of cementum. The layer of cementum is thin close to the cemento-enamel junction[20] (20 to 50 μm), while at the apex it may be 200 to 300 mm thick.

Histology and Composition

Histologically, a distinction is made between acellular and cellular cementum. On the surface of acellular cementum, the cells of the periodontal membrane are separated from the calcifying cementum by a 3 to 5 μm-wide zone of precementum or cementoid with densely packed collagen fibrils.[19] The prevailing fiber orientation is perpendicular to the surface (Fig. 4-1) and most mineral crystals are oriented in the direction of the fibers. Most of the acellular cementum is uniform in structure, with fine collagen fibrils that do not show a distinct Sharpey's fiber pattern. These fibrils join into distinct fibers after they enter the periodontal membrane. Cellular cementum is characterized primarily by the presence of embedded cells (cementocytes), or lacunar spaces, or canaliculi from degenerated or dead cells.[3,24]

Physiology

The function of cementum is to transmit occlusal forces to the periodontal membrane in the form of pull on the fiber structures, and to resist pressure against the root surface. The fiber attachment to the cementum is maintained by a very slow, continuous deposition of new cementum anchoring new fibers (fig. 4-2A), or after injury to the cementum, by resorption and repair with new fiber attachment.[5,9] There is a

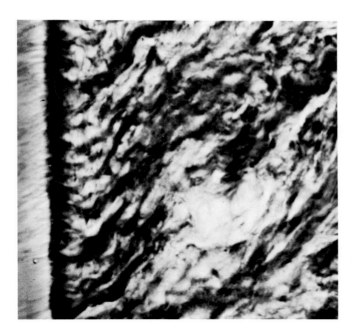

Fig. 4-1. Longitudinal section of human tooth. Attachment of oblique periodontal fibers into the cementum. Note how the coarse wavy fiber bundles in the periodontal membrane are dispersed into finer fibrils, which enter the cemental surface.

tendency for cemental deposition to even out irregular root surfaces and root depressions (Fig. 4-2, B).

Radioautographic studies indicate a very slow renewal rate of cementoblasts,[8] and an equally slow collagen turnover in the periodontal membrane close to the cementum,[11,23] much slower than the turnover close to the alveolar bone. It has been observed that the fibers entering the cementum are the last collagen fiber structures in the periodontium to lose their collagen characteristics during trauma from occlusion,[17] disuse atrophy,[17] and scurvy.[25]

Evidence of resorption and repair is commonly found on the root surfaces of practically all functional teeth.[6] It has been known for a long time that resorption of cementum can be induced by trauma from occlusion.[9,16] Reparative cementum may form on both dentinal and cemental surfaces (Fig. 4-3) at a much faster rate than the normal continuous formation of cementum. The biologic inductive mechanism of cemental repair is unknown. Independent of pulp vitality, repair cementum may form and become attached to dentin and cementum after apiectomies or after periodontal treatment.[2]

Hypercementosis or cemental spurs may form in response to heavy functional demands, but for unknown biological reasons, rapid cementogenesis may also occur during nonfunction. In bifurcations of molars, irregular cementum without functional arrangements of fiber structure and globular calcification is often seen associated with ectopic enamel (Fig. 4-4).

Cementum may be torn loose from the surface of a tooth by undue pull on periodontal fibers. Such cemental "tears" are most likely to be observed at the level of the alveolar crest or at the apex of teeth as a result of trauma from occlusion (Fig. 4-5).

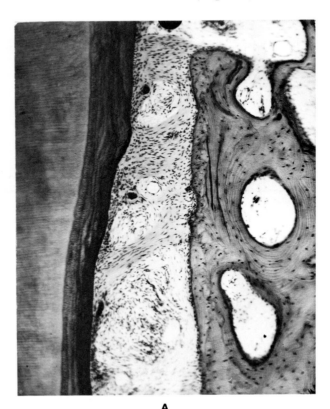

A

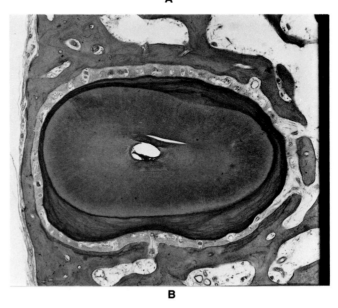

B

Fig. 4-2. *A*, Longitudinal section of human tooth. The cementum has a lamellated structure from continuous deposition. *B*, Cross-section of maxillary bicuspid root. Note uneven deposition of cementum resulting in lessened concavity of the furcation grooves.

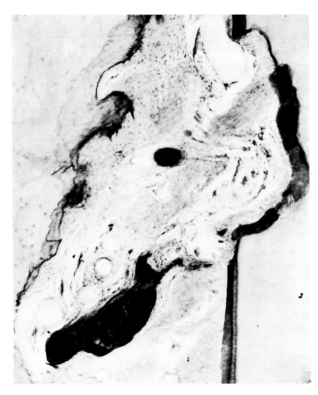

Fig. 4-3. Longitudinal section of human tooth. Traumatic tear with reparative cementum over dentine and old cementum. The piece of tooth that had been torn loose is now surrounded by periodontal membrane (*bottom*).

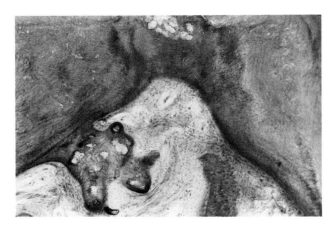

Fig. 4-4. Thick layers of cellular and irregular cementum in furcation of mandibular molar.

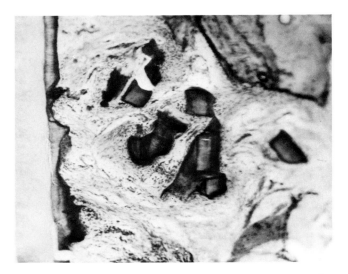

Fig. 4-5. Cemental tears at the level of the alveolar crest. Excessive occlusal wear indicated bruxism. Note repair on tooth surface and embedded particles of cementum in the periodontal membrane.

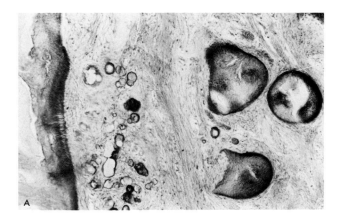

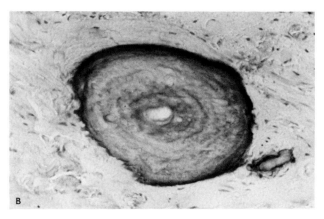

Fig. 4-6. *A,* Irregular cementicles and dystrophic calcification in gingiva, slightly coronal to the alveolar crest. *B,* Typical cementicle with lamellated structure from periodontal membrane of nonfunctioning tooth.

Small bodies of a calcified cementum-like substance (Fig. 4-6) may be found in the periodontal membrane as cementicles. These may be free cementicles unattached to the tooth, or attached or embedded cementicles associated with the root cementum. It has been suggested that these structures are either calcified Malassez epithelial rests or calcified thrombi in small blood vessels.[13] Neither of these theories has been proved.

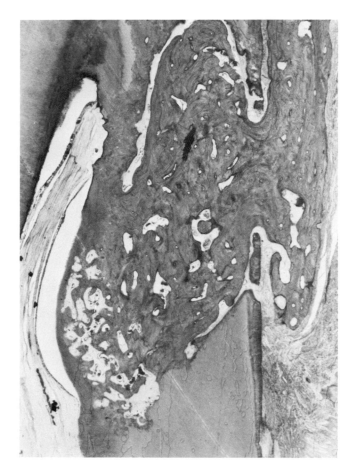

Fig. 4-7. Longitudinal section of maxillary central incisor and labial alveolar crest. The tooth had functioned as a single abutment for a five-unit fixed bridge. There are root resorption and ankylosis with bone, which has some histological resemblance to cementum.

During healing of severe trauma (Fig. 4-7) or reimplantation of teeth, cementum and alveolar bone may fuse and obliterate the periodontal space. Such a fusion is called *ankylosis*. This is apparently an abnormal repair process, which is often followed by progresive root resorption and eventually by loss of the tooth.

ALVEOLAR BONE

The alveolar process is the bony extension of the mandible and the maxilla surrounding the roots of the teeth. Within the alveolar process is the alveolar bone, a thin plate of lamellated bone that provides housing and attachment for the teeth. The alveolar bone is joined both morphologically and functionally to the alveolar process or supporting bone.[20]

Anatomy

The alveolar process develops with the alveolar bone during root formation of the teeth and grows as the teeth erupt. However, true functional morphology is not gained until the teeth engage in occlusal func-

tion. The coronal border of the alveolar bone (the alveolar crest) extends to approximately 1 mm. from the cementoenamel junction of the teeth on both the buccolingual and interproximal aspects. Thus, the alveolar crest has a scalloped or crescent-shaped appearance buccally and lingually, while the interproximal bone contour varies from convex in the anterior region to almost flat in the molar areas.

The anatomy of the alveolar processes depends to a great extent upon the position and alignment of the teeth.[7] With the teeth in extreme buccal or lingual version, the alveolar process may be extremely thin or even partially missing on that side of the teeth. A local area in which the labial or lingual bone is missing,

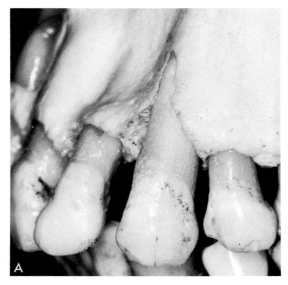

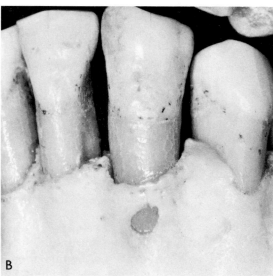

Fig. 4-8. *A,* Dehiscense; a labial or lingual cleft can be seen on the alveolar process where the root surface is not covered by bone. *B,* Fenestration, indicating a window-like labial or lingual lack of bone coverage over the root of a tooth.

creating a V-shaped defect in the bone, is called a *dehiscence* (Fig. 4-8, A). If there is a marginal ring of labial or lingual bone around the coronal part of the root, but some root surface not covered by bone apically to the crestal bone, the area without bone covering is called *fenestration* (Fig. 4-8, B). Dehiscence and fenestration are found associated with extreme buccal or lingual versions of teeth and occur in approximately 20% of all teeth.[22] Both the alveolar bone and the supporting bone will become thicker and denser with increased functional demands,[4] and thinner with lack of function.

The alveolar bone plate is perforated to allow for communication of nerves and blood vessels between the periodontal membrane and the marrow spaces. There are a greater number of perforations for the posterior than for the anterior teeth, and also more perforations in the cervical than in the middle and apical thirds of the periodontium.[1] However, in roentgenograms, the alveolar bone plate appears as a continuous radiopaque line around the roots of the teeth and is called *lamina dura*.

Histology and physiology

Because of the unique functional demands and ever-changing positions of the teeth associated with physiological mesial drift and compensating eruption, a high degree of adaptability is required of the alveolar bone,[21] and continuous growth must take place at the alveolar crest (Fig. 4-9). Three cell types are found associated with bone: osteoblasts, osteocytes, and osteoclasts. Whether these cells can be transformed

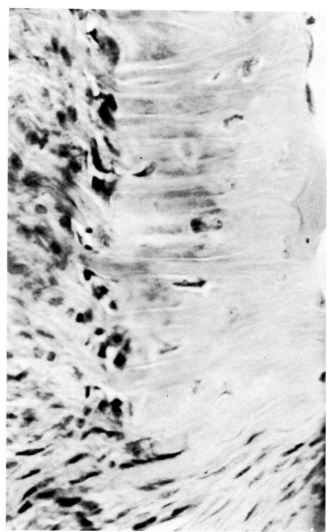

Fig. 4-10. Labial alveolar crest from functioning maxillary central incisor. Heavy collagen fiber bundles (Sharpey's fibers) are entering the newly formed bone. On the surface of the alveolar crest, the fibers are tangentially attached to the crest or they run almost parallel to the bone (*bottom*).

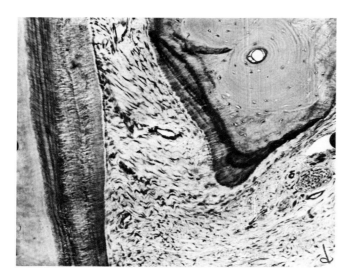

Fig. 4-9. Longitudinal section through tooth and alveolar crest. The tooth had been exposed to heavy occlusal function. Note continuous growth of alveolar crest and cementum as indicated by the presence of cementoblasts and osteoblasts and the lamellated structure on the surface of both bone and cementum.

from one type to another, or whether they represent different cell types of separate origin, is still debatable.[12] The cellular components of bone undergo changes related to aging.[24] The red bone marrow is replaced by fatty marrow. Aging osteoblasts may cease matrix production.[24] The organic component of calcified bone is almost entirely collagen.[14]

The main collagen fiber structure of the alveolar bone consists of Sharpey's fibers that enter the bone from the periodontal membrane (Fig. 4-10). If the alveolar bone is sectioned parallel to the periodontal surface and slightly under the surface, the Sharpey's fibers appear as circular structures; some of the fibers are fully calcified. The calcified tissues between the embedded periodontal fibers contain layers of fibers that are oriented parallel to the surface of the bone, but there are often also some fibrils with a random orientation entwining the Sharpey's fibers. Calcification on the surface of the bone often occurs between the fibers rather than within them.

Although bone physically is rigid, it is constantly undergoing remodeling in response to changes in functional demands and for the purpose of homeostasis of the blood calcium content. The biological mechanisms initiating and maintaining these homeostatic metabolic processes, and the role of the alkaline phosphates in the process of mineralization, are not fully understood.

According to all indications of cellular and metabolic activity, there is a highly developed field for biologic adaptation on the interphase between the alveolar bone and the periodontal membrane. In contrast, the relatively stable collagen of the mature periodontal fibers and the cementoblasts has only a minimal potential for adaptive physiological changes.

REFERENCES

1. Birn, H.: The vascular supply of the periodontal membrane, J. Periodont. Res. 1:51, 1966.
2. Frank, R., et al.: Gingival reattachment after surgery in man: An electron microscopic study, J. Periodont. 43:597, 1972.
3. Furseth, R.: A microradiographic and electron microscopic study of the cementum of human deciduous teeth, Acta Odont. Scand. 25:611, 1967.
4. Glickman, I., and Smulow, J.B.: Buttressing bone formation in the periodontium, J. Periodont. 36:365, 1965.
5. Gottlieb, B.: Biology of the cementum, J. Periodont. 13:13, 1942.
6. Henry, J.L., and Weinmann, J.P.: The pattern of resorption and repair of human cementum, J.A.D.A. 42:270, 1951.
7. Hirschfeld, I.: A study of skulls in the American Museum of Natural History in relation to periodontal disease, J. Dent. Res. 5:241, 1923.
8. Kenney, E.B., and Ramfjord, S.P.: Cellular dynamics in root formation of teeth in rhesus monkeys, J. Dent. Res. 48:114, 1969.
9. Kronfeld, R.: Biology of the cementum, J.A.D.A. 25:1451, 1939.
10. Listgarten, M.A.: A light and electron microscopic study of coronal cementogenesis, Arch. Oral Biol. 13:93, 1968.
11. McHugh, W.D., and Zander, H.A.: Cell division in the periodontium of developing and erupted teeth, Dent. Pract. 15:451, 1965.
12. Melcher, A.H.: Biological processes in resorption, deposition, and regeneration of bone. In S.S. Stahl, In Periodontal Surgery. Biologic Basis and Technique, edited by S. S. Stahl. Springfield, Il.: Charles C. Thomas, 1976.
13. Mikola, O.J., and Bauer, W. H.: Cementicles and fragments of cementum in the periodontal membrane, Oral Surg. 2:1063, 1949.
14. Miller, E.J., and Martin, G.R.: The collagen of bone, Clin. Orthop. 59:195, 1968.
15. Neiders, M.E., et al.: Electron probe microanalysis of cementum and underlying dentin in young permanent teeth, J. Dent. Res. 51:122, 1972.
16. Orban, B.: Resorption and repair of the surface of the root, J.A.D.A. 15:1768, 1928.
17. Ramfjord, S.P., and Kohler, C.A.: Periodontal reaction to functional occlusal stress, J. Periodont. 30:95, 1959.
18. Selvig, K.A.: An ultrastructural study of cementum formation, Acta Odont. Scand. 22:105, 1964.
19. Selvig, K.A.: Studies on the Genesis, Composition and Fine Structure of Cementum, Oslo: Universitietsforlaget, 1967.
20. Sicher, H., and Bhaskar, S. N.: Orban's Oral Histology and Embryology, 7th ed, St. Louis: C. V. Mosby Co., 1972.
21. Soni, M.M.: Quantitative study of bone activity in alveolar and femoral bone of the guinea pig, J. Dent. Res. 47:584, 1968.
22. Stahl, S.S.: Cantor, M., and Zwig, E.: Fenestration of the labial alveolar plate in human skulls, Periodontics. 1:99, 1963.
23. Stallard, R.E.: The utilization of H^3 proline by the connective tissue elements of the periodontium, Periodontics 1:185, 1963.
24. Tonna, E.A.: Factors (aging) affecting bone and cementum, J. Periodont. 47:267, 1976.
25. Waerhaug, J.: Effect of C-avitaminosis on the supporting structure of the teeth, J. Periodont. 29:87, 1958.

5

PHYSIOLOGY AND DEFENSE MECHANISMS OF THE DENTOGINGIVAL JUNCTION

The continuity of the epithelium is considered to be an important protective barrier to foreign agents, including bacteria, their toxic products, and antigenic substances. This continuity is lost with the eruption of teeth, and another anatomic and functional dentogingival complex of tissues is required to provide an effective interface between hard and soft tissues and local and systemic defense mechanisms.

DENTO-GINGIVAL JUNCTION

The dento-gingival junction (DGJ) is the mechanism that takes on the function of the protective barrier. This function had been provided by a continuous mucosa prior to the penetration of the teeth into the oral cavity. The sealing junction between the epithelium and the adjoining tooth surface is the most vulnerable component of periodontal health. Besides the anatomical structural barrier, a dynamic defense system is active at the DGJ. Of particular importance are the gingival sulcus and the junctional epithelium.

The gingival sulcus

The gingival sulcus has been defined as "a shallow groove between the tooth and the gingiva, extending from the free surface of the junctional epithelium [sulcus bottom] to the gingival margin" (Fig. 5-1).[33] Thus, the gingival sulcus is a histological phenomenon that cannot be assessed clinically by probing or by any other presently available method.

In germ-free animals,[1] or following prolonged perfect plaque control,[20] there appears to be no gingival sulcus, and the junctional epithelium extends to the free gingival margin, with a very narrow zone of sulcular epithelium at the gingival margin. However, such conditions do not exist in clinically healthy gingiva in average persons[47] or animals,[22] in which some sulcus depth can almost always be observed histologically. The average histological sulcus depth in humans has been reported to be 0.2 to 0.7 mm.[15,28] It appears that this depth can be reduced to 0 by prophylaxis followed by perfect chemical plaque control,[46] whereas with conventional toothbrushing there will be at least a shallow sulcus. Therefore, it is possible that the sulcus depth is related to the level of plaque on the tooth surface[33] and the mechanical effects of tooth cleaning procedures.[46] Thus, the bottom of the sulcus may move up or down depending on those conditions.

Both the junctional and the oral sulcular epithelium undergo continuous turnover of cells with surface shedding. The renewal or turnover time of specific epithelial structures depends on how the basic data are processed.[25] If mitotic activity is related to surface area, the junctional epithelium has a very high turnover and shedding rate, since the surface area of the junctional epithelium in the normal gingival sulcus is very small compared to the area of basal cells.[21] It has been suggested that the renewal time for junctional epithelium in primates is about 5 days,[33] while for oral

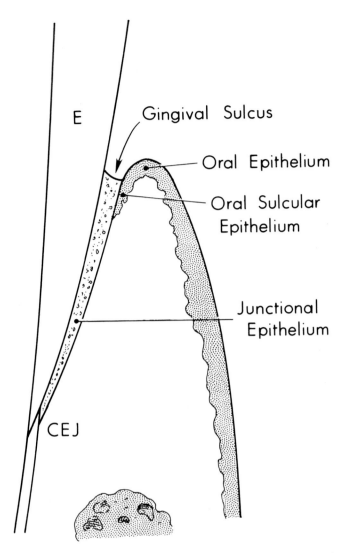

Fig. 5-1. Schematic representation of dento-gingival junction and gingival sulcus.

Labels in figure: E, Gingival Sulcus, Oral Epithelium, Oral Sulcular Epithelium, Junctional Epithelium, CEJ

gingival epithelium it is 8 to 10 days. The most important clinical consideration is the very high rate of shedding of junctional cells, expressed as number of exfoliated cells per unit of surface area. This rate has been calculated to be 50 to 100 times faster than for oral gingival epithelium. This means that degenerating surface cells, covered and sometimes invaded by bacteria, are expelled at a fast rate, and it also means that superficial epithelial tears are eliminated readily. Thus, the high rate of turnover of junctional and sulcular epithelium, as well as the connective tissue of the periodontium, are important aspects of the defense mechanism.

Physical aspects of dentogingival junction. Only minimal mechanical or physical force is required to penetrate to the base of the junctional epithelium. Such mechanical separation does not necessarily split the epithelial attachment to the teeth, but often makes a separation between junctional cells slightly away from the tooth surface.[23,39]

It appears that in unanesthetized humans, routine clinical probing will extend to the connective tissue attachment in the presence of various degrees of gingival inflammation.[23,29,35] The penetration of the probe may be slightly beyond the bottom of the junctional epithelium in cases of active destructive periodontitis with degenerated connective tissues apically to the epithelial attachment.[31] Routine scaling will also split the junctional epithelium and extend to the connective tissue attachment.[30] In cases of healthy gingiva, the probing may end within the junctional epithelium, thus precluding an accurate clinical assessment of the connetive tissue attachment in humans and in animals after treatment.[2,7]

Because the separation of the junctional epithelium from the tooth is often intercellular,[17,43] enzymatic action upon intercellular substances may be of great significance in deepening of the gingival sulcus. Along with bacterial hyaluronidases and collagenases,[44] lysosomal enzymes from polymorphonuclear cells[38] may be active in weakening cell adhesion and thereby reducing the physical strength of the dentogingival junction.

The initial epithelial changes of DGJ separation are widening of the intercellular spaces and increased permeability before actual cell detachment occurs. Electron-microscopic features of initial separation between epithelial cells include widening of the intercellular spaces, opening of tight junctions, and decreased number of desmosomes.[32]

Gingival fluid and functions. Since it was first demonstrated that fluid could pass from the blood into the gingival sulcus in animals[4] and humans,[5] a large number of investigations regarding this gingival fluid have appeared. The gingival fluid contains most of the components of the blood serum, including functionally active neutrophils and components of the complements of the complement system.

The complement system is activated during gingival inflammation. Activation results in the generation of substances that enhance phagocytosis and destruction of bacteria and perpetuate the inflammatory response. Complement components also contain antibodies specific for determinants of bacteria present in periodontal pockets. Complement components may be involved in bone resorption associated with tissue destruction.

Also of great interest in the etiology of periodontal disease and gingival defense is the fact that foreign matters and fluids may pass from the gingival sulcus into the underlying connective tissue.[20] Relatively large albumin molecules,[41] antigens, and a number of enzymes may penetrate the junctional and sulcular epithelium.[6] It also appears that several enzymes such as histamine,[9] hyaluronidase,[27] and horseradish peroxidase,[26] may increase the intercellular spaces and make the epithelium more penetrable to bacterial toxins or other noxious substances. Because bacteria commonly present in bacterial plaque may produce such enzymes,[37] it has been suggested that the gingival defense may be lowered by these bacterial enzymes as they make the junctional and sulcular epithelium penetrable to substances that would not otherwise be able to penetrate.

The permeability of the epithelium in the gingival sulcus may also be increased by release of lysosomal enzymes from neutrophils.[40]

The neutrophils present in the gingival fluid transmigrate from the gingival plexus of vessels through the junctional epithelium to the gingival sulcus and oral cavity. The bases for the migration of neutrophils are chemotactic substances in dental plaque and saliva. These functionally active neutrophils are the first line of defense at the dento-gingival junction. Although the enzymes produced by the neutrophils in response to bacterial challenge may produce damage to the tissues, as well as kill bacteria, the damage is contained by control mechanisms and repaired quickly because of the rapid turnover of the periodontal tissues.

The amount of gingival fluid flow is related to vascular permeability in the so-called crevicular plexus.[10,11,12] Along the junctional epithelium, the subepithelial vessels are parallel to the surface and are made up mostly of venules rather than capillaries. The venules have a greater disposition toward increased permeability than do capillaries and arterioles, and they are more susceptible to hemorrhage, thrombosis, and allergic injury. There is a marked tendency toward permeability of the crevicular plexus vessels following mechanical and chemical injury.[11,12,13,14]

The gingival fluid flow is increased by masticatory function, contact stimuli of the tooth, and toothbrushing.[4,5] The role of tooth and gingival movements with pulse pressure in the expulsion of foreign material from the sulcus has not been assessed.[18] It seems reasonable that the tonus of healthy collagenous gingival fibers will tend to move foreign material out of the sulcus. This mechanism of sulcular cleaning is effective against a smooth tooth surface, such as intact enamel, but the roughness found associated with subgingival margins of dental restorations[42] and exposed cementoenamel junctions will interfere with expulsion of bacteria and toxic products. Even intact exposed cementum has roughness corresponding to the Sharpey's fiber attachment.[34] This roughness may enhance bacterial retention. The cemental surface may also absorb toxins, which then cannot be expelled by the normal sulcular defense mechanisms. Thus, the gingival defense system is by far the most effective in maintenance of normal anatomical relations between the intact tooth and the gingiva when the junctional epithelium contacts only enamel.

The junctional epithelium and the epithelial attachment complex seem to be sterile under physiological conditions,[19,32] and, if infected by injury, they regain sterility by natural defense mechanisms.[39] It thus appears that the junctional epithelium provides a seal that prevents bacteria normally present in the gingival sulcus from penetrating along the tooth surface to the connective tissue attachment.

SUMMARY

The mechanisms of defense of the dento-gingival junction involve tissues that provide for delivery of humoral and cellular responses to potentially destructive bacteria, their toxins, and antigenic substances. Mechanisms of defense also include an unusually high turnover rate of tissue; this tissue, when damaged, is quickly repaired. The anatomical continuity provided by the junctional epithelium, and the functional characteristics of the junctional epithelium that allow the passage of active neutrophils to the site of injurious agents, involve lines of defense that are generally highly effective. In chapter 7, the conditions under which defenses are no longer effective and the onset of disease occurs are discussed.

REFERENCES

1. Amstad-Jossi, M., and Schroeder, H. E.: Age-related alterations of periodontal structures around the cemento-enamel junction and of the gingival connective tissue composition in germ-free rats, J. Periodont. Res. 13:76, 1978.
2. Armitage, G. C., Svanberg, G. K., and Löe, H.: Microscopic evaluation of clinical measurements of connective tissue attachment levels, J. Clin. Periodontol. 4:173, 1977.
3. Attström, R., and Egelberg, J.: Emigration of blood neutrophils and monocytes into the gingival crevices, J. Periodont. Res. 5:48, 1970.
4. Brill, N., and Krasse, B.: The passage of tissue fluid into the clinically healthy gingival pocket, Acta Odont. Scand. 16:322, 1958.
5. Brill, N., and Björn, H.: Passage of tissue fluid into human gingival pockets, Acta Odont. Scand. 17:11, 1959.
6. Caffesse, R. G., and Nasjleti, C. E.: Enzymatic penetration through intact sulcular epithelium, J. Periodont. 47:391, 1976.
7. Caton, J., and Zander, H. A.: Osseous repair of an infrabony pocket without new attachment of connective tissues, J. Clin. Periodontol. 3:54, 1976.
8. Cimasoni, G.: Crevicular Fluid Updated, Basel: S. Karger, 1983.
9. Egelberg, J.: Diffusion of histamine into the gingival crevice and through the crevicular epithelium, Acta Odont. Scand. 21:271, 1963.
10. Egelberg, J.: The blood vessels of the dento-gingival junction, J. Periodont. Res. 1:163, 1966.
11. Egelberg, J.: Permeability of the dento-gingival blood vessels. I. Application of the vascular labeling method and gingival fluid measurements, J. Periodont. Res. 1:180, 1966.

12. Egelberg, J.: Permeability of the dento-gingival blood vessels. II. Clinically healthy gingivae, J. Periodont. Res. 1:276, 1966.
13. Egelberg, J.: Permeability of the dento-gingival blood vessels. III. Clinically inflamed gingivae, J. Periodont. Res. 1:287, 1966.
14. Egelberg, J.: Permeability of the dento-gingival blood vessels. IV. Effect of histamine on vessels in clinically healthy and chronically inflamed gingivae, J. Periodont. Res. 1:297, 1966.
15. Gargiulo, A. W., Wentz, F. M., and Orban, B. J.: Dimensions and relations of the dento-gingival junction in humans, J. Periodont. 32:261, 1961.
16. Genco, R. J. and Slots, J.: Host responses in periodontal diseases, J. Dent. Res. 63:441, 1984.
17. Henning, F. R., and Zander, H. A.: Method for studying limits of gingival crevice and relative strength of epithelial attachment, J. Dent. Res. 42:653, 1963.
18. Körber, H. H.: Periodontal pulsation, J. Periodont. 41:382, 1970.
19. Lindhe, J., and Mansson, U.: The bacteriologyy of the gingival crevices of erupting human incisors, J. Periodont. Res. 1:14, 1966.
20. Lindhe, J., and Rylander, H.: Experimental gingivitis in young dogs, Scand. J. Dent. Res. 83:314, 1975.
21. Listgarten, M. A.: Normal development, structure, physiology and repair of gingival epithelium, Oral Sci. Rev. 1:3, 1972.
22. Listgarten, M. A., and Ellegaard, B.: Experimental gingivitis in the monkey, J. Periodont. Res. 8:199, 1973.
23. Listgarten, M. A., Mao, R., and Robinson, P. J.: Periodontal probing and relationship of the probe tip to periodontal tissues, J. Periodont. 47:511, 1976.
24. Löe, H., and Holm-Pedersen, P.: Absence and presence of fluid from normal and inflamed gingivae, Periodontics 3:171, 1965.
25. Löe, H., and Karring, T.: A quantitative analysis of the epithelium-connective tissue interphase in relation to assessment of the mitotic index, J. Dent. Res. 48:634, 1969.
26. McDougall, W. A.: Pathways of penetration and effects of horseradish peroxidase in rat molar gingiva, Arch. Oral Biol. 15:621, 1971.
27. Murphy, P. J., and Stallard, R. E.: An altered gingival attachment epithelium, Periodontics. 6:105, 1968.
28. Orban, B., and Kohler, J.: Die physiologische Zahnfleischtasche, Epithelansatz und Epitheltiefenwucherung, Z. Stomatol. 22:353, 1924.
29. Pedersen, G.: Exact method for clinical measurement of loss of periodontal attachment, Scand. J. Dent. Res. 85:414, 1977.
30. Ranfjord, S. P., and Kiester, G.: The gingival sulcus and the periodontal pocket immediately following scaling of teeth, J. Periodont. 34:401, 1963.
31. Saglie, R., Johansen, J. R., and Flötra, L.: The zone of completely and partially destructed periodontal fibers in pathological pockets, J. Clin. Periodontol. 47:281, 1976.
32. Schroeder, H., and Listgarten, M. A.: The Fine Structure of the Developing Epithelial Attachment of Human Teeth, Basel: S. Karger, 1971.
33. Schroeder, H. E.: Histopathology of the gingival sulcus, T. Lehner. In The Borderland Between Caries and Periodontal Disease, ed. London: Academic Press, 1977.
34. Selvig, K. A.: Ultrastructural changes in cementum and adjacent connective tissue in periodontal disease, Acta Odont. Scand. 24:459, 1966.
35. Sivertson, J. F., and Burgett, F. G.: Probing of pockets related to the attachment level, J. Periodont. 47:281, 1976.
36. Skougaard, M.: Cell renewal with special reference to the gingival epithelium, Adv. Oral Biol. 4:261, 1970.
37. Söder, P. O., and Nord, C. E.: Determination of hyaluronidase activity in dental plaque material, J. Periodont. Res. 4:208, 1969.
38. Taichman, N. S.: Mediation of inflammation by the polymorphonuclear leukocyte as a sequela of immune reactions, J. Periodont. 41:228, 1970.
39. Taylor, A. C., and Campbell, M. M.: Reattachment of gingival epithelium to the tooth, J. Periodont. 43:281, 1972.
40. Thilander, H.: The effect of leukocytic enzyme activity on the structure of the gingival pocket epithelium in man, Acta Odont. Scand. 21:432, 1963.
41. Tolo, K.: A study of permeability of gingival pocket epithelium to albumin in guinea pigs and Norwegian pigs, Arch. Oral Biol. 16:881, 1971.
42. Waerhaug, J.: Effects of rough surfaces upon gingival tissue, J. Dent. Res. 35:323, 1961.
43. Weinreb, M. W.: The epithelial attachment, J. Periodont. 31:186, 1960.
44. Weis, L., and Kapes, D. L.: Observation on cell adhesion and separation following enzyme treatment, Exp. Cell Res. 41:701, 1966.
45. Wilson, A. G., and McHugh, W. D.: Gingival exudate. An index of gingivitis? Dent. Pract. Dent. Rec. 21:261, 1971.
46. Wolfram, K., et al.: Effect of tooth cleaning procedures on gingival sulcus depth, J. Periodont. Res. 9:44, 1974.
47. Zachrisson, B. U., and Schultz-Haudt, S. O.: A comparative histological study of clinically normal and chronically inflamed gingivae from the same individuals, Odont. Tidskr. 76:179, 1968.

6

CLASSIFICATION, MEASUREMENT, EPIDEMIOLOGY, AND NATURAL HISTORY OF PERIODONTAL DISEASES

Several issues are brought together in this chapter because they relate to each other. For example, epidemiology requires some form of measurement, and a study of the natural history of disease depends on epidemiological methods. An outline or classification of the nature of periodontal diseases should establish the vocabulary necessary to discuss these various issues.

Concepts of classification, epidemiology, measurement, and natural history reflect attempts to explain the nature and control of periodontal diseases. Questions that require further clarification include the following: Is gingivitis an initial stage of periodontitis, and, if so, under what conditions does it convert to destructive peridontitis? Are there ways to predict such a change or to measure the activity of periodontal lesions? Are various forms of periodontal disease specific bacterial infections? Is the natural history of adult periodontitis that of a chronic infective process that is episodic, site-specific and characterized by quantal, localized losses of attachment? Is it possible, considering the inadequacy of present methods of measurement, to use prevalence data about adult periodontitis from epidemiological and clinical studies as incidence data? Can cross-sectional data be analyzed to provide reliable information on the natural history of periodontitis? Are host responses site-specific, so that disease activity at individual sites will vary in accordance with differences in systemic and local defense mechanisms and with differences in the numbers and species of pathogenic and "protective" microorganisms at these sites? Is periodontitis age-dependent? Is periodontitis the major cause of tooth loss (by extraction) in adults? What are the risk factors in periodontal disease? Is gingivitis a disease? Is it a dental health problem? What is the magnitude of destructive periodontitis in the United States?

Of the three major surveys of periodontal disease conducted by the National Institute of Dental Research, only the first two have been reported and reevaluated in great detail. The data from these studies, which were published in 1965[50] and 1979,[51] have been reinterpreted a number of times, and the various interpretations reflect innovative ways of reassessing the data. These and other studies have demonstrated the importance of epidemiologic data.

CLASSIFICATION OF PERIODONTAL DISEASES

Classifications of periodontal diseases vary according to opinions regarding the etiology of the diseases and to the emphasis placed upon clinical and histopathological findings.[38,42,81,82] Controversial areas that influence classification include the kind of data needed to accept that (1) gingivitis is or is not a disease; (2) specific bacteria or immune responses cause specific forms of destructive periodontal disease; (3) specific systemic factors cause periodontitis or influence its progress; (4) periodontal manifestations of dermatologic disorders are or are not forms of periodontal disease and do or do not significantly influence the progress of periodontal diseases; and (5) loss of attachment can or cannot progress in the absence of inflammation. These are only a few of the issues that must be resolved in order to reach a consensus on the classification of periodontal diseases.

In most forms of destructive periodontal disease, the pathobiologic phenomena that occur are immune and nonimmune inflammatory responses to injury from bacterial plaque. The associated loss of attachment and supporting structures, and the development of periodontal pockets, reflect the varying degrees of adequacy of host defenses, bacterial virulence, and other local and systemic factors that may influence the symbiotic balance between host and microbes.

There are still not enough data to classify periodontitis as a series of specific infections, especially if one desires to provide a diagnosis of various site-specific bacteria in the same mouth. The classification of periodontitis into adult and childhood/juvenile forms points up the advances in our understanding of the disease, although it must be admitted that placing adult periodontitis into a separate category seems much less difficult than categorizing such other forms of juvenile periodontitis, prepubertal periodontitis, and rapidly progressing periodontitis.

Older reports on classification of periodontal diseases by the Committees on Nomenclature of the American Academy of Periodontology have not been widely used, although their division of inflammatory lesions into gingivitis and periodontitis is still generally accepted. However, until data is available to define precisely the etiology of periodontal diseases, it is unlikely that any classification of peridontal diseases will reflect other than an incomplete picture and the need for simplicity or convenience. New classifications of periodontitis will continue to be presented,[31,84] but cannot be considered final for a number of reasons, including insufficient diagnostic criteria, uncertainty about disease activity and the role of the host locally to various specific bacteria, retrospective kinds of data about the patient, and the complexity of histopathologic changes. The classification of periodontal diseases given in table 6-1 is a simple and convenient way of categorizing periodontal diseases, one which recognizes the inflammatory basis for clinical and histologic manifestations and reflects the possibility that systemic and local factors may modify the host's responses to bacteria and their products.

The local factors, including bacteria, their products, and antigens, are discussed in chapter 8; intrinsic or systemic modifying factors of the inflammatory response are presented in chapter 9; and the relationship of occlusion to periodontal disease is given in chapter 10.

The details of the clinical characteristics of gingivitis are given in chapter 12, and the histopathology of gingivitis and periodontitis is discussed in chapter 7. Therefore, only a brief consideration of gingivitis and periodontitis will be presented here.

Gingivitis refers to the inflammatory response of the gingiva to local irritants such as dental plaque. Such inflammatory lesions are called *simple gingivitis* when no specific unusual modifying factors are present and there is no marked gingival enlargement.

If there is marked enlargement or hyperplasia, and known or suspected local or systemic modifying factors are present, the gingival inflammatory response is classified as *complex gingivitis*. The name of the modifying factor is used in designating the disease: *pregnancy gingivitis*, for example. Gingival hyperplasia associated with mouth breathing is termed *mouth-breathing gingivitis*. *Allergic gingivitis* occurs in some individuals who use a particular type of chewing gum.[52] *Acute necrotizing ulcerative gingivitis* (NUG), referred to in the past as *Vincent's infection* or *trench mouth*, is an acute inflammatory disease characterized principally by an acute necrotizing ulcerative process. It is also considered a complex form of gingivitis.

Traumatic gingivitis refers to direct injury to the gingiva from physical agents, drugs, chemicals, or thermal agents. Causes include improper toothbrushing, aspirin burn, phenol excharization, or burns from hot foods.

Gingival recession or *gingival atrophy* may be related to aging or to traumatic injury, such as that caused by improper toothbrushing or, inadvertently, by the dentist (iatrogenic). Gingival atrophy usually refers to atrophic tissues in elderly patients.

A *periodontal abscess* is an acute inflammatory lesion characterized by a focal accumulation of pus in the periodontium. It usually occurs in a pathologically deepened gingival crevice or a periodontal pocket when foreign agents such as food debris and microorganisms become lodged in the tissues.

Trauma from occlusion refers to progressive injury to the supporting structures of the teeth as a result of occlusal dysfunction. Occlusal factors are considered a modifying factor but not an initiating factor in inflammatory periodontal disease.

Simple periodontitis (including chronic inflammatory disease, adult periodontitis, and chronic destructive periodontal disease) refers to an inflammatory lesion of the periodontium in which the development of peridontal pockets (formed by apical migration of epithelial attachment and loss of alveolar bone) occurs, but the response of the tissues is not adversely influenced by systemic factors or intrinsic disease.

Table 6-1. Classification of periodontal diseases

Gingivitis
  Simple
  Complex
    Gingival hyperplasia
    Necrotizing ulcerative
    Traumatic
    Gingival atrophy/recession
Trauma from occlusion
Periodontitis
  Simple
  Complex
    e.g., prepubertal, juvenile

Complex Periodontitis refers to destructive periodontal disease involving loss of attachment in epithelial and connective tissue, and loss of supporting bone, in association with known or suspected local or systemic factors that interfere with the defense mechanisms normally involved in effectively meeting the microbial challenge of dental plaque. Included are destructive diseases of the supporting periodontal structures in which the responses of the host have been adversely affected by specifiable or by obscure intrinsic factors such as, in early-onset periodontitis, genetic and/or molecular neutrophil defects. Prepubertal, juvenile, and rapidly progressing periodontitis are discussed in chapter 13.

The majority of cases of periodontal disease can be accounted for by what is known as the *gingivitis/adult periodontitis complex*, which includes all forms of simple gingivitis and simple periodontitis. This complex is, in general, an inflammatory response to bacterial plaque on the teeth, and no detectable disturbance in the host's defence mechanisms is presently known to occur. A number of disturbances may affect the periodontium and influence periodontal therapy (Table 6-2).

Table 6-2. Outline of diseases, states, or agents that may affect the periodontium and complicate periodontal therapy

Herpes simplex	Chédiak-Higashi syndrome
Chickenpox	Diabetes mellitus
Heavy metals	Erythema multiforme
Scleroderma	Lichen planus
Dialysis	Radiation
Hypophosphatasia	Neoplasia
Leukemia	Scurvy
Acatalasia	Down's Syndrome
Palmar-plantar hyperkeratosis	Cyclic neutropenia
Benign mucous membrane pemphigoid	Pregnancy, puberty

EPIDEMIOLOGY OF PERIODONTAL DISEASES

Descriptive epidemiology refers to large-scale studies of the distributions and determinants of states of health in human populations.[106] Descriptive and clinical epidemiological studies are conducted to determine the various aspects of the prevention and control of disease. Large descriptive epidemiologic studies on the severity of gingivitis and periodontitis have been conducted throughout the world, and analyses of the data have led to ideas concerning etiologic factors, prevalence, and the natural history of periodontal diseases. Much of the data are highly aggregated, and events have not always been linked to persons, place, and time. *Social epidemiology* has been defined as including those behavioral, cultural, and economic factors associated with the development and progression of disease and with maintenance of health.[13]

Clinical epidemiology is the application of epidemiological principles and methods to problems encountered in clinical dentistry.[29] Its emphasis is on health-seeking behaviour, referral patterns, diagnostic approaches, treatment choices and outcomes, and technological evaluations. Major objectives are optimization of diagnosis and treatment of disease, and health-resource allocation. The clinician requires some skill in clinical epidemiology in order to make decisions based on often uncertain information that may be expressed in terms of probabilities, or on information estimated on the basis of the clinician's past experience with similar disease states.

Incidence refers to the number of cases of disease that occur in a given period of time per unit of population; for example, 50 cases of measles occurring for every 10,000 children in 1 year. The period of time involved is referred to as the *rate*. *Prevalence* refers to the number of cases of disease found at a particular time regardless of time of onset. Prevalence is a function of both incidence and duration of disease; thus, one may speak of the incidence of acute necrotizing ulcerative gingivitis and the prevalence of periodontitis. Although it is generally not possible to estimate incidence from age-specific prevalence, a statistical model has been proposed to estimate incidence from age-specific prevalence using *cross-sectional data*.[56]

Cross-sectional data are observations obtained for individuals in the same age group and/or at the same time. *Longitudinal data* are observations of the same individuals repeated over time so that causal inferences may be drawn in relation to the temporal sequence of events. The *cohort effect* refers to variations in health status that arise from the different causal factors to which each birth cohort (group) is exposed.[54] Generally, data from cross-sectional studies cannot be used to differentiate between age-effect and cohort effect and therefore to determine the putative association of periodontitis with age. Thus, both risk factors and disease are ascertained at the same time. But, insofar as periodontitis can be considered a nonreversible disease, the nature of age as a risk factor can be estimated using cross-sectional data.

In epidemiological studies of the state of health, the effect of disease is the dependent variable and the cause of disease is the independent variable. In clinical practice, the effect is naturally of particular interest to the patient and dentist; it is what the dentist seeks to address with periodontal therapy. In doing so, he thus speaks to change the dependent variable.

Experimental unit

Many of the principles and methods used in descriptive epidemiology, including the measurement of disease and analysis of data, are used in clinical epidemiological studies and clinical trials.[18] There is uncertainty about what constitutes the appropriate fundamental experimental unit—patient, tooth, or other specific sites—and whether a particular statistical model can account for the possibly inappropriate use of a particular experimental unit; for example, the use of multiple sites in the same patient as independent entities.[45] This uncertainty causes several problems.

The problems in the conduct of epidemiological studies and clinical trials involve (1) the apparently discontinuous nature of periodontitis, which is characterized by seemingly random onsets at individual sites in the dentition, with sporadic exacerbations of the disease and extended periods of remission; and (2) lack of an accurate measure of periodontitis progress or activity.

The first problem suggests that periodontitis is seldom generalized throughout the mouth, neither in terms of active disease nor in severity of past effects. To pool information (in other words, to average all the measurements of diseases) from all sites—whether active or inactive and with or without loss of attachment—may not provide a clear statement about the periodontal status of a patient or a population.

If the "site-specific" or "burst" model of periodontitis[102] is correct, then the significance of the findings of a number of epidemiological studies of periodontitis and clinical trials is open to question because of those studies' use of pooled information. This problem is apparent in evaluating therapeutic outcomes. Most sites that are measured would be inactive according to the "burst" model and would not be able to respond to therapy, thereby swamping active disease sites and any therapeutic effects that may be present.[43] Attempts to treat individual sites (for example, attachment level at a specific site) as experimental units, rather than taking the patient as the statistical sampling unit (which requires using the summary or average mouth score for all sites), have been questioned. Although it has been suggested that individual sites exhibit characteristics of statistically independent events and are only minimally host-specific, evidence does not provide much support for that concept. When properly monitored, sites within the same mouth will show association, and site behavior over time will therefore not be random and unpredictable.[43]

OBSERVATIONS

Valid and reliable data about the status of the periodontium and etiological factors in periodontal diseases are desired in epidemiological studies, clinical trials, and even in clinical practice. *Valid measures* of periodontal disease should accurately depict the state of the periodontium relative to disease. *Reliable observations*, when repeated, are expected to provide essentially the same data. Furthermore, the observations (measurements) to be made should be appropriate (valid) for the questions being asked. In view of recent perspectives on periodontal diseases, the questions being asked cannot be adequately answered by past epidemiological studies. In those studies, the observations were often directed only at providing information on the prevalence of disease in different populations that were at possible risk for various potential etiologic factors in periodontal disease. Unfortunately, given the various methods of observation and the differences among different observers, severity data for gingivitis and periodontitis is difficult to compare and assess.

A correlation or conjunction between two variables is not sufficient evidence to conclude that one variable, such as plaque, causes an effect on another variable, such as gingivitis.[5] In this case, it is first necessary to establish that plaque causes gingivitis. This has been done in experiments in which plaque was removed and in which gingivitis then disappeared.[59] With the return of plaque, the gingivitis also returned. Specific characteristics of the plaque, such as bacteria, have yet to be identified. The relationship among plaque, its removal, and gingivitis can be demonstrated with replicability and predictability. Although precise cause-and-effect relations may not be determined from descriptive epidemiologic surveys, it may be possible to plan experiments to deal more directly with cause and effect and to identify specific organisms.

Although the presence of periodontal disease is in itself a significant finding, it is also necessary to assess the severity of the disease. While gingivitis may be reversible through removal of local irritants (plaque and calculus), and destructive periodontitis currently is not reversible for the most part, it is obvious that severity data on sites of destructive periodontal disease are very important for an understanding of the natural history of the disease and for its prevention. Whether the destructive process is active at the time of prevalence assessment cannot be determined on the basis of either field survey methods or laboratory techniques currently available.

Measurement of periodontal status

The measurement of clinical and epidemiological correlates of periodontal diseases and health is generally accomplished by scales referred to as *nominal*, *ordinal*, and *interval*.[29]

Nominal data refers to phenomena that can be categorized but that are without inherent order.

Ordinal data refers to periodontal data that is ordered on the basis of diagnostic criteria, but for which the sizes of the intervals are not specified (e.g., none, some, more, most). Such data may be expressed as numbers 0, 1, 2, etc.; however, the true size of the interval between none, some, more, and most, in terms of quantity (of plaque or gingivitis), is not known.

Where the size of an interval is known and can be measured in such physical units as millimeters, grams, etc., the data are ordered and are referred to as *interval data*. Although measurement error is a consideration, using a probe having millimeter markings to measure attachment level provides interval data.

When there is a true zero point, the scale is called a *ratio* scale. This scale has had limited application in clinical measurement, even though data acquired with it may be related to gain and loss of attachment.

The use of ordinal data in statistical analyses requires the use of nonparametric tests because such data are not isomorphic to the structure of arithmetic.[4] For example, on an ordinal scale, a grade of 4 gingivitis is not necessarily two times a grade of 2. The numerical expressions for ordinal-scaled assessments of the severity of gingivitis and the quantity of plaque or gingivitis are generally called *indices*, or *indexes*. The indices discussed here do not provide information on active disease sites in periodontitis.

Index measurements

The measurement of gingivitis and periodontitis has generally been accomplished by methods of observation that are insensitive to disease activity. These methods measure only effects of disease. They do not reflect recent findings, which suggest that, at any one time in chronic destructive periodontitis, most sites in the mouth are inactive, while only a few (3.5%) are active.[32] Repeated measurements retrospectively indicate disease activity at the clinical or epidemiological level of assessment.

Many indices have been developed. They were used first for epidemiological surveys and then for clinical trials, and even for monitoring individual patients. Indices for gingivitis, plaque, calculus, periodontal disease, and treatment need have been used, discarded, and reevaluated for a number of reasons. The search continues for indices that can satisfy the conditions in the field and in the laboratory as far as simplicity, reproducibility, and analysis, yet provide the maximum amount of information consistent with the data reduction desired. It is most desirable that the index permit direct comparisons among epidemiological studies of different populations by different investigators.[16] Such requirements have yet to be realized in practice.

Gingivitis. One of the first successful numerical systems for recording gingival heath was the *PMA index*.[100] Each area of the gingiva—papillary (P), mar-

ginal (M), and attached (A)—was considered to be involved sequentially from P to A and thus could be used to measure the severity of the disease. The severity of inflammation in each area was graded on a scale from 0 to 4. These scores were added and the average value for the total number of teeth scored was given in PMA units per person. Initially, only the labial gingivae of the mandibular six anterior teeth were scored, but a number of modifications were later introduced. All the teeth could be scored, data could be presented without reference to severity (units scored as 0 or 1), and all scores for PMA units could be added and the sum taken as representing the status of the individual. This index was initially intended primarily for the assessment of gingivitis in children and is no longer in use.

Commonly used indices of gingivitis are the *gingival index*,[58] the *papilla bleeding index*,[98] and the *sulcus bleeding index*.[72] Although bleeding may be an important aspect in these indices, the gingival index may not utilize the bleeding component. A comparison of the gingival index with the modified papilla bleeding index suggests the bleeding index may be more sensitive than the gingival index to early gingivitis, but there is little agreement over the criteria for measurement and the standards to be employed.

The gingival index (GI),[58,59] based on a scale of 0 to 3, has been used in a number of clinical studies to assess inflammation. A score of 1 indicates mild inflammation, with no bleeding on probing and only slight change in color and edema. A score of 2 indicates moderate inflammation with redness, edema, glazing, and bleeding on probing. A score of 3 indicates severe inflammation, marked redness, edema, ulceration, and a tendency to spontaneous hemorrhage. The mesial, distal, buccal, and lingual surfaces are scored separately. The linearity of the GI index has not been tested; the index is similar in this respect to the PMA index and most other indices. It has been widely used in clinical trials and in some epidemiological studies.

The papilla bleeding index (PBI) is an index that is sensitive enough to be used for monitoring individual patients.[101] The PBI is a modification of the sulcus bleeding index (SBI), which was not limited to bleeding but also considered color, edema, and ulceration. The PBI is based on bleeding following gentle probing of the interdental papilla: 0 = no bleeding, 1 = single bleeding point, 2 = several bleeding points at the gingival margin (or fine line of blood), 3 = interdental triangle filled with blood, and 4 = profuse bleeding. The PBI has been modified to use a timed appearance of bleeding; 0 = no bleeding in 30 seconds of probing; 1 = bleeding between 3 and 30 seconds; 2 = bleeding within 2 seconds of probing; 3 = bleeding immediately upon probing. The sum of these scores, divided by the number of papilla examined, is the PBI. Control of uniform probing pressure is a problem in using this index.

Gingival crevicular fluid measurement has been used as an index of gingival inflammation for clinical trials and individual patients, but is not practical for epidemiological studies involving field conditions or large numbers of subjects. Variation in collection of the fluid requires careful evaluation.[19]

There is no universally accepted index of gingivitis. Several reports dealing with gingivitis indices have provided insight into current concepts of measuring gingivitis and their application to clinical epidemiologic studies.[7,10,110]

Periodontitis. The *periodontal index* (PI)[97] is of historical interest. It was used widely for early epidemiological surveys.[91-97] It is based on a nonlinear scale of 0, 1, 2, 6, 8, in which the criteria for scoring are weighted heavily in favor of destructive periodontal disease. A score of 0 is based on the absence of overt inflammation and loss of function due to destruction of supporting structures. A score of 1 (mild gingivitis) is given when there is an overt area of inflammation in the free gingiva, but does not circumscribe the tooth. A score of 2 (gingivitis) requires that inflammation completely circumscribe the tooth, without any apparent break in the epithelial attachment. A score of 6 (gingivitis with pocket formation) is given when the epithelial attachment has been broken and there is a pocket.

There is no interference with normal masticatory function, no increase in tooth mobility, and no drifting. A score of 8 indicates advanced destruction with loss of masticatory function. The tooth may be loose, may have drifted, may sound dull on percussion with a dull instrument, and may be depressible in its socket. Because the index is nonlinear, average scores for the same individual and for a population are not arithmetic averages and may show more or less severity than actually exists.

The *periodontal disease index* (PDI),[89] like the PI index, is a composite index, in that gingivitis and periodontitis are scored on the same scale. However, it is not necessary to use the composite score. The gingivitis aspect of the PDI may be used to score gingivitis (scale of 0 to 3), and the destructive aspects of periodontitis may be scored on basis of level of attachment (scale of 4 to 6), which is measured with a periodontal probe. A score of 0 indicates the absence of disease. A score of 1 indicates mild to moderate inflammation not extending all around a tooth. A score of 3 indicates severe gingivitis with marked redness, a tendency to bleed, and ulceration. When the attachment is apical to the cementoenamal junction but not by more than 3 mm, a score of 4 is given. A score of 5 is given when the attachment is greater than 3 mm but not more than 6 mm apical to the cementoenamel junction. A score of 6 is given when the attachment is more than 6 mm apical to the cementoenamel junction. Only six teeth are scored, but the results have been found to be representative of the whole mouth.[46,53,85,90] Scoring the right maxillary first molar, left central incisor, left first premolar, left mandibular first molar, right central incisor, and right first premolar takes only a few minutes. The gingivitis part of the index has been used in a modified form in many clinical trials. The epithelial attachment part of the index has been modified in numerous clinical trials, and the composite index (PDI) has been used in several epidemiological surveys,[8,17,21,87,88] and has been extensively studied.[46,49,53,79,85]

Periodontal probing

The clinical measurement of periodontitis is directed primarily toward evaluating the position of the level of attachment with the cementoenamel junction. Episodic loss of attachment and an increase in attachment following therapy at various sites in the mouth can be evaluated with repeated periodontal probing. However, where changes are small and rapid, as well as sporadic, detection by probing may be inadequate.

Data-pooling all sites in the mouth to arrive at one number, as several epidemiological indices have done,[29,58,97] may lead to the interpretation that periodontal disease is a slow, continuous process throughout the mouth. Such may be the case without contradicting the concept of periodontitis as an intermittent disease occurring sporadically at different sites in the mouth.[62]

Composite index scores of periodontal disease reflect the use of the individual patient as the experimental unit. The acceptance of a discrete, episodic, and site-specific natural history of periodontitis requires statistical analysis that can become increasingly complex. Maintaining the identities of both the subject and specific sites as experimental units is a problem.

Non-clinical measurement of periodontal status

Indicators of active sites of periodontitis have yet to be developed and accepted. It is also not possible to identify what subjects may be at risk for periodontitis. In effect, present indices and probing of attachment levels are not indicators of periodontal disease activity. The criteria being measured are inadequate to indicate such activity. A wide range of studies have addressed this problem in relation to saliva, plaque constituents, gingival crevicular fluid, enzymes, specific bacteria, and immunologic products. None of these specimen sources has provided the dental practitioner with a precise clinical correlate of periodontal disease activity.[27] However, there has been progress in finding analytic techniques for measuring the activity of periodontal diseases, and perhaps also for measuring susceptibility. The areas being considered are (1) specific bacteria and their products; and (2) responses of the host to injurious agents, including those produced by the host's own cells: for example, neutrophils and products of tissue injury.

The detection of disease-associated bacteria in subgingival plaque using dark-field microscopy has met with limited success. Highly specific polyclonal and monoclonal antisera to such suspected pathogens as *Bacteroides gingivalis* and *Actinobacillus actinomycetemcomitans (A.a.)* have been developed, and methods for the identification of these bacteria by ELISA immunofluorescence and flow cytometry have been improved. The use of DNA probes is also possible, but none of these sophisticated methods have been accepted as reliable indicators of current disease. Bacterial assessment may ultimately be useful for choosing modes of treatment, classifying diseases, and determining patient and site vulnerability, although microbial methods of identification do not now appear to be candidates for sole indicators of active disease.

Correlations between local antibody response and local disease activity are being explored. A correlation between elevated serum antibody titers and periodontal diseases, such as that between localized juvenile periodontitis and the antibody to *A.a.*, and that between acute necrotizing ulcerative gingivitis and the antibody to *Bacteroides intermedius* and medium-sized spirochetes, has been demonstrated, but the meaning of the correlation has yet to be clarified. Other correlates of host response include complement levels, prostaglandins, and interleukins.

Gingival crevicular fluid and products of tissue injury are being explored, but no markers have been developed to indicate active periodontitis. Multiple profiles (local antibody, PGE, enzyme and tissue product analyses) may provide the sought-for markers.

Radiographs

In several studies, radiographic techniques have been evaluated or advocated for the assessment of periodontal disease.[11,23,30,66,108] In one longitudinal study, in which the relationships among radiographic bone height, pocket depth, and attachment level were compared over a 4-year period, a high correlation was found between initial and subsequent measurements of radiographic bone level, pocket depth, and attachment level.[49] Although interproximal attachment levels can be estimated with a fair degree of accuracy, and radiographs can be used for comparison of changes in interproximal bone height over time, absolute values in millimeters cannot be obtained. The use of radiographic techniques in epidemiological field stud-

ies is limited by the conditions under which the study is to be made and by the need and value of those techniques compared to the value of repeated measurements of the attachment level made with a periodontal probe. The use of radiographic methods to evaluate patients, even in clinical trials, has yet to be accepted widely. Repeat radiographs showing bone loss reflect retrospectively the presence of disease. It has been suggested that subtraction radiography may be a precise method of measuring localized bone lesions of periodontitis.

Indices for plaque, calculus, oral hygiene

Several indices for plaque, calculus, and oral hygiene have been developed[35,54,58,89,90,111] and used in a number of clinical studies.[35,58,89] All these indices are nonlinear, using nominal or ordinal scales.[90] Calibration of scoring error cannot be determined directly in an index in which removal of the plaque with a probe is necessary.[45,48] Currently used indices estimate the amount of plaque present in terms of area of tooth covered and thickness of plaque covering the area. True measurement of the amount of plaque present on the teeth is not feasible for epidemiological studies and is feasible only for limited clinical epidemiological studies.

So many indices have been developed and used without determination of their reproducibility and validity that there seems to be a new index or a modification of an old one for almost every publication with a need for an index. Recently, (1985) the Council on Dental Therapeutics suggested two plaque-assessing methods as acceptable indices for the estimation of cleaning ability. However, those recommendations should not deter the researcher from choosing a plaque index carefully, basing his choice on the objectives of the study, the size of the population, the period of the study, and the type and extent of the change anticipated.[28] In addition, the index's degree of linearity, validity, scoring error and reproducibility should be established. It should also be remembered that an index treats all plaque as undifferentiated; it treats the mass as if it consisted etiologically of nonspecific bacteria.

Calculus indices have been developed for epidemiological studies,[71,89] as well as for clinical trials. However, until the recent interest in "calculus-preventing" dentifrices, such indices[109] received very little attention. In clinical trials, their value is generally, by design, limited. In these trials, prevention of plaque is the primary goal, the idea behind them being that preventing plaque prevents calculus.

The *simplified oral hygiene index* (OHI-S) has been widely used in a number of surveys and clinical trials.[35] The criteria are related to an oral debris score and a calculus score, which when added together make up the OHI-S. The oral debris scoring system is based on the amount of soft foreign matter loosely attached to the tooth. A score of 0 indicates no debris present. A score of 1 indicates soft debris covering not more than ⅓ of the tooth surface, or the presence of extrinsic stains without debris, regardless of surface area covered. A score of 2 indicates soft debris covering more than ⅓, but not more than ⅔, of the exposed tooth surface. The surfaces examined are the facial surfaces of the upper first molars and the upper right and lower left incisors, and the lingual surfaces of the lower first molars. Calculus is scored as for plaque, except that individual subgingival flecks are scored as 2 and a continuous, heavy band of subgingival calculus is scored as 3. This index has the disadvantage of being a composite one, dealing with both calculus and plaque in the same index.

The *plaque index* (PL.I) uses a 0 to 3 scoring scale.[58,59,60] A score of 0 indicates no plaque adjacent to the gingiva (Fig. 6-1). A score of 1 indicates plaque adhering to the free gingival margin and adjacent tooth surface. Plaque can be detected only when a probe is run across the tooth surface. A score of 2 indicates a moderate accumulation of soft deposits within the gingival pocket, on the gingival margins and/or the adjacent tooth surface, that can be seen without staining or use of a probe. A score of 3 indicates an abundance of soft debris within the gingival pocket or on the gingival margin and adjacent tooth surface. Calibration of observations cannot be made directly. Although this index is weighted toward plaque adjacent to or in contact with the gingiva, its linearity has not been established.[45] The PL.I. has been used to study the relationship between early gingivitis and early plaque formation, and is used chiefly in conjunction with the gingival index (GI).

All indices tend to be nonlinear, to have unknown validity, and to be designed for a homogenous disease process.[20,53,79] Measurement error has a significant impact upon how data can be analyzed and interpreted.

Tooth mobility

The use of tooth mobility as a parameter of periodontal disease is discussed in chapter 11. Several methods for determining tooth mobility are complex and beyond the scope of epidemiological studies.[73,80] Simple tests of mobility have been used and appear reliable;[55] however, correlation with loss of supporting structures is less than direct.

PREVALENCE OF GINGIVITIS

Gingivitis in children. The prevalence of gingivitis in children aged 5 to 11 years has been reported to vary from 9% to 85%, depending on age, location, and criteria used in the studies.[103] In one study, the prevalence of gingivitis was found to be 5%, 14%, 17%, and 9% in U.S. children aged 2, 3, 4, and 5 years, respectively.[5] In another study of children aged 6 to 11 years, 13.6% had gingivitis.[51] In a study using the PMA index of 32,000 children aged 5 to 17 years, 53% were found to have gingivitis.[68] A study using the PI index of 22,000 children aged 5 to 14 years showed 21% with gingivitis.[96] In a sample of Chicago children aged 12 to 17 years, about 40% had gingivitis. Concern about the range between these studies has led to the question of whether the data reflect measurement error or whether they represent true population differences. These questions have yet to be answered.

These data on prevalence reflect different populations, the use of different indices and different observers, as well as different measurement errors. In addition, the data can refer to average mouth scores, or to gingivitis/no gingivitis. Thus, the true nature of gingivitis and how it is related to permanent tooth eruption, plaque, and dental caries, may be obscured by irrelevant scores. Whether gingivitis has a prevalence of 15% or 85% may have significant bearing on

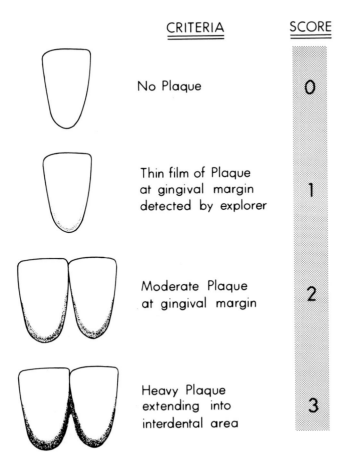

CRITERIA	SCORE
No Plaque	0
Thin film of Plaque at gingival margin detected by explorer	1
Moderate Plaque at gingival margin	2
Heavy Plaque extending into interdental area	3

Fig. 6-1. The plaque index (PL.1)[60] See text.

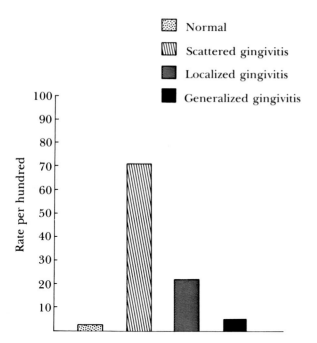

Normal

Scattered gingivitis

Localized gingivitis

Generalized gingivitis

Fig. 6-2. Prevalence of periodontal disease of primary teeth as determined by periodontal disease index (PI) scores, Tecumseh, Michigan, 1960. (Jamison, 1960.)[47]

health care concerns. The questions of whether gingivitis is a disease or not, and what the relationship of gingivitis is to the development of periodontitis, are both fundamental and unresolved.

When gingivitis is viewed in terms of averages taken from less than the whole mouth or of absence or presence, as shown in figure 6-2, the data can be interpreted differently than by concluding, for example, that 95% of children aged 5 to 14 years had gingivitis.[47] Considering gingivitis on the basis of site-specific lesions should provide even more insight into the prevalence of gingivitis in a population. The significance of gingivitis has been questioned,[13] as has epidemiologic data on the prevalence of gingivitis in children under 11 years of age,[103] because of the need to translate epidemiologic data into requirements for dental care and supply of dentists. Such estimates of trends require accurate data. In addition, when average mouth scores for gingivitis, or gingivitis/no gingivitis scores, are reported, it is difficult to assess whether and to what extent specific kinds of gingival lesions precede periodontitis or whether gingivitis may not be a harbinger of destructive periodontis. Certainly better epidemiologic as well as clinical data are needed. The differences in tissue responses between children and adults must be considered. By what criteria should the inflammatory response to erupting teeth be judged as normal or as gingivitis? The answer to that question requires a number of research ap-

proaches. If site-specific data were to be considered, some of the discrepancies in reported prevalences would disappear.

The prevalence of acute necrotizing ulcerative gingivitis (NUG) has not been clearly determined, due to the limited use of a random population by most reports. The incidence in the United States appears to vary from as little as 0.2% to somewhat more than 2.0%. An increased incidence is seen in children with Trisomy 21 (mongolism). Few children have NUG before adolescence or puberty.

Gingivitis in teenage populations. The prevalence of gingivitis after 11 years of age to about 17 years of age appears to be less than the prevalence seen during the mixed dentition period. However, the prevalence may reach 90% in some teenage groups.[107] Generally speaking, the epidemiologic data for prevalence of gingivitis in teenage populations suffers from several of the same interpretation problems as that for children, but the confusion surrounding eruption of teeth and the impact of puberty is not present.

Gingivitis in adults. The prevalence of gingivitis in adults is often presented in relation to age, usually from age 20 to age 70. The prevalence of gingivitis in adults has been reported to range from 75 to 95%,[39,58] and up to 100% in persons 30 years of age and older. In a comprehensive cross-sectional national study covering the period of 1971-74, approximately 50% of dentate adults in the U.S. had no gingivitis.[51] The reasons for these reported differences in prevalence have not been clarified, although it has been hypothesized that there was a reduction in gingivitis from the time of a previous study[50] in the period from 1960 to 62.[23] It has been suggested that in these studies gingivitis was underestimated. The significance of the differences between these studies is more than academic in relation to planning future treatment and manpower needs, and to putative decreases in prevalence of gingivitis.

Prevalence of periodontitis. The prevalence of adult periodontitis in the United States has been conservatively estimated to be approximately 10% at 20 years of age, 35% at 50 years, and 55% at 70 years of age.[34,41,77] However, these data may not reflect the apparent decrease in advanced periodontitis that in the past led to loss of teeth. Recent data challenge the concept of age relationships and universality of destructive periodontal disease.[13,39,41]

Destructive periodontitis is uncommon in children,[47] as shown in figure 6-3. It has been reported that as much as 6% of teenage youths may have some degree of periodontitis.[76] The prevalence of localized juvenile periodontitis is probably less than 0.1%. Periodontal pockets are seen in a few children before the age of 13 years.[8,17,47,88] Populations with poor oral

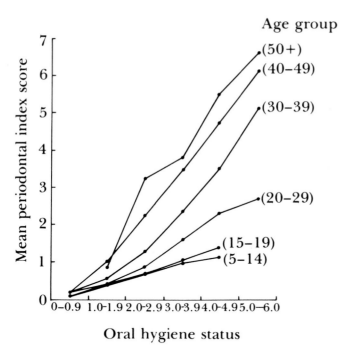

Age group

Fig. 6-3. Mean periodontal index scores of 2365 persons by age groups and oral hygiene status, Burma, 1961. (Littleton, 1964.)[59]

hygiene appear to be most severely affected.[63,89] In some countries, the prevalence of adult periodontitis reaches 100% after 40 years of age.[65] Irrespective of the accuracy of these prevalence figures, it has been believed that ultimately periodontitis accounts for the majority of tooth loss in adults.[22,65,84] However, because in many studies indices are expressed as group means, cross-sectional data are interpreted as if they were longitudinal, and frequency distributions are not given, it is very likely that the prevalence of periodontitis severe enough to result in tooth loss has been over-estimated for 18 to 65-year-old adults in the U.S.

The variation in prevalence data is due partly to differences in diagnostic criteria and to averaging attachment levels or using composite scores for whole mouth assessments. If the criterion for the presence of periodontitis is attachment level more than 3 mm apical to the cementoenamel junction, such averaging will swamp specific sites with a greater loss of attachment than 3 mm.

Epidemiologic studies are difficult to find that give an accurate picture of site-specific prevalence without losing the identity of the person as the experimental unit, and that provide information on severity that can be used to determine treatment needs, manpower requirements and etiologic factors.

The results of a survey conducted by the National Institute of Dental Research from February 1985 to April 1986 of more than 15,000 working population and about 5,000 senior citizens indicated that only 4.2% of the working population aged 18-65 were edentulous, but of senior citizens aged 65 and older, almost 42% were edentulous. On periodontal probing, 6% of sites in employed persons showed some bleeding, while in seniors 10% showed evidence of gingivitis. In the employed population, 7.56% of the people had at least one site with 6 mm or more attachment loss, whereas the figure was nearly 34% for senior citizens. These data suggest chronic destructive periodontal disease may not be the major reason for tooth loss in the adult 18-65-year-old population. This preliminary conclusion follows the 1979 NIDR survey data, which indicated that the rate of tooth extraction is declining in the United States,[51] and another report that suggests that advanced periodontal disease is not a major cause of tooth loss.[6] The actual major cause appears to be caries, especially in lower socioeconomic-class populations.

Before 20 years of age, tooth loss due to destructive periodontal disease does not occur frequently.[44] It increases after that time, especially in populations at risk.[62] Thus, with increasing age, 13-to-15 years and upward, the percentage of individuals with bone loss and periodontal pockets increases.[8,99] After 25 to 30 years of age, there appears to be an increase in the prevalence of destructive periodontal disease.[47,57,65] Bone resorption reaches a plateau at ages 40 to 50, but this may be due to extraction of the teeth that are most severely involved.[99] The interpretation of epidemiologic data, which suggests a reduction in periodontitis for 18-65-year-old individuals, seems to imply that more attention will have to be paid to disease in the 65-year-plus population, and that treatment needs may be less than anticipated in the 18-65-year-old groups because of increased personal and professional care, and possibly because of widespread use of antibiotics and low levels of fluoride.

DESIGN AND ANALYSIS

The design of epidemiologic studies and clinical trials requires sophisticated approaches, not only because of the complexity of periodontal disease but because of less than precise methods for assessing the state of the disease. Problems in identifying the sampling unit, the detection of a small percentage of sites changing over time, measurement errors and the choice of appropriate statistical methods appear to be resolvable, but have become increasingly more difficult.

Recent concerns about the design and analysis of epidemiologic studies have focused on the experimental unit. As already indicated, if the site is the unit of observation, but the subject or patient the unit of analysis, how can the swamping effect of the large number of inactive sites be dealt with in terms of epidemiologic and statistical approaches? It is unlikely that sites behave independently, and attempts to justify statistical models of site-to-site and time-to-time independence in relation to the discrete biological burst model may lead to misleading results.[43] These problems were discussed in detail at a Conference on Clinical Trials in Periodontal Diseases.[18]

EPIDEMIOLOGIC RELATIONSHIPS RELEVANT TO THE PREVALANCE AND/OR SEVERITY OF PERIODONTAL DISEASES

A number of host and environmental factors have been considered as being possibly related to gingivitis. These include age, oral hygiene, sex and sex-related factors, puberty, pregnancy, smoking, fluorides, and intake of antibiotics. Among all epidemiological factors, oral hygiene is most closely correlated with gingivitis.[103]

Oral hygiene and age. As already indicated, the prevalence and severity of bone loss appears to increase with increasing age, and in some populations, virtually everyone shows some evidence of bone loss by middle age.[33,57,65,91] The association with age does not necessarily reflect the aging process per se, but may reflect the length of time that local irritants, such as plaque and calculus, have affected the periodontium. Because of practicing poorer oral hygiene than do younger individuals, older persons may run a higher risk of periodontitis. This has yet to be demonstrated.

It has been suggested that about 90% of the variance in PI scores could be explained after the influences of age and oral hygiene have been estimated.[92] On the basis of a study in Burma,[57] it was concluded that the simultaneous effects of age, debris, and calculus account statistically for 2/3 of the variance in periodontal index (PI) scores for persons with gingivitis only as well as for persons with destructive periodontal disease. However, the correlation between plaque index scores and gingivitis index scores has been found to be somewhat less than what is implied. Linear correlations vary from 0.44 to 0.87, depending on the population studied.[5,50,51] The differences may relate to certain bacteria in the plaque. The relationship of PI scores to a number of variables in the HANES (1971-74) data[53] was found to be highest for OHI-S scores, indicating that the oral hygiene index was the strongest predictor of the periodontal index.[14]

In figure 6-4, age and oral hygiene status are compared. Note that the mean periodontal index score for the 5-to-14 year-old group with a oral hygiene score of 4.0 to 4.9 units is about 1 unit, and the mean periodontal index for the 50+ age group with the same oral hygiene score (4.0 to 4.9) is about 5.5 PI units. Mean PI scores in persons of equivalent age increase consistently with each progression to a group with a higher OHI-S score. When groups with equivalent

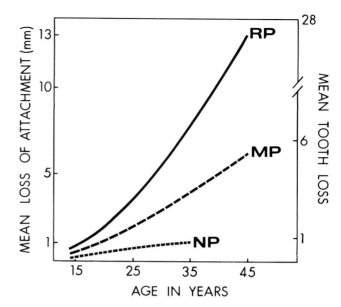

Fig. 6-4. Graphical representation of periodontal status and tooth loss in relation to age in years. RP = rapidly progressive adult periodontitis; MP = moderately progressive; and NP = nonprogressive periodontitis (After Löe et al., 1986.)

oral hygiene index scores are compared, PI scores tend to increase with age, but probably reflect the result of the presence of long-term irritants rather than simply aging. Older people with inadequate oral hygiene may be more at risk of destructive periodontal disease than those with good oral hygiene.

Although the association between periodontal disease and age is consistent for most groups of people, individual and group exceptions do occur. In a study of over 5000 people from Ecuador and Montana, a steady increase in calculus and periodontal destruction was demonstrated from 5 to 50+ years of age.[35] However, some middle-aged primitive Ecuadoran tribesmen who had extensive deposits of calculus and debris had only marginal gingivitis.[33] Such exceptions to the relationship among age, periodontal disease, and oral hygiene indicate the possibility of other differences being present, including differences in the bacterial composition of plaque, intrinsic host responses, or both. Although differences among groups in the prevalence and severity of periodontal disease tend to disappear in groups comprised of individuals of comparable age and oral hygiene status,[35,56,87] recent concepts of periodontal disease stress changes in specific sites, in which the amount of plaque and severity of disease are not always highly correlated. Many older individuals, among whom gingivitis is widespread, do not have significant destructive periodontitis.

Socioeconomic, ethnic and geographic factors. The association among periodontal disease, education, and socioeconomic status has been studied in several surveys. In general, as formal education decreases, the prevalence and severity of periodontal disease increase.[11,94,95,113] As income increases, periodontal status improves.[70] Such differences have been attributed to differences in oral hygiene and dental care.[112]

Data comparing the prevalence of gingivitis in black people and white people indicate that the prevalence and severity of disease is greater in black populations.[95,96] This difference may be due to such cofactors as oral hygiene, socioeconomic status and access to dental care. When education, dental care, and oral hygiene were comparable, no clear-cut differences were observed.[95] When populations in Norway,[12] Ceylon,[113] Burma,[57] and other areas are studied, differences in oral hygiene account for the greater prevalence of periodontal disease found in some Asians compared to that found in some Scandinavians. Thus, although the prevalence and severity of periodontal disease is greater in some Asian[36,65] and African countries than in the United States and Europe,[65,99] such differences do not reflect an inherent adverse racial or geographical factor in the causation of periodontal disease.

Sex factors. Most epidemiologic surveys consistently report that the prevalence of gingivitis is lower in females than in males.[11,51] The figures in one study were 80% for females and 88% for males.[65] The sex-related factor appears to be absent in some third-world countries; in a few instances, the severity is worse in females. Differences can usually be explained by females' practicing better oral hygiene and/or by the effects of pregnancy.

An increase in gingival inflammation has been shown to occur during pregnancy, independent in some instances of quantitative changes in plaque.[40] A correlation between gingivitis index scores and blood progesterone during pregnancy has suggested that increased gingival blood capillary permeability makes the dentogingival complex more sensitive to bacteria and other irritants.[40] The role of increased numbers of *Bacteroides intermedius* has yet to be determined, and a relative deficiency of IgA in some pregnant women has to be more fully evaluated.

On the basis of several epidemiologic studies, there appears to be an increase in the prevalence of gingivitis related to hormonal changes at puberty, both in males and females.[22,68] The magnitude of this effect is open to question because of the problems associated with diagnostic standards for prepubertal gingivitis.

Other factors. Generally, the use of antibiotics has been considered as a factor in relation to reports of a reduction in periodontal disease. However, it has not been possible to link a reduction (which has not been proved) in periodontal disease to increased antibiotic consumption.[41]

A demonstrated relationship has not been substantiated between a putative reduction in the prevalence of gingivitis and intake of fluoride (antibacterial effect). Studies of children, youths, and adults have not shown that a difference exists in mean gingivitis scores between fluoridated and nonfluoridated communities.[75,104]

It has been shown that the long-term use of tobacco has an effect on periodontal health. Smokers at all ages tend to have higher periodontal index scores than do nonsmokers.[102]

Epidemiological studies of the relationships between vitamin levels and the prevalence and severity of periodontal disease have been reported for Alaska,[93] Ethiopa, and Burma.[57] No substantial relationship was found between vitamin levels and the severity of periodontal disease.

NATURAL HISTORY OF PERIODONTAL DISEASE

Gingivitis. The sequence of events leading from a clinically apparent normal gingiva to gingivitis has been determined from a number of epidemiologic and clinical studies. Although the transition from gingivitis to periodontitis is not clearly understood, several aspects of gingivitis suggest the complex nature of the process. This process will be considered in chapter 7, which deals with pathogenesis.

Gingivitis is reversible, at least to the extent that high gingivitis scores at some sites will change to lower scores or to 0 when plaque control is instituted. Interestingly, some sites do not change, and there may be less change with high scores than with low scores, or vice versa.[83]

On the basis of structural and functional changes at the dento-gingival junction (formation of a gingival pocket and conversion of junctional epithelium to pocket epithelium), gingivitis has been considered to be a disease. Whether or not the inflammation associated with permanent tooth eruption should be scored as gingivitis has yet to be determined, or at least to be agreed upon for epidemiologic and clinical studies.

Based on present epidemiological data, gingivitis begins with the eruption of the primary dentition, although prevalence and severity are probably low and principally related to the eruption of teeth. In one study, the prevalence of gingivitis was 5% at the age of 2 years and increased during the next few years to about 10% by 5 years of age. It was reported in the Health and Examination Survey (HES),[50] and the Health and Nutrition Examination Survey (NHANES)[51] for the periods 1960-62 and 1971-74 respectively, that only 13.6% suffered from gingivitis. However, there is some agreement that gingivitis prevalence in children increases to the age of 11-to-12 years where it may be as high as 70-80%. Other studies report high prevalence figures for 3-5 year-old children, e.g., 50 to 95%.[47,69]

After 11 years of age, at which age there is a peak,[22,69] there is a decline in prevalence through much of the teenage years to 17 years of age.[107] The HES and NHANES data has been evaluated to determine if there was a trend in the prevalence of gingivitis between the time of the first and second survey.[23]

The possibility of a true decline has been questioned[103] and considered,[25] but studies on the basis of relationships among gingivitis and smoking, income, education, oral hygiene, dental care, and use of antibiotics seem to support the decline.[103] By the age of 20 years, the prevalence has increased to 75%, and by 30 years and older, some gingivitis is present in all adults.[65]

Periodontitis. The onset of periodontitis has been considered to begin during adolescence and to have a linear progression throughout life. However, recent perspectives on the disease process suggest that adult periodontitis may have a discrete, episodic and site-specific natural history, exhibiting sporadic, acute exacerbations that cause quantal, localized losses of attachment.[43] Indices are methodologically capable of detecting such changes if composite scores are used. In the interpretation of epidemiologic data consisting of infrequent observations, the results of a slow continuous destructive process would appear to be the same as those of a process characterized by sporadic exacerbations interspersed with periods of extended remission. If the "burst" model of disease progress and attachment loss is valid, and cannot merely be explained by changes due to chance events arising from measurement error, then new approaches to epidemiologic studies and analysis will be required to establish the natural history of periodontitis. Present clinical epidemiologic data fit the concept of periodontitis as an intermittent chronic disease.

The natural history of periodontal disease in man may be expressed in terms of initiation, rate of progress, and consequent loss of teeth. Such a history should be based on prospective studies of populations which have not been exposed to preventive programs, systemic drugs (e.g., antibiotics), or other factors known to influence the disease. The population should be geographically stable, at risk for the disease (i.e., periodontitis), and capable of being monitored over sufficient time for tooth loss to occur. Comparisons of data for different populations require careful consideration of methods of analysis.

A few longitudinal studies have been conducted,[41,62,64] but studies on the total sequence of events have been virtually nonexistent, except for the one conducted in Sri Lanka.[62] In contrast to the study in Sri Lanka, where dental care was almost nonexistent (few caries), as well as oral hygiene, a study of Norwegian students and academicians with excellent oral hygiene was conducted.[63] The Norwegian group av-

eraged an annual loss of attachment of 0.1 mm., whereas the Sri Lankan group averaged 0.2 to 0.3 mm/year.[61,62,63] Because of the severity of the disease, the latter data have been said to describe the unnatural history of periodontal disease.[34]

Based upon interproximal loss of attachment and tooth loss in the Sri Lankan study, three groups were identified: a group (RP) with rapidly progressing disease (8%); a group (MP) characterized by moderately progressing disease (80%); and a group (NP) characterized by nonprogressing disease (10%). The data relative to attachment loss and tooth mortality are shown graphically in figure 6-4.

In the RP group at 25 years of age, the mean loss of attachment was 4.5 mm and mean tooth loss was 5.9 teeth. The mean rate of periodontal destruction for all teeth was 0.5 mm/year and mean annual rate of tooth loss was 0.40. In the MP group, the mean loss of attachment at 25 years of age was about 1.8 mm and tooth loss was 0.10 tooth/year. However, at 35 years of age, the mean loss of attachment was 3.9 mm, with tooth mortality unchanged at approximately 0.1 tooth/year. In the NP group, even at age 30-35 years, the mean loss of attachment was approximately 1 mm and the rate of 0.05 mm/year continued on toward 40 years of age. Tooth loss was inconspicuous and did not seem to increase. These data differ significantly from those given for studies of other populations,[34] such as that of the United States. This difference indicates again that the severity of disease varies considerably among individuals and that the prevalence and severity of periodontitis vary from one population to another.

The data from various studies do differ about the prevalence and severity of adult periodontitis, and views on the pattern of disease may be changing from the views held previously. It had been generally thought that a rapid increase in the prevalence of periodontitis occurred from about 15 to 20 years of age to about 30 to 40 years of age, and that after 40 years of age the disease steadily increased with age to one degree or another in all subjects and was the primary cause of loss of teeth with increasing age. The progress of the disease, viewed on a general basis, was considered to be slow and progressive. However, it is now thought that loss of attachment may vary among sites in one person as well as among different people, and may occur at different rates. That the prevalence and severity of the disease do not increase linearly with age has a number of implications. One is that there is a need to find ways of determining susceptibility to disease; another is that ways of delivering appropriate health care for the increasing number of older people in the population need to be found. All of the characteristics of periodontitis may not be seen in individual patients. Not all people or teeth or tissues are at equal risk. The reinterpretation of data from prior epidemiologic studies suggests that the prevalence of periodontitis in terms of severity has been overestimated. Some periodontitis may be present in most adults, but the prevalence of periodontitis severe enough to lead to tooth loss may be relatively low.

SUMMARY

Epidemiologic data suggests that gingivitis is prevalent in childhood and remains so among adults in all populations; that destructive periodontitis is uncommon before 15 years of age and perhaps only a relatively small percentage of the U.S. population has periodontitis severe enough to lead to tooth loss; that the severity of periodontitis does not increase linearly with age and the effect of age may be minimal when good oral hygiene is maintained; that susceptibility varies among individuals and between populations; that variations in gingivitis and periodontitis are associated with different defensive responses to plaque, to different levels of plaque and to different compositions of plaque; that gingivitis does precede periodontitis but does not always progress to periodontitis; that the severity of gingivitis may not parallel that of periodontitis; and that differences in destructive periodontal disease associated with such factors as race, gender, and socioeconomic status tend to disappear when the level of oral hygiene is considered.

Clinical or descriptive epidemiologic data currently does not clarify the concept of the "burst" theory of attachment level change; does not indicate that gingivitis and periodontitis are unrelated; does not provide conclusive evidence of a secular decrease in gingivitis; does not point to a precise method of indicating who in the population is susceptible to tooth loss due to periodontitis; does not predict precisely what to anticipate as a population ages; and does not clarify markers for the transition from reversible gingivitis to destructive periodontitis. Social epidemiology does not at this time provide clear answers on what behavioral, socioeconomic, and cultural factors may be associated with the development and progression of periodontitis.

There is no well-accepted method for the assessment of the extent and severity of periodontal disease for epidemiologic studies. The PI and PDI methods, which express a single mean index score of disease severity, do not provide information on the extent or distribution of the disease. An index such as the extent and severity index (ESI), with the appropriate statistic,[16] suggests the possibility of and need for indices that are simple to use and that permit direct comparisons among epidemiologic studies of different populations conducted by different investigators.

Methods of measurement and analysis of data for classical or descriptive epidemiologic studies have been used for clinical epidemiologic studies and clinical trials. The trend in evaluating gingivitis is to use an index of bleeding, and in assessing periodontitis to relate attachment level to the CEJ with a periodontal probe. Severity and extent of gingivitis and periodontitis have become necessary data for acceptable detailed epidemiological research as well as for clinical trials. At the present time, traditional clinical criteria are not adequate to determine active disease sites or, quantitatively, the response to therapy. However, there are no objective indicators of disease that provide more specific data than clinical measures of bleeding and attachment levels. Even so, there is considerable evidence that nonclinical objective methods can be developed.

REFERENCES

1. Albino, J.E., et al.: A comparison of six plaque scoring methods for assessing oral hygiene, J. Periodont. 49:419, 1978.
2. Allen, E.F.: Statistical study of the primary causes of extraction, J. Dent. Res. 23:453, 1944.
3. Anerud, A., et al.: The natural history of periodontal disease in man. Changes in gingival health and oral hygiene before 40 years of age, J. Periodont. Res. 14:526, 1979.
4. Ash, G.M.: Isomorphism of biologic ordinal scale measurements and arithmetic of parametric statistical methods, Thesis, Kalamazoo College, Michigan, 1971.
5. Ash, M.M., et al.: Correlation between plaque and gingivitis, J. Periodont. 34:424, 1964.
6. Bailit, H.L., et al.: Is periodontal disease the primary cause of tooth extraction in adults? J. Am. Dent. A. 114:40, 1987.
7. Barnett, M.L., et al.: The modified papillary bleeding index: Comparison with gingival index during the resolution of gingivitis, J. Prev. Dent. 6:135, 1980.
8. Basu, M.K., and Dutta, A.N.: Report on prevalence of periodontal disease in the adult population of Calcutta by Ramfjord's technique, J. All-India Dent. A. 35:187, 1963.
9. Beck, J.D., et al.: Risk factors for various levels of periodontal disease and treatment needs of Iowa, Community Dent. Oral Epidemiol. 13:93, 1985.
10. Bollmer, B.W., et al.: A comparison of 3 clinical indices for measuring gingivitis, J. Clin. Periodontol. 13:392, 1986.
11. Björn, H. and Holmberg, K.: Radiographic determination of periodontal destruction in epidemiological research, Odontol. Revy 17:232, 1966.
12. Brandtzaeg, P., and Jamison, J.C.: A study on periodontal health and oral hygiene in Norwegian Army recruits, J. Periodont. 25:302, 1964.
13. Burt, B.A., et al.: Periodontal disease, tooth loss, and oral hygiene among older Americans, Community Dent. Oral Epidemiol. 13:93, 1985.
14. Burt, B.A., et al.: Diet and Dental Health, a Study of Relationships, United States, 1971-74. National Center for Health Statistics, Vital and Health Statistics. Series II, No. 225. DHHS Pub. No. (PHS) 82-1645. Public Health Service, Washington, D.C., U.S. Government Printing Office, 1982.
15. Capello, J.A.: Correlation between plaque and gingivitis, Thesis, The University of Michigan, 1973.
16. Carlos, J.P., et al.: The extent and severity index: A simple method for use in epidemiologic studies of periodontal disease, J. Clin. Periodontol. 13:500, 1986.
17. Chawla, T.N., et al.: Prevalence of periodontal disease in urban Lucknow (India) using the Ramfjord technique, J. All India Dent. A. 35:151, 1963.

18. Chilton, N.W.: Conference on clinical trials in periodontal diseases, J. Clin. Periodontol. 13:May, 1986.

19. Cimasoni, G.: Crevicular Fluid Updated, Basel: S. Karger, 1983.

20. Coyne, D.: An analysis of calculus indices, Thesis, The University of Michigan, 1970.

21. Curilovic, Z.: Die Epidemiologie parodontaler Erkrankungen bei schweizer Jugendlichen und prognostische Konsequenzen, Zurich, Switzerland: University of Zurich, 1977.

22. Curilovic, Z., et al.: Gingivitis in Zurich schoolchildren. A reexamination after 20 years, Schweiz Monatsschr. Zahnheilk. 87:801, 1977.

23. Douglass, C., et al.: National trends in the prevalence and severity of the periodontal disease, J. Am. Dent. A. 107:403, 1982.

24. Dunning, J.M., and Leach, L.B.: Gingival-bone counts: A method for epidemiological study of periodontal disease, J. Dent. Res. 39:506, 1960.

25. Douglass, C.: Discussion: Epidemiology of gingivitis, J. Clin. Periodontol 13:367, 1986.

26. Ennever, J., et al.: The calculus surface index method for scoring clinical calculus studies, J. Periodont. 32:54, 1961.

27. Fine, D.H. and Mandel, I.D.: Indicators of periodontal disease activity: An evaluation, J. Clin. Periodontol. 13:533, 1986.

28. Fishman, S.L.: Current status of indices of plaque, J. Clin. Periodontol. 13:371, 1986.

29. Fletcher, R.H., et al.: Clinical Epidemiology—The Essentials, Baltimore: Williams and Wilkins, 1982.

30. Fröhlich, E.: Comparison between anatomical and radiographic interpretation of marginal pariodontal disease, Parodontologie 12:89, 1958.

31. Genco, R.J.: Progress in periodontal research, Findings from the Periodontal Disease Clinical Center, State University of New York at Buffalo, Northeast Society of Periodontists Bulletin 11:5, 1981.

32. Goodson, J.M., et al.: Patterns of progression and regression of advanced destructive periodontal disease, J. Clin. Periodontol. 9:472, 1982.

33. Greene, J.C., and Suomi, J.D.: Epidemiology and public health aspects of caries and periodontal disease, J. Dent. Res. (Special Issue C) 56:20, 1977.

34. Greene, J.C.: Discussion: Natural history of periodontal diseases, J. Clin. Periodontol. 13:441, 1986.

35. Greene, J.C., and Vermillion, J.R.: The simplified oral hygiene index, J.A.D.A. 68:7, 1960.

36. Gupta, O.P.: Epidemiological study of periodontal disease in Trevandrum, India, J. Dent. Res. 43:876, 1964.

37. Haffajee, A.D., et al.: Clinical parameters as predictors of destructive periodontal disease activity, J. Clin. Periodontol. 10:257, 1983.

38. Hine, M.D., and Hine, C.L.: Classification and etiology of periodontal disturbances, J.A.D.A. 31:1297, 1944.

39. Hugoson, A., and Jordon, T.: Frequency distribution of individuals aged 20-70 years according to severity of periodontal disease, Community Dent. Oral Epidemiol. 10:187, 1982.

40. Hugoson, A.: Gingival inflammation and female sex hormones. A clinical investigation of pregnant women and experimental studies in dogs, J. Period. Re. 5:7 (Suppl), 1970.

41. Huges, J.T., et al.: Natural History of Dental Diseases in North Carolina (1976-77), Durham: Carolina Academic Press, 1982.

42. Hyman, H.: Survey Design and Analysis, New York: Free Press, 1955.

43. Imrey, P.B.: Considerations in the statistical analysis of clinical trials in periodontitis, J. Clin. Periodontol. 13:517, 1986.

44. Interdepartmental Committee on Nutrition for National Defense, Manual for Nutrition Surveys. Republic of Vietnam Nutrition Survey. U.S. Government Printing Office, Washington, D.C., July 1960.

45. Jackson, P.A.: A qualitative evaluation of the Silness and Löe plaque index, Thesis, Ann Arbor: The University of Michigan, 1970.

46. Jamison, J.C.: Some comparisons of two methods of assessing periodontal disease, Am. J. Public Health 53:1102, 1963.

47. Jamison, J.C.: Prevalence and severity of periodontal disease in a sample of a population, Thesis, The University of Michigan, 1960.

48. Judge, S.P.: Intra- and inter-examiner reliability for scoring plaque and gingivitis, Thesis. Ann Arbor: The University of Michigan, 1973.

49. Kelly, G.P.: Relationships of radiographic bone height, pocket depth and attachment level in a longitudinal study of periodontal disease, Thesis, The University of Michigan, 1973.

50. Kelly, J.E., and Van Kirk, L.E.: Periodontal disease in adults, United States 1960-62. National Center for Health Statistics, Vital and Health Statistics. Series 22, No. 12, PHS Pub. No. 2000, Public Health Service, Washington, D.C., U.S. Government Printing Office, 1965.

51. Kelly, J.E., and Harvey, C.R.: Basic data on dental examination findings of persons 1-74 years, United States 1972-74. National Center for Health Statistics, Vital and Health Statistics. Series 11, No. 214. DHEW Pub. No (PHS) 79-1662. Public Health Service, Washington, D.C., U.S. Government Printing Office, 1979.

52. Kerr, D.A., et al.: Idiopathic gingivostomatitis, Oral Surg. 32:402, 1971.

53. Kjome, R.L.: Effects of tooth sample selection on the periodontal disease index, Thesis, The University of Michigan, 1975.

54. Last, J., ed. A Dictionary of Epidemiology, New York: Oxford University Press, 1983.

55. Laster, L., et al.: An evaluation of clinical tooth mobility, J. Periodont. 46:603,1975.

56. Leske, M.C., et al.: Estimating incidence from age-specific prevalence in glaucoma, Am. J. Epidemiol. 113:606, 1981.

57. Littleton, N.W.: The epidemiology of periodontal disease in Burma, Thesis, The University of Michigan, 1964.

58. Löe, H.: The gingival index, the plaque index, and the retention index systems, J. Periodont. 38:610, 1967.

59. Löe, H, et al.: Experimental gingivitis in man, J. Periodont. 36:177, 1965.

60. Löe, H., and Silness, J.: Periodontal disease in pregnancy. I. Prevalence and severity, Acta Odont. Scand. 21:533, 1963.

61. Löe, H., et al.: The natural history of periodontal disease in man. Tooth mortality rates before 40 years of age, J. Periodont. Res. 13:563, 1978.

62. Löe, H., et al.: Natural history of periodontal disease in man, J. Clin. Periodontol. 13:431, 1986.

63. Löe, H., et al.: The natural history of periodontal disease in man, J. Periodontol. 49:607, 1978.

64. Lyons, H., et al.: Report of the Nomenclature and Classification Committee, J. Periodont. 30:74, 1959.

65. Marshall-Day, C.D., et al.: Periodontal disease: Prevalence and incidence, J. Periodont. 26:185, 1955.

66. Marshall-Day, C.D., and Shourie, K.Z.: A roentgenographic survey of periodontal disease in India, J.A.D.A. 39:572, 1949.

67. Marthaler, T.M., et al.: A method for the quantitative assessment of plaque and calculus formation, Helv. Odontol. Acta 5:39, 1961.

68. Massler, M., et al.: Epidemiology of gingivitis in children, J.A.D.A. 45:319, 1952.

69. Massler, M., et al.: Occurrence of gingivitis in suburban Chi-

cago school children, J. Periodont. 21:146, 1950.

70. Mobley, E., and Smith, S.H.: Some social and economic factors relating to periodontal disease among young Negroes, J.A.D.A. 66:486, 1963.

71. Mühlemann, H.R., and Villa, P.: The marginal line calculus index, Helv. Odontol. Acta 11:175, 1967.

72. Mühlemann, H.R., and Muzor, Z.S.: Gingivitis in Zurich school children, Helv. Odontol. Acta 2:3, 1958.

73. Mühlemann, H.R.: Periodontometry, a method for measuring tooth mobility, Oral Surg. 4:1220, 1951.

74. Mühlemann, H.R.: Psychological and chemical mediators of gingival health, J. Prev. Dent. 4:6, 1977.

75. Murray, J.J.: Gingivitis in 15-year old children from high fluoride and low fluoride areas, Arch. Oral Biol. 14:951, 1964.

76. National Center for Health Statistics. Periodontal disease among youths 12-17 years. United States, Vital and Health Statistics. Series II, No. 141. DHEW Pub. No. (HRA) 74-1623. Health Resources Administration, Washington, D.C., U.S. Government Printing Office, June 1974.

77. National Center for Health Statistics. Related dental findings in adults by age, race, and sex. United States, 1960-62, Vital and Health Statistics. Series 11, No. 7. DHEW Pub. No. (HRA) 74-1274. Health Resources Administration, Washington, D.C., U.S. Government Printing Office, August 1973.

78. National Center for Health Statistics. Periodontal disease and oral hygiene among children. United States, Vital and Health Statistics. Series 11, No. 117. DHEW Pub. No. (HSM) 72-1060. Health Services and Mental Health Administration. Washington, D.C., U.S. Government Printing Office, June 1972.

79. Naylor, G.G.: Correlation among the Ramfjord plaque index, the Ramfjord gingivitis index, and dry weight plaque, Thesis, The University of Michigan, 1974.

80. O'Leary, T.J., and Rudd, K.D.: An instrument for measuring horizontal tooth mobility, USAF School of Aerospace Medicine TDR 63-8, August 1963.

81. Orban, B.: Classification and nomenclature of periodontal diseases, J. Periodont. 13:88, 1942.

82. Orban, B.: Classification of periodontal disease, Parodontologie 3:159, 1949.

83. Page, R.C.: Gingivitis, J. Clin. Periodontol 13:356, 1986.

84. Page, R.C., and Schroeder, H.E.: Periodontitis in man and other animals. A comparative review, Basel: S. Karger, 1982.

85. Palacios, J.: Isomorphism of the periodontal disease index and linear transformations, Thesis, The University of Michigan, 1971.

86. Ralls, S.A., and Cohen, M.E.: Problems in identifying "bursts" of periodontal attachment loss, J. Periodontol 57:746, 1986.

87. Ramfjord, S.P., et al.: Epidemiological studies of periodontal disease, Am. J. Public Health 58:1713, 1968.

88. Ramfjord, S.P.: The periodontal status of boys 11 to 17 years old in Bombay, India, J. Periodont. 32:237, 1961.

89. Ramfjord, S.P.: Indices for prevalence and incidence of periodontal disease, J. Periodont. 30:51, 1959.

90. Ramsey, N.: An evaluation of the arithmetic validity of clinical indices, Thesis, The Univerisity of Michigan, 1969.

91. Russell, A.L.: Epidemiology of periodontal disease, Int. Dent. J. 17:282, 1967.

92. Russell, A.L.: International nutrition surveys: A summary of preliminary dental findings, J. Dent. Res. 43:233, 1963.

93. Russell, A.L., et al.: Periodontal disease and nutrition in Eskimo Scouts of the Alaska National Guard, J. Dent. Res. 40:604, 1961.

94. Russell, A.L.: A social factor associated with the severity of periodontal disease, J. Dent. Res. 36:922, 1957.

95. Russell, A.L., and Ayers, P.: Periodontal disease and socio-economic status in Birmingham, Ala, Am. J. Public Health 50:206, 1960.

96. Russell, A.L.: Some epidemiological characteristics of periodontal disease in a series of urban populations, J. Periodont. 28:286, 1957.

97. Russell, A.L.: A system of classification and scoring for prevalence surveys of periodontal disease, J. Dent. Res 35:350, 1956.

98. Saxer, U.P., and Muhlemann, H.R.: Motivation und Aufklärung, Schweiz. Mschr. Zahnheilk 85:905, 1975.

99. Schei, O., et al.: Alveolar bone loss as related to oral hygiene and age, J. Periodont. 30:7, 1969.

100. Schour, I., and Massler, M.: Prevalence of gingivitis in young adults, J. Dent. Res. 27:733, 1948.

101. Silness, J., and Löe, H.: Periodontal disease in pregnancy. II. Correlation between oral hygiene and periodontal condition, Acta Odont. Scand. 22:121, 1964.

102. Socransky, S.S., et al.: New concepts of destructive periodontal disease, J. Clin. Periodontol. 11:21, 1984.

103. Stamm, J.W.: Epidemiology of gingivitis, J. Clin. Periodontol. 13:360, 1986.

104. Stamm, J.W., and Banting, D.W.: Comparison of root caries prevalence in adults with lifelong residence in fluoridated and nonfluoridated communities, J. Dent. Res. 59:407 (Abstract), 1980.

105. Suomi, J.D., and Barbano, J.P.: Patterns of gingivitis, J. Periodont. 39:71, 1968.

106. Susser, M.W.: Causal Thinking in the Health Sciences. Concepts and Strategies of Epidemiology, New York: Oxford University Press, 1973.

107. Sutcliffe, P.: A longitudinal study of gingivitis and puberty, J. Periodont. Res. 7:52, 1972.

108. Theilade, J.: An evaluation of the reliability of radiographs in the measurement of bone loss in periodontal disease, J. Periodont. 31:143, 1960.

109. Turesky, S., et al.: Reduced plaque formation by the chloromethyl analogue of Vitamin C, J. Periodontol. 41:41, 1970.

110. Varma, A.O.: Discussion: A procedure for evaluating the reliability of a gingival index, and a comparison of 3 clinical indices for measuring gingivitis, J. Clin. Periodontol. 13:396, 1986.

111. Volpe, A.R., and Manhold, J.H.: A method of evaluation of the effectiveness of potential calculus inhibiting agents, N.Y. State Dent. J. 7:289, 1962.

112. Waerhaug, J.A.: Epidemiology of periodontal disease—review of literature. In World Workshop in Periodontics, ed. S.P. Ramfjord et al., 182. Ann Arbor, Michigan: The University of Michigan, 1966.

113. Waerhaug, J.: Prevalence of periodontal disease in Ceylon. Association with age, sex, oral hygiene, socio-economic factors, vitamin deficiencies, malnutrition, betal and tobacco consumption and ethnic group. Final report, Acta Odont. Scand. 25:205, 1967.

114. Weski, O. Parondontopathien Zahnheilkunde, Berlin: Herman Meusser, 1924.

7

Concepts of the pathogenesis of gingivitis and periodontitis have been developed through clinical and microscopic observations, including human and animal studies, and through the use of ultrastructural, histometric, and biochemical methods. However, the sequence of events in the transition from a normal periodontium to the characteristic lesion of chronic destructive (adult) periodontitis has not been precisely determined. The development of a gingival pocket and its transition to a periodontal pocket is still the subject of considerable research. A number of difficult questions about bacteriologic and histopathologic changes associated with the disease remain to be answered.

Consideration of etiologic factors is presented in chapters 8, 9, and 10, and details of the host response are presented in chapter 9.

PROGRESSION OF PERIODONTAL DISEASE

Here is an oversimplified view of the course of development of adult periodontitis, from inception to periodontal pocket: first, gingivitis occurs in response to bacterial plaque on the teeth; then a gingival pocket occurs; and finally, there may be a transformation from gingivitis to periodontitis upon the formation of a periodontal pocket.

The pathogenesis of periodontal disease has been described in four distinct stages: (1) colonization, (2) invasion, (3) destruction, and (4) healing.[22] It has been suggested that the transition from gingivitis to periodontitis results from a localized periodontal infection in which pathogenic subgingival bacteria, especially in a host with compromised peripheral defenses, invade the tissues from bacterial plaque extending apically along the root surface. Although there is some evidence for the presence of bacteria in severe, advanced cases of periodontitis, invasion of tissues in adult periodontitis has not been demonstrated through experiments or through morphological observation, either because of technical difficulties or because invasion does not occur.[41,67] Indirect forms of bacterial injury endotoxins, antigens, enzymes and immune responses have also been suggested as etiologic factors.

The clinical signs and symptoms and histopathologic changes in periodontitis are not easily correlated with the infrequent, localized, seemingly independent and sporadic episodes of acute inflammation that have been proposed to occur in chronic destructive periodontitis.[80] This relationship is difficult to assess, inasmuch as no test, diagnostic procedure, or criterion of absolute disease activity is available at this time. Also, such variation in the rate of disease progress among individuals and sites in an individual (for example, attachment loss may occur rapidly but with intermittent quiescent periods) has been questioned on the basis of measurement and analysis errors.[58]

If attachment loss occurs rapidly but infrequently at different sites, the time frame increment for the detection of active disease would have to be small but frequent; otherwise, probability suggests that only inactive sites will be detected. Thus, ideas about chronic destructive periodontal disease may reflect a retrospective view of the accumulated effects of an acute, possibly microabscessing inflammation that has occurred at unknown times in the past.

Furthermore, shifts in microbiota cannot be directly related to disease activity and may only reflect a need for a more suitable ecologic niche for certain bacteria that are not necessarily involved in active disease. Although shifts in microbial composition in pockets with increased depths is a general trend at different reconstructed stages of adult periodontitis, there is insufficient consistency in microbial composition at probability-defined inactive sites of disease to implicate any specific bacteria or combinations of bacteria as etiologic agents of chronic destructive periodontitis, or for any specific bacteria connected with episodic changes in attachment.[41]

Variations in the progress of periodontal disease can be viewed in relation to local perturbations in the inflammatory response that occur because of the nature of the challenge of the injurious agent and/or because of disturbances in the defense mechanism itself.

INFLAMMATION AS A DEFENSE MECHANISM

The health of a biological system is dependent upon complex, highly coordinated, more or less universal mechanisms that maintain the functional integrity of the system. Because biological systems are open systems[12] (that is, they are inseparable from the external environment and do not maintain unique stationary levels) biological homeostasis refers to a steady state in a dynamic system. But there may be more than one, or even an infinite number, of possible homeostatic levels in an open system, which is a system that exhibits only the constancy of constant change. Thus, homeostatic systems are in dynamic equilibrium with their environment, and the cellular constituents are in a state of continuous construction and destruction. The mechanisms involved in homeostasis include immune and nonimmune inflammatory responses.

The biological system, including the periodontium, can be considered to be dependent upon homeostatic and self-monitoring controls that involve the impact of macromolecular coded information on cell receptors, these cell receptors, depending on the circumstances, are stimulated to give synthesizing, proliferative, or destructive signals to the cells. Although such homeostatic communication signaling is accepted for the control of immune mechanisms,[10] or nonspecific biological systems,[6] it is not unusual to consider inflammation only from the standpoint of a disease mechanism.[93]

A number of inflammatory mechanisms have been implicated as having the ability to mediate injury, despite the primarily protective nature of these responses. The presence of macro- and microabscesses associated with the containment of injurious agents attest to the destructive potential of these agents and the self-monitoring control of the inflammatory mechanisms.

Clinical implications

Another aspect of inflammation as a defense mechanism is the ability of the host to repair destruction of tissues, but not to completely restore unique structures such as the attachment apparatus of the teeth beyond certain limits without some help (hopefully) from guided tissue regeneration.

The use of anti-inflammatory agents to control the inflammatory process (and hopefully its destructive aspects), and the use of antibiotics to control putative invasion of bacteria, are the subjects of rigorous research. The design of studies, including measurement of sites and analysis of the data, requires special care if the natural history of adult periodontitis is not that of a gradual disease progression, but that of an episodic disease occurring independently at various sites in the mouth and characterized by long periods of remission interspersed with short periods of disease activity. This view of chronic destructive periodontal disease requires the resolution of several analytic problems in order to validate a clinical therapy. In effect, the inferential analysis will require the patient, rather than individual sites in the patient's mouth, to be the experimental unit, because sites within the same patient may not respond independently.

Pathogenesis

The pathogenesis of the inflammatory lesion begins with the local response of the gingival tissues to injury from bacteria and their products or antigens when the balance between the normal resident microbial population and the structural, (e.g., intact epithelial barrier) and functional defensive mechanisms (e.g., neutrophils and macrophages) are changed. Change can take the form of changes in the amount and/or composition of plaque and/or quantitative/qualitative changes in the function of polymorpholeukocytes.

It has not been possible to definitely distinguish between the normal state of gingival tissues and the initial stage of gingivitis, probably because injury is not present in this first stage. The presence of a few scattered inflammatory cells, predominantly T cells and a few B cells and plasma cells, reflects the ongoing cellular surveillance and response to bacterial and other exogenous products that may pass through the relatively permeable junctional epithelium. However, such a clean picture is seldom observed in human subjects because there are very few instances in which plaque-free teeth are present.

Where there is a normal host/bacterial balance, a clinically healthy gingiva may be characterized by a lymphocyte-rich infiltrate in the subepithelial connective tissues and by polymorphonuclear leukocytes (PMNs) in the junctional epithelium, even in the presence of plaque. With a shift in favor of bacteria, a clinical gingivitis may be evident. These changes may fluctuate so that aperiodic exacerbations of gingivitis occur in relation to changes in host defenses and plaque mass.

If the inflammatory response becomes intensified because of a significant shift in the balance of host response/bacterial injury toward the microbial side, there is an increase in PMNs, and plasma cells may become the dominant cells in the subepithelial connective tissues. As the inflammatory response becomes more severe, the proportion of T cells decreases and B cells and plasma cells increase, with concomitant destruction of collagenous fibers.

The shift from a predominantly T cell infiltrate to a B cell infiltrate appears to be related to the formation of a *gingival pocket*. A gingival pocket has been described as a pathologically altered gingival sulcus lined, to a variable extent, with pocket epithelium.[50] Once a gingival pocket has formed, gingivitis can no longer be reversed with supragingival tooth cleaning.

The transition from the gingival pocket to a periodontal pocket may occur in the presence of even temporarily compromised peripheral defenses of the host.[67]

On the basis of currently available evidence, it is possible to use a simple model (Fig. 7-1) to describe the sequence of events in the development of inflammatory periodontal disease. The response to injury is inflammation, the character and severity of which may be modified by systemic factors, such as peripheral defenses, and/or the amount and composition of bacterial plaque.

As indicated in Figure 7-1, injury to the gingiva resulting from the presence of plaque leads to gingivitis. The nature and severity of the inflammatory response will depend on the nature of the plaque and the modification of the response by specific or unusual intrinsic or systemic host factors. It does not appear that the disease necessarily progresses to periodontitis.[46,84,85,86] Intrinsic local and systemic factors may account for the wide spectrum of susceptibility to the disease among individuals and for the varying extent of the disease from one area of the mouth to another.

TRANSITION OF GINGIVITIS TO PERIODONTITIS

The concept that chronic destructive periodontitis is an extension of gingivitis into the supporting structures is based on the observation that gingivitis is a precursor of periodontitis, and on the relationship that experimental gingivitis studies have established between plaque and gingivitis. However, experimental periodontitis in dogs does not invariably result in a loss of attachment,[38] and it may be present for long periods of time in humans without resulting in destructive periodontitis, even with long-term accumulation of plaque.[43,53,69]

On the basis of existing evidence, two concepts of the development of periodontitis are evident. The first concept holds that destructive periodontal disease is a sequel to chronic gingivitis, and thus the gingivitis-periodontitis relationship is a continuum of the inflammatory process, involving first the gingiva and then the deeper supporting structures. The second concept holds that the causative agent or the response of the host differs with time, individuals, teeth, and species.

In the first concept, the plaque may be composed of nonspecific bacteria or bacterial products that reach a level and duration of injury sufficient to cause destructive periodontal disease; or, the concept may involve immune responses wherein plaque would be the source of antigens that continuously challenge the gingiva. In the 2nd concept, periodontitis develops at some time in response to specific microorganisms or when a systemic modifying factor adversely affects the normal protective mechanisms of the host in the presence of specific bacteria. For example, a destructive process may result from a change in flora to anaerobic collagenolytic organisms because of the development of conditions favorable to the growth of such organisms in deep gingival crevices. Neither of the two concepts mentioned would necessarily preclude the possibility of either mechanism being involved in the pathogenesis of periodontitis, or the possibility that the disease progression is sporadic, with periods of extended remission[26,32] or cyclic changes in the degree of inflammation.[31,53]

HISTOPATHOLOGY OF PERIODONTAL DISEASE

The histopathology of the earliest stages of gingivitis

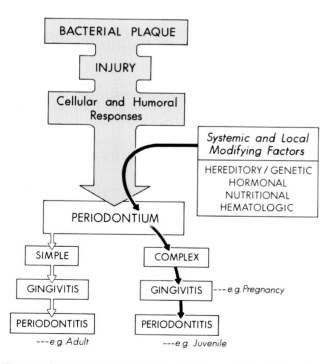

Fig. 7-1. Pathogenesis of periodontal disease. Injury to the gingiva causes an inflammatory response which may be specifically or unusually modified by intrinsic local or systemic factors. The extent and severity of the response will depend on the nature of the injurious agent and the modifying factors.

has been specifically described on the basis of studies of experimental gingivitis in animals[42,68] and humans,[45,52,97] and of studies of the natural history of periodontal disease in dogs.[40] A study model of the pathogenesis of inflammatory periodontal disease has been divided into *initial, early, established, and advanced* stages.[53] Such subdivisions do not necessarily relate to the sequence of clinical events in the pathogenesis of the disease; however, placing the emphasis on the transition from a normal gingiva to gingivitis, and from gingivitis to periodontitis, may facilitate the development of a better understanding of the pathogenesis of periodontal disease.

Normal gingiva

In the clinically healthy gingiva (Fig. 7-2), as defined by a gingival index score of 0, polymorphonuclear leukocytes and lymphocytes are found in the junctional epithelium.[5,42,75] In addition, the subjacent connective tissue may show a small number of scattered chronic inflammatory cells.[5,73,98] The gingiva is characterized by a shallow gingival sulcus. However, in the dog model, in which there is such intense and scrupulous control of plaque that the gingival index score is 0 and gingival fluid is absent, inflammatory infiltration may be absent.[2,5,65] However, it may not be possible to obtain complete reduction in all animals, nor perhaps in humans.[2,57] In order to describe the first alterations considered to be due to disease, it is helpful to describe the histological features of an infiltrate-free gingiva (Fig. 7-3). Possibly, very early changes from normalcy merely reflect homeostatic aspects of the host's defensive mechanisms.

In several studies, clinical normalcy in dogs has been characterized by the absence of gingival sulcular fluid flow[2,40,44] and by a small number of sulcular leu-

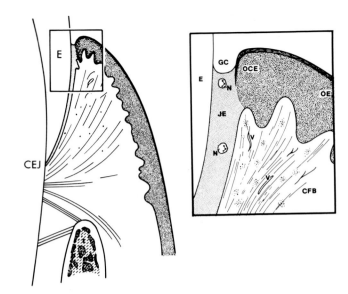

Fig. 7-3. Schematic representation of healthy gingiva after experimental reduction of plaque. Clinically the color, form, density, and attachment are consistent with a normal gingiva. The gingival crevicular fluid (GCF) is essentially normal. There are only a few neutrophils (N) present in the junctional epithelium (JE). The blood vessels (V) are flat, and dense collagen fiber bundles (CFB) are well defined throughout the tissues. E, enamel; OCE, oral crevicular epithelium; OE, oral epithelium; GC, gingival crevice; CEJ, cementoenamel junction.

kocytes.[2,4,5,68] It has been found that the gingival sulcus is often absent, especially where plaque control has been achieved by chemical inhibitors.[53]

The histological features of the healthy dog gingiva include junctional epithelium several cells thick, without rete pegs, and highly oriented subepithelial collagen fiber bundles.[2,55] In both dogs and humans, a few isolated leukocytes may be found in the junctional epithelium and in the adjacent connective tissue.[2,57,68,72,73] There is no inflammatory infiltrate, although a small number of isolate neutrophilic granulocytes, macrophages, and lymphocytes is present. In one study, immunoblasts were practically absent in the dog's healthy gingiva.[2] The junctional epithelium is in contact with the enamel, and in this respect is similar to the dentogingival tissues in erupting human teeth.[85] The dentogingival blood vessels subjacent to the junctional epithelium consist of a flat plexus of vessels[13,81] surrounded by and embedded in dense collagen fiber bundles.[2]

GINGIVITIS

A very early stage of plaque-associated gingivitis in humans has been characterized by an increased flow of gingival fluid[44] and the increase of leukocyte migration through the junctional epithelium into the oral

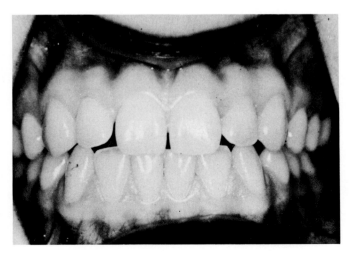

Fig. 7-2. Clinically healthy gingiva. It has a uniform pale pink color, and there is no bleeding on probing of shallow gingival sulci. Tissues are firm and dense.

cavity via the gingival sulcus.[71,75,91] The histopathological changes that occur in the human gingiva when plaque is allowed to return after plaque and gingivitis indices have been at zero levels for 28 days have been described.[57] The earliest change (Fig. 7-4), occurring by the 2nd to 4th day of plaque accumulation, is vasculitis involving the plexus of vessels subjacent to the junctional epithelium.[57,81] There is an acute exudative inflammatory response involving increased numbers of polymorphonuclear leukocytes, some loss of perivascular collagen, and the beginning of an inflammatory infiltrate in humans[57] and dogs.[39,68] These changes may occur within the first few days, but the gingiva will still appear to be clinically healthy. The plaque index (PI)[45] in the human study[57] was scored 1.29 by the 2nd day and 2.29 by the 8th day.

In the initial stage of subclinical gingivitis, there is a migration of polymorphonuclear leukocytes into the junctional epithelium and gingival sulcus.[3,40,68,82,92] The increased permeability of the vessels,[13,57,81] increased amounts of gingival fluid,[13] fibrin deposition,[53,68] and increase in inflammatory cells[40,68] are due to the inflammatory response brought about by substances in the accumulating dental plaque. Such substances include chemotactic agents that attract polymorphonuclear leukocytes to the site of the plaque. These changes involve the junctional epithelium and the most coronal part of the gingival connective tissues.

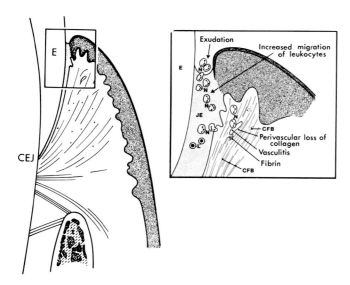

Fig. 7-4. Schematic representation of experimental gingivitis. Acute exudative inflammatory response developing two to four days following plaque accumulation. There is increased exudation of crevicular fluid; greater number of neutrophils (N) in the junctional epithelium (JE); perivascular loss of collagen; fibrin deposition; vasculitis; and rete peg formation in the junctional epithelium. The collagen fiber bundles (CFB) are not altered. The inflammatory response is limited to the tissues subjacent to the most coronal aspect of the junctional epithelium. E, enamel; L, lymphocytes.

The changes in the junctional and oral sulcular epithelium include a separation of the epithelial cells and an apical shift of the bottom of the sulcus. The change in the junctional and oral sulcular epithelium becomes more obvious with the deepening of the gingival sulcus and the transition to a gingival pocket, the sulcus becoming lined with variable degrees of pocket epithelium.[74]

In experimental dog gingivitis, the changes that occur in the most coronal connective tissues adjacent to the gingival sulcus after 4 days of plaque accumulation consist of a decrease in collagen density around the blood vessels. The collagen content of the connective tissue is 56%, and the cells present include neutrophils, small lymphocytes, and immunoblasts. Similar changes occur in humans in the initial stage of gingivitis, but the cellular infiltration appears to be more apical in humans than in dogs.[57]

The initial changes in the development of gingivitis after 2 to 4 days of plaque accumulation include vasculitis of the vessels subjacent to the structural epithelium; reduction of perivascular collagen; extravascular deposition of proteins, including fibrin; gingival fluid exudation; and migration of leukocytes into the junctional epithelium.[53]

After 4 to 7 days of plaque accumulation in experimental gingivitis in humans,[57] there is an infiltration of large numbers of lymphoid cells into the connective tissue. These lymphoid cells make up about 75% of the cells in the infiltrate in the inflamed area.[71] Only a few plasma cells are present at this time. The area of inflammation adjacent to the base of the gingival crevice increases, and collagen loss reaches 60 to 70%.[57,71] The fibroblasts in the area are larger than those in adjacent noninflamed tissues and are closely associated with lymphoid cells.[57,71,78,86] Macrophages or monocytes make up about 2% of the cells.

It has been suggested that the character of the infiltrate and the tissue changes is consistent with delayed hypersensitivity.[34,57] The features of early gingivitis can be induced by applying a sensitizing antigen to the marginal gingiva.[95]

The gingival crevicular fluid and the number of leukocytes increase and reach a maximum between 6 to 12 days after the onset of clinical gingivitis.[40] The quantity of fluid is apparently related to the size of the area of inflammation in the connective tissue.[39,63,68]

The junctional epithelium contains an increased number of polymorphonuclear leukocytes, especially from the basal layers of the surface layers (Fig. 7-5). Increased numbers of monocytes, especially lymphocytes, are found at the inflammatory site. The cells in the crevicular fluid are still mainly neutrophils.[3]

Changes in the junctional epithelium are associated with alterations in the connective tissue in early gingivitis. Rete peg formation from oral crevicular epi-

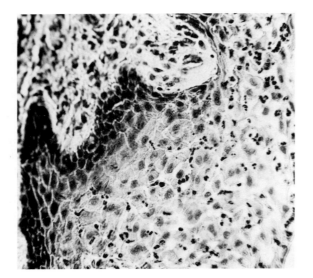

Fig. 7-5. *A,* Low power view of inflammatory infiltrate in crevicular epithelium.

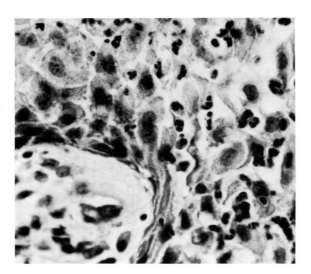

Fig. 7-5. *B,* High power view, showing presence of numerous neutrophils (PMN).

thelium and junctional epithelium may occur at this time.[39,57]

The features of gingivitis that occur 4 to 7 days after plaque accumulation begins[57] include an infiltration of mononuclear cells, especially lymphocytes; further reduction of collagen fibers; alteration of fibroblasts, especially those at the site of the acute inflammation subjacent to the junctional epithelium; and proliferation of the basal layers of the junctional epithelium.[53] These changes, described as early gingivitis, are in addition to those already present in the initial stages of experimental gingivitis.

Within 2 to 4 weeks after the beginning of plaque accumulation, the gingivitis has become established (Fig. 7-6) and is characterized by a predominance of

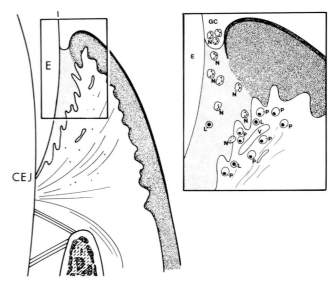

Fig. 7-6. Schematic representation of chronic gingivitis. In spontaneous or naturally occurring gingivitis, or after two to four weeks of plaque accumulation in experimental gingivitis, the histological characteristics include preponderance of plasma cells (P); loss of collagen fibers; proliferation of junctional epithelium; and, not shown, presence of extravascular immunoglobulins. Ulceration and lateral extension of the pocket epithelium occur. Active chronic inflammation may involve the free gingival fibers, and the junctional epithelium may extend slightly apical to the cementoenamel junction (CEJ). E, enamel; N, neutrophils; L, lymphocytes; GC, gingival crevice.

plasma cells (Fig. 7-7) within the connective tissues.[39,57,97]

The gingival lesions (Fig. 7-8) showing the predominance of plasma cells have been described as chronic or established gingivitis.[16,49,53,89,98] Even so, the manifestations of acute inflammation persist from the initial stages of the inflammatory reaction. The plasma cells are present in the initial area of inflammation as well

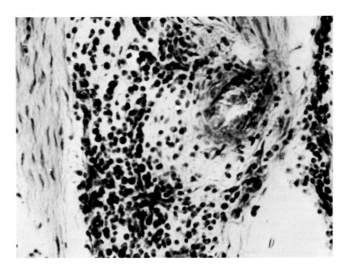

Fig. 7-7. Chronic gingivitis. Inflammatory infiltrate with plasma cells occurring predominantly between dense fiber bundles.

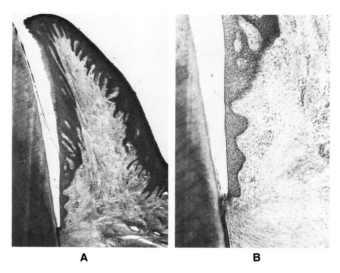

Fig. 7-8. Chronic gingivitis. *A,* Low power view, showing general alteration and thickening of the crevicular epithelium. *B,* High power view, showing lateral extension of junctional epithelium and development of subjacent inflammatory infiltration. Epithelium does not extend apical to the cementoenamel junction.

as in clusters adjacent to vessels and between fibers in the deeper connective tissues (Fig. 7-9). The plasma cells range from immature to degenerating forms.[18] There are lymphocytes still present, altered fibroblasts, and neutrophils. Macrophages are common, and mast cells have been reported in substantial numbers.[18,54] A loss of collagen becomes extensive, involving a larger volume of the gingiva. Scar tissue and fibrosis may occur at the edge of the gingival lesion.

Several changes occur in the junctional and oral crevicular epithelium in chronic gingivitis; some have been marked and have led to the use of the term *pocket epithelium.*[98] Changes include lack of continuity of the external basal lamina, and extension (Fig. 7-10) of the junctional epithelium apical to the cementoenamel junction.[38,53] There is no bone loss, and no bacteria can be seen between the epithelial cells or in the connective tissues.[18]

PERIODONTITIS

The response of the host to dental plaque is inflammation of the gingiva. The character and severity of

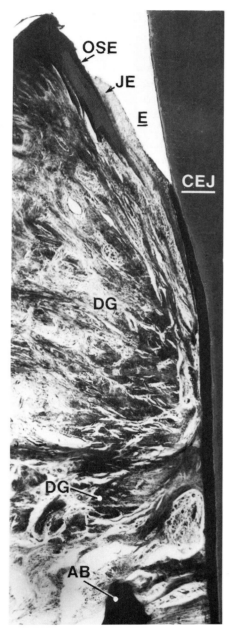

Fig. 7-10. Extension of epithelium apically to cementoenamel junction (CEJ). E, enamel space; OSE, oral sulcular epithelium; JE, junctional epithelium; DG, dento-gingival periodontal fibers; AB, alveolar bone.

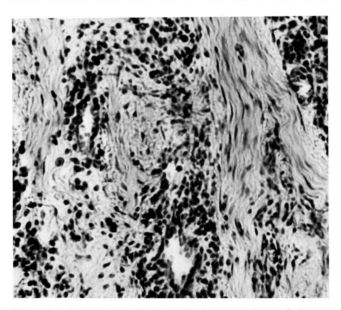

Fig. 7-9. Inflammatory infiltrate, with large numbers of plasma cells adjacent to vessels and between connective tissue fibers.

the inflammatory response appears to be dependent upon the nature of the plaque present, the duration of the presence of plaque, and the response of the host. There is a rather predictable response of the gingiva to plaque injury: the development of chronic gingivitis, which may persist for long periods of time without progression to periodontitis.[29,31,38,85,86] However, the transition from an established lesion[53] or chronic gingivitis to an advanced lesion or periodontitis with bone loss and pocket formation is not predictable, although it is possible to artificially induce the development of a periodontal lesion consistent with the histopathological characteristics of naturally occurring destructive periodontal disease.[31,36,69] On the basis of clinical and histological evidence, gingivitis precedes the transition to periodontitis.

Many of the features of periodontitis have been described in the past, including its clinical features[17,23,27,90] and its epidemiological,[59,64,85] histological,[1,8,16,19,24,25,27,33,49,66,89,99] and ultrastructural characteristics.[20,21,48,70,76,87] Characteristics of periodontitis that have been described (fig. 7-11) include the presence of periodontal pockets; varying degrees of ulceration, suppuration, loss of gingival and periodontal fibers, gingival fibrosis, fibrosis of the marrow spaces; and bone loss. Clinical changes include a loss of attachment level; alterations in color, form, and density of the

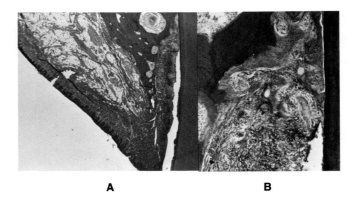

Fig. 7-12. Periodontitis. *A,* Low power view, showing palatal aspect of the periodontium, with an intrabony pocket present. *B,* High power view, showing bone resorption and dense inflammatory infiltrate.

tissues, including varying degrees of hyperplasia and recession; bleeding with slight trauma; exudation, which may be frank pus; increased tooth mobility and drifting of teeth; and loss of teeth. Unlike the initial phase of gingivitis, in which the clinical features appear normal, the tissues in periodontitis reflect to varying degrees the state of the periodontium on observation, which includes periodontal probing and radiographic evaluation; however, the activity of the disease may not necessarily be reflected in the clinical characteristics, since they may only reflect the disease's history.

In periodontitis, the inflammatory infiltrate is no longer related to the tissues subjacent to the base of the gingival crevice, as it is in gingivitis; instead, it extends apically and laterally to form a band around the teeth (Fig. 7-12). In addition to acute vasculitis, chronic inflammation with resulting fibrosis is present. The dense inflammatory infiltrate consists of plasma cells, lymphocytes, and macrophages. Plasma cells may be present in clusters deeper in the connective tissue around blood vessels and between the remaining collagen fibers. Unlike in early gingivitis, in periodontitis, many of the lymphocytes in the advanced lesion have membrane-associated immunoglobulins, and many plasma cells have cytoplasmic immunoglobulin.

The junctional epithelium is located apically to the cementoenamel junction (Fig. 7-13), and strands of pocket epithelium extend apically into the connective tissues and apically along the root surface.[38,54,69] The junctional epithelium forms the base of the periodontal pocket and is attached to the root surface. The cemental surface coronal to the attachment may show fragments of fibers embedded in the cementum or clefts where fibers had been present. Plaque and calculus are also present on the root surface, and the tissues are in contact with the plaque except for poly-

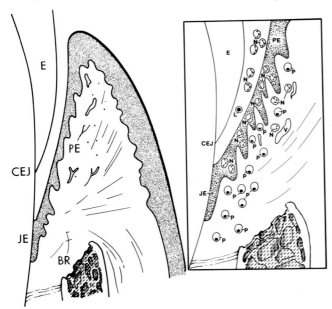

Fig. 7-11. Schematic representation of periodontitis. Extension of lesion into the periodontal membrane, with loss of alveolar bone (BR) and formation of periodontal pocket. Lymphocytes (L) and macrophages are present but plasma cells (P) predominate. Much of the normal dense collagen fiber bundles have been destroyed and replaced with granulation tissue, fibrosis, or scar tissue. Active chronic inflammation may extend throughout the lesion, and the junctional epithelium (JE) is apical to the cementoenamel junction (CEJ). E, enamel; N, neutrophils; V, vessels; PE, pocket epithelium.

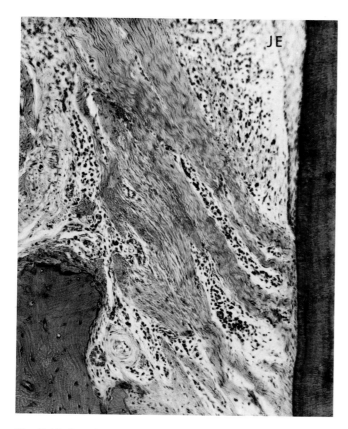

Fig. 7-13. Junctional epithelium (JE) present on cementum, with inflammatory infiltrate extending between the collagen fibers.

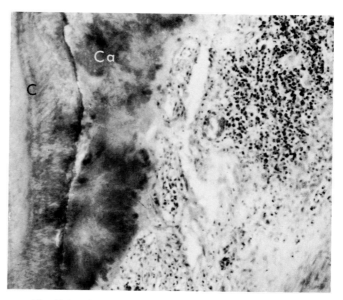

Fig. 7-14. Calculus (Ca) on the cemental (C) surface.

bly.[31,53,96] During an acute exacerbation, frank pus may be a prominent feature of the crevicular exudate; however, there is little evidence of tissue necrosis except in the presence of an abscess.

Often overlooked in histopathological evaluations is the reparative phase of the inflammatory process. Granulation tissue, fibrosis, and scar tissue relates to

morphonuclear leukocytes (Fig. 7-14) interposed between plaque and tissues.

The normal architecture of the structural components of the gingival tissues is altered, and collagen destruction in the zone of dense inflammatory infiltration is almost complete, but fibrosis may be present in the adjacent areas. Although the fiber bundles of the gingiva are disorganized and lost, the transseptal fiber bundles are continuously regenerated in advance of the lesion or represent the residual collagen fibers that traverse the alveolar bone. The transseptal fibers remain in the presence of bone loss and appear to separate the inflammatory infiltrate from the remaining alveolar bone (Fig. 7-15).

Bone resorption (Fig. 7-16, A) appears to be related to extensions of the inflammatory infiltrate around the blood vessels that enter the alveolar crest and, to a lesser extent, to those extensions that involve the periodontal membrane and periosteum.[1,31,49,79,94] With the loss of alveolar bone proper, fibrosis of the marrow occurs (Fig. 7-16B). The resorption of bone is mediated by osteoclasts.[1,31,79]

It has become evident that periods of acute exacerbations of the disease may occur. With periods of quiescence and active destructive disease, the histological appearance of the lesion may vary considera-

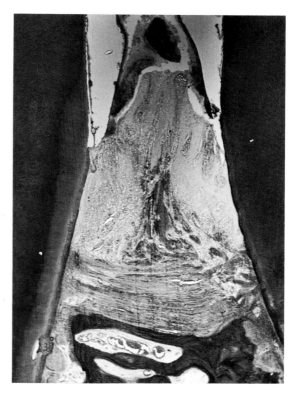

Fig. 7-15. Transeptal fibers remaining in the presence of bone loss.

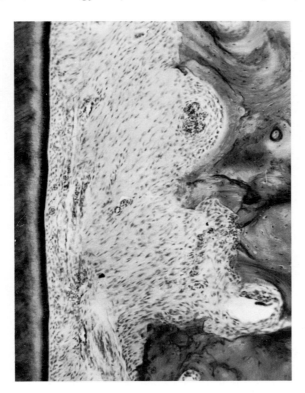

Fig. 7-16. *A,* Bone resorption and bone formation.

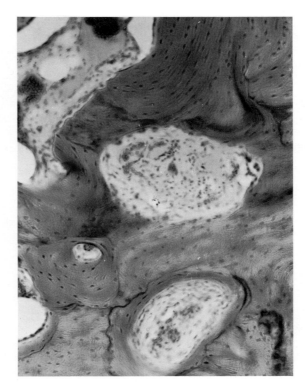

Fig. 7-16, cont'd *B,* Fibrosis of marrow spaces apical to bone loss associated with periodontitis.

repair and are important aspects of the host's response to injury. The virtual absence of pain in the development is related to the nature of the tissue changes present.

SUMMARY

The pathogenesis or development of inflammatory periodontal disease begins with the response of the gingiva to plaque on the teeth. On the basis of microscopic or ultrastructural observations of the gingiva, and except in the experimental model, in which plaque is prevented from forming, it is unlikely that the gingiva is free of some evidence of the inflammatory changes in the gingiva, although the clinical features still suggest a healthy gingiva.

In the experimental model in the dog, the signs of health include the absence of significant gingival sulcus, the virtual absence of gingival crevicular fluid, and a comparatively small number of polymorphonuclear leukocytes in the crevicular fluid. Histologically, the junctional epithelium is in contact with the enamel everywhere, there are no rete pegs, and only a few inflammatory cells are present between the junctional epithelial cells and within the subjacent connective tissue. These characteristics of a model healthy gingiva are used as the baseline for studying changes related to the accumulation of dental plaque and transition from a gingival sulculus to a gingival pocket, the precursor of a periodontal pocket.

The initial changes in the healthy gingiva of a dog are evident 2 to 4 days following the beginning of plaque accumulation. The principal changes are an acute exudative inflammation with vasculitis, gingival fluid exudation, extravascular fibrin, some loss of perivascular collagen, and the beginning of an inflammatory cell infiltrate in the junctional epithelium. These changes have been referred to as *initial gingivitis*[53] and under less than experimental conditions may not be observed.[53]

Within 4 to 7 days following the start of plaque accumulation in the human experimental model, there is an accumulation of large numbers of lymphoid cells in the connective tissue; these cells make up 75% of the total infiltrate population. Collagen loss reaches 60 to 70% with cytoplasmic alterations in the fibroblasts. At this time there is some proliferation of the junctional epithelium, the acute exudative inflammation still persists, and the quantity of gingival fluid continues to increase. These features of early gingivitis[53] have been considered to constitute an important stage in the pathogenesis of inflammatory periodontal disease.

Under experimental conditions in humans, a preponderance of plasma cells is present in the connective tissues 2 to 3 weeks after plaque has begun to accumulate. Collagen loss is still continuing, but no bone loss is present. The junctional and oral crevicular epithelium may proliferate, and so-called "pocket epithelium" may form. The inflammatory response centers on the base of the gingival crevice. Features of the acute exudative inflammation persist in the lesion. These changes are consistent with *chronic* or *established* gingivitis[53] and have been described by a number of investigators.

At some point, chronic gingivitis may progress to periodontitis, which is characterized by varying degrees of bone loss, loss of attachment, pocket formation, tooth mobility, and loss of teeth. The characteristics of chronic gingivitis are also present in periodontitis. Active chronic inflammation, characterized by continued loss of collagen fibers, fibrosis, granulation tissue, and an inflammatory infiltrate of plasma cells, is present throughout the tissues, but periods of quiescence and exacerbation of the inflammatory process occur. Granulation tissue, fibrosis, scarring, dense cellular infiltration, collagen loss, and bone loss indicate the discontinuous nature of the disease loss, and findings of variations within a mouth and among subjects and relative to the progression of chronic destructive periodontitis.[26,30]

The presence of neutrophils in the gingival sulcus and junctional epithelium suggests that neutrophil chemotaxis is an important aspect of the protective mechanism of the host. Dental plaque substances and some bacteria are chemotactic factors for neutrophils. Tissue changes and the accumulation of neutrophils suggest that lysosomal enzymes may be released from neutrophils and may contribute to tissue damage as well as to tissue defense. Gingival fluid also contains complement fragments, which could mediate chemotaxis, but leukocyte migration still occurs with complement inhibition. Chemotaxis may occur directly from bacteria and from the neutrophils themselves. Although the potential for damage exists, there is no body of evidence to indicate that the overall biological significance of neutrophil function is not protective.

The predominantly lymphocytic infiltration has suggested that cellular immunity may play a significant role in the development of destructive periodontal disease. Humoral immunity has also been implicated in the pathogenesis of periodontal disease. Changes in the tissues consistent with the histopathological features of periodontitis have been demonstrated in studies of immune responses.[37,60] However, several studies indicate that immune factors exert a protective effect during the earliest stage of gingivitis.

The mechanism related to the loss of collagen in gingivitis and periodontitis is not clear, but several possibilities have been suggested. Decreased collagen production has been proposed,[56] but the rapidity of the process points more to a destructive process mediated by the host. Bacterial collagenase does not appear to be present in sufficient quantities in the tissues, but collagenase produced by macrophages could be involved in collagen breakdown when these cells are activated either by endotoxin or by the macrophage activating factor, which is produced by stimulated lymphocytes.[62] However, inhibitor systems for collagenase also exist,[15] and are probably important in the control of the activity of this enzyme. The homeostasis of the tissues may be influenced by humoral immune responses, resulting in the formation of immune complexes, and by cellular immune responses, resulting in the activation of macrophages by lymphocytes.

There are several mechanisms that have potential for bone resorption in periodontal disease. The immune mechanisms suggested are a lymphokine, which is called the osteoclast activating factor (OAF); the prostaglandin E2 (PGE2); and less probably, the action of endotoxin. The presence and significance of PGE2 and OAF in human periodontal disease have not been clarified.

Epidemiologic evidence for the progression of gingivitis to adult periodontitis has been demonstrated.[43] Although gingivitis precedes periodontitis, it does not necessarily proceed to periodontitis. The circumstances surrounding the progression of gingivitis to periodontitis have not been clarified, but several possibilities have been suggested, including specific and nonspecific bacterial injury, immune responses, and unusual intrinsic modifying factors.

REFERENCES

1. Akiyoshi, M., and Mori, K.: Marginal periodontitis: A histologic study of the incipient stage, J. Periodont. 38:45, 1967.
2. Attström, R., et al.: Clinical and stereologic characteristics of normal gingiva in dogs, J. Periodont. Res. 10:115, 1975.
3. Attström, R.: Studies on neutrophil polymorphonuclear leukocytes at the dento-gingival junction in gingival health and disease, J. Periodont. Res. 6:(suppl. 8), 1971.
4. Attström, R., and Egelberg, J.: Presence of leukocytes within the gingival crevices during developing gingivitis in dogs, J. Periodont. Res. 6:110, 1971.
5. Attström, R.: Presence of leukocytes in crevices of healthy and chronically inflamed gingiva, J. Periodont. Res. 5:42, 1970.
6. Black, M.M., and Wagner, B.M.: Dynamic Pathology. Structural and Functional Mechanisms of Disease, St. Louis: C.V. Mosby Co., 1964.
7. Borel, J.F.: Studies in chemotaxis, Int. Arch. Allergy Appl. Immunol. 39:247, 1970.
8. Box, H.E.: Studies in Periodontal Pathology, Toronto: University of Toronto Press, 1924.
9. Brandtzaeg, P.: Local formation and transport of immunoglobulins related to the oral cavity, In Host Resistance to Commensal Bacteria, ed. T. McPhee. Edinburgh: Churchill Livingstone, 1972.
10. Burnet, F.M.: Immunology, Aging, and Cancer, San Francisco: W.H. Freeman and Co., 1976.
11. Cowley, G.: Tissue reaction to factors producing periodontal disease—a review. In The Prevention of Periodontal Disease, ed. J.E. Eastoe et al. London: Henry Kingston Publishers, 1971.
12. Drabkin, D.L.: Imperfections: Biochemical phobias and metabolic ambivalence, Perspect. Biol. Med. 2:476, 1959.

13. Engelberg, J.: The topography and permeability of vessels at the dento-gingival junction in dogs, J. Periodont. Res. 2:(suppl. 1), 1967.
14. Egelberg, J.: The blood vessels of the dento-gingival junction, J. Periodont. Res. 1:163, 1966.
15. Eisen, A.Z., et al.: Inhibition of human skin collagenase by human serum, J. Lab. Clin. Med. 75:258, 1970.
16. Fish, E.W.: Parodontal disease: The pathology and treatment of chronic gingivitis, Br. Dent. J. 58:531, 1935.
17. Fox, J.: The Natural History and Disease of the Teeth, Part II. London: E. Cox, 1823.
18. Freedman, H.L., et al.: Electron microscopic features of chronically inflamed human gingiva, J. Periodont. Res. 3:313, 1968.
19. Fullmer, H.M.: A histochemical study of periodontal disease in the maxillary alveolar precess of 135 autopsies, J. Periodont. 32:206, 1961.
20. Garant, P.R., and Mulvihill, J.E.: The fine structure of gingivitis in the beagle. III. Plasma cell infiltration of the subepithelial connective tissue, J. Periodont. Res. 7:161, 1971.
21. Gavin, J.R.: Ultrastructural features of chronic marginal gingivitis, J. Periodont. Res. 5:19, 1970.
22. Genco, R.J., et al.: 1985 Kreshover Lecture: Molecular factors in influencing neutrophil defects in periodontal disease, J. Periodont. Res. 12:1379, 1986.
23. Glickman, I., and Smulow, J.B.: Periodontal Disease: Clinical, Radiographic and Histopathologic Features, Philadelphia: W.B. Saunders, 1974.
24. Goldman, H.M.: The behavior of transseptal fibers in periodontal disease, J. Dent. Res. 36:249, 1957.
25. Goldman, H.M.: The relationship of the epithelial attachment to the adjacent fibers of the periodontal membrane, J. Dent. Res. 23:177, 1944.
26. Goodson, J.M., et al.: Patterns of progression and regression of advanced destructible periodontal disease, J. Clin. Periodontol. 9:472, 1982.
27. Gottlieb, B., and Orban, B.: Zahnfleischentzündung and Zahnlockerung. Berlin: Berlinische Verlagsanstalt (G.M.B.H.), 1933.
28. Grant, D.A., and Orban, B.: Leukocytes in the epithelial attachment, J. Periodont. 31:87, 1960.
29. Greene, J.C., and Suomi, J.D.: Epidemiology and public health aspects of caries and periodontal disease, J. Dent. Res. 56:(Special Issue C) C20, 1977.
30. Haffajee, A.D., and Socransky, S.S.: Attachment level changes in destructive periodontal disease, J. Clin. Periodontol. 13:461, 1986.
31. Heijl, L., et al.: Conversion of chronic gingivitis to periodontitis in squirrel monkeys, J. Periodont. 47:710, 1976.
32. Hoover, D.R., and Lefkowitz, W.: Fluctuations in marginal gingivitis, J. Periodont, 36:310, 1965.
33. Hopewell-Smith, A.: Pyorrhea alveolaris—mits pathohistology. I. Preliminary note. II. Concluding remarks, Dent. Cosmos 53:397, 981, 1911.
34. Horton, J.E., et al.: A role for cell-mediated immunity in the pathogenesis of periodontal disease, J. Periodont. 45:351, 1974.
35. Imrey, P.B.: Considerations in the statistical analysis of clinical trials in periodontitis, J. Clin. Periodontol. 13:517, 1986.
36. Kennedy, J.E., and Polson, A.M.: Experimental marginal periodontitis in squirrel monkeys, J. Periodont. 44:140, 1973.
37. Levy, B.M., et al.: Adjuvant induced destructive periodontitis in nonhuman primates. A comparative study, J. Periodont. Res. 11:54, 1976.
38. Lindhe, J., et al.: Plaque induced periodontal disease in beagle dogs, J. Periodont. Res. 10:243, 1975.
39. Lindhe, J., et al. A clinical and stereologic analysis of the course of early gingivitis in dogs, J. Periodont. Res. 9:314, 1974.
40. Lindhe, J., et al.: Experimental periodontitis in the beagle dog, J. Periodont. Res. 8:1, 1973.
41. Listgarten, M.A.: Pathogenesis of periodontitis, J. Clin. Periodontol. 13:418, 1986.
42. Listgarten, M.A., and Ellegaard, B.: Experimental gingivitis in rhesus monkeys, J. Periodont. Res. 8:199, 1973.
43. Löe, H., et al.: Natural history of periodontal disease in man. Rapid, moderate, and no loss of attachment in Sri Lankan laborers 14 to 46 years of age, J. Clin. Periodontol. 13:431, 1986.
44. Löe, H., and Holm-Pedersen, P.: Absence and presence of fluid from normal and inflamed gingiva, Periodontics 3:171, 1965.
45. Löe, H., et al.: Experimental ginigivitis in man, J. Periodont. 36:177, 1965.
46. Lövdal, A., et al.: Incidence of manifestations of periodontal disease in light of oral hygiene and calculus formation, Acta Odont. Scand. 56:21, 1958.
47. Manor, A., et al.: Bacterial invasion of periodontal tissues in advanced periodontitis in humans, J. Periodontol. 55:567, 1984.
48. Mazzalla, W.J., and Vernick, S.H.: The ultrastructure of normal and pathologic human gingival epithelium, J. Periodont. 39:5, 1968.
49. Melcher, A.H.: The pathogenesis of chronic gingivitis. I. The spread of the inflammatory process, Dent. Pract. Dent. Rec. 13:2, 1962.
50. Muller-Glauser, W., and Schroeder, H.E.: The pocket epithelium: a light and electron microscope study, J. Periodontol. 53:133, 1982.
51. Page, R.C., and Schroeder, H.E.: Periodontitis in man and other animals. A comparative review, Basel: S. Karger, 1982.
52. Page, R.C.: Gingivitis, J. Clin. Periodontol. 13:345, 1986.
53. Page, R.C., and Schroeder, H.E.: Pathogenesis of inflammatory periodontal disease. A summary of current work, Clin. Invest. 33:235, 1976.
54. Page, R.C., et al.: Host tissue response in chronic inflammatory disease. IV. The periodontal and dental status of a group of aged great apes, J. Periodont. 46:144, 1975.
55. Page, R.C., et al.: Collagen fiber bundles of the normal marginal gingiva, Arch. Oral Biol. 19:1039, 1974.
56. Page, R.C., and Schroeder, H.E.: Biochemical aspects of the connective tissue alterations in inflammatory gingival and periodontal disease, Int. Dent. J. 23:455, 1973.
57. Payne, W.A., et al.: Histopathologic features of the initial and early stages of experimental gingivitis in man, J. Periodont. Res. 10:51, 1975.
58. Ralls, S.A., and Cohen, M.E.: Problems in identifying "bursts" of periodontal attachment loss, J. Periodontol. 57:746, 1986.
59. Ramfjord, S.P., et al.: Epidemiological studies of periodontal diseases, Am. J. Public Health 58:1713, 1968.
60. Ranny, R.R., and Zander, H.A.: Allergic periodontal disease in sensitized squirrel monkeys, J. Periodont. 41:13, 1970.
61. Ritchey, B., and Orban, B.: The periodontal pocket, J. Periodont. 23:199, 1952.
62. Rizzo A.A., and Mitchell, C.T.: Activation of latent collagenase by microbial plaque, J. Periodont. Res. 9:81, 1974.
63. Rudin, H.J., et al.: Correlation between sulcus fluid rate and clinical and histological inflammation of the marginal gingiva, Helv. Odont. Acta 14:2, 26, 1970.
64. Russell, A.L.: Epidemiology of periodontal disease, Int. Dent. J. 17:282, 1967.
65. Rylander, H., and Lindhe, J.: Experimental gingivitis in dogs. A morphometric study, Scand. Div., I.A.D.R. Abstract No. 65, 1974.

66. Schroeder, H.E., and Attström, R.: Pocket formation: An hypothesis. In The Borderland Between Caries and Periodontal Disease II, ed. W.T. Lehner and G. Cimasoni, London: Academic Press, 1980.
67. Schroeder, H.E.: Discussion: Pathogenesis of periodontitis, J. Clin. Periodontol. 13:426, 1986.
68. Schroeder, H.E., et al.: Initial gingivitis in dogs, J. Periodont. Res. 10:128, 1975.
69. Schroeder, H.E., and Lindhe, J.: Conversion of stable established gingivitis in the dog into destructive periodontitis, Arch. Oral Biol. 10:775, 1975.
70. Schroeder, H.E.: Ultrastructure des lesions gingivales precoces, Rev. Fr. Odonta-stomatol. 20:103, 1973.
71. Schroeder, H.E., et al.: Correlated morphometric and biochemical analysis of gingival tissue in early chronic gingivitis in man, Arch. Oral Biol. 18:899, 1973.
72. Schroeder, H.E.: Transmigration and infiltration of leukocytes in human junctional epithelium, Helv. Odont. Acta 17:6, 1973.
73. Schroeder, H.E., et al.: Structural constituents of clinically normal and slightly inflamed dog gingiva; A morphometric study, Helv. Odont. Acta 17:70, 1973.
74. Schroeder, H.E., and Listgarten, M.A.: Fine structure of the developing epithelial attachment of human teeth, Monographs in Developmental Biology. Vol. 2. Basel: S. Karger, 1971.
75. Schroeder, H.E.: Quantitative parameters of early human gingival inflammation, Arch. Oral Biol. 15:383, 1970.
76. Selvig, K.A.: Ultrastructural changes in cementum and adjacent connective tissue in periodontal disease, Acta. Odont. Scand. 24:459, 1966.
77. Simpson, D.M., and Avery, B.E.: Histopathologic and ultrastructural features of inflamed gingiva in the baboon, J. Periodont. 45:500, 1974.
78. Simpson, D.M., and Avery, B.E.: Pathologically altered fibroblasts within lymphoid infiltrates in early gingivitis, J. Dent. Res. 52:1156, 1973.
79. Soames, J.V., et al.: The progression of gingivitis to periodontitis in the beagle dog: A histological and morphometric investigation, J. Periodont. 47:435, 1976.
80. Socransky, S.S., et al.: Concepts of destructive periodontal disease, J. Clin. Periodontol. 11:21, 1984.
81. Söderholm, G., and Attström, R.: Vascular permeability during initial gingivitis in dogs, J. Periodont. Res. 12:395, 1977.
82. Stern, I.B.: Electron microscopic observations of oral epithelium, Periodontics 3:224, 1965.
83. Suomi, J.D., et al.: Marginal gingivitis during a sixteen week period, J. Periodontol. 42:268, 1971.
84. Suomi, J.D., et al.: A follow-up study of former participants in a controlled oral hygiene study, J. Periodont. 44:662, 1973.
85. Suomi, J.D., et al.: The effect of controlled oral hygiene procedures on the progression of periodontal disease in adults: Radiographic findings, J. Periodont. 2:562, 1971.
86. Suomi, J.D., et al.: The effect of controlled oral hygiene procedures on the progression of periodontal disease in adults. Results after third and final year, J. Periodont. 42:152, 1971.
87. Takarada, H., et al.: Ultrastructural studies of human gingiva. II. The lower part of the pocket epithelium in chronic periodontitis, J. Periodont. 45:155, 1974.
88. Takarada, H., et al.: Ultrastructural studies of human gingiva. I. The upper part of the pocket epithelium in chronic periodontitis, J. Periodont. 45:30, 1974.
89. Talbot, E.S.: Interstitial Gingivitis or So-Called Pyorrhea Alveolaris, Philadelphia: S.S. White Dental Mfg. Co., 1899.
90. Talbot, E.S.: Pyorrhea alveolaris, Dent. Cosmos 28:689, 1886.
91. Theilade, E., et al.: Experimental gingivitis in man. II. A longitudinal clinical and bacteriological investigation, J. Period. Res. 1:1, 1966.
92. Thilander, H.: The effect of leukocytic activity on the structure of the gingival pocket epithelium in man, Acta Odont. Scand. 21:431, 1963.
93. Thomas, L.: Inflammation as a defense mechanism. (eds): In The Inflammatory Process, ed. B.W. Zweifach et al. Vol. 3, New York: Academic Press. 1974.
94. Weinmann, J.P.: Progress of gingival inflammation into the supporting structures of the teeth, J. Periodont. 12:71, 1941.
95. Wilde, G., et al.: Host tissue response in chronic periodontal disease. VI. The role of cell-mediated hypersensitivity, J. Periodont. Res. 12:179, 1977.
96. World Workshop in Periodontics. Ed. S.P. Ramfjord, D.A. Kerr, and M.M. Ash. Ann Arbor, Michigan: The University of Michigan, 1966, pp. 120-121.
97. Zachrisson, B.W.: A histologic study of experimental gingivitis in man, J. Periodont. Res. 3:11, 1969.
98. Zachrisson, B.W., and Schultz-Haudt, D.S.: A comparative histological study of clinically normal and chronically inflamed gingiva from the same individuals, Odont. Tidskr. 76:179, 1968.
99. Znamensky, N.E.: Alveolar-pyorrhea. Its pathological anatomy and its radical treatment, Br. Dent. J. 23:585, 1902.

8

ETIOLOGY OF PERIODONTAL DISEASE—PLAQUE, CALCULUS, AND IATROGENIC FACTORS

There is general agreement that the most frequent cause of gingivitis is the accumulation of microbial plaque on or at the cervical region of the teeth. At the time of eruption of the teeth, especially of the permanent dentition, the nature of the inflammatory response must be considered as a part of the immunologic, ecologic and structural adjustments being made by the host at the local as well as the systemic level. Many factors, from malposed teeth to neutrophil function, may interfere with plaque control via local and systemic mechanisms.

On the basis of available evidence, it is reasonable to state that all presently known intrinsic local and systemic defense mechanisms operating at the dentogingival junction can be compromised by disturbed intrinsic factors (humoral/cellular) and/or extrinsic factors (decreased plaque control). These factors then lead to functional and structural changes in the dentogingival function, which increase its susceptibility to the destructive challenge of opportunistic bacteria. Modifying factors include systemic and local disturbances in defense mechanisms. These disturbances enhance the opportunity of bacteria to successfully challenge the dentogingival barrier.

The most likely cause of periodontitis is microbial plaque. Trauma from occlusion, hormonal factors, and neutrophil dysfunction are capable of modifying unfavorably the defense of the host.

Classification of etiologic factors. For convenience in discussion, the causes of inflammatory periodontal diseases are often divided between initiating and modifying factors. The modifying factors are further divided between local (extrinsic) and systemic (intrinsic) factors (Table 8-1). The initiating factors are responsible for causing the disease and the modifying factors for altering either the inflammatory response or the initiating factor.[54] The extrinsic factors originate locally and the intrinsic factors are systemic in origin. Because

Table 8-1. Etiological factors in inflammatory periodontal disease

Initiating Factors
Bacterial plaque, calculus
Mouthbreathing
Eruption of Teeth
Modifying Factors
Local
Malocclusion
Mouthbreathing
Food impaction
Dental morphology
Soft tissue factors
Dental-iatrogenic
Traumatic occlusion
Systemic
Hormonal status
Nutrition
Drugs
Stress and emotion
Aging
Systemic diseases
Genetic anomalies

extrinsic and intrinsic factors are related, the convenience of using these different categories should not overshadow the importance of interrelating the factors whenever possible and appropriate. Systemic factors are discussed in Chapter 9.

The cause of gingivitis and periodontitis is considered to be primarily bacterial substances in dental plaque,[19,29,108] but the response of the host and the consequences of intrinsic host-related factors are also important in the pathogeneses of inflammatory periodontal disease. Although the response is dependent in most individuals on the presence of particular toxigenic and antigenic products, in some individuals the nature and severity of the periodontal response will also depend upon other factors, such as defects in the white blood cells and genetic anomalies. Systemic factors, host resistance, and immunologic factors in periodontal disease are discussed in Chapter 9.

Infection The nature of periodontal disease seems reasonably clear i.e., it is an infection caused by somewhat uncertain mixture of microbes via uncertain mechanisms. It is not uncommon to see adult periodontitis described as a chronic infectious process, a bacterial infection, a local infectious disease, a mixed infection, an infective process, and an inflammatory disease associated with various microbial types. However, except for acute necrotizing ulcerative gingivitis (ANUG), the nature of the inflammatory response in gingivitis, especially in children (up to 11 years), still begs the question in recent literature as to whether or not gingivitis is a disease, let alone a site-specific disease or an infection. The differences in response between the tissues of children and adults to the presence of plaque cannot be explained simply on the basis of age, infection/no infection, or disease/no disease.

Infection sometimes means that bacteria have caused overt signs of damage; in other instances, their mere presence in a site normally sterile is sufficient to indicate that an infection is present, with or without signs of disease or damage. When the signs of disease occur at a site where a variety of indigenous flora exists normally without causing damage, an infection is said to be present if 1 or more of the strains of microbes present takes an opportunity to cause damage.

The old concept that a sterile gingival sulcus reflects a healthy gingiva, and that the mere presence of bacteria there reflects an infection, was an oversimplification of more difficult diagnostic problems concerning the borderland between disease activity and no disease. The signs and symptoms of gingivitis (as well as of periodontitis) are well established by convention; however, the determination of whether or not disease or an infection exists depends on philosophical descriptions of "life outside the range of normal"; on whether there has been an inadequate adaptation to changes in external and internal environment; and on whether there is a deviation from or interruption in normal structure or function. Attempts to locate and identify the earliest structural and functional changes using microscopic, ultrastructural, immunologic, biochemical, bacteriologic and clinical parameters have not led to meaningful determinants of disease/no disease or of disease activity. Whether or not an infection exists is dependent upon: (1) the detection of microbes in an otherwise sterile tissue site; or (2) the presence of bacterial species (or a specific microbe) which reproducibly precede and cause tissue damage of a detrimental change of function.

Normally, bacteria are not present in living tissues except on a transient basis; transient bacteria are associated with toothbrushing, eating and other normal functions. The presence of scattered bacteria does not demonstrate bacterial invasion. Circumstances of the location would require localized microcolonies to be present or morphologically homogenous microorganisms representing 1 or more invading bacterial species to be disseminated in the periodontal tissues.[67] The evidence for tissue invasion is weak and verification is extremely difficult.[102]

For apparently unknown reasons, gingivitis is not categorized as a local infectious disease (except for ANUG), whereas periodontitis is commonly described in this way. The concept that attachment loss does not occur for the most part without meaningful precursor gingivitis might be strengthened if the conversion from gingivitis to periodontitis were to be based on evidence of a site-specific infection by opportunistic bacteria in pre-existing gingival inflammations and subsequent loss of attachment, and if these conditions could be shown to correspond reproducibly with mixed, predominantly anaerobic species of bacteria. There does not appear to be sufficient consistency in the composition of microbiota at diseased sites to implicate any of the microbes that are strongly associated with adult periodontitis as likely etiologic agents of adult periodontitis.[67]

INITIATING FACTORS

Extrinsic initiating factors of inflammatory periodontal disease include plaque, calculus, mouthbreathing, and various types of mechanical trauma. There is no convincing evidence that there are intrinsic initiating factors for inflammatory periodontal disease.

Dental plaque

The term *plaque* was first used in a dental context in 1898 by G.V. Black to describe the feltlike mass of microorganisms over carious lesions.[11] It has since been defined as the soft, tenacious material found on tooth surfaces, which is not readily removed by rinsing with water,[15] and as a soft concentrated mass consisting mainly of a large variety of bacteria held together in an intermicrobial substance.[116] However, these definitions are limited, as there is considerable variation in the structural, bacteriologic, and biochemical composition of the plaque.

Dental plaque is a highly organized ecologic unit consisting of masses of bacteria imbedded in an amorphous matrix consisting of macromolecules synthesized by proliferating bacteria, as well as constituents of the crevicular fluid (Fig. 8-1). *Materia alba* is an adventitious creamy-white loose accumulation of microorganisms, cell debris, and food residues that can be removed with a stream of water (Fig. 8-2).

Microorganisms that inhabit the surface of the teeth and soft tissues make up the indigenous or normal

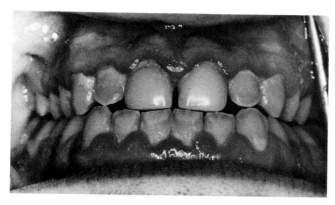

Fig. 8-1. Dental plaque on all surfaces of the teeth.

microflora. There is a balance between the host and the relatively innocuous microflora, which, in some instances, can even be beneficial by acting as a deterrent to the establishment of pathogens or opportunistic microbes.

The development of the indigenous microflora begins at birth and continues in accordance with the general principles that govern ecologic processes elsewhere. The ability of bacteria to colonize the surface of a tooth depends upon a number of factors, but of considerable importance is the specific ability of bacteria to attach to a tooth and/or to other microorganisms. The characteristic of *adherence* provides the mechanism by which some types of bacteria can attach to and colonize certain surfaces, whereas others cannot do so or compete in those sites with other bacteria.

The *ecologic determinants* of plaque include (1) *environmental factors* such as diet, ph, PO2, CO2 and

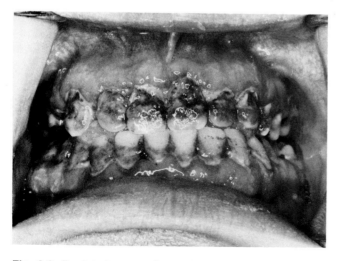

Fig. 8-2. Dental plaque and materia alba formed in complete absence of home care.

other (Fig 8-3); (2) *microbial interactions*—interbacterial adherence, competition for substrates; and (3) *host factors*—saliva, crevicular fluid, adherence, and immune defense. Plaque microbial ecology reflects complex dynamic ecosystems in which patent selective forces regulate bacterial colonization. The *virulence* factors possessed by bacteria include (1) the capacity to colonize specific sites; (2) the ability to evade the host's defenses; and (3) the capacity to cause injury to the tissues.

The formation of dental plaque reflects the accumulation of bacteria already present in the oral cavity. Its formation is highly dependent upon specific attachment mechanisms, including (1) ability to adhere specifically to pellicle; and (2) the ability of bacteria to adhere to each other.

Pellicle. The earliest deposit to form on the cleaned surface of a tooth has been called the "acquired pellicle."[73] It is derived primarily from the saliva,[3] and is the first evidence of plaque development.[78,98] The formation of a biological film or pellicle is a prerequisite for adhesion of formed elements, such as bacteria or cells. Such thin multilayers of natural complex polymers form spontaneously on solids found in biological fluids including saliva, seawater, lakes, and streams.

The pellicle is a structureless, acellular film of glycoproteins that becomes visible within 2 hours following a prophylaxis with pumice or a equivalent abrasive. In addition, after this time, the organic layer has a remarkable uniformity of thickness (0.1 to 0.7) and continuity of its border.[109] It is composed primarily of glycoproteins adsorbed selectively to the surface of hydroxyapatite crystals from the saliva.[20,40,68,75] Other proteins include antibodies, lactoferrin, and transferrin.

Formation of plaque. Plaque begins to form soon after the development of the pellicle with bacterial colonization. Such colonization is dependent upon such factors as availability of nutrition and of oxygen, and the ability of microorganisms to adhere to specific surfaces. The rate of plaque formation following its removal is largely dependent upon oral hygiene measures (Fig 8-4). There is a shift in the composition of the bacterial flora along with an increase in thickness of plaque that has been ascribed to (1) specific adherence, (2) bacterial aggregation, and (3) changes in growth conditions such as anaerobiosis and nutritional interactions between bacteria.

Bacterial colonization. Early colonizers of the pellicle are mainly gram-positive cocci and rods, but soon other bacteria aggregate to the 1st colonizers to form scattered colonies. Subsequently, large coherent masses of plaque form in the absence of oral hygiene measures. Thus, in experimental gingivitis, initiated by having subjects refrain from practicing oral hygiene measures, the indigenous gram-positive flora prolif-

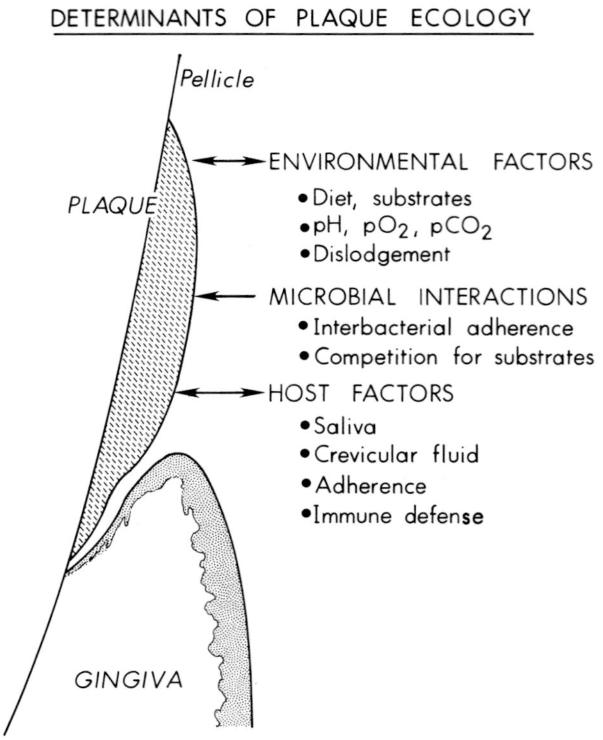

DETERMINANTS OF PLAQUE ECOLOGY

Pellicle

PLAQUE

→ ENVIRONMENTAL FACTORS
• Diet, substrates
• pH, pO₂, pCO₂
• Dislodgement

→ MICROBIAL INTERACTIONS
• Interbacterial adherence
• Competition for substrates

→ HOST FACTORS
• Saliva
• Crevicular fluid
• Adherence
• Immune defense

GINGIVA

Fig. 8-3. Ecologic determinants of plaque.

erate and an increasing number of gram-negative cocci and rods appear during the first 2 days of plaque formation. The cultivable cocci and rods that predominate are streptococci (e.g., *A. naeslundii* and *A. viscosus*), and *Rothia dentocariosa*.[80]

In the next 2 to 4 days of plaque accumulation, there is a proliferation of fusobacterium and filamentous bacteria as well as of others already present. From 4 to 9 days, the composition becomes more diverse, with considerable variation between subjects, depending on the development of gingivitis. However, specific species of *Actinomyces*, *Streptococcus*, *Fusobacterium*, *Veillonella*, and *Treponema* appear to be reproducibly associated with the development of gingivitis in young adults.[80]

The subgingival flora associated with a generally healthy gingiva is composed primarily of *Actinomyces*, *Streptococcus*, and *Veillonella* species. The initial colonization of the subgingival area is by *Bacteroides gingivalis*, a species almost absent from healthy sulci. There is a shift of the percentage distribution of various groups of cultivable bacteria from a healthy gingival sulcus (40% *Streptococcus*, 40% *Actinomycees*, 20% anaerobic gram-negative rods) to advanced periodontitis (5% *Streptococcus*, 15% *Actinomycees*, and 80% gram-negative rods). The bacteria at healthy sites are predominantly non-motile, gram-positive facultative cocci and rods with *Streptococcus* and *Actino-*

mycetes species predominating, whereas the bacteria associated with gingivitis and periodontitis are more complex, with increasing proportions of motile, gram-negative and anaerobic species, including *B. intermedius*, *B. gingivalis*, *Actinobacillus actinomycetemcomitans* (*A.a.*) and spirochetes.[66] The complexity of the spirochetal flora increases with disease. Most of the spirochetes have not been cultivated successfully, and taxonomic diversity is extensive. Most appear to be treponemes, but a large number have yet to be named and described.

There is not sufficient evidence to implicate specific shifts in the bacterial flora or specific bacteria (singly or in groups) as indicators or etiologic agents of adult periodontitis.[67] However, a proposed specific concept for the pathogenesis of destructive periodontal disease has received support.[27,106] For example, *Bacteroides gingivalis* has been implicated as a major pathogen in severe forms of adult periodontitis, *B. intermedius* and intermediate-sized spirochetes in ANUG, *Actinobacillus actinomycetemcomitans* with localized juvenile periodontitis, *B. intermedius* with pregnancy, gingivitis, and capnocytophaga species and *A.a.* with advanced periodontitis of juvenile diabetics. Such bacterial associations remain to be clarified in relation to specific defects in host defense.

Mechanisms of colonization. Bacteria attach to host tissues with a remarkable degree of specificity through a complex recognition system, perhaps analogous to the mechanisms involved in antigen-antibody reactions; i.e., "lock and key dovetailing of surface molecules." The adherence of bacteria occurs in a specific interaction in which macromolecules (adhesions) on the surface of bacteria bind to complementary structures (ligands) on the surfaces of the host's tissue.

Adhesions, which are often present in filamentous surface appendages such as pili or fimbriae, are thought to involve lectinlike and/or hydrophobic ligands. Thus, bacteria have on their surface carbohydrate-binding proteins that serve to bind the microorganism to corresponding glycoconjugates on the surface of the host's tissues. The site of attachment is called a *binding site,* and the molecules with which the adhesions interact on the host are called *receptors.*

After the initial colonization of the pellicle by adhesion-ligand mechanisms has taken place, further buildup of plaque may occur as a result of aggregations of bacteria, or of interbacterial binding of specific pairs of different bacterial species that benefit from such an ecologic interaction. The cell-cell interaction with bacterial coaggregation of actinomycetes and gram-negative organisms such as bacteroids have suggested to some investigators the possibility that actinomycetes may be a marker for transition from gram-positive plaque microflora to one with predominant gram-negative species.

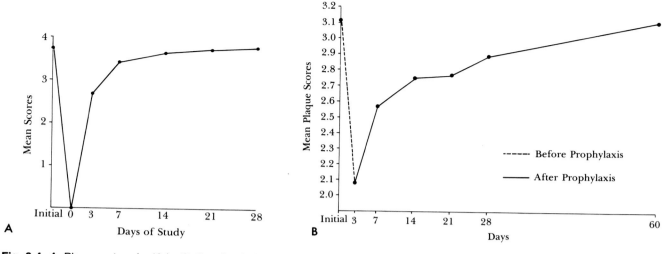

Fig. 8-4. *A,* Plaque return in 40 institutionalized children. Initial scores (scale of 0 to 5) were again reached about one week after prophylaxis at day 0. *B,* Return of plaque after prophylaxis in 80 adult subjects. Plaque scores based on a scale of 0 to 5.

Antiplaque influences. Negative influences on bacterial adherence can affect the colonization of oral tissues. Salivary glyoproteins, lysozyme, mucins, and secretory IgA are thought to interfere with adherence mechanisms and/or to cause bacterial agglutination.

Dietary lectins may cause bacterial aggregation. Human milk is an example. It is suggested that such factors as lactoferrin lysozyme and bacteriocidins influence bacteria negatively. However, the significance of lactoferrin in milk, saliva, tears, and neutrophils to plaque ecology has to be clarified. Much the same can be said about lysozyme and about bacteriocidins. Bacteriocidins are capable of inhibiting the growth of competing bacteria.

Bacterial products in plaque. Enzymes such as collagenase, proteases, hyaluronidase, chondroitin sulfatase, neuraminidase, and β-glucuronidase are probably produced by bacteria as well as by lysosomes of the body cells. The substrates of these enzymes are components of the connective tissue, ground substance, and intercellular epithelial substance, and theoretically could be affected by small amounts of the enzymes under natural conditions. However, the experimental effects of these enzymes[105,112] may differ significantly from those in the natural situation, where small concentrations of a mixture of enzymes would be found.[12] Also, it does not appear likely that bacterial enzymes would reach the connective tissue in sufficient quantity to cause breakdown of collagen fibers.

Several cytotoxic and chemotactic substances are produced by bacteria in dental plaque, including products of metabolism and of lysis of bacterial cells and extracellular substances synthesized by bacteria. Ammonia, sulfide, amines, indole, skatole, organic acids, polysaccharides, and certain glycans could damage the epithelium and initiate an inflammatory reaction in the connective tissues. However, the actual role of these cytotoxic substances in periodontal inflammation is not known. The release of lysosomal enzymes from macrophages and leukocytes could be stimulated by these plaque substances, and thus could be indirectly responsible for the loss of supporting structures in periodontal disease. The concentration of such cytotoxic, chemotoxic, and chemotactic substances in plaque, and their presence and action in the tissues, have not been determined.

It is also possible that enzymes, glycans, extracellular polysaccharides, and other bacterial products may act as antigens and lead to immunological reactions, including both cell-mediated and humoral hypersensitivity.[28,43,82,83]

Response to plaque. Immune and nonimmune inflammatory responses may occur in the presence of bacteria and bacterial products (including antigens) in dental plaque. These responses include the inflammatory responses involving vascular and cellular components, as well as activation of (1) the secretory-mucosal immune system, (2) the neutrophil-antibody-complement system, (3) the lymphocyte-macrophage system, and (4) immune regulation. Immune responses to plaque include antibodies, complement activation, polymorphonuclear leukocyte killing, activation of macrophages, and release of lymphokines by plaque-sensitized T and B lymphocytes.

It has been suggested that several events herald a change from gingivitis to destructive periodontitis: (1) conversion of a predominantly T cell infiltrate to a B cell infiltrate;[103] (2) shift of microbial composition from predominantly non-motile, gram-positive facultative cocci and rods to more motile, gram-negative and anaerobic species; (3) shift from one immunologic profile to another;[67] and (4) transition of a gingival sulcus to a gingival pocket as characterized by pocket epithelium.[102] None of these responses has been shown to be useful in demonstrating active periodontitis. Defenses of the host are described in Chapter 9.

Diet and plaque. Several studies suggest that the consistency, composition, and microflora of the plaque, and its tendency to mineralize, are related to the chemical composition and physical consistency of the diet,[12] even though it is not necessary for food to be taken into the mouth for plaque to form.[18,44] The vigorous or excessive chewing of hard or coarse foods does not seem to affect the amount of plaque at gingival margins and approximal areas.[8,18,44,64,126] A number of studies have been conducted on the potential relationship of the intake of sugars and the quantity of plaque;[14,23,24,38] however, the effects do not appear to be clinically significant. Individual variations are present and little attempt has been made to study the plaque in specific sites that might be possible to relate to disease. There is probably a relationship between masticatory patterns and the movements of the tongue and cheeks with incisal and occlusal limitation of growth of plaque, but the cervical areas of the teeth, the gingival margin, and most of the attached gingiva do not receive physical stress from food.[126] There is some evidence that diet may influence slightly the quantitative proportions of the microorganisms in plaque,[53,99] but the significance of such differences is not currently apparent.

DENTAL CALCULUS

The mineralization of dental plaque to form calculus (Fig. 8-5) occurs in vivo in humans. However, the presence of microorganisms does not appear to be necessary—a white crystalline structure resembling calculus has been reported in germ-free animals.[38] Despite the evidence, it would be an error to regard the formation of calculus as independent of the presence and metabolic activity of plaque microorganisms.

Composition and formation. The composition of calculus varies considerably among individuals and even within individuals. The organic content constitutes about 12% of the calculus,[85] and includes protein, carbohydrates, lipid fractions, and various types of non-vital microorganisms, especially of the filamentous type, such as liptothrix. The inorganic component is mostly calcium phosphate, which is present as amorphous material and in a crystalline form. The crystalline form includes hydroxyapatite [$(Ca_{10}(PO_4)_6(OH)_2$], about 20% and octocalcium phosphate $Ca_4HPO_4(PO_4)_25H_2O$), about 50%. Brushite [$(CaHPO_4 \cdot 2H_2O)$], whitlockite [$Ca_3(PO_4)2$], and magnesium make up the remaining percentages.[101] Whitlockite (WH) is abundant in subgingival calculus, and brushite is found only in supragingival calculus attached to mandibular anterior teeth.

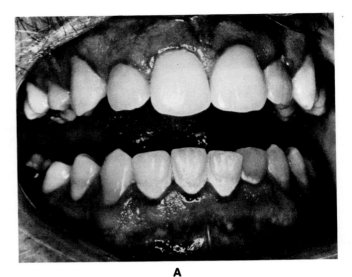

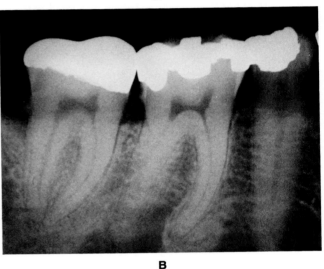

Fig. 8-5. *A,* Calculus formation on the labial surfaces of the mandibular incisors. *B,* Calculus seen radiographically on the distal surfaces of molars.

Dental calculus is preceded by plaque formation,[36,118,130] but the mechanisms of its mineralization have not been determined. Calcium phosphate crystals can be detected in the plaque matrix, within some bacteria, and in the pellicle. Clinically, several aspects of calculus formation have been noted: the better the oral hygiene the less the calculus formed, but variations are great when oral hygiene is not good. Although the rate of calcium formation (Fig. 8-6) varies greatly among individuals, the relation of such differences to oral hygiene, diet, rate of salivary flow, and systemic disease has not been demonstrated clearly. For unknown reasons, possibly involving bacterial flora, children form less calculus than adults. The greater amount of calculus on the facial surfaces of the maxillary molars and the lingual surfaces of the mandibular incisors has been related to the proximity of the orifices of the salivary glands.

Several theories for the formation of calculus have been suggested in the past. None has been accepted singly or in combination as providing an adequate explanation of the mechanisms of calculus formation. These theories generally relate to changes in the pH of saliva or plaque, phosphatase action, and seeding via bacteria.

One theory proposes that saliva may become more alkaline with a loss of carbon dioxide and enhance the precipitation of calcium phosphate. The presence of carbonic anhydrase, which is produced by plaque or salivary bacteria, could cause the breakdown of a complex ion of carbon dioxide and calcium phosphate, which tends to keep phosphate in solution. The breakdown would then allow calcium phosphate to be precipitated.[22] Another theory involves the possibility of saliva becoming more alkaline because of the formation of ammonia by oral bacteria. Plaque can break down urea rapidly to give rise to ammonia and carbon dioxide. Another theory on the mineralization of plaque relates to the formation of seeding substances produced by bacteria or by intercellular crystalization. In the latter instance, the seeding could occur in viable organisms or because of the presence of dead microorganisms.[36,94,95,101]

During the initial phase of calcification, octacalcium phosphate (OCP) or brushite form, and the plaque is gradually hydrolyzed into hydroxyapatite (OHA) and/ or whitlockite (WH). Thus, the bacteria and matrix of supragingival plaque are calcified, with OCP forming first, and then transformed into OHA. If the pH is low and the Ca/P ratio is high, brushite is formed initially and transformed into OHA or WH in an early stage of calcification that is related to NH_4 produced by plaque bacteria.[17] In the presence of Mg^{2+}, Zn^{2+}, and CO_3^{2-}, tissue fluid, and under anaerobic conditions, whitlockite is formed as the main component of subgingival calculus.

The role of calculus in the pathogenesis of periodontal disease may be the same as that of plaque, with the addition of the physical effects of a rough, hard substance acting as a foreign body in contact with soft tissues. There is no evidence that calculus causes physical irritation when the teeth move during mastication or toothbrushing. It seems probable that large deposits of subgingival calculus could interfere with cell migration and crevicular fluid flow, but the concept has not been demonstrated scientifically.

There is no dentifrice with significant biologic preventative qualities. Commercial products are available that have been reported to be effective based on studies in which very slight but statistically significant differences were found between calculus index scores of individuals using the active dentifrice and individuals using a placebo dentifrice.

STAINS

Pellicle and plaque may be stained by food products, including tea and coffee, by tobacco tars, by the products of chromogenic bacteria, and by metallic particles. Such extrinsic staining may be prevented by good oral hygiene measures. Brown, black, green, and orange stains are seen frequently in children with poor oral hygiene, but the relationship or chromogenic bacteria has not been substantiated in many instances. Black stain or "metabolic" stain found adjacent to the free gingival margin may be difficult to eliminate because plaque may be scanty and rough surfaces may be present. Metallic salts may be an occupational hazard, and staining of the teeth may be extensive unless adequate home care procedures and frequent professional care are instituted. Stains on the teeth caused by tobacco tars may be brown to black, depending on oral hygiene and amount of smoking done. Tobacco tars and heat may cause chemical and thermal injury and exaggerate periodontal disease. The identification of the cause of a particular stain may be difficult, but most stains may be removed if not located in development grooves, porous areas, and cracks in the enamel. Such staining is common in heavy smokers. Intrinsic stains include those due to developmental disturbances, such as fluorosis and tetracycline staining. Extrinsic stains are not significant factors in the etiology of periodontal disease, but may be a significant esthetic problem for the patient.

LOCAL MODIFYING FACTORS

Local or extrinsic modifying and predisposing factors in the etiology of chronic inflammatory periodontal disease include malocclusion, food impaction, overhanging margins, rough surfaces of teeth and restorations, dental prosthesis, unilateral mastication, smoking, diet (soft, sucrose present), abnormal gin-

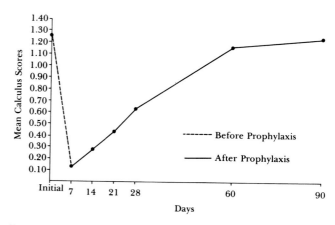

Fig. 8-6. Rate of calculus return after prophylaxis in 80 adult subjects. Scores are based on Ramfjord calculus index of 0 to 3.

gival-dental contours and relationships, and trauma from occlusion. These factors influence or modify inflammatory periodontal disease, usually by increasing the plaque on the tissues, but traumatic occlusion may act by altering the inflammatory response.

Malocclusion

The relationship between malocclusion and periodontal disease is secondary to initiating factors (those that directly cause injury); i.e., malocclusion may predispose to plaque accumulation because of related mouthbreathing, impinging overbite, crowding of the teeth, partially erupted or malposed teeth, and crossbite with unilateral mastication. A discrepancy between the size of the teeth and the bony support may predispose to periodontal disease and gingival recession, especially in the presence of dehiscence and fenestration.[4,42,88] However, facial malpositioning of teeth and dehiscence and fenestration are not accepted as initiating factors in periodontal disease.[5,127]

A number of parameters of malocclusion have been correlated with periodontal disease,[13,22,37] but a positive correlation between classes of malocclusion and periodontal disease has not been found.[25,26]

No correlation has been found between open bite and the severity of periodontal disease,[1] and conflicting results have been reported for the effect of crossbite on periodontal health.[37,77] Traumatic occlusion, trauma to the soft tissues from appliances, and oral hygiene problems may occur in the treatment of malocclusion and influence the status of the periodontium unfavorably.

Mouthbreathing

The role of mouthbreathing as an etiologic factor in periodontal disease has been confused by a number of conflicting reports.[46,55,68,114] The frequent association of mouthbreathing with malposed and crowded maxillary anterior teeth presents a problem in accurately differentiating the effects of mouthbreathing from those of crowding (Fig. 8-7). Although mouthbreathing may be associated with anterior open bite or failure to maintain a lip seal, drying of the anterior gingivae may not occur because of full coverage of the gingiva by the lips. Gingivitis may not be a significant problem in such instances when reasonable oral hygiene is maintained. Mouthbreathing may or may not be a significant predisposing factor, and each individual must be evaluated separately.[47] Infrequently, specific treatment for anatomical defects of allergy may be necessary to relieve nasal obstruction. In a few instances, orthodontic treatment may be indicated for periodontal treatment to be successful.

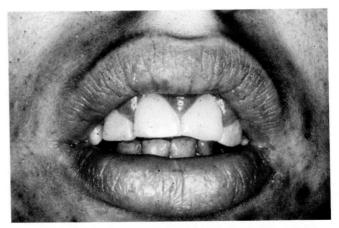

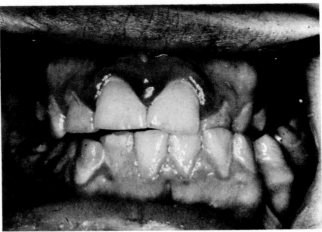

Fig. 8-7. Mouthbreathing with associated gingivitis.

Food Impaction

Injury to the gingiva may occur with "stepping" of marginal ridges; in the presence of inadequate interproximal contacts, related either to drifting of teeth or to faulty dental restorations; with contacts that are slightly open; and with malposed teeth or loss of centric stops, especially between anterior teeth. Food impaction may also be related to other "plunger cusp" effects. It may occur where mesial and distal cusp ridges make an acute angle so that food is forced into an embrasure and into the interproximal area.

Food impaction may result from faulty centric stops. For example, in a patient without third molars, the restoration of a maxillary first molar may be faulty because the distal lingual cusp does not make contact with the mesial marginal ridge of the mandibular second molar. Because of a lack of such contact, there is often a drifting distally of the second molar. This problem occurs especially if there is bruxism and no freedom for protrusive movement is provided for between the distal cusp ridge of the distal buccal cusp of the maxillary first molar and the mesial cusp ridge of the mandibular second molar. In such instances, the initial complaint of the patient may be food impaction at the lingual interproximal area between the first and second mandibular molars.

Food impaction may not occur invariably in what appear to be defective interproximal contacts and marginal ridge relationships.[59,84] When present, food impaction is a symptom of a problem that requires a proper diagnosis and definitive treatment; symptomatic treatment with dental floss and other periodontal home care aids are not sufficient.

Dental Morphological Factors

Two anatomical factors relating to tooth morphology have been considered as predisposing factors in periodontal disease: (1) radicular extension of the enamel into furcation areas; and (2) an anomaly of the maxillary lateral incisors and occasionally the central incisors. The presence of a distopalatal or palatal groove has been suggested to predispose the plaque accumulation and formation of narrow periodontal pockets.[21,62] This groove is sometimes mistaken for a root fracture when the patient has vague complaints.

A normal morphological feature that is a consistent problem in periodontal instrumentation is the presence of the deep mesial fossa just apical to the interproximal contact area and marginal ridge on maxillary first premolars. Plaque and calculus in this area are frequently missed during instrumentation, and flossing in the area is often ineffective.

A number of studies have considered the extension of enamel into the furcation area,[120] but there are conflicting reports on the significance of the projections as predisposing factors in periodontal disease.[2] Their status as contributory etiological agents has not been determined.[88]

Soft Tissue Factors

The anatomical factors of the gingiva that have been considered to be predisposing causes include inadequate width of attached gingiva, inadequate vestibular depth, frenular attachments, and retromolar and palatogingival protuberances.

It has been found that there is a persistent flow of crevicular fluid, and thus some inflammation present, when there is less than 2 mm of keratinized gingiva (with 1 mm of attached gingiva), even with plaque-free surfaces.[57] However, there is evidence that such mucogingival features are not frequently a problem unless there is clinical evidence that plaque cannot be controlled.[76]

The presence of frenula and muscle attachments has not been proved to pull the free gingival margin from the tooth,[90] and thus to lead to plaque accumulation and pocket formation. However, such anatomical features have been linked to periodontal problems due to displacement.[35] A frenulum should be considered to be a significant factor only when interference with plaque control occurs and periodontal problems persist.

The idea that vestibular depth is important as an etiologic factor in periodontal disease has not been supported,[7] and even shallow vestibular fornices are compatible with gingival health.[125] In some instances, vestibular depth might be related to a frenulum or muscle attachment and the width of the attached gingiva. However, attempting surgically to deepen the vestibular depth only because it appears too shallow for adequate oral hygiene apparently has little justification.

Restorative Dentistry

The relationship between restorations and inflammatory periodontal disease may be due to the problems existing from cervical carious lesions, from trauma at the time of preparing the teeth to receive the restorations, and/or from faulty contours, margins, and occlusal relations of the restorations. The periodontal aspects of restorative dentistry are discussed in chapter 27, and the occlusal aspects in chapter 10. A comprehensive consideration of restorative dentistry and periodontics has also been discussed elsewhere.[91]

Carious lesions may extend beyond the level of attachment and require that the preparation involve some loss of attachment. A lack of careful instrumentation may also cause a loss of attachment, but this form of injury may be reversible, provided that the margins of the restorations are well adapted to the marginal outline of cavity or crown preparations.[115]

The form of restorations, especially where margins end on root surfaces or close to the level of attachment, is seldom precisely the form which was present prior to loss of the tooth structure. Thus, the position of the margins and crown contours on the facial, lingual, and approximal surfaces has been the subject of a number of studies. It has been found that excessive axial crown contours tend to enhance plaque accumulation and gingival inflammation.[41,81,89,97,129]

There is no acceptable evidence that buccal and lingual contours have to be "adjusted" or given extra "deflective" contour to prevent food from being driven into the sulcus.[6,129] Because of greater plaque accumulation, too much contour appears to be more detrimental to periodontal health than lack of contour.

The relationship between marginal adaptation of restorations and periodontal health has been studied extensively and a positive relationship between the severity of periodontal disease and faulty margins has been reported.[9,10,119] It is assumed that the faulty margins act as sites for the retention of bacterial plaque, and thus cause the increase in inflammatory response rather than being simply mechanical irritation.

The location of the margins of restorations has been studied in relation to placement at the base of the crevice,[113] between the base and the free gingival margin,[41,48,79,121] at the free gingival margin,[74] and occlusally or incisally to the free gingival margin. In general, subgingival placement of margins is more detrimental to periodontal health than placement in a supragingival position,[51] but not always. The retention of plaque as related to roughness of the margin, exposure of cement, and trauma during tooth preparation is a factor in the problem of marginal placement and periodontal health. When possible, restorations should be delayed until the hygiene phase has been established so that the margins of the restorations can be placed correctly in relation to the free gingival margin. The indications for subgingival placement of the margins of restorations are discussed in chapter 27.

The type of restorative material appears to have little bearing on gingival inflammation, provided that the removal of plaque is adequate.[58,110,123,124] However, restorative materials differ in porosity, roughness, and retentive potential for plaque,[61,128] and some, such as glazed porcelain,[50] may present less of a problem than other materials. Provisional restorations that are poorly fitting and porous can do permanent damage.[16]

SUMMARY

The etiology of periodontal disease may be considered on the basis of *initiating* and *modifying* factors,[54] and both groups may be further divided into factors of *extrinsic* and *intrinsic* origin, although there are no known intrinsic initiating factors. Systemic modifying factors are discussed in chapter 9.

Extrinsic initiating factors in chronic inflammatory periodontal disease principally include dental plaque and its microbial flora, which cause the largest proportion of all periodontal diseases. Inflammatory periodontal disease does not occur in the absence of injurious (initiating extrinsic) local factors, but, once initiated, may be modified by certain intrinsic factors.

Dental plaque is an accumulation of bacteria, bacterial products, salivary proteins, and lectins from ingested foods. However, such an accumulation is not an amorphous mass, but rather a highly organized bacterial ecologic unit that differs in composition among sites and individuals.

Bacterial plaque begins with the adherence specifically of various indigenous oral microbes to selected dental surfaces, some via a thin film (pellicle) that soon covers a tooth after cleaning. Also, plaque grows by specific interbacterial adherence by coaggregation of one bacterium with another. Further colonization and growth occurs by concurrent processes of cell multiplication and attachment of new organisms. There is a shift from predominantly gram-positive coccal forms to a complex population including filamentous organisms, gram-negative cocci, vibrios and spirochetes. Closely associated with the development of gingivitis, the development of plaque mass and composition is modified by abrasive and washing forces, including toothbrushing.

Calculus may be considered to be mineralized or calcified plaque. It is almost always covered by plaque. The role of calculus in the etiology of periodontal diseases has been considered to be similar to that of dental plaque. It has been suggested that the role of calculus in the pathogenesis of periodontal disease may have been exaggerated in the past. However, if calculus is considered to be calcified plaque, its prevention and removal are as important as that of plaque.

A number of predisposing factors contribute to the retention of plaque or cause direct injury to the tissues, as in food impaction. Mouthbreathing and dental trauma may also be considered as initiating factors. The most significant predisposing or local modifying factors are those that cannot be controlled by specific measures in an oral hygiene program; included are faulty margins of restorations, destruction of attachment during cavity preparation, and food impaction.

REFERENCES

1. Alexander, A.G. Habitual mouth breathing and its effect on gingival health, Parodontologie 24:49, 1970.
2. Andrews, N.H. Periodontal significance of cervical enamel projections, J. Can. Dent. Assoc. 41:50, 1975.
3. Armstrong, W.G. Origin and nature of the acquired pellicle, P. Roy. S. Med. 61:923, 1968.
4. Batenhorst, K., et al. Tissue changes resulting from facial tipping and extrusion of incisors in monkeys, J. Periodont. 45:660, 1974.
5. Beagrie, G., et al. Tooth position and anterior bone loss in skulls, Br. Dent. J. 129:471, 1970.
6. Becker, C.M. and Kaldahl, W.B. Current theories of crown contour, margin placement and pontic design, J. Prosthet. Dent. 45:268, 1981.
7. Bergenholtz, A., and Hugoson, A. Vestibular sulcus extension surgery in cases with periodontal disease, J. Periodont. Res. 2:221, 1967.
8. Bergenholtz, A., et al. Den plaqueavlägsnande förmägen hos nägre mundhygieniska hjälpmedel, Sven. Tandläk. Tidskr. 60:447, 1967.
9. Björn, A.L., et al. Marginal fit of restorations and its relation to periodontal disease, J. Periodont. 43:415, 1972.
10. Björn, A.L., et al. Marginal fit of restorations and its relation to periodontal bone level. Part II. Crowns, Odont. Revy 21:337, 1970.
11. Black, G.V. Dr. Black's conclusions reviewed again, Dent. Cosmos 40:440, 1898.
12. Bowen, W.H. Nature of plaque, Oral Sci. Rev. 9:3, 1975.
13. Buckley, L. The relationship between malocclusion and periodontal disease, J. Periodont. 43:415, 1972.
14. Carlsson, J., and Egelberg, J. Effect of diet on early plaque formation in man, Odont. Rev. 16:112, 1965.
15. Dawes, C., Jenkins, G.N., and Tonge, C.H. The nomenclature of the integuments of the enamel surface of teeth, Br. Dent. J. 115:65, 1963.

16. Donaldson, D. Gingival recession associated with temporary crowns, J. Periodontol. 44:691, 1973.
17. Driessens, F.C.M., et al. On the physiochemistry of plaque calcification and the phase composition of dental calculus, J. Periodont. Res. 20:329, 1985.
18. Egelberg, J. Local effect of diet on plaque formation and development of gingivitis in dogs. I. Effects of hard and soft diets, Odont. Rev. 16:31, 1965.
19. Ellison, S.A. Oral bacteria and periodontal disease, J. Dent. Res. (Suppl. 2) 49:198, 1970.
20. Ericson, T. Adsorption to hydroxyapatite of proteins and conjugated proteins from human saliva, Caries Res. 1:52, 1967.
21. Everett, F., and Kramer, G. The disto-lingual groove in the maxillary lateral incisor: A periodontal hazard, J. Periodont. 43:352, 1972.
22. Fehr, F.R. von Der, and Brudevold, F. In vitro calculus formation, J. Dent. Res. 39:1041, 1960.
23. Folke, L.E.A., et al. Effect of dietary sucrose on quantity of plaque, Scand. J. Dent. Res. 80:529, 1972.
24. Fry, A.J., and Grenby, T.H. The effects of reduced sucrose intake on the formation and composition of dental plaque. A group of men in the Antarctic, Arch. Oral Biol. 17:873, 1972.
25. Geiger, A., et al. Relationship of occlusion and periodontal disease. Part VIII. Relationship of crowding and spacing to periodontal destruction and gingival inflammation, J. Periodont. 45:43, 1974.
26. Geiger, A., et al. Relationship of occlusion and periodontal disease. Part V. Relation of classification of occlusion to periodontal status and gingival inflammation, J. Periodont. 43:330, 1974.
27. Genco, R.J., et al. 1985 Kreshover Lecture: Molecular factors influencing neutrophil defects in periodontal disease, J. Dent. Res. 65:1379, 1986.
28. Genco, R.J., et al. Antibody mediated effects of periodontium, J. Periodont. 45:330, 1974.
29. Genco, R.J., Evans, R.T., Ellison, S.A. Dental research in microbiology with emphasis on periodontal disease, J.A.D.A. 78:1016, 1969.
30. Gibbons, R.J. Adherent interactions which may affect microbial ecology in the mouth, J. Dent. Res. 63:378, 1984.
31. Gibbons, R.J. Adhesions of bacteria to the surface of the mouth. In Microbial Adhesion to Surfaces, ed. R.C.W. Berkeley et al. Society of Chemical Industry, London, Chichester: Ellis Horwood, Ltd., 1980.
32. Gibbons, R.J., and van Joute, J. On the formation of dental plaque, J. Periodont. 44:347, 1973.
33. Gibbons, R.J., and Nygaard, M. Interbacterial aggregation of plaque bacteria, Arch. Oral Biol. 15:1397, 1970.
34. Gilmore, N., and Sheiham, A. Overhanging dental restorations and periodontal disease, J. Periodont. 42:8, 1971.
35. Glickman, I. Clinical Periodontology, 4th ed. Philadelphia: W.B. Saunders Co., 1972.
36. Gonzales, F., and Sognnaes, R.F. Electron microscopy of dental calculus, Science 131:156, 1960.
37. Gould, M., and Picton, D. The relation between irregularities of teeth and periodontal disease, Br. Dent. J. 121:20, 1966.
38. Guggenheim, B. Extracellular polysaccharides and microbial plaque, Int. Dent. J. 20:257, 1960.
39. Gustafsson, B.E., and Krasse, B. Dental calculus in germ free rats, Acta Odont. Scand. 20:134, 1962.
40. Hay, D.I., et al. The adsorption of salivary proteins by hydroxyapatite and enamel, Arch. Oral Biol. 12:937, 1967.
41. Herlanda, R.E., et al. Forms, contours and extensions of full coverage in occlusal reconstruction, Dent. Clin. North Am. Vol. 147, March 1962.
42. Hirschfeld, I. A study of skulls in the American Museum of Natural History, J. Dent. Res. 4:241, 1923.
43. Horton, J.E., et al. A role for cell-mediated immunity in the pathogenesis of periodontal disease, J. Periodont. 45:351, 1974.
44. Howitt, B.F., et al. A study on the effects upon the hygiene and microbiology of the mouth of various diets without and with the use of the toothbrush, Dent. Cosmos 70:757, 1928.
45. Jacobson, L. Mouthbreathing and gingivitis, J. Periodont. Res. 8:269, 1973.
46. Jacobson, L., and Linder-Aronson, S. Crowding and gingivitis: A comparison between mouthbreathers and nonmouthbreathers, Scand. J. Dent. Res. 80:500, 1972.
47. James, W., and Hastings, S. Discussion of mouthbreathing and nasal obstruction, P. Roy. S. Med. 25:1343, 1932.
48. Johnson, J.F., et al. Modern Practice in Crown and Bridge Prosthodontics, 3rd ed. Philadelphia: W.B. Saunders Co., 1971.
49. Kani, T., et al. Microbeam X-ray diffraction analysis of dental calculus, J. Dent. Res. 62:92, 1983.
50. Kaqueler, J.C., and Weiss, M.B. Plaque accumulation on dental restorative materials, I.A.D.R. Abstract No. 615, March 1970.
51. Karlsen, K. Gingival reactions to dental restorations, Acta Odont. Scand. 28:895, 1970.
52. Keenan, M.P., et al. Effects of cast gold surface finishing on plaque retention, J. Prosthet. Dent. 43:168, 1980.
53. Kelstrup, J., et al. Bacteriological, electron microscopical, and biochemical studies on dento-gingival plaque of Moroccan children from an area with low caries prevalence, Caries Res. 8:61, 1974.
54. Kerr, D.A., and Ash, M.M. Oral Pathology. Philadelphia: Lea and Febiger, 1971.
55. Kleinberg, I., et al. Effect of air drying on rodent oral mucous membrane. A histologic study of simulated mouthbreathing, J. Periodont. 32:38, 1961.
56. Kraus, F.W., et al. The acquired pellicle: Variability and subject-dependence of specific proteins, J. Oral Pathol. 2:165, 1973.
57. Lang, M., and Löe, H. The relationship between the width of keratinized gingiva and gingival health, J. Periodont. 43:623, 1972.
58. Larato, D.C. Influence of silicate cement restorations on gingiva, J. Prosthet. Dent. 26:186, 1971.
59. Larato, D.C. Relationship of food impaction to intrabony lesions, J. Periodont. 42:237, 1971.
60. Larato, D. Alveolar plate fenestrations and dehiscences of the human skull, Oral Surg. 29:816, 1970.
61. Laurell, L., et al. The effect of different levels of polishing amalgam restorations on plaque retention and gingival inflammation, Swed. Dent. J. 7:45, 1983.
62. Lee, K., et al. Palato-gingival grooves in maxillary incisors, Br. Dent. J. 124:14, 1968.
63. Leach, S.A. The acquired integuments of the teeth, Br. Dent. J. 122:537, 1967.
64. Lindhe, J., and Wicén, P.O.. The effects on the gingivae of chewing fibrous foods, J. Periodont. Res. 4:193, 1969.
65. Lindhe, J., and Koch, G. The effect of supervised oral hygiene on the gingiva of children. Lack of prolonged effect of supervision, J. Periodont. Res. 2:215, 1967.
66. Listgarten, M.A. Structure of the microbial flora associated with periodontal disease and health in man. A light and electron microscope study, J. Periodont. 49:1, 1976.
67. Listgarten, M.A. Pathogenesis of periodontitis, J. Clin. Periodontol. 13:418, 1986.
68. Lite, T., et al. Gingival pathosis in mouthbreathers, Oral Surg. 8:382, 1955.
69. Löe, H., et al. Two years oral use of chlorhexidine in man.

I. General design and clinical effects, J. Periodont. Res. 11:135, 1976.

70. Löe, H., and Schiott, C.R. The effect of mouth rinses and topical applications of chlorhexidine on the development of dental plaque and gingivitis in man, J. Periodont. Res. 5:79, 1970.

71. Löe, H. A review of the prevention and control of plaque. In Dental Plaque, ed. W.D. McHugh. Edinburgh: E. & S. Livingstone, 1970.

72. Löe, H., Theilade, E. and Jensen, S.B. Experimental gingivitis in man, J. Periodont. 36:177, 1965.

73. Manly, R.S. A structureless recurrent deposit on teeth, J. Dent. Res. 22:479, 1943.

74. Marcum, J.S. The effect of crown margin depth on gingival tissues, J. Prosthet. Dent. 17:479, 1967.

75. Mayhall, C.W. Concerning the composition and source of the acquired enamel pellicle of human teeth, Arch. Oral Biol. 15:1327, 1970.

76. Maynard, J., Jr., and Oshsenbein, C. Mucogingival problems: prevalence and therapy in children, J. Periodont. 46:543, 1975.

77. McCombie, F., and Stothard, D. Relationship between gingivitis and other dental conditions, J. Can. Dent. Assoc. 30;506, 1964.

78. Meckel, A.H. The nature and importance of organic deposits on dental enamel, Caries Res. 2:104, 1967.

79. Minker, J.S. Simplified full coverage preparations, Dent. Clin. N. Amer. 9:355, 1965.

80. Moore, W.E.C., et al. Bacteriology of experimental gingivitis in young adult humans, Infect. Immun. 38:651, 1982.

81. Morris, M.L. Artificial crown contours and gingival health, J. Prosthet. Dent. 12:1142, 1962.

82. Nisengard, R.T. The role of immunology in periodontal disease, J. Periodont. 48:505, 1977.

83. Nisengard, R. Immediate hypersensitivity and periodontal disease, J. Periodont. 45:343, 1974.

84. O'Leary, T., et al. Interproximal contact and marginal ridge relationships in periodontally healthy young males classified as to orthodontic status, J. Periodont. 46:6, 1975.

85. Osuoji, C.I., and Rowles, S.L. Studies on the organic composition of dental calculus and related calculi, Calcif. Tissue Res. 16:193, 1974.

86. Page, R.C. Gingivitis, J. Clin. Periodontol. 13:345, 1986.

87. Paunio, K. The role of malocclusion and crowding in the development of periodontal disease, Int. Dent. J. 23:420, 1973.

88. Pennel, B.M., and Keagle, J.G. Predisposing factors in the etiology of chronic inflammatory periodontal disease, J. Periodont. 48:517, 1977.

89. Perel, M.L. Axial crown contours, J. Prosthet. Dent. 25:642, 1971.

90. Palcek, M., et al. Significance of the labial frenum attachment in periodontal disease in man. Part I. Classification and epidemiology of the labial frenum attachment, J. Periodont. 45:891, 1974.

91. Ramfjord, S.P. Periodontal aspects of operative and restorative dentistry. In Principles and Practice of Operative Dentistry, ed. G.T. Charbeneau, Philadelphia: Lea and Febiger, 1975.

92. Richter, W.A., and Veno, H. Relationship of crown margin placement to gingival inflammation, J. Prosthet. Dent. 30:157, 1973.

93. Risnes, S. The prevalence and distribution of cervical enamel projections reaching into the bifurcation on human molars, Scand. J. Dent. Res. 87:413, 1974.

94. Rizzo, A.A., et al. Calcification of oral bacteria, Ann. N.Y. Acad. Sci. 109:14, 1963.

95. Rizzo, A.A., et al. Mineralization of bacteria, Science 135:439, 1962.

96. Ruzicka, F. Structure of sub-and supragingival dental calculus in human periodontitis, J. Periodont. Res. 19:317, 1984.

97. Sackett, B.P., and Gildenhuys, R.R. The effect of axial crown over-contour on adolescents, J. Periodont. 47:320, 1976.

98. Saxton, C.A. Scanning electron microscope study of formation of dental plaque, Caries Res. 7:102, 1973.

99. Schamschula, R.G., and Barnes, D.E. The Lactobacillus flora of saliva and plaque in primitive peoples in Papua, New Guinea, Aust. Dent. J. 15:28, 1970.

100. Scheinin, A., and Makinen, K.K. The effect of various sugars on the formation and chemical composition of dental plaque, Int. Dent. J. 21:302, 1971.

101. Schroeder, J.E. Formation and Inhibition of Dental Calculus, Berne: Hans Huber, 1969.

102. Schroeder, H.E. Discussion: Pathogenesis of periodontitis, J. Periodont. Res. 13:426, 1986.

103. Seymour, G.J. and Greenspan, J.S. The phenotypic characterization of lymphocyte subpopulations in established human periodontitis, J. Periodont. Res. 14:39, 1979.

104. Slots, J. The predominant cultivable microflora of advanced periodontitis, Scand. J. Dent. Res. 85:114, 1977.

105. Smith, F.N., and Ramfjord, S.P. Hyaluronidase applied to the gingiva of rhesus monkeys, J. Periodont. 44:361, 1973.

106. Socransky, S.S. Microbiology of periodontal disease—present status and future considerations, J. Peridontol. 48:497, 1977.

107. Socransky, S.S., et al. New concepts of destructive periodontal disease, J. Clin. Periodontol. 11:21, 1984.

108. Socransky, S.S. The relationship of bacteria to the etiology of periodontal disease, J. Dent. Res. (Suppl. 2) 49:203, 1970.

109. Sönju, T., et al. Electron microscopy, carbohydrate analyses and biologic activities of the proteins absorbed in two hours to tooth surfaces in vivo, Caries Res. 8:113, 1974.

110. Sotres, L.S., et al. A histologic study of gingival tissue response to amalgam, silicate, and resin restorations, J. Periodont. 40:543, 1969.

111. Suomi, J.D., et al. The effect of controlled oral hygiene procedures on the progression of periodontal disease in adults: Results after third and final year, J. Periodont. 42:152, 1971.

112. Stallard, R.E., and Awwa, I.A. The effect of alterations in external environment on the dentogingival junction, J. Dent. Res. 48:671, 1960.

113. Stein, R.S., and Glickman, I. Prosthetic considerations essential for gingival health, Dent. Clin. North Am. 4:77, 1960.

114. Sutcliffe, P.L. Chronic anterior gingivitis—an epidemiological study in school children, Br. Dent. J. 125:47, 1960.

115. Taylor, A.C., and Campbell, M.M. Reattachment of gingival epithelium to the tooth, J. Periodontol. 43:281, 1972.

116. Theilade, E., and Theilade, J. Role of plaque in the etiology of periodontal disease and caries, Oral Sci. Rev. 9:23, 1976.

117. Theilade, E., et al. Experimental gingivitis in man. II. A longitudinal clinical and bacteriologic investigation, J. Periodont. Res. 1:1, 1966.

118. Theilade, J., and Schroeder, H.E. Recent results in dental calculus research, Int. Dent. J. 16:205, 1966.

119. Trott, J.R., and Sherkat, A. Effect of Class II amalgam restoratives on health of the gingiva: A clinical survey, J. Can. Dent. Assoc. 30:766, 1964.

120. Tsatsas, B, et al. Cervical enamel projections in the molar teeth, J. Periodont. 44:312, 1973.

121. Tylman, S.D. Theory and Practice of Crown and Fixed Partial Prothodontics, 6th ed. St. Louis: C.V. Mosby Co., 1970.

122. Vonesh, E.M, Correlation between extensive orthodontic treatment and periodontal disease. Thesis, The University of Michigan, 1968.

123. Waerhaug, J. Effect of rough surfaces upon gingival tissue, J. Dent. Res. 35:323, 1956.
124. Waerhaug, J., and Zander, H.A. Reaction of gingival tissues to self-curing acrylic restoratives, J.A.D.A. 66:513, 1963.
125. Ward, V. The depth of the vestibular fornix in the mandibular anterior region in health, J. Periodont. 47:651, 1976.
126. Wilcon, C.E., and Everett, F.G. Friction on the teeth and the gingiva during mastication, J.A.D.A. 66:513, 1963.
127. Wingard, C., and Bowers, G. The effects on facial bone from facial tipping of incisors in monkeys, J. Periodont. 47:450, 1976.
128. Wise, M.D., and Dykema, R.W. The plaque retaining capacity of four dental materials, J. Prosthet. Dent. 33;178, 1975.
129. Yuodelis, R.A., et al. Facial and lingual contours of artificial complete crown restorations and their effects on the periodontium, J. Prosthet. Dent. 29:61, 1973.
130. Zander, H.A., et al. Mineralization of dental plaque, Proc. Soc. Exp. Biol. (N.Y.) 103:257, 1960.

9

ETIOLOGY OF PERIODONTAL DISEASES—HOST DEFENSES AND SYSTEMIC FACTORS

The defenses of the host against injurious agents are made by an array of central and peripheral networks consisting of tissues, cells, and molecules or chemical mediators. Any inherent (genetic) or functional disturbance of these systems of defense may provide opportunities for microorganisms to cause injury to the host. Often the mechanisms underlying such disturbances have been unknown and simply described as those "systemic factors" that modify host defenses to bacterial dental plaque. The importance of systemic factors in modifying host defenses has been demonstrated in a number of diseases in which the number and/or functions of polymorphonuclear leukocytes (PMNs, neutrophils) have been decreased. However, the relationship between periodontitis and systemic diseases other than those involving neutrophil dysfunction is not always clear.

The defensive mechanisms involved in protection of the host, and expressed locally as inflammation, involve specific and nonspecific interactions between cells and molecules inside and outside the immune system. Bidirectional communication may modify many of the protective, reparative, and potentially destructive aspects of the host's defenses. Such communication rests with a number of molecules (e.g., lymphokines and cytokines) expressed in a variety of lymphoid tissues both constitutively and in response to different stimuli.

Rapid advances in molecular biology make it necessary to constantly update most concepts of host defenses, especially in relation to repair and immune defenses. An understanding of immune defenses is important for evaluating the etiology and pathogenesis of a rapidly progressive periodontitis associated with AIDS: AIDS-virus-associated periodontitis AVAP).[226] It is probable that the causative factor relates in some way to the deficient immune system.

Concepts to explain variations in severity of peri-odontal disease by modification of the host's defenses have often been nonspecific. However, the evidence is rapidly accumulating to implicate specific mechanisms by which host responses could be modified, especially as related to neutrophil function and/or modulation of activities of the cells of the periodontium by soluble mediators released by immune cells.

The ways in which the defenses of the host are viewed in relation to destruction in periodontitis may be based upon several seemingly unrelated concepts. In general, such concepts tend to specify which host defenses are primarily involved in the protective and destructive aspects of periodontitis.

ETIOLOGIC FACTORS AND HOST DEFENSES

Concepts of the development of chronic inflammatory periodontal disease and destruction of supporting structures emphasize that bacteria cause damage (1) *directly*, through the release of toxins, enzymes, and metabolic products, and (2) *indirectly*, by triggering host-mediated mechanisms that activate complement and mediators of inflammation, suppress the immune system, and induce dysfunction of defensive cells, including immune and nonimmune cells. This paradigm has several variations regarding microbial pathogenesis, etiologic factors, and how damage occurs.

Variations in ideas about etiologic factors and host defenses relate to several areas of uncertainty: (1) whether microbial etiology is specific[189] or nonspecific;[210] (2) whether bacterial metabolic products, such as toxins and enzymes (some of which appear to be able to permeate sulcular and junctional epithelium to reach subepithelial tissues), alone cause the kind of tissue damage seen in chronic destructive periodontal disease, *or* whether such products, because they are often antigenic, may also indirectly cause damage by evoking potentially destructive immune responses;[33,72,80,120,121,122,138] (3) whether the damage to the tissues results inadvertently from protective immune responses evoked by the dental plaque products (directly by several types of immune cells and/or indirectly by modulation of the activity of the supporting tissues by soluble mediators released by the host's immune cells),[43] or whether the damage results primarily from the action of defensive cells (such as neutrophils) dedicated to the prevention of bacterial invasion even at the expense of the host;[54] (4) whether bacterial invasion does[3,52,168,169,172] or does not[108,170] occur; (5) whether factors other than bacteria and/or defective or over-reactive host defenses are of etiologic significance; In other words, whether there are inherent and/or acquired molecular defects in cells other than those involved in innate and acquired immunity, including progenitor cells of the periodontal membrane (periodontosis?),[221] alveolar bone (negative bone factor?),[59] and cementum (cementopathia?);[147] and (6) whether systemic disease,[17,31,75,117] nutritional states,[2,71,100] or general metabolic disturbances[40,153] are of significance in the modification of chronic inflammatory periodontal disease.

The conclusion that host defenses against injurious agents may be potentially damaging as well as beneficial comes from observations that defensive mechanisms used to inhibit or destroy bacteria or their products may inadvertently cause damage to the host's own tissues. Differentiating the damage caused by the infectious agent from that attributed to the defense mechanism may be difficult, if not impossible. The view that the host's protective mechanisms are dedicated to the prevention of bacterial invasion even at the expense of destroying the periodontium[54] should be kept in proper perspective.

The controversy over the specific[189] and non-specific[210] microbial etiology of periodontal diseases has a bearing on determining how the host responds to an infectious agent. If a single pathogenic species is the cause of inflammatory periodontal disease, as is the case in an infectious disease such as tuberculosis, then the pathogenesis of the infection, the histopathologic mechanisms, the correlation between the presence of the bacteria and disease activity, and the response of the host might be more specific. But suspected periodontal pathogens (spirochetes, streptococci, actinomyces, gram-negative, anaerobic rods of the *Bacteroides melanogenious* group, including such species as *B. melanogenious*, *B. gingivalis*, and *B. intermedius*, and facultatively, anaerobic, gram-negative rods of the genera *Capnocytophaga*, *Eikenella*, and *Actinobacillus*) are all members of the normal oral flora.[210] As suggested by Theilade,[210] several organisms fulfill some of the criteria set up by Socransky for determination of a periodontal pathogen,[192] including altered immune response, possession

of virulence factors, and animal pathogenicity. Accordingly, the elimination of the suspected species without otherwise changing the plaque should cure the disease, although this may not be possible when dealing with indigenous bacteria.

The non-specific microbial theory suggests that the amount of plaque may reach a point at which the combined virulence of the bacteria present causes disease. Some of the virulence factors responsible for periodontal destruction are present in all the organisms. Differences of opinion exist regarding the composition of plaque. Some suggest that the plaque will cause disease regardless of its composition, while other opinions suggest that the virulence of several species may be enhanced when host resistance is decreased, but that no one organism is responsible for the disease. Local and systemic differences in host resistance, rather than differences in microflora, may explain variations among sites in the same individual and among individuals in relation to the severity of disease. Thus, different combinations of subgingival organisms have various virulence factors that promote colonization of pockets, inhibit or destroy host defenses, and initiate inflammation. In this respect, different combinations of indigenous bacteria have enough potential to cause the gingivitis-periodontitis progression of disease in the periodontium.

The presence of bacteria within gingival tissues has been a matter of controversy off and on for years. Special interest in the junctional, pocket and sulcular epithelium as portals of entry for microorganisms has continued to lead researchers to postulate the existence of bacteria in diseased gingival tissues. However, the evidence is weak and bacterial invasion is enormously difficult to verify.[179]

The subgingival bacterial colonization involved in the etiology of periodontitis begins first with supragingival plaque and an associated gingivitis. The extension of supragingival plaque apically is accompanied mainly by gram-negative rods and spirochetes, and perhaps by loss of hemidesmosomes between junctional epithelium and the tooth structure. The reasons for apical movement of the bacteria and the ability to evade host defenses are still not determined. The virulence factors that have been suggested to contribute to the pathogenesis include ability to adhere to and colonize the tooth surface; factors causing inflammation and tissue destruction; an ability to evade or prevent effective host mechanisms; and a susceptible host.[188] The question of invasion of subgingival tissues remains to be settled.

The foregoing factors suggest that the host/pathogen relationship in inflammatory periodontal disease reflects a breakdown of symbiosis between host and indigenous microbes, apparently at different sites and times in the same individual. In addition, it seems that inflammatory periodontal diseases are caused primarily by bacterial products in gingival pockets. If any bacteria are capable of invading the subgingival tissues and evading host defenses, they must be the same bacteria found predominating in pockets. Bacteria found in tissues have not been found to actively invade, survive and multiply there.[108,210] In any case, the defensive mechanisms of the host must effectively localize bacteria and bacterial products before or during the early invasive processes.

HOST DEFENSES

The defensive responses of the host to bacteria, their metabolic products, and antigens involve mechanisms ranging from the structural and functional barrier of the dentogingival junction to complex inflammatory and immune reactions. Obviously, these responses may operate in sequence, in unison, or in combination to eliminate or neutralize agents potentially capable of causing disease.

A number of disturbances may result in defective defense mechanisms, and bacteria may be able to respond to and overcome the host's defenses. The majority of protective mechanisms are positive, although, in a few instances, regulation may be defective or the defensive response simply nonbeneficial at a certain site and time in a particular host.

MECHANISMS OF DEFENSE

The defenses of the host involve both nonspecific and specific immunity, including (1) the structural and functional barrier of the gingiva and dentogingival junction; (2) inflammation—vascular and nonspecific cellular responses; (3) specific humoral and cellular responses; and (4) healing—repair and regeneration. Both inflammatory mechanisms and immune responses are active at the plaque-gingival interface. One of the prime functions of the immune response is to activate the inflammatory response. Complex linkages between the two kinds of responses exist.

Nonspecific immunity includes innate defensive mechanisms such as the intact skin and mucosa, soluble factors on the surface of the mucosa or in the gingival sulcus that interfere with bacterial adherence or colonization, and phagocytes and natural killer cells. Specific or adaptive immunity includes cellular (lymphocytes) and humoral (antibody) immune responses, as well as some of the phagocytic functions.

Structural and Functional Barriers

A major area of concern regarding the defense of the periodontium against bacteria and their products is the dentogingival attachment. The dentogingival junction and gingiva both act as physical and functional barriers to the entry of foreign agents into the sub-

epithelial tissues. The continuity of the dentogingival junction and gingiva is highly effective in preventing bacterial invasion, but, without the functional aspects of these tissues, it is unlikely that the physical barrier alone would be sufficient to prevent infection.

Functional barriers that involve the saliva and crevicular fluid, and act in concert with the functional aspects of the structural continuity barrier, include transmigrating neutrophils, the rapid turnover of junctional epithelium, the flushing action of crevicular fluid, neutrophils in the crevicular fluid, the constant sloughing of keratinized gingival and junctional epithelial cells, and the secretory-immune system. These mechanisms are generally effective in preventing entry of microorganisms and their metabolites into the subepithelial connective tissues. If bacteria cross the barrier, as with transient bacteremia, the microbes are eliminated locally or from the blood stream without injury, unless the homeostatic host/microbe balance is upset.

Another of the mechanisms operating against bacterial invasion by the various bacterial species that make up the usual microflora of plaque is the facilitation of competition between bacteria and the inhibition of growth of new invaders by the metabolic products of resident flora. For example, gram-negative rods and spirochetes are not able to form plaque without gram-positive species to help them.[187] The mechanisms by which the integrity of the dentogingival junction is broken down by local factors are not clear, nor is it clear under what circumstances a putative "opportunity" is created by which certain bacteria can cause chronic destructive periodontal disease. The presence of supportive nutrients, such as hemin, proteins and fatty acids, in the gingival exudate in relation to inflammation may provide an advantage for periodontopathic bacteria. Thus, "opportunistic" infections could occur because of a breakdown in local self-regulating microbial population control (amount and composition of plaque), especially with diseases involving ontogenetic or acquired defects in the number and/or function of cells (such as neutrophils) involved in defense.

The nature of the junction between soft and hard tissues, and of the relationships between those tissues, is unique in the body. The possibility of regeneration and repair is limited except under a few circumstances; significant reattachment of periodontal fibers into diseased root surfaces is not a common sequence in the natural history of chronic destructive periodontal disease. In the reparative phase of inflammation, the healing of highly specialized tissues may not be ideal because of fibrosis and scar formation with loss of some function. Such changes may compromise a site such as the dentogingival junction and make it more susceptible to further injury. Root surface changes and apically directed growth of epithelium make normal repair and regeneration difficult or impossible.

In addition to the epithelial barrier itself, host defenses of the gingival sulcus and pocket include antibacterial action of phagocytes, secretory and gingival fluid immunoglobulins, and other antimicrobial substances in the gingival exudate, such as lysozyme and complement. Because of mechanisms that impair the host's defenses, these mechanisms are not always successful.[188,204] Some bacteria produce proteolytic and glycosaminoglycan-hydrolyzing enzymes that degrade the epithelial barrier and allow toxic and antigenic substances to reach the subepithelial tissues and provoke inflammation and damage to the tissues.[188]

Inflammation

Inflammation is a local reaction of tissues to injury. Injury most commonly consists of bacterial infection with demonstrable tissue damage. Without the inflammatory response, microbes could enter the tissues after breaching the integrity of the skin, mucosa, or dentogingival junction and become established sufficiently to cause further damage (injury). Thus, without the reparative aspects of inflammation and regeneration, the continuity of the dentogingival junction cannot be maintained. That repair and regeneration are limited in restoring an efficient microbial barrier at the dentogingival junction may account for the apparent episodic, site-specific variation in chronic destructive periodontal disease.[60,191] The significance of repair has been reflected in attempts to guide regeneration for the restitution of lost attachment.[46,62,141,143,154,195] Very little information is available about the healing phase of periodontal diseases.[53]

The normal host defense mechanisms eliminate microbes without allowing meaningful damage to the host. Actual invasion by bacteria, as is reflected by proliferation and dissemination of morphologically homogenous populations, has not been demonstrated,[108] except in acute necrotizing ulcerative gingivitis and perhaps in some severe forms of periodontitis.[3,52,169] Conclusive evidence for bacterial invasion in adult periodontitis has yet to be presented. However, a number of potentially injurious mediators of inflammation produced by bacteria have been implicated as etiological factors in periodontal disease (Table 9-1).

Response to injury is a much more complex subject than the definition of inflammation. It is a complex and interrelated sequence of events involving vascular and cellular events, which include coagulation and enzyme systems that complement the response. In response to injury, white blood cells (polymorphonuclear leukocytes (PMNs)) and tissues produce chemical substances that mediate and control inflammatory as well as immune mechanisms. Endogenous mediators (Table 9-2) that effect the sequence of complex cellular and molecular interactions in inflammation include substances that cause increased vascular permeability, enhance clotting mechanisms, and influence the attraction of defensive cells to the site of injury. They also include the engulfing of foreign substances by the defensive cells, as well as the immune responses.

Vascular responses

The reactive changes in periodontal disease begin with the injury and the initial vascular response, in which there is increased permeability of the microcirculation (arterioles, capillaries, venules, veins). With increased vascular permeability, the constituents of the plasma, including blood serum, red cells, white cells and fibrin, cross the vessel walls. Biochemically active substances that may mediate these changes in vascular permeability are the vasoactive amines histamine and serotonin. Histamine is released from mast cells and serotonin from blood platelets. Prostaglandins (PGE_2) are also involved in increased vascular permeability. The mediators of vascular change also include kinins and plasma-protein fractions of complement. In addition to immune and nonimmune inflammatory responses, fibrinolytic, kinin, and clotting systems mediate inflammation and tissue damage and interact to maintain the vascular system and limit the spread of infection.

Components of Inflammatory and Immune Responses

The functions of the components of inflammatory and immune responses overlap and are not easily sep-

Table 9-1. Exogenous mediators of inflammation from bacterial sources

Organic acids:	e.g., lactic, formic
Cytotoxins:	e.g., NH_3, indole, amines, H_2S
Endotoxins:	Lipopolysaccharides
Enzymes:	e.g., proteases, collagenases

Table 9-2. Some endogenous mediators of inflammation

Category	Major mediators
Vasoactive amines	Histamine
	5-hydroxytryptamine
Lymphocyte products	Migration inhibitory factor (MIF)
	Mitogen factors
	Lymphotoxin
Lysosomal components	Cationic proteins
	Acid proteases
Acidic lipids	Prostaglandins
Complement	C3, C5 fragments C567 complex
Kinin system	Bradykinin
Clotting	Fibrinopeptides

arated. Some cells (e.g., phagocytes and certain of the lymphocytes) and soluble factors (e.g., complement, lysozyme, etc.) may not be involved in specific reactions to each particular infectious agent; however, some cells (e.g., T-lymphocytes) and products (e.g., antibodies) of B cells that are components of adaptive acquired immunity do respond specifically to each infectious agent and remember it so as to prevent reinfection at a later time. That nonspecific innate and specific adaptive immunity to microbial invasion are defensive mechanisms is an important consideration in understanding the overlapping of the nonspecific and specific microbial etiologic concepts of inflammatory periodontal diseases.

Cellular components. The cellular components of non-specific immunity against bacteria include (1) *phagocytes* (neutrophils, monocytes, and macrophages), which are considered a part of innate immunity; and (2) *lymphocytes* (T cells), which mediate specific adaptive immune responses. Also participating in the inflammatory response are mast cells, eosinophils and basophils. These cells contain a multilobed nucleus and primary and secondary granules. In some cells the granules stain red (eosin), others stain blue (basic), and others do not take up stain (neutral), hence the use of the names *eosinophil, basophil,* and *neutrophil* to describe these polymorphonuclear cells.

Neutrophils constitute 50 to 60% of total white cells and about 90% of the polymorphi. Polymorphonuclear leukocytes (PMNs, neutrophils) are attracted to the site of injurious agents by chemotactic factors and infectious agents. The neutrophils are principally phagocytic and their primary known role is the prevention of bacterial invasion by the localization and killing of bacteria.[157,161,165,199] Some of the granules in neutrophils contain lysozyme, others contain perioxidase and acid phosphatase, and still others contain alkaline phosphatase as well as other enzymes. Mixtures may occur. Most enzymes in granules are more involved with digestion of microbes that have already been killed than in actual killing. Killing of bacteria in neutrophils occurs principally either as a result of oxidants (O_2-dependent killing) or as a consequence of cationic proteins (O_2-independent killing).[50]

Eosinophils generally constitute no more than 3 to 5% of the leukocytes in normal, non-allergic individuals. Although eosinophils may function as phagocytes, their primary function appears to be related to immunity to helminth infections.[23]

Basophils reflect less than 0.2% of the leukocytes. The basophil and mast cells contain vasoactive amines. The granules of mast cells contain serotonin (5-HT), heparin, histamine, and proteases.[23,164] Basophils and mast cells may be indistinguishable from one another in a number of their properties. Mast cells produce major arachidonic acid metabolites, leukotrienes, and prostaglandin.[21]

Mast cell activation may be produced by injury or immunologic stimuli such as antigens, which lead to the release of granule-associated mediators (histamine, heparin, proteolytic enzymes, chemotactic factors) into intercellular spaces. Also, plasma membrane changes allow phospholipase A_2 to cleave arachidonic acid from membrane phospholipids. The metabolism of arachidonic acid by the cyclo-oxygenase pathway results in the formation of prostaglandins and thromboxane, and other mediators (e.g., chemotactic factor) by the lipoxygenase pathway.[164] These preformed and newly formed mediators of the vascular responses may also induce the cellular infiltrate, including neutrophils and mononuclear cells.

Monocyte/macrophages. Monocytes represent a pool of circulating white blood cells that migrate to organs and tissues to become macrophages. A network of these phagocytic tissue macrophages is found in central lymphoid tissues (thymus and bone marrow), and in peripheral lymphoid tissues such as the spleen, tonsils, liver, lymph nodes, and gastrointestinal tract (e.g., Peyer's patches). The primary function of these cells includes the removal of particulate matter (antigen, bacterium) by phagocytosis, and the presentation of antigen (e.g., bacteria and their products) to antigen-sensitive lymphocytes. This network of antigen-presenting cells (APC) will be considered in relation to the immune response.

Lymphocytes. There are at least two kinds of lymphocytes, both of which arise from primary lymphoid tissue: T cells, which differentiate initially in the thymus, and B cells, which differentiate in bone marrow (Fig. 9-1). They serve different functions. Another population of non-T, non-B cells *(null cells)* differentiate along unknown lines. The lymphocytes become committed in the primary lymphatic organs to behaving as B cells or particular types of T cells, and to reacting with specific antigens. During their development, these cells acquire specific antigen receptors that commit them to antigenic specificity (In other words, to recognizing only one or two antigens). These committed lymphocytes enter the circulation and enter secondary or peripheral lymphoid tissues (spleen, lymph nodes, and diffusely in other tissues), where they encounter antigens and complete their differentiation into mature forms, including regulator T cells and effector T and B cells. More specifically, these forms include T-helper cells (T_H), T-suppressor cells (T_S) and T-cytolytic cells (T_C), and B cells.[135] Thus, following binding by specific antigens in peripheral lymphoid tissues, the T and B cells proliferate and differentiate as clones into effector cells (e.g., T cells with cytotoxic and other functions or antibody-producing plasma cells from B cells) and into memory

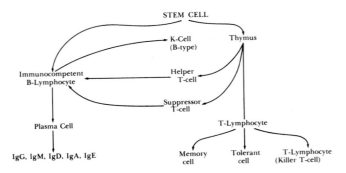

Fig. 9-1. Cellular elements of the immune system.

cells that recirculate through the tissues and lymphoid tissues as a means of surveillance for bacteria (Fig. 9-1).

The T helper cells help other cells. They help T_C cells to become functional, macrophages to be highly active, and B cells to form antibodies. Soluble mediators of cell-mediated functions include lymphokines released by antigen-stimulated lymphocytes. Lymphokines are produced by both T and B cells.[33] Similar factors produced by non-lymphocytic cells, such as normal macrophages, fibroblasts and keratinocytes, are classed generally as cytokines.[33] The general term "cytokine" is replacing the more restricted term "lymphokine", i.e., neither the production of, nor the effects of molecular signaling "kines" are restricted to lymphoid cells. Lymphokines and cytokines are soluble mediators by which cells communicate with each other. Some of the many that have been classed as lymphokines include macrophage-inhibiting factor (MIF), macrophage-activating factor (MAF), chemotactic factor (CF), interferons, osteoclast-activating factor (BCGF), a B cell differentiating factor (BCDF), and BCDF-2, which is the same as human B_2 interferon.[180]

Cytokines include interleukin-1 (IL-1), produced by macrophages,[122] B cells and epithelial cells, and interleukin-2. Interleukin-1 induces T_H cells to produce and release interleukin-2, which together with specific antigen activates T cells to release lymphokines or become cytotoxic. Interleukin-1 has been demonstrated to be present in crevicular fluid,[122] and should be considered in relation to immune-mediated connective tissue and bone changes in periodontal disease. Disrupted epithelium can be a potent source of IL-1 production. Thus, there is potential for modulation of inflammation and immune reactions by epithelia.[122] Interleukin-3 is the growth factor for mast cells and Interleukin-4 is the complementary DNA for human B-cell stimulating factor 1.

Histocompatibility complex. All species contain a gene segment called the *major histocompatibility complex* (MHC). In humans, this gene cluster is referred to as *histocompatibility leukocyte antigen*

(HLA) and is present on chromosome 6. The MHC or HLA gene cluster is encoded for molecules that are involved in the initiation, stimulation, and suppression of the immune response.[164] The histocompatibility complex restricts the recognition of antibody by lymphocytes. Inasmuch as lymphocyte activation and blast transformation are controlled by HLA, an association between HLA and various diseases, including juvenile periodontitis, has been considered.[53]

Most subsets of lymphocytes do not recognize antigen molecules directly but require the antigen to be presented by an antigen-presenting cell (APC). The APC must present to the T cell at least two molecules—the antigen and one of the histocompatibility molecules.[135,164] Class I molecules regulate the interaction between cytolytic T cells and target cells bearing a virus or tumor antigen; class II molecules regulate the interaction between helper T cells and the antigen-presenting cell.

All living cells have molecules imbedded in their surface that are uniquely specific. These molecules have genetically determined "recognition" markers of biologic individuality. For this reason, humoral defenses mediated by antibodies can recognize bacteria as unwanted invaders.

Complement. Complement is a complex of proteins (C1 through C9) found in normal blood serum in an inactive form (Fig. 9-2). Complement cooperates with antibodies to destroy (lyse) certain bacteria, increase capillary permeability, and recruit phagocytic cells at the site of inflammation. The activation of the complement system may be an important immunopathologic mechanism against the initiation and progression of periodontal disease. There are two pathways

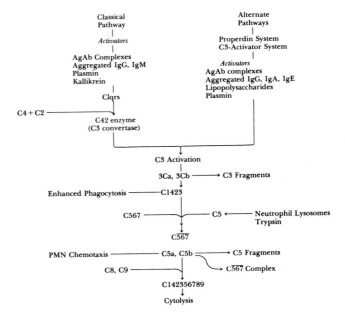

Fig. 9-2. Complement activation.

involved in the activation and cascade of reactions: (1) the *direct*, or *classical*, pathway, which is activated as a consequence of antigen reacting with antibody, or other actions involving plasmin, kallikrein and trypsin complex related to inflammation and clotting mechanisms; and (2) the *alternate*, or *properdin*, pathway, which is not dependent upon antibody but serves a cytolytic function that may be required to combat bacterial infection before an antibody response is expressed. Conversely, *B. gingivalis* may be capable of destroying the hemolytic activity of the complement components C3, C4 and factor B.

The components of the classical pathway are the 1st component (C1), which is the recognition unit, an activation unit (C4, C2, C3), and the membrane unit (C5 thru C9). Activation triggers the cascade of reaction from C1 thru C9 that ends with lysis of the bacterial cell membrane. The activation of complement (complement fixation) sets into motion the cascade, which continues until activity in a particular serum sample is no longer demonstrable.

Complement activation results in a number of biological activities associated with C proteins or their fragments. The principal activities include (1) histamine release from mast cells and increased vascular permeability—C3a, C5a; (2) neutrophil (PMN) chemotaxis—C3a, C5a, C567; (3) opsonization (immune adherence) and enhanced phagocytosis by neutrophil leukocytes and macrophages—C3b, C5b; (4) membrane damage and destruction of gram-negative bacteria, lysis of red blood cells—C3, C9; and (5) activation of B-lymphocytes—C3b.[135,164]

Potentially, the complement activation could be responsible for tissue damage through the attraction of leukocytes that inadvertently release excess lytic enzymes, as well as for complement-mediated lysis of tissue cells. The products of kinin-like activity following complement activation, while chemotactic for neutrophils (PMNs) and macrophages, are toxic to fibroblasts. Thus, factors released from the phagocytes may result in breakdown of collagen and connective tissue ground substance and of repair (fibrogenesis). However, there is no direct evidence that complement is not adequately controlled, or that destructive periodontitis reflects a defective complement mechanism.

Kallikrein-kinin system. Kinins are vasoactive substances released during injury and involved in acute inflammation. The prototype of the kinins is bradykinin.[223] Enzymes capable of forming kinins are kininogenases and include kallikreins. As a result of injury, the Hageman factor (Fig. 9-3) activates clotting and the formation of plasmin. These activated factors are responsible for the conversion of the proenzyme kallikreinogen into kallikrein, which is an enzyme capable of splitting kinins from kininogen. The proenzyme is present in the neutrophil. The kallikrein-kinin

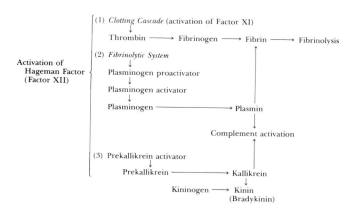

Fig. 9-3. Kinin, clotting, fibrinolytic and complement systems.

system is one of the nonspecific mechanisms involved in immunity.[164]

Bacterial lipopolysaccharide (LPS), which is a gram-negative bacterial endotoxin, has been shown to be capable of penetrating healthy sulcular epithelium and initiating an inflammatory response mediated by the kallikrein-kinin system[128] (Fig. 9-3). Once in the gingival tissues, LPS may be directly toxic, induce macrophages to produce collagenase, activate complement by classical and alternate pathways,[131,132] act as a polyclonal B cell activator, and induce bone resorption. LPS activates the Hageman factor, which then activates the clotting system and the plasma kallikrein-kinin system.[128,131]

Prostaglandins. Prostaglandins are fatty acids (sometimes referred to as cellular hormones) that are produced by many cells, including macrophages, fibroblasts, and eosinophils.[89,116] They have been implicated as mediators of acute and chronic inflammation,[60,97,129,208] bone resorption,[94,148,158] and immune reactions.[77,112] Prostaglandins are present in elevated concentrations in inflamed gingival tissues.[97] Prostaglandins may also induce chemokinesis in phagocytes.

The sequential activation of histamine, kinins, prostaglandins, and archidonic acid metabolites via the lipooxygenase pathway has been suggested to be involved in the progression of gingival inflammation;[85,89] in other words, to contribute to the activation of inflammatory mediators characteristic of chronic inflammatory lesions, not just to the earlier phases of acute inflammation.

Several studies, using the rationale that non-steroidal anti-inflammatory drugs (NSAIDS) inhibit prostaglandin formation, have explored the potential of NSAIDS for the treatment of gingival inflammation and bone loss in periodontitis.[47]

Antibodies. *Antibodies* are a group of proteins named *immunoglobulins* (Ig). A basic structure is common to all the classes of Ig (Fig. 9-4). There are five classes: IgA, IgG, IgM, IgD, IgE. IgA is involved in

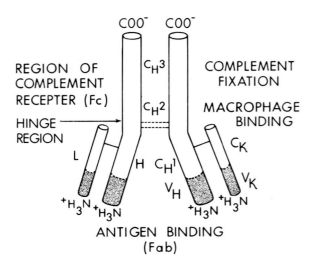

Fig. 9-4. Prototypic structure for an IgG antibody molecule. Antigen binding is associated with Fab regions and Fc regions with complement fixation.

the prevention of bacterial adherence. IgG functions as an antitoxin and as an opsonin (meaning that it coats foreign agents to facilitate their elimination). IgM is involved in complement activation (fixation) and is important for agglutination (clumping) of bacteria. IgD is considered to be involved in immune tolerance, which is a state in which agents normally considered to be antigenic fail to cause an immune response. Antibodies are produced by plasma cells located in lymph nodes and spleen. Serum contains mostly IgG, some IgA and IgM, and minute amounts of IgE and IgD. The main immunoglobulin in secretions is IgA. Secretory IgA is different than serum IgA.

Antibodies are Y-shaped (Fig. 9-5), bifunctional molecules having one region involved with antigen binding (Fab) and another region (Fc) that mediates binding to tissues, including macrophages. Fc also activates via the Clq component of the complement system (Fig. 9-2). Macrophages, neutrophils, and all other cells of the mononuclear-phagocyte system have Fc receptors. Recognition of bacteria may occur via Fc receptors and the C3b receptor component of the classical complement pathway.

The immune system is capable of recognizing specifically thousands of different antigens. Antigen molecules each have a set of antigenic determinants called *epitopes*. The epitopes on one antigen are generally different from those on another, but their molecular shapes are recognized by the antibodies and cells of the specific immune system. Each lymphocyte is only capable of recognizing 1 specific antigen, and thus the proportion of lymphocytes recognizing a particular antigen is small. However, by clonal selection, in which antigen binds to those few cells that can recognize it, B cells are induced to proliferate and mature into antibody-producing cells and longer-lived memory

cells. These cells have the same specificity for antigen as do the cells induced to proliferate. Antibodies interfere with bacterial functions and interact with other systems in the development of the immune response. However, bacterial destruction requires synergistic action with phagocytes.

Elevated levels of antibodies directed specifically to antigens of such bacteria as *A.a.* are found in saliva, serum, and gingival crevicular fluid in many patients with localized juvenile periodontitis (LJP).[53,160]

Neutrophil function/dysfunction. The successful elimination of a microorganism by a neutrophil, the first line of cellular defense, requires that the neutrophil reach the site of potential or beginning infection, recognize the invader, and then interiorize, kill, and digest the infectious agent.[70] This broad sequence of events requires migration to and the elimination of the microorganisms. Defects in chemotaxis, phagocytosis, and bacterial killing have been related to periodontal disease. Defects in the functions of migration and killing may be expressed as congenital and acquired diseases[23,156] (Table 9-3). Although it has been reported that individuals with quantitative and/or qualitative neutrophil disorders are susceptible to periodontal disease,[22,55,124,157,214,216] such a linkage is not always present.[13,96] However, chemotactic defects in blood neutrophils do occur.[218,219]

Defects in function relate to the neutrophil itself, to mediators of neutrophil function, or to leuko-

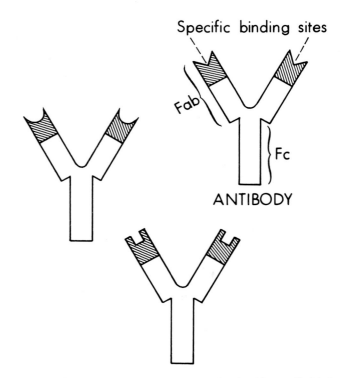

Fig. 9-5. Schematic representation of antibody with specific binding sites.

Table 9-3. Some disturbances involving neutrophil number or function

Agranulocytosis
Cyclic neutropenia
Localized juvenile periodontitis
Down's syndrome
Chronic granulomatous disease
"Lazy leukocyte" syndrome
Microtubule assembly defects (Chédiak-Higashi syndrome)
Defect in activation of membrane oxidase system
Inhibition of migration and phagocytosis
Hyperosmolarity secondary to diabetes
Ethanol intoxication
Papillon-Lefevre syndrome
Glycoprotein receptor defect

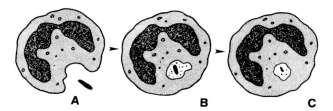

Fig. 9-6. *A,* Bacterium being engulfed in neutrophil after making contact. *B,* Closure of cell membrane around microbe. *C,* Destruction of bacterium in the cell membrane-lined vacuole.

aggressive properties of bacteria that allow them to evade the neutrophil-antibody-complement system.[53] Such pathogens as black-pigmented *Bacteroides* and *Actinobacillus* produce toxins and other factors that kill or reduce the function of neutrophils.[54,188] These aspects are discussed later in this chapter and in chapter 13.

As indicated in Table 9-3, a number of disturbances relate to the importance of the neutrophil in the host's defenses, including such uncommon diseases as Chédiak-Higashi syndrome,[209] chronic granulomatous disease,[32] glycoprotein receptor CR3 defect,[211] Papillon-LeFèvre syndrome,[51,57] and "lazy leukocyte" syndrome.[6]

The migration of neutrophils in the tissues occurs by random migration or by direct response to chemotactic stimuli. Chemotactic agents include fragments from activation of complement (e.g., C5a), products of activated mast cells, macrophages, and lymphocytes, proteins from coagulation and activation of kinin pathway, and products of infectious agents. Proof of most chemotaxins in lacking, but a number of synthetic agents are used in in vitro and in vivo tests, including the synthetic peptide N-f Met-Leu-Phe (FMLP), which is similar to bacterial chemotaxins and natural chemotaxins such as leukotriene B and C5a.

The normal neutrophil has a large number of receptors for FMLP, but there is a reduced number of available binding sites in localized juvenile periodontitis (LJP).[53] The reduced receptor density in LJP correlates with a reduced rate of chemotaxis.

Phagocytosis is the ability of a neutrophil (and macrophage) to surround and internalize the bacterium within a phagosome (Fig. 9-6). Ultimately, almost all bacteria are killed by phagocytic cells, but not all organisms are killed by the same mechanisms.[165,199]

The process of eliminating microbes can be considered to begin with recognition by the neutrophil of the microbe and attachment of the neutrophil to the microbe. At the site of inflammation, phagocytes recognize foreign or infectious microorganisms. Sometimes the attachment is enhanced if the bacterium has been opsonized by C3b complement. In effect, phagocytes use opsonins to facilitate adhesion to and internalization of bacteria. Thus, phagocytosis is facilitated if the antigen has been coated with antibody (IgG and IgM immunoglobulins) and complement (C36) so that antigen can be bound via Fc and C3 receptors on its surface (Fig. 9-7).

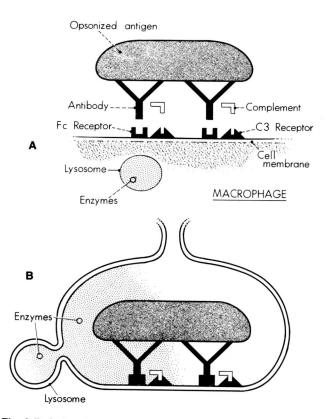

Fig. 9-7. *A,* Attachment of opsonized bacterium (antigen) via cell membrane receptors (Fc and C3). *B,* After attachment the bacterium (or bacterial substance) is internalized by microtubular action to invaginate the cell membrane and surround the microbe. The invaginated membrane forms a vacuole and fuses with enzyme-laden lysosomes. The lysosomal enzymes digest the bacterium.

The surface of a phagocyte contains two binding sites or receptors for opsonins: the Fc receptor, which binds IgG and IgM antibodies, and the C3 receptor, which attaches to the C3 component of complement. When attachment of the antigen (bacterium) occurs, a number of responses occur, including phagocytosis. Particulate matter is engulfed into the cytoplasm by invagination of the cell membrane and formation of a cell-membrane-lined vacuole (phagosome). Adjacent lysosomes (cytoplasmic vesicles filled with digestive substances) fuse with the phagosome and discharge the enzymes into it, thus forming a phagolysosome, where the infectious agent is killed by a battery of microbicidal mechanisms.

Killing mechanisms. Neutrophils have a number of ways of killing bacteria,[93,165] including the ability to reduce oxygen to superoxide, hydrogen peroxide and other O_2 reduction products, as well as proteins that remain active under anaerobic conditions.[50]

Cationic proteins, which are present in neutrophils and some macrophages, are active in the early alkaline phase of phagocytosis. In contrast to non-oxygen-dependent killing, the microbicidal effects of the products of oxidative metabolism have in the past been considered to be important. In the neutrophil, hydrogen peroxide is generated following a respiratory burst, and, in the presence of myeloperoxidase and halide, bacteria are halogenated, with resulting disruption of cell walls.

The effectiveness of the host to kill bacteria depends in part on the type of bacterial wall, on whether it is gram-positive, gram-negative, mycobacterial, or spirochetal. The ability of the host to damage the proteins and polysaccharides in bacterial cell walls is an important aspect of the host's defenses. Although proteins and polysaccharides in the outer surface of a bacterium act as targets for the antibody response, destruction of bacteria ultimately requires phagocytic cells.

All bacteria have an inner cell membrane and a peptidoglycan wall. Gram-negative bacteria have an outer lipid bilayer in which lipopolysaccharide (LPS) is sometimes found. Lysomal enzymes and lysozyme are active against the peptidoglycan layer, and cationic proteins and complement are effective against the outer lipid bilayer of gram-negative bacteria.

Gingival fluid. It has been recognized for some time that the neutrophil is the first line of defense against infectious agents, not only in the tissues but against plaque bacteria in gingival crevices.[8,9,161,224,225] The chemotactic substances produced by dental plaque bacteria and present in saliva produce a chemical gradient across normal junctional epithelium and connective tissues. As neutrophils migrate from the vessels of the gingival plexus, they are guided by the chemotactic gradient into the gingival sulcus, where they are func-

tional. Other protective mechanisms are also present in the gingival fluid.

Fragments of components of the complement system that can mediate chemotaxis[224] are present in the gingival fluid, as are most of the substances present in the blood serum. In patients with localized juvenile periodontitis, cleavage products of C3, C3 proactivator, and C4 are present in the gingival fluid.[174] Complement activation is important for the initiation of the inflammatory response and the enhancement of phagocytic activity.[4] Antibodies present in gingival fluid come from plasma cells in the gingiva, and others come from the blood plasma. Some of the antibodies may be specific for periodontopathic bacteria present in periodontal pockets. Much of the immunoglobulin produced by gingival plasma cells is nonsense antibody resulting from polyclonal activation,[145,148] but some of the immunoglobulin reacts specifically with periodontopathic bacteria.[145] The lack of specific antibody titer increases in adult periodontitis may be due in part to comparing a generalized increase in antibody titer to an increase in specific antibody titers.

Juvenile periodontitis

Many of the studies of neutrophil function/dysfunction relate to localized juvenile periodontitis (LJP) because it is considered to be a model of neutrophil function.[217] The most consistent abnormality in LJP is depressed in vitro chemotaxis of peripheral blood neutrophils.[53,171,215,216] The LJP abnormality has not been related to random migration nor to adherence, but is due to a lack of response to the chemotactic gradient. The migratory cytoskeletal apparatus is intact in LJP neutrophils.

In LJP, there may be a genetically determined defect in the expression of surface glycoprotein-100 (GP-100); in other words, GP-100 may regulate chemotactic receptor density. There is also a reduced density of C5a receptors.[217] These factors do not account for all the chemotactic defects in LJP,[218] as chemotaxis is also modulated by serum factors and bacteria.[171]

Depressed neutrophil chemotaxis in LJP occurs in about 70% of the cases in which neutrophil function is tested.[53] Several other functions that have been tested include phagocytosis, oxygen consumption, ATP energy utilization, lysozyme release, adherence and deformity, random migration, and chemotactic defect; but of these, only phagocytosis seems to be defective.[202] The locomotory defect appears to be a true chemotactic defect, manifested as a reduced ability of neutrophils to respond to a gradient of chemotactic factor, and not a result of humoral factors acting on normal cells.[49,53,98,215] The locomotory defect in LJP is constant, even into adulthood.[53] It is not reversed by successful elimination of clinically obvious active disease.[202]

AIDS

The relationship between polymorphonuclear leukocyte function and the etiology of periodontal diseases of HIV-infected persons has not been clarified. The chemotactic response to C5a has been reported to be depressed in drug addicts with AIDS.[155] However, supporting evidence for functional differences in phagocytosis and chemotaxis in relation to peripheral neutrophils has not been reported. In relation to the rapid destruction in AIDS virus-associated periodontitis (see chapter 13), it has been suggested that an enhanced neutrophil response to periodopathic bacteria could be responsible.[226] Although the etiology of AVAP is unclear, it is likely that the compromised immune system is involved. The possibility of a shift in oral bacteria and opportunistic pathogens being involved has not been determined.

Summary: The neutrophil is the predominant cell of the acute inflammatory response and the first line of defense against microbial invasion. Neutrophils are phagocytic, and this capacity is relevant to both the prevention and cause of some diseases. Many clinical disturbances are associated with defective leukocyte chemotaxis and other abnormalities of the immune response, but in some clinical disturbances only abnormal chemotactic responsiveness of the leukocyte can be identified.

There is little doubt that susceptibility to infection is related to defective neutrophil function, including dysfunction residing in the neutrophil and defects in mediators of neutrophil function. Such defects involving neutrophil function are related to the migration phenomena, the killing cascade, or both.[23] Clinical disturbances may be associated with cellular defects in chemotaxis (e.g., juvenile periodontitis), chemotactic factors (e.g., deficiency of C1, C4, C2, etc.), and inhibitors of granulocytes or chemotactic factors (e.g., alcoholism and cirrhosis).[156,157] Derangement of phagocytosis, independent of related functions such as locomotion, secretion, and bactericidal mechanisms, may have specific consequences. The recognition and response of neutrophils to microorganisms may be enhanced by interaction with serum factors (e.g., opsonins). The virulence of specific bacteria may be related to failure of neutrophils to recognize the bacteria, the ability of bacteria to produce a cell surface that prevents recognition, and microbial deception of both opsonins and neutrophils.[199]

Defective neutrophil function in localized juvenile periodontitis has been reported to be related to chemotactic factors and reduced phagocytosis. Although the defect may be related to a reduced number of receptor cites for chemotactic factors on the surfaces of neutrophils, receptors for phagocytosis (e.g., c3b) do not appear to be reduced in number. The chemotactic receptors (e.g., fMLP and C5a) and phagocytic receptor (C3b) mediate specific granule release and superoxide anion production. Many questions remain to be answered, but there is general agreement that chemotaxis and phagocytosis are in some way compromised by defective neutrophil function.[215]

The possibility that specific bacteria, such as *Actinobacillus actinomycetemcomitans* (*A.a.*), may be the most important causative agent in LJP, and the specific mechanism by which *A.a.* may uniquely take advantage of the defect in neutrophils in this type of periodontitis, has yet to be clarified.

Dysfunction of the neutrophil barrier caused by extrinsic microbial factors and/or by intrinsic mechanisms can have a significant role in severe and rapid progressive periodontal disease. The possibility that tissue damage is mediated by enzymes or lysozyme (e.g., cationic protein) produced by neutrophils (and macrophages) requires further clarification.

IMMUNE RESPONSES

In addition to those host defenses involving neutrophil functions and antimicrobial enzymes that have been described already, the immune system has responses that contribute specifically to the elimination of foreign and potentially injurious agents. The harmful foreign agent or antigen (Ag) can be distinguished as a nonself substance by immunocompetent cells. Some of these cells are B cells, which form specific antibody (Ab) to protect against defensive mechanisms, and others are T cells, which mediate a number of defensive mechanisms, including cytotoxic actions against target cells. These humoral and cell-mediated immune responses are collectively called specific immune responses (SIR). SIR can be divided conceptually into the *afferent* response, which relates to action involving the formation of antibodies and "immune" lymphocytes, and the *efferent* response, which relates to the exertion of actions by antibodies and effector lymphocytes.

Evidence is available for the concept that the accumulation of subgingival bacterial plaque elicits a systemic immune response locally. The development of the immune response may begin when an antigen gains entrance into the body via the skin, mucosa or crevicular/junctional epithelium and in association with the inflammatory response. The defenses of the host prior to, during, and subsequent to such entrance will vary depending on many factors, including the type of antigen (e.g., type of microorganism). Some of the injurious agents reach lymphoid tissue or lymph nodes, where macrophages or antigen-presenting cells become attached to the antigen and present that antigen to lymphocytes in order to stimulate a specific immune response against it.

The concept of a local immune response in the gingiva has been difficult at times to explain because of the common opinion that the gingiva contained no lymphoid tissue. However, a relationship between foci of gingival lymphoid cells and organized lymphoid tissue in lymph nodes has been considered. One possibility suggested is that plaque antigen diffuses or is transported by antigen-binding cells to the focus of lymphoid cells, where T and B cells' interactions may relate to effector cells and soluble mediators with the potential for modifying the periodontium. This route may be subsidiary to the essential role in the immune response played by regional lymph nodes.

Specific immune response

Conceptually, the specific immune response (SIR) is divided into three major categories of response: (1) humoral; (2) cell-mediated immunity (CMI); and (3) a combination of (1) and (2).[135] The sequence of events leading up to humoral response and CMI involves interactions among B and T lymphocytes and, as accessory cells, macrophages and dendritic cells. The reticular or dendritic cells of the lymphoreticular organs, which have little if any phagocytic capability, include dendritic cells (DCs), interdigitating reticular cells (IDCs), and Langerhans' cells (LCs).[135] These cells are antigen-presenting cells.

Humoral immune response

The humoral immune response involves the synthesis of antibodies against antigen; specifically, against periodontopathic bacteria or their products. The formation of antibody takes place as a result of the response of B cells, which undergo a sequence of developmental changes leading to the formation of the plasma cell (Fig. 9-8). Plasma cells are the progeny of antigen-stimulated B cells and are capable of synthesizing and secreting immunoglobulins. They develop at extravascular sites at such places as lymph nodes, beneath mucocutaneous surfaces, and sites of microbial injury in relation to the presence of foreign agents.

Antibodies act in a number of ways in defense of the host, including enhancement of phagocytosis, cell lysis in relation to complement, precipitation of soluble antigens, and agglutination of particulate matter. Antibodies also interfere with or neutralize the normal functions of enzymes and toxins. The actions of antibodies are essentially beneficial.

B Cell Activation. The activation of B cells and their differentiation into plasma cells generally requires an interaction with T lymphocytes; in other words, the response to the antigen requires that both T cells and B cells recognize the antigen. In contrast to these T dependent antigens (TD-Ags), a small number of T independent antigens (TI-Ags) may produce antibody independently of T cell help. This is of particular interest because of the antigenic determinants of lipo-

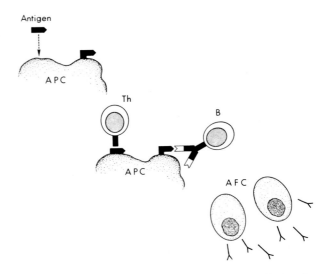

Fig. 9-8. Antibody response occurs when T dependent antigen (TD-Ag) is processed by an antigen-presenting cell (APC) and presented to T_H cells and B cells. The T_H cells provide help to B cells, which are stimulated to proliferate and become antibody-forming cells (AFC).

polysaccharides in dental plaque. Thus, although these TI-Ags induce pure humoral responses—induce B cells to form antibodies without the assistance of helper (T_H) cells—[135] many TI-Ags possess the ability at high concentrations to activate B cell clones that are not specific for that antigen. This is called polyclonal B cell activation.[164]

After B cell activation, binding of antigen, and cooperative interaction with T cells and macrophages or accessory antigen-presenting cells, B cells proliferate and differentiate into plasma cells that secrete antibody molecules of the same antigen specificity as the B cell, and as a rule the same Fc portion. Both B and T cells are activated when they bind antigen in the presence of accessory cells.

Lymphocyte transformation. Both B cells and thymus-dependent lymphocytes in chronically inflamed gingival tissues may in part be sensitive to plaque antigens, possibly with specific surface antibody. Sensitized lymphocytes activated by an appropriate antigen will, on encountering the antigen again, respond by transformation to blast cells; lymphokines are elaborated. These lymphokines are potentially capable of regulating constructive as well as destructive aspects of inflammation. A lymphocyte transformation reaction assay has been suggested as an in vitro method of studying the relationship of cellular immune responses to the periodontal status.[80,81] However, a number of problems in methodology do exist, and clinical correlates of periodontal disease severity and activity have not been determined. Inasmuch as in vitro correlates of cell-mediated immunity are not specific for T cell activity, interest has developed in the measurement of antibodies in the serum, saliva, and crevicular fluid, in order to determine the presence of increased antibody levels in response to specific microorganisms.

Serum antibodies. It is probable that lymphoid tissues have to react almost constantly with antigen from transient bacteria and their products at the dentogingival junction as well as elsewhere (indigenous flora of intestines, skin, etc.). Such stimulation is probably related to the usual concentration of antibodies in serum and *natural antibodies* (Igs that react with Ags but to which the host has had no known prior exposure). The level of antibodies in the peripheral circulation generally reflects the level of antibodies produced by the overall humoral immune response.

Antibody-mediated immunity. The formation of antibody that binds to antigen results in complement fixation and the formation of an antigen-antibody complex. This AgAb complex is then phagocytized by neutrophils. By these mechanisms, most gram-positive organisms and some gram-negative bacteria are rapidly killed. The rapid ingestion of organisms depends on opsonization by antibody and complement. Humoral immunity is also effective against bacteria that release toxins.

Cell-mediated immune response

As implied by the term *cell-mediated immunity* (CMI), the immune mechanism is mediated by cells, by at least two subsets of T lymphocytes. Unlike the humoral response, which can be evoked by either TI or TD antigens, the CMI response can only be elicited by TD antigens[135] (Fig. 9-9).

The CMI response is mediated by (1) T lymphocytes expressing the surface antigen OKT4 and involved in antimicrobial CMI, and (2) precursor T lymphocytes that express the antigen OKT8 and become cytotoxic cells.[135] Thus, T cells of CMI include those that mediate a number of functions via lymphokines and those that function as killer cells in antitissue immunity.

Lymphokines. Lymphokines are polypeptitide products of activated lymphocytes. Unlike antibodies their chemical composition is not determined by the stimulating antigen. They can be grouped into 3 main categories:[33] (1) those that modulate the inflammatory response, such as migration inhibition factor (MIF), macrophage activation factor (MAF), macrophage chemotactic factor (MCF), at least one chemotactic factor for each type of granulocyte, leukocyte-inhibitory factor (LIF), etc.; (2) those that cause cell proliferation, such as mitogenic factors or activators; and (3) those that damage target cells, such as lymphotoxins. Thus lymphokines may influence macrophages, lympho-

cytes, granulocytes and other cells, and may contribute to bone resorption, destroy tissues while destroying bacteria, and activate fibroblasts. Fibroblastic activation may contribute to collagen formation and healing in the reparative phase of inflammation. The term "lymphokine" is yielding to the term "cytokine" because the original term related only to substances functioning as molecular signals between immunocompetent cells.

Direct cell-mediated lymphocytotoxicity has been related to lymphocytes of the OKT4 lineage.[43] In vitro target cells include fibroblasts, epithelial, and endothelial cells. Antibody-dependent, cell-mediated cytotoxicity has been reported to occur in chronic inflammatory periodontal disease. Cytotoxic lymphocytes and lymphotoxin (soluble mediator),[73] which may

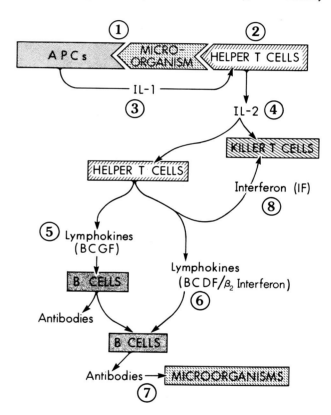

Fig. 9-9. Communication via lymphokines occurs in the activation of T cells by antigen-presenting cells (APC). Coupling *(1)* of the antigen (microorganism) with the helper T cell *(2)* and APC via cell surface receptors (including class II MHC) results in the production of interleukin-1 (IL-1) by APC *(3)*. The activated helper T cell is stimulated to elaborate IL-2 *(4)*, which in turn stimulates other antigen-activated cells to proliferate. These helper T cells secrete a lymphokine called B-cell growth factor (BCGF), which causes B cells to multiply *(5)*. Yet another lymphokine, B-cell differentiating factor *(6)*, initiates the production of antibodies *(7)*. The helper T cells also produce a lymphokine called gamma interferon, which has a number of effects, including augmentation of natural killer cell activity *(8)*, and activation of macrophages and endothelial cells.

be produced by B cells, can be locally damaging to target cells in the periodontium.

Cellular immune mechanisms that may modify the host do not necessarily cause cell death but may result only in impaired function. Soluble mediators may influence fibroblastic proliferation and collagen synthesis, and may relate to differences between the types of collagen found in normal and inflamed gingiva.[137] Interleukin-1 may influence fibroblastic proliferation, as may macrophages which are induced to produce fibroblast-activating factor and Interleukin-1 by lipopolysaccharide and T cells. Lymphocytes may be induced to release lymphokines by agents which stimulate macrophages.

Given the possibility of both inhibitory and stimulatory effects on collagen production by fibroblasts, due to different mediators from the same stimulated lymphocytes,[73,219] and the heterogeneity of the fibroblast population in the periodontium, the effects of cellular and soluble mediator components of the local immune response on the supporting tissues may vary considerably.[43] It has been hypothesized that available evidence suggests that macrophage-derived enzymes[219] and complement[97] play key roles in the interaction between dental plaque and host defenses.[43]

A causative role for lymphokines in disease has not been established; however, an insufficient or excessive production of lymphokines may contribute to diseases having an infectious or autoimmune disease origin.

Antigen-presenting cells. The cellular response in CMI to an appropriate antigen (Ag) involves presentation of antigen to T cells by an antigen-presenting cell (APC), which can be an IRC or an LC.[135] These types of reticular cells are not classical histiocytes or inflammatory macrophages, but do express large amounts of HLA-DR antigens (i.e., class II major histocompatibility complex antigens). It has been suggested that the principal accessory cells involved in CMI are the Langerhans' cells of the skin and gingiva. Class II major histocompatibility complex (MHC) antigens have their largest expression on APCs. Thus there is an interaction among helper and suppressor lymphocytes, APCs, and the expression of Class II MHC antigens within the periodontium. This interaction may be of importance to inflammation and immune responses.

The cells concerned in the humoral response to TD-Ags, B-cells, T_H cells and macrophages appear to require contact, except for B cell activation of T cell factors from activated T_H cells. Macrophages process antigen and present it to immunocompetent lymphocytes (Fig. 9-9). The accessory cell activities of macrophages in CMI and humoral responses are similar.

Dendritic cells (DCs) appear to play important roles in specific immune responses (SIRs).[135,183] DCs generally possess IaAg (I-region Ags) of MHC and complement (C3b) receptors. In generic usage, IDCs are designated as interdigitating dendritic cells and LCs as Langerhans' dendritic cells. DCs are antigen-retaining cells and LCs are accessory cells for the CMI response. Langerhans' dendritic cells are present in squamous epithelium, where their processes interdigitate to form a chain above the basal layer. They probably serve there as the principal accessory cell for the development of delayed hypersensitivity. LCs appear to be able to induce T cells that resist T_S cells. It has been suggested that LCs may make a major contribution to immunologic defense of the skin and mucosa, the principal agency being CMI.[197]

Immune regulation

It has become increasingly clear that components of the immune system, and probably of the nonspecific immune system as well, effect their individual ends through an extensive information network dedicated to self-homeostasis.[183] The control or regulation of such a homeostatic network (or networks) is important to understand in order to differentiate between perturbations in the network due to elimination of foreign antigens and perturbations due to defects in the information-regulatory network(s). How the vast communications complex, which links cells inside and outside of the immune system together and provides links with cells of the neuro-endocrine systems, is regulated at the cellular and molecular level requires further clarification.

Perturbations in these homeostatic networks generally reflect responses associated with the elimination of foreign substances (antigen). However, defects in the information-regulatory networks that link cells within and outside the immune system may be reflected in an inadequate, inappropriate, or exaggerated form of immune response resulting in an increased susceptibility to infection and, potentially, tissue damage.

Hypersensitivity. When a perturbation in the immune system resulting from the presence of an antigen is beneficial, the term *immune response* is used; if the result is harmful, the term *hypersensitivity* is used. Hypersensitivity reactions may be related to circulating antibodies (immediate hypersensitivity) or to delayed responses (delayed hypersensitivity), which occur where there is no circulating antibody involved but where lymphocytes and macrophages are associated with the response. Humoral and cellular responses may have a degree of interdependence.

Summary of immune defenses

Secretory-mucosal immune system. Secretory-mucosal immune defenses are provided by the function

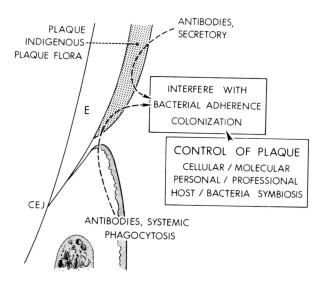

Fig. 9-10. *Secretory-mucosal immune defenses* and other factors involved in plaque control and pathogenicity limit the development of periodontal disease.

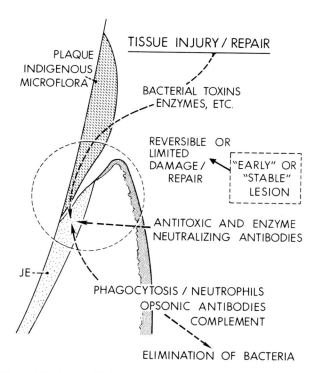

Fig. 9-11. *Neutrophil-Antibody-Complement defenses* are probably operational in conjunction with the secretory-mucosal immune defenses at all times, but may be increasingly involved prior to and during active periods of disease.

of secretory immunoglobulin (sIgA) in the saliva and by those immune mechanisms which operate at the

level of the crevicular fluid and junctional epithelium (Fig. 9-10). The relative importance of humoral (antibody), cellular (neutrophil), and structural barriers to infectious agents has not been resolved, but the defensive role of the neutrophil against infectious agents potentially capable of destruction is suggested in juvenile periodontitis. There is a growing list of "new" diseases associated with defects in neutrophil function or in the mediators of neutrophil function.

Saliva contains a number of components that contribute to host defenses, including antibodies; lysozyme, which at times functions as an enzyme to break down cell wall structures; and lactoperoxidase, which can inhibit bacterial enzyme transport systems.

Neutrophil-antibody-complement system. Vascular and cellular responses particularly involving neutrophils may not require specific immune mechanisms. However, the phagocyte may not recognize the infectious agent, either because complement is not activated, so that attachment occurs via C3b, or because the bacteria do not have a suitable receptor for phagocytosis. Under these circumstances, the *neutrophil-antibody-complement axis* (Fig. 9-11) is used. Through it, a mechanism is provided for attaching the neutrophil to the infectious agent via antibody and complement (Fig. 9-12).

Lymphocyte-macrophage system. In the past, much attention was given to the possibility that immune factors, including the lymphocyte-macrophage system (Fig. 9-13), could be subverted to cause directly the tissue damage seen in periodontitis. In addition to the direct cytotoxic and proteolytic effects of subgingival plaque, the indirect effects of the response of the host's immune system to the continued presence of plaque (antigens) were also implicated as causative factors in destructive periodontal disease. Thus, immunologic phenomena were strongly considered in the etiology of periodontal disease, as the results of immunologic deficiency, regulatory disturbance, or hypersensitivity. Such concepts suggest that immune responses have the potential to inadvertently exert destructive as well as protective effects (Fig. 9-14).

The basis for the belief that immune mechanisms might be responsible for some of the destructive effects of periodontal disease comes from evidence that bacteria, bacterial parts, chemotactic factors, and other plaque products penetrate the junctional epithelium and provoke a protective immune response.

Inflammatory-immune response linkages. The principal cells of the inflammatory response involve granulocytes, while the most prominent cells of the immune response are lymphocytes and macrophages or antigen-presenting cells. However, such a differentiation may provide an erroneously rigid view of the immune system. The inflammatory and immune sys-

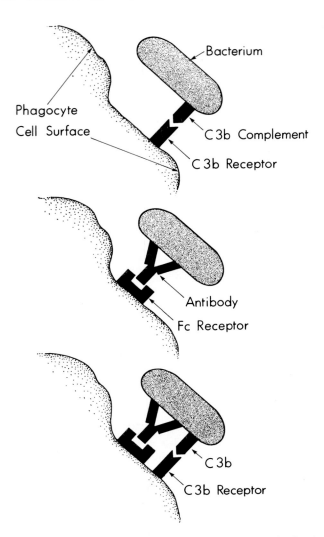

Fig. 9-12. Phagocytic activity is enhanced by opsonization by complement mediated by C3b bound to the surface of infectious agents and C3b receptors, as well as by binding of the microorganism "coated" with antibody to Fc receptors on the bacterium. Binding is greatly enhanced via both Fc receptors and C3b receptors (after Riott et al.[164]).

tems communicate and interact with each other via immunoglobulins (antibodies) and such chemical mediators as lymphokines and cytokines.

In addition to these links between immunologic and inflammatory mechanisms are the complement, kinin, coagulation, and fibrinolytic systems, which have already been described briefly. Also discussed briefly was the importance of the linked group of genes in the immune system called the major histocompatibility complex (MHC), especially class II antigens, which are important regulators and stimulators of immune responses.

In addition to binding antigen, the antibody molecule can interact with inflammatory cells and soluble mediators to modulate such biological mechanisms as

phagocytosis, cell lysis, and secretion of substances from neutrophils, macrophagen, and other cells. These antibodies may have a specific property of binding unique antigens and a nonspecific property of interacting with inflammatory cells and/or soluble serum components such as complement.

Immune responses and periodontal disease

The importance of neutrophils in defense has already been discussed, and it has been indicated that the function of the cells at the dentogingival junction is to engulf foreign injurious agents and partially degrade them by internalization and enzymatic digestion. However, inasmuch as neutrophils cannot recognize "foreignness," and their function is dependent upon an interaction of antibody and complement with the foreign agent, the inflammatory-immune linkage is readily apparent. It has been suggested that the damage associated with chronic inflammatory periodontal disease is related to immunologic injury; in other words, that the antigens of indigenous plaque bacteria cause a hypersensitivity reaction rather than a protective immune response. Immunologic injury is now generally spoken of in terms of inappropriate immunoregulation of immune and inflammatory responses.

Immune responses to dental plaque. Immune responses to bacteria and their products in dental plaque have been related to antibody responses to specific and nonspecific antigenic or mitogenic substances, to lymphoproliferative response and lymphokine production, and to immunohistologic features of developing plaque-induced gingivitis. Such responses have been studied in relation to periodontal therapy and cross-sectional evaluations of normal and diseased tissues.

Antibody response. The manifestations of an immune response in the gingiva to bacteria and/or their products may be reflected in the circulating blood as well as in the periodontal tissues. The specificity of the response has been related to generally good correlations between microbiologic findings in adult periodontitis and serum antibody levels.[133] Although a correlation between levels of circulating antibodies and severity of periodontal disease has been found,[54] elevated levels of serum antibody to specific bacteria are not always found.

With the highly sensitive enzyme-linked immunoabsorbent assay (ELISA), which can detect antibody of different classes simultaneously, elevated *Bacteroides gingivalis* antibody levels are often but not consistently found in adult periodontitis.[206] The same is true for antibodies to *Actinobacillus actinomycetemcomitans* in localized juvenile periodontitis. The results are much more variable with other potential per-

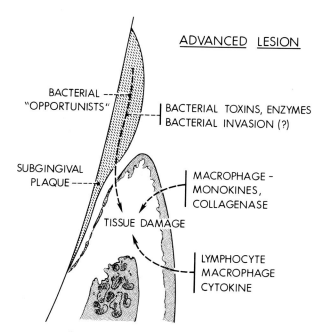

ADVANCED LESION

BACTERIAL "OPPORTUNISTS"

BACTERIAL TOXINS, ENZYMES
BACTERIAL INVASION (?)

SUBGINGIVAL PLAQUE

MACROPHAGE - MONOKINES, COLLAGENASE

TISSUE DAMAGE

LYMPHOCYTE MACROPHAGE CYTOKINE

Fig. 9-13. The outcome of interactions between microorganisms and host defenses may reflect tissue damage secondary to attempts to control microbial injury. The cellular infiltrate, fibrosis and bone loss in the advanced lesion of adult periodontitis or chronic inflammatory periodontal disease suggests retrospectively only the potential for an inadequate defense by the lymphocyte-macrophage system. As a consequence of genetic and/or systemic factors, blocking of phagocytic activity, and/or disturbances of immuno-regulatory control, tissue damage may occur at one time or another generally, or at selected local sites on teeth.

iodontopathic-related organisms that have been evaluated.

Similar variations in correlations occur between antibody response and clinical improvement of periodontal lesions following local therapy. It has been suggested that bacteria may exert an immunorepressive effect that may increase with higher bacterial loading, thus explaining an increased level of antibody following periodontal therapy.[206]

Specificity of the immune response in periodontal disease has received some support from the finding of specific antibody in gingival fluid, sometimes more than is found in the serum.[45] However, reactive antibodies may not necessarily imply specificity of induction.[183]

Large numbers of immunoglobulin-producing plasma cells in diseased periodontal tissues reflect nonspecific antibody that does not react specifically with antigenic determinants of plaque bacteria or altered tissue components.[26] It has been suggested that much of the immuglobulin produced by plasma cells in the gingiva is nonsense antibody resulting from

polyclonal activation.[145,148] However, some specificity in immune responsiveness to oral bacteria does exist.[145]

Lymphoproliferative response. In vitro studies of peripheral blood mononuclear cells from patients with periodontal disease have indicated that these circulating cells respond to antigens from plaque bacteria by proliferation and lymphokine production.[73,811,82,83] Although several studies seem to indicate a correlation between the magnitude of lymphoid cell responsiveness and the severity of periodontal disease, other investigators have not found such a relationship. Thus, there has been some question of how well such in vitro techniques reflect a relationship between peripheral cells and the severity of such highly localized lesions in vivo. This technique problem has been partially answered by the development of monoclonal antibodies that allow the interactions to be studied in situ.[84]

Another in vitro reaction thought to reflect an in vivo correlate of immunoregulation is the autologous mixed lymphocyte reaction (AMLR). A depressed spontaneous proliferation of peripheral blood lymphocytes in patients with advanced periodontal disease has been suggested to be evidence of a possible defect in immunoregulation of chronic inflammatory periodontal disease.[183]

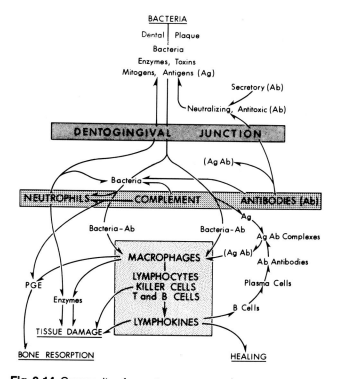

Fig. 9-14. Composite of secretory-mucosal immune system, neutrophil-antibody-complement system, and the lymphocyte-macrophage system in dental plaque/host interactions.

There is some evidence that lymphoproliferative responses to some putative periodontopathic bacteria may be depressed in patients with periodontal disease. Suppression of both T and B cells to extracts of bacteria have been demonstrated.[186] There is some evidence that depressed AMLR tends to return to normal after periodontal therapy of advanced disease. This evidence has been interpreted by some investigators to indicate that plaque bacteria may influence immunoregulatory mechanisms. Several components of dental plaque, such as LPS, LTA, dextran, and levan, have immunosuppressive as well as adjuvant effects.

Lymphocyte activation. Differentiation of lymphocytes in the gingival tissues is brought about by bacterial substances in dental plaque. Of particular interest has been the issue of whether the activation of lymphocytes relates specifically to bacterial antigens or nonspecifically to bacterial polyclonal activators such as lipopolysaccharides from gram-negative bacteria.

The concept of polyclonal activation of B cells requires that significant amounts of Ig with a broad spectrum of antigenic specificities to plaque-related and nonplaque-related antigens be produced in the gingiva, and that little or no immune complex should be expected. If B cell activation is monoclonal, specific antibody will be produced in the gingival tissue, and the deposit of immune complex should be expected.[144] If the immune complex is present, complement may be activated and neutrophils and monocytes may maintain the inflammatory response and cause some tissue destruction. When lymphocyte activation occurs in vitro, the use of a specific antibody results in a proportion of responding cells so low that data analysis is difficult.

Activation of lymphocytes, whether by mitogens or antigens, results in the production of lymphokines, including lymphotoxin, osteoclastic-activating factor, and chemotactic factor, that have been implicated in the mechanisms of destructive periodontal disease.[144] The production of lymphokines by T cells reflects a part of the concept that, in the pathogeneses of periodontal disease, T lymphocytes have an important role in delayed hypersensitivity.

A number of in vitro studies using peripheral blood cells have provided some support for the concept that polyclonal B cell activation is of importance in the pathogenesis of progressive periodontal disease,[183,185] but a protective role for T cell-mediated mechanisms has been suggested as well.[196]

Polyclonal B cell activation and induced immunoglobin production in humans is regulated by T cells. The control of the B response, whether specific, polyclonal, or polyclonal augmentation of a specific response, is mediated by T cells.[29] Therefore, the regulatory influence of T_H and T_s lymphocytes, interacting in concert with feedback, feedforward, and amplification networks, may play a significant role in immunoregulation of chronic inflammatory disease. In this respect, the emphasis is not on potential destructive mechanisms, but upon self-homeostatic control networks operating both systemically and locally at cellular and molecular levels for the benefit of the host. Thus, the picture of total immunity involves control of tissues, cells, and soluble mediators in and outside the immune system, even the behavior of supporting structures of teeth.

Immunohistology. The histologic features associated with the changes in the periodontium associated with experimental accumulation of plaque have been discussed in chapter 7. The resulting lesions have been described,[8,146,149,176] and, on the basis of the sequence of events, have been separated into *initial, early* and *established* stages of gingivitis, with periodontitis as the *advanced* stage.[146,149] Such a separation is a matter of convenience for discussion. There are few long-term studies.[151,185]

The early lesion of plaque-induced gingivitis is characterized by an infiltrate in which small, medium, and large lymphocytes and macrophages predominate, along with small numbers of plasma cells.[151,175,176] The morphologic features of the early lesion[146,176] are consistent with delayed hypersensitivity.[145,222] Typical lesions have been created in animal gingiva sensitized to skin contact antigens and then challenged at the gingival margin with the same antigen.[222] A specific T cell mechanism has been suggested.[39,231] The duration of the early lesion has not been definitely determined; it may persist for long periods of time.[149]

The established gingival lesion seems to reach a stable state and may remain there for days, weeks, or years, but may at some time or some place in the mouth develop into periodontitis.[178] The most prominent cell in the junctional and pocket epithelium is the neutrophil. The established lesion is characterized by a predominance of plasma cells and B lymphocytes. Macrophages are present in the lamina propria of the pocket wall, and plasma cells are located at the periphery. As the severity of the gingivitis increases, the proportion of T cells decreases and that of B cells and plasma cells increase.

In early studies of chronic inflammatory periodontal disease, the infiltrate was described as consisting of large numbers of immunoglobulin-producing plasma cells[26] (subsequently identified as predominantly B cells).[112] Gingivally confined lesions were found to be largely lymphocytic,[112] and the stable lesion was thought to be T cell in nature.[39,231] It was postulated that the change from a stable lesion to a progressive lesion reflected the conversion from a predominantly T cell response to a response consisting of large numbers of B cells.[185] Such a conversion has been suggested to support the concept of a specific immune response; in other words, the idea that lesions of adult periodontitis should be considered as B cell lesions. This concept has been challenged because of the long period of time that B cell lesions can be stable before becoming destructive.[146] The possibility has been suggested that the cause of the conversion of a stable lesion[185] to an aggressive one is a change in the microbial flora or an infection of the gingival tissue.[145] Of course, it has not been possible to determine at the time whether a lesion is active, and destruction can only be determined retrospectively.

Humoral and cell-mediated aspects of local immune responses to dental plaque

The concept of the protective nature of immune responses has regained ascendancy[206] after the renewal of interest in the destructive mechanisms associated with neutrophil function,[55] especially as these mechanisms relate to localized juvenile periodontitis (LJP). However, there have been several modifications of the concept that immune mechanisms play a significant role in the pathogenesis of periodontal disease. The emphasis has changed from viewing chronic inflammatory periodontal disease (CIPD) as simply the reflection of inadvertent damage resulting from a provoked, protective humoral and/or cell-mediated immune response. CIPD is now viewed as also being a reflection of detrimental changes in the periodontium resulting from immunologically driven modification of host tissue behavior.[43] Much more emphasis is now placed upon the immunoregulatory aspect of chronic inflammatory periodontal disease[183] and upon the fundamental linkage of immune and inflammatory mechanisms, both of which normally function in a state of successful homeostasis.

Concepts of immune injury

The role of humoral and/or cell-mediated immunity in chronic destructive periodontal disease has been related in the past to the potential of immune responses to produce damage via hypersensitivity reactions. The potential for direct damage was attributed to microorganisms with the ability to induce the disease and to immunomodulating agents capable of enhancing or suppressing the immune response.[101] Conceptually, either response could occur in relation to antigenic stimulation, whether a single specific antigen or several nonspecific antigens were present. Even the immune responses to a single causative periodontopathic organism might modulate the defenses of the host and the behavior of supporting tissues at the cellular and molecular level.

Hypersensitivity. It has been suggested that all types of hypersensitivity reactions may be attributed to bacterial plaque.[101] These reactions include *imme-diate* or antibody-mediated hypersensitivity reactions (Coombs and Gell types I, II, III), and *delayed* or cell-mediated (type IV) hypersensitivity reactions mediated primarily by T cells and macrophages. But it has been proposed that these reactions, although acting inappropriately and sometimes causing inflammation and tissue damage, are expressions of beneficial immune responses. In addition to bacteria, the principal mitogenic plaque substances suggested to be involved in these reactions are such potent biologic materials as lipopolysaccharides (LPS) from gram-negative bacteria, dextrans, and levans. These substances are able to penetrate junctional and crevicular epithelia.

Antibody-mediated reactions. Because of IgE immunocytes present in chronically inflamed gingiva, it has been proposed that gingivitis may reflect an aspect of an immediate reagin-mediated hypersensitivity reaction. The IgE immunoglobulin has affinity for most cells, which are found widely in the gingiva and release inflammatory mediators upon degranulation. Antigen-antibody reactions involving IgE can cause mast cell degranulation.[164] Although local anaphylactic reactions might be possible,[183] the amount of IgE in the gingiva does not support the possibility that this kind of immune response has a major role in adult periodontitis.

The local inflammatory response to antigen-antibody complexes involving IgG or IgM, especially within vessel walls, is a form of immediate hypersensitivity (Arthus reaction) that may result in complement activation. Although initially protective, subsequent phagocytosis of the complex could potentially lead to lysosomal release and tissue damage. Large numbers of polymorphonuclear leukocytes are related to this kind of reaction. The role of such reactions in destructive periodontal disease has not been established.

Conceptually, lesions due to cytotoxic type hypersensitivity might involve the formation of immune complexes that can activate the complement system. Responses might then occur in low-grade chronic infection where there is weak antibody response and deposition of complexes in the tissues, or in autoimmune disease where the continued production of autoantibody to a self-antigen leads to prolonged immune complex formation and tissue deposition. Tissue damage appears to occur when polymorphs attempt to phagocytose tissue-trapped complexes and when lysosomal enzymes are released and cause tissue damage. The acceptance of this type of hypersensitivity in chronic destructive periodontal disease has not been established.

Cell-mediated reactions. Cell-mediated hypersensitivity or delayed hypersensitivity reactions are initiated by cells rather than by antibody. Because lymphocytes and plasma cells predominate in human periodontitis,[146] these cells have been suggested to play a role in the pathogenesis of periodontal disease.[33,72,222] The early lesion[176] already described has histologic features consistent with the lesions of delayed hypersensitivity.[145,222]

Discussion over the protective and destructive aspects of immune responses has led to a large number of investigations about the immunopathological reactions brought about by neutrophils, lymphocytes, and macrophages, and the potential role of those reactions in the destructive aspects of periodontal disease. The protective nature of the immune response is generally accepted, especially in relation to the neutrophil.[53,54] However, the potential role of cellular and soluble mediator components of the local immune response in modifying host tissue behavior has yet to be clarified.[43,183]

The type of cellular infiltrate (lymphocytes),[151,178,185] and increased blastogenesis of peripheral lymphocytes when stimulated with plaque antigens,[113,121,146,150] have suggested that cellular immunity is involved in the pathogenesis of periodontal disease.[101,138,183,222]

The concept of direct damage by provoked protective immune responses operating under conditions of hypersensitivity has not been strongly supported for several reasons.[113] These reasons include the finding that B cells as well as T cells produce lymphokines; that the predominate cellular infiltrate in chronic inflammatory disease is composed of B cells and plasma cells; that established lesions in which B cells and plasma cells predominate can form and remain stable for indefinite periods without progression; and that B cell activity is not essential in some animals for severe forms of periodontitis to occur.[146,149,178] In the case of delayed hypersensitivity reactions, T cells and macrophages are the predominant cells.[113] Therefore, it has been suggested that T cells and cell-mediated hypersensitivity may play a role in the development of the early lesion, a mild, reversible gingivitis in which tissue damage is almost negligible.[144,222]

Because of conflicting evidence and the nature of the inflammatory infiltrate, it seems unlikely that delayed hypersensitivity mechanisms, as now understood, can account for the fibrosis and bone resorption that occur in chronic destructive periodontal disease. Although it is thought that these processes may be the consequence of the activities of granulocytes, B lymphocytes, or plasma cells,[222] it has been suggested that cellular and soluble mediator components of the local immune response to plaque may have a role in the pathogenesis of chronic destructive periodontal disease.[43]

Immunoregulation of periodontal disease

Although it is generally agreed that immunological mechanisms are involved in the pathogenesis of periodontal disease,[183] the regulation of such mechanisms is far from clear. Interactions among plaque bacteria, their products, and the immune system are generally regulated in such a way as to prevent injury and inadvertent damage to the host. Such regulation of the immune and inflammatory response at the macro- and micro-environmental level requires a vast network of communicating cells and mediators with functions ranging from enhancement to suppression of the immune response. The existence of helper (T4-positive) and suppressor (T8-positive) lymphocytes, and the expression of class II major histocompatibility complex (MHC) antigen, which is involved in the initiation, stimulation, and suppression of the immune response,[164] suggest the widespread nature of the network involved in the regulation of these interactions.

Although class II MHC antigens are found on a number of different cell types, their largest expression is found on antigen-presenting cells (APCs).[183] These interdigitating reticulum cells are thought to play a role in presenting antigen to T cells, and to be involved in the initial formation of a perivascular inflammatory lesion in experimental gingivitis.

The rather constant 14:T8 (T_H:T_S) ratio of 2:1 in experimental gingivitis, the probable involvement of APCs perivascularly, the 2:1 ratio for helper-suppressor lymphocytes in gingivitis (stable lesion) in children, and the development of perivascular lesions in the gingiva that are similar to the controlled delayed-type hypersensitivity reaction in the skin, have been suggested as providing support for the concept of immunoregulatory control of chronic inflammatory periodontal disease.[183] The depression of T4:T8 ratio has been proposed to reflect a local immunoregulatory imbalance in adult periodontitis.

The importance of immunoregulatory T cells in the progression of periodontal disease remains to be ascertained.[101] The concept of a central role for T cell control in periodontal disease, and of an imbalance in such control being related to the progression of periodontal disease, is based upon the interpretation of a number of studies.[183]

Studies in germ-free animals of the change from T cell to B cell-dominated lesions in periodontal disease have suggested the role of T cells in regulating the B cell response.[207] The results of other studies[231] have been taken to support the concept that progressive periodontal disease is primarily a B cell lesion and that T cells have a regulatory role in controlling the B cell response.[183]

Interactive bacterial-immunologic regulatory responses include suppression of both T and B cell function,[186] including suppression induced by *A.a.* and mediated by suppressor T cells. A modulatory effect of periodontopathic bacteria on the adherence of polymorphonuclear leukocytes has been reported.[181]

Repeated mucosal presentation of ingested bacterial antigens may be capable of modulating the systemic immune response elicited locally via an oral tolerance phenomenon. *Oral tolerance* is a state of systematic unresponsiveness resulting from presentation of antigen orally via ingestion or inhalation.[101] The possibility of such oral tolerance being related to subgingival periodontopathic antigens and to the development or progression of chronic inflammatory periodontal disease has not been established.

Concepts of local immunoregulatory imbalance as a factor in the progression of periodontal disease include a wide range of potential mechanisms for cellular regulation of chronic disease, as well as molecular regulatory interactions such as that involving the role of interleukin-1 (IL-1) in antigen presentation to T cells.[122] The activity of IL-1 in immune and non-immune mechanisms is widespread, and probably homologous to osteoclast-activating factor.

Interferon (IFN_2), prostaglandin E_2 (PGE_2), and IL-2 constitute an immunomodulatory circuit with a number of activities. These activities include control of antibody production, regulation of class II MHC antigen expression and antigen presentation, and augmentation of polymorphonuclear leukocyte activity.[41,182,183] IFN_2 is produced by activated T cells. The possibility that an IFN_2-PGE_2 regulatory loop operates locally has been suggested, but remains speculative.[183]

The possibility of an immunoregulatory defect being present in periodontal disease has been suggested, on the basis of depressed spontaneous proliferation of peripheral blood lymphocytes in advanced periodontitis, and using spontaneous proliferation as a measure of autologous mixed lymphocyte reaction (AMLR) and AMLR as an in vitro correlate of immunoregulation.

In summary, the regulation of the interactions among the cells and soluble mediators inside and outside the immune system with bacteria and their products involves complex self-homeostatic networks dedicated to the protection of the host. Local responses to antigenic and mitogenic substances are generally successful, and, even in the presence of chronic injury, the gingival response may stabilize for long periods of time. The possibility that progressive periodontal lesions may occur as a consequence of local immunological imbalance remains enigmatic; however, phenomenologic cellular and molecular mechanisms to support such a concept have been reported.

HEALING, REPAIR, REGENERATION

The features of active chronic inflammatory periodontal disease reflect ongoing injury and repair in a microenvironment determined primarily at the cellular and molecular level by host/microbial interactions. The general features of tissue change relate to the stage and severity of the disease.

Aside from a cellular infiltrate consistent with ulceration of the crevicular epithelium, or those changes already described for lesions developing in relation to plaque accumulation (initial, early, established, advanced, and stable or progressive lesions), the most prominent changes relate to the conversion of morphologically distinct arrangements of dense connective tissue into progressively less distinct connective tissue patterns with loss of attachment to teeth and bone and to bone marrow fibrosis. The cellular and molecular determinants of these kinds of change are largely speculative, although the potential mechanisms for destruction and repair have provided a number of paradigms for discussion.

With the partial or total resolution of nonspecific chronic inflammation, repair is ongoing and fibrosis is related to macrophages. However, in delayed hypersensitivity triggered by specific antigen, other mechanisms for mediating the fibroblastic response may contribute to the process of repair. As already discussed, T lymphocytes produce lymphokines, which activate macrophages and which also may directly influence fibroblast behavior.[176] Thus, the lymphocyte, through soluble mediators, can directly influence the activation and proliferation of fibroblasts and collagen synthesis, or amplify the influence on fibroblast behavior through macrophage participation.

The repair process, which involves the control of injury, recruitment and activation of fibroblasts, collagen synthesis, fibrosis, and scar tissue, is the consequence of a wide range of interactions between cells and soluble mediators. Control mechanisms for healing may involve similar processes and the same cells that are involved in destructive processes.

Regeneration

The repair of gingival soft tissues following therapeutic procedures that cause injury, including scaling and root planing, curettage, gingivectomy, flaps, and grafts, is described in detail in later chapters. Generally, the data suggest a consistent rate of re-epithelization, 7 to 14 days following surgery, and a range of 10 to 30 days for connective tissue organization and maturation.[195] In addition to repair of injured supporting tissues, of particular interest is the complete restitution of the attachment apparatus lost as a consequence of periodontal disease. Complete restitution of form and function involves regeneration of the periodontium.

Regeneration may be considered to consist of (1) complete reversal of changes in the junctional epithelium, (restoration of histologic, anatomic and functional characteristics of the gingival sulcus with the presence of a shallow groove between the tooth and a normal healthy gingiva); (2) new attachment of the principal fibers of the periodontal membrane into newly formed normal cementum (periodontal membrane connective tissue attachment); and (3) restoration of alveolar bone to normal form and height. Such complete regeneration is the ultimate goal of corrective periodontal therapy.

As used here, the term *new attachment* refers to any connective tissue attachment obtained coronal to the apical extent of root planing.[79] *Reattachment* refers to the reunion of connective tissue to the root surface in the presence of preserved periodontal membrane,[79] and can take place when root surfaces have not been curetted or injured.[95] Complete removal of all inserted collagen from all root surfaces is not easily accomplished. Several techniques have been devised for complete denudation and preparation of the root surface for new connective tissue attachment. "Healing by scar" may take place often.[195]

By whatever mechanism loss of attachment occurs in relation to etiologic agents in destructive periodontal disease, reattachment of connective tissue to a diseased root surface does not occur predictably. Apparent rapid healing or attachment gain described in the "burst" theory[191] of attachment level change in periodontitis[60] has been questioned,[159] such repair has not been described histologically.

In terms of so-called "regenerative" procedures that involve root planing,[194,226] healing occurs via a long junctional epithelium virtually without predictable new attachment.[107,143,194,195,232] Although healing may be considered clinically acceptable, it cannot be considered ideal, as the goal of regeneration is not reached. At best, it is considered to be repair.[232] Thus, before a new attachment can occur, the epithelium must first be excluded from the root surface[24] without root resorption or ankylosis occurring.

Recently it has been proposed that new connective tissue attachment can occur on previously diseased roots, provided that the cells populating the healing surface are of the proper origin and potential.[119] Cells derived from the periodontal membrane are the only ones capable of producing new cementoblasts, cementum, and principal fibers.[64] Cells from epithelium, gingival connective tissue and bone are not.[74,118] Although total exclusion of the epithelium may allow regeneration of the attachment,[24] whenever epithelial migration is retarded, the potential for root resorption is increased,[74] and whenever periodontal membrane is present, there is a reduction in ankylosis.[141]

The use of Millipore filter material to cover the crestal bone and tooth surface coronal to the cementoenamel junction does prevent both epithelium and gingival connective tissue from colonizing the surface.[11,143] The use of Millipore filter membrane does facilitate the formation of new attachment on root surfaces previously exposed to plaque. Gore-tex membrane has also been used.[28,62,63] It may be slightly more biocompatible, because new cementum may be deposited. Non-resorbable membrane (Gore-tex) is effective in blocking the proliferation of the epithelium and gingival connective tissue while allowing proliferation of cells from the periodontal ligament.[28] In general, new attachment is related to the problem of guiding the growth of periodontal membrane granulation tissue.

Evidence has been presented for the use of citric acid and fibronectin as adjuncts to conventional periodontal therapy. They may be used to enhance new connective tissue attachment in sites where exogenous fibronectin has been applied.[190] Fibronectin (FN) is a glycoprotein widely distributed throughout the body. Cellular FN is a component of fibrillar, extracellular structure and basement membranes. FN mediates cellular adhesion, acts as a nonspecific opsonin, promotes cell motility during wound healing, and promotes macrophage activity. It may mediate cell-matrix interactions and promote cellular adhesion to substrates by binding to collagen.

In summary, the use of a membrane filter placed over denuded root surfaces can prevent all periodontal tissues except those of the periodontal membrane from making contact with the root. Thus, healing can occur with substantial amounts of new connective tissue attachment (formation of new cementum with insertion of collagen fibers) and without root resorption or ankylosis. Therefore, on the basis of the principle of guided tissue regeneration,[63] some predictability for restitution of the attachment apparatus can be demonstrated using Millipore filter or Gore-tex membrane. However, all the goals for regeneration of the supporting structures have yet to be ultimately satisfied by practical clinical procedures.

OTHER SYSTEMATIC MODIFYING FACTORS THAT MAY INFLUENCE LOCAL DEFENSES

Host defense mechanisms may be compromised by known and unknown factors, including hormones, nutrition/diet, hematologic disturbances, and drugs.

Hormonal Factors

The nature and severity of the inflammatory response of the periodontal tissues to local irritants such as plaque bacteria and their products may be influenced by hormonal factors during puberty, pregnancy, and probably during menopause. Endocrine secretions by the pituitary, thyroid, and parathyroid glands are potentially capable of altering the state of the periodontium, but there is insufficient evidence that such potential influences specifically alter host defenses to plaque bacteria.

Sex hormones

Gingivitis that occurs during puberty has been referred to as pubertal gingivitis, and gingivitis during pregnancy as pregnancy gingivitis. These forms of gingivitis are possibly related to changes in the plaque microbiota and to hormonal imbalance. They are discussed in detail in chapter 12, which deals with gingivitis. The mechanism by which hormonal imbalance acts as an intrinsic modifier of inflammation has not been determined, but experimental evidence suggests that a raised level of progesterone could affect the function and permeability of the vessels of the cervical plexus.[77] *B. intermedius* has been associated with pregnancy gingivitis. The effects of progesterone on the microvasculature indicate that an existing inflammation can be aggravated by increased levels during pregnancy.[40,105,127] If a relationship between puberty and gingivitis is not accounted for by the presence of plaque[200] and variations in its bacterial composition (the most likely influence), then the role of hormones in puberty gingivitis may be similar to that in pregnancy gingivitis.

Diabetes

There are conflicting data on the prevalence and severity of periodontal disease in diabetic patients compared to normal individuals, and on whether diabetes has any relationship at all to periodontal disease.[17,31,75]

Diabetic patients have an increased susceptibility to infection, especially those whose diabetes is poorly controlled. Multiple periodontal abscesses may occur in diabetic patients following deep scaling if prophylactic measures are not taken. Although diabetes mellitus may, when it is severe or poorly controlled, act as a modifying factor in periodontal disease, the pattern of relationship is inconsistent. Patients with juvenile onset diabetes may or may not demonstrate severe bone loss, and the adult onset type of disease does not appear to affect the initiation or progress of periodontal disease. *Capnocytophaga* species and *A.a.* have been found to be associated with advanced periodontitis in juvenile diabetics (see chapter 13).[117,140]

Other hormones

The effects of endocrine secretions on the periodontium have been studied in animals,[153] but the effects of disturbances of thyroid, adrenal, pituitary, and parathyroid hormones on the initiation and progression of existing human periodontal disease have not been demonstrated. If such hormones are a factor in periodontal disease, they are modifying factors, not initiating factors.

Nutrition/Diet

The effects of severe malnutrition on the periodontium have been studied extensively in animals, but only a few controlled human studies have investigated the relationship between nutritional deficiencies and periodontal disease. Malnutrition may result from a deficiency of specific food elements in the diet, or from defective utilization, processing, or storage of nutrients in the diet. Although it is possible to affect the growth, development, and metabolic activities of the periodontium through nutrition deficiencies, the clinical and histological evidence suggests that the effect on periodontal disease is indirect, modifying existing disease rather than initiating periodontal disease. Thus, deficiency states do not influence the inflammatory response if no local factors, such as plaque and calculus, are present to initiate the inflammation.

Some parts of the world have severe nutritional problems, such as kwashiorkor, and in some areas, severe periodontal disease, such as necrotizing ulcerative gingivitis, occurs in 3-year-old children. Frank nutritional deficiencies from a lack of nutrients in the diet are quite unusual in the United States. When present, they are usually mutliple deficiencies secondary to such problems as alcoholism, ulcerative colitis, and neoplasia.

The role in periodontal health of food consistency in the diet does not appear to be significant. On the basis of the relationship between plaque and gingivitis, and the failure to establish an effect on plaque accumulation even when coarse foods are chewed excessively, it does not appear that consistency of diet has any bearing on periodontal disease in humans.

Vitamins, proteins, minerals

Vitamin C is important for the maintenance for collagen, cell respiration, blood sugar level, and capillary integrity. A deficiency of vitamin C sufficient to cause scurvy is rare in the United States and other developed countries. So-called subclinical deficiencies, when levels of ascorbic acid are measured by the whole blood or leukocyte-platelet method of determination, have not been shown to cause periodontal disease.[36]

In humans, frank scurvy is characterized by hemorrhagic diathesis, increased susceptibility to infection, and impaired wound healing. The severity of an existing gingivitis or periodontitis will be increased, but not caused, by a deficiency of vitamin C. Although an ascorbic acid-free diet in certain animals results in increased tooth mobility, hemorrhage, and decreased connective tissue, present evidence does not demonstrate a positive correlation between the presence and severity of periodontal disease and plasma or serum ascorbic acid levels.[100,228] Even when subjects develop scurvy, gingival changes fail to develop except in the presence of existing gingivitis.[326] Animal studies do not demonstrate unique oral lesions in riboflavin deficiencies.[2]

Except in extreme deficiency states, it is unlikely that undernourished individuals will reflect periodontal changes consistent with periodontal disease, irrespective of deficiencies in proteins, minerals, and vitamins. Severe nutritional deprivation states involving proteins and ascorbic acid may be associated with more severe periodontal disease, but have not been shown to initiate periodontitis.

Hematologic Disturbances

Except for the qualitative and/or quantitative disturbances in neutrophils already discussed, blood dyscrasias do not result in periodontal disease. In the absence of bacterial plaque and disturbances in neutrophil function, patients with hemorrhagic diatheses and anemias do not have more periodontal disease than normal individuals. Bleeding and control of hemorrhage may make control of plaque more difficult in patients with bleeding disorders. The periodontal problems associated with aplastic anemia are similar to those with acute leukemia, but other anemias involving only red blood cells do not relate to gingival changes outside those due to bacterial plaque. Gingivitis has been related to hypogammaglobulinemia.[16]

Drugs

No drugs have been confirmed as capable of initiating periodontitis, but several may be of significance in modifying the host's response to dental plaque. A number of drugs are capable of causing hyperplastic gingivitis. Hyperplastic gingivitis is discussed in detail in chapter 12.

Gingival hyperplasia is a side-effect of such drugs as phenytoin (Dilantin)[1,5,12] and sodium valproate[203] (Depakene), which are anticonvulsants; nifedipine (Procardia), which is an anti-anginal medication;[99,110] and cyclosporine (originally termed "Cyclosporin-A"), which is an immunosuppressant used to treat type-I diabetes mellitus, to prevent organ transplant rejection, and to treat autoimmune disorders.[166]

SUMMARY

The interactions between potential pathogenic bacteria and host defenses are reflected in specific and nonspecific responses, both locally and systemically. Such interactions involve cellular and molecular factors produced by and/or influenced by components of the inflammatory response and immune system (Fig. 9-14). The overall response is protective, although tissue damage may occur either inadvertently or as a result of self-homeostatic mechanisms. Although many basic mechanisms of systemic and local responses have been clarified, some key questions have yet to be answered.

Although bacteria are considered to be the principal etiologic agents in chronic inflammatory periodontal disease, there is no convincing evidence that bacterial invasion is primarily responsible. Rather, bacteria produce damage via the release of toxins, enzymes and metabolic products, which trigger host-mediated destruction by the activation of complement and mediators of inflammation, by the suppression of the immune system, and/or by causing dysfunction or avoidance of defense cells. Systemic disorders may also influence the quantitative and qualitative aspects of defense.

The repair and regeneration of periodontal tissues during and after active periodontal disease appears to be regulated in part by a number of integrated mechanisms involving chemical mediators produced by some of the cells of the immune system and of the periodontal membrane. The formation of new attachment requires that epithelium must first be excluded from a tooth surface from which irritants have been removed. Cells derived from the periodontal membrane are the only ones capable of producing new cementoblasts, cementum, and principal fibers.

Systemic modifying factors that may influence host defenses are reflected principally in disturbances of neutrophil function; however, the known systemic factors that compromise the periodontal status are relatively few. The relationship between hormonal imbalance and pregnancy or puberty gingivitis is not well understood. Except in severe nutritional states, nutrition and diet do not appear to be significant factors in modifying local defenses.

REFERENCES

1. Aas, E.: Hyperplasia gingivae diphenylhydantoinea, Acta Odont. Scand. 21:Suppl. 34, 1963.
2. Afonsky, D.: Oral lesions in niacin, riboflavin, pyridoxine, folic acid and pantothenic acid deficiencies in adult dogs, Oral Surg. 8:867, 1955.
3. Allenspach-Petrzka, G.E., and Guggenheim, B.: Bacterial invasion of the periodontium: An important factor in the pathogenesis of periodontitis? J. Clin. Periodontol. 10:609, 1983.
4. Allison, A., et al.: Activation of complement by alternate pathway as a factor in the pathogenesis of periodontal disease, Lancet 2:1001 1976.
5. Angelopolous, G.P., and Goaz, P.W.: Incidence of diphenyl hydantoin gingival hyperplasia, Oral Surg. 34:898, 1972.
6. Arnold, R.M., and Hoffman, D.L.: Oral management of lazy leukocyte syndrome—a case report, Quintessence Int. 10:9, 1979.
7. Arnold, R.R., et al.: A bactericidal effect for human lactoferrin, Science 197:263, 1977.
8. Attström, R., and Egelberg, J.: Presence of leukocytes within the gingival crevices during developing gingivitis, J. Periodont. Res. 6:110, 1971.
9. Attström, R.: The roles of gingival epithelium and phagocytosing leukocytes in gingival defense, J. Clin. Periodontol. 2:25.
10. Aukhil, I., et al.: Periodontal wound healing in the absence of periodontal ligament cells, J. Periodontol. 58:71, 1987.

11. Aukhil, I., et al.: An experimental study of new attachment procedure in beagle dogs, J. Periodont. Res. 10:643, 1983.
12. Babcock, J.R.: Incidence of gingival hyperplasia associated with Dilantin therapy in a hospital population, J.A.D.A. 71:1447, 1965.
13. Baer, P.M.: The neutrophil: Progression of disease: An update and critical review, J. Periodontol. 7:137, 1983.
14. Bandilla, K.K., et al.: Immunoglobulin classes of antibodies produced in the primary and secondary responses in man, Clin. Exp. Immunol. 5:627, 1969.
15. Barnett, M.L., et al.: The prevalence of periodontitis and dental caries in a Down's syndrome population, J. Periodontol. 57:288, 1986.
16. Barrickman, R., et al.: Gingivitis in hypogammaglobulinemia, J. Periodont. 44:171, 1975.
17. Bernick, S., et al.: Dental disease in children with diabetes mellitus, J. Periodont. 46:241, 1975.
18. Beumer, J., et al.: Childhood hypophosphatasia and the premature loss of teeth, Oral Surg. 35:63, 1973.
19. Beumont, R.H., et al.: Relative resistance of long junctional epithelium adhesions and connective tissue attachments to plaque-induced inflammation, J. Periodontol. 55:213, 1984.
20. Bissada, N.F., et al.: Neutrophil functional activity in juvenile and adult onset diabetic patients with mild and severe periodontitis, J. Periodont. Res. 17:500, 1982.
21. Bloom, G.D.: Structural and biochemical characteristics of mast cells. In The Inflammatory Process, ed. B.W. Zweifach et al. 2nd ed., Vol. I. New York: Academic Press, 1973.
22. Bodey, G.P., et al.: Quantitative relationships between circulating leukocytes and infections in patients with acute leukemia, Ann. Intern Med. 64:328, 1966.
23. Boggs, D.R., and Winkelstein, A.: White Cell Manual. 4th ed. Philadelphia: F.A. Davis Company, 1983.
24. Björn, H.: Experimental studies on reattachment, Dent. Pract. Dent. Reconst. 11:351, 1961.
25. Bowers, G.M., et al.: Histologic evaluation of new attachment in human intrabony defects: A literature review, J. Periodontol. 53:509, 1982.
26. Brandtzaeg, P., and Tolo, K.: Immunoglobulin systems of the gingiva. In The Borderland Between Caries and Periodontal Disease, ed. T. Lehner. London: Academic Press, 1977.
27. Brandtzaeg, P., and Kraus, F.W.: Autoimmunity and periodontal disease, Odont. Tidskr. 73:282, 1965.
28. Caffesse, R.G., et al.: New attachment achieved by guided tissue regeneration in beagle dogs, J. Dent. Res. 66:280 (Special Issue) abst. no. 1391, 1987.
29. Carpenter, A.B., et al.: T cell regulation of polyclonal B cell activation induced by extracts of oral bacteria associated with periodontal diseases, Infect. Immun. 43:326, 1984.
30. Cogen, R.B., et al.: Leukocyte function in the etiology of acute necrotizing ulcerative gingivitis, J. Periodontol. 54:402, 1983.
31. Cohen, D., et al.: Diabetes mellitus and oral periodontal disease: Two year longitudinal observations, Part I. J. Periodont. 41:709, 1970.
32. Cohen, M.S., et al.: Phagocytic cells in periodontal defense. Periodontal status of patients with chronic granulomatous disease of childhood, J. Periodontol. 56:611, 1985.
33. Cohen, S.: The roll of cell-mediated immunity in the induction of inflammatory responses, Am. J. Pathol. 88:502, 1977.
34. Cole, K.L. et al.: The autologous mixed lymphocyte reactions (AMLR) using periodontal lymphocytes, J. Dent. Res. 65:473 (abst.), 1986.
35. Cole, R.T., et al.: Connective tissue regeneration to periodontally diseased teeth. A histological study, J. Periodont. Res. 15:1, 1980.
36. Crandon, J.H., et al.: Experimental human scurvy, N. Engl. J. Med. 223:353, 1940.
37. Cutress, T.: Periodontal disease and oral hygiene in Trisomy 21, Arch. Oral Biol. 16:1345, 1971.
38. Daly, C.G., et al.: Bacterial endotoxin: A role in chronic inflammatory disease, J. Oral Pathol. 9:1, 1980.
39. Davenport, R.H., et al.: Histometric comparison of active and inactive lesions of advanced periodontitis, J. Periodontol 53:285, 1982.
40. Deasy, M., et al.: The effect of estrogen, progesterone, and cortisol on gingival inflammation, J. Periodont. Res. 7:111, 1972.
41. Demaeyer, E., and Demaeyer-Guignard, J.: Immunomodulating properties of interferons, Phil. Trans. R. Soc. Lond. B. 299:77, 1982.
42. Derenzis, R.A., and Chen, S.: Ultrastructural study of cultured human gingival fibroblasts exposed to endotoxin, J. Periodontol. 54:86, 1983.
43. Dolby, A.E.: Cellular and soluble mediator components of the local immune response to dental plaque, J. Clin. Periodontol. 13:928, 1986.
44. Dunn, C.J., et al.: An appraisal of the interrelationships between prostaglandins and cyclic nucleotides in inflammation, Biomedicine 24:214, 1976.
45. Ebersole, J.L., et al.: Gingival crevicular fluid antibody to oral microorganisms. I. Method of Collection and Analysis of Antibody, J. Periodont. Res. 19:124, 1984.
46. Edwards, R.G., et al.: Repair of the dentogingival interface. Dent. Pract. 19:301, 1969.
47. Eiattar, R.M.A., et al.: Arachidonic acid metabolism in inflamed gingiva and its inhibition by anti-inflammatory drugs, J. Periodontol. 55:536, 1984.
48. Eisen, H.N.: Immunology. An Introduction to Molecular and Cellular Principles of the Immune Responses, New York: Harper & Row, 1974.
49. Ellegaard, B., et al.: Neutrophil chemotaxis and phagocytosis in juvenile periodontitis, J. Periodont. Res. 19:261, 1984.
50. Elsbach, P., and Weiss, J.: A reevaluation of the roles of the O_2-dependent and O_2-independent microbial systems of phagocytes, Rev. Infect. Dis. 5:843, 1983.
51. Farzim, I., and Edalat, M.: Periodontosis with hyperkeratosis palmaris et plantaris (the Papillon-Lefevre syndrome), J. Periodont. 45:316, 1974.
52. Frank, R.M.: Bacterial penetration in the apical pocket wall of advanced human periodontitis, J. Periodont. Res. 15:563, 1980.
53. Genco, R.J., et al.: Molecular factors influencing neutrophil defects in periodontal disease, J. Dent. Res. 65:1379, 1986.
54. Genco, R.J., and Slots, R.J.: Host responses in periodontal diseases, J. Dent. Res. 63:441, 1984.
55. Genco, R.J., and Mergenhagen, S.E.: Summary of a workshop on leukocyte function in bacterial diseases with an emphasis on periodontal disease, J. Infect. Dis. 139:604, 1979.
56. Genco, R., et al.: Antibody-mediated effects on the periodontium, J. Periodont. 45:330, 1974.
57. Giasanti, J., et al.: Palmar-plantar hyperkeratosis and concomitant periodontal destruction (Papillon-Lefevre syndrome), Oral Surg. 36:40, 1973.
58. Giddon, D.B., et al.: Acute necrotizing ulcerative gingivitis in college students, J.A.D.A. 68:381, 1964.
59. Glickman, I.: Clinical Periodontology, Philadelphia: W.B. Saunders Co., 1953, pp. 501-511.
60. Goodson, J.M., et al.: Patterns of progression and regression of advanced destructive periodontal disease, J. Clin. Periodontol. 9:472, 1982.
61. Goodson, J.M., et al.: Prostaglandin E_2 levels and human periodontal disease, Prostaglandins 6:81, 1974.
62. Gottlow, J., et al.: New attachment formation as the result of controlled tissue regeneration, J. Clin. Periodontol. 11:494, 1984.

63. Gottlow, J., et al.: New attachment formation in the human periodontium by guided tissue regeneration. Case reports, J. Clin. Periodontol. 13:604, 1986.

64. Gould, T.R.L., et al.: Migration and division of progenitor cell populations in periodontal ligament after wounding, J. Periodont. Res. 15:20, 1980.

65. Goultschin, J., and Shoskan, S.: Inhibition of collagen breakdown by diphenylhydantoin, Biochim. Biophys. Acta 631:188, 1980.

66. Hall, B.K., and Squier, C.A.: Ultrastructural quantitation of connective tissue changes in phenytonin-induced gingival over-growth in the ferret, J. Dent. Res. 61:942, 1982.

67. Hanes, P.J., et al.: Cell and fiber attachment to demineralized dentin from normal root surfaces, J. Periodontol. 56:752, 1985.

68. Hausman, E.: Potential pathways for bone resorption in human periodontal disease, J. Periodont. 45:338, 1974.

69. Hinmann, J.W.: Prostaglandins, Ann. Rev. Biochem. 41:161, 1972.

70. Hirsch, J.G.: Neutrophil leukocytes. In The Inflammatory Process, ed. B.W. Zweifach et al. Vol. 1. New York: Academic Press, 1973.

71. Hojer, J.A.: Studies in scurvy, Acta Pediat. (Suppl.) 3:119, 1924.

72. Horton, J.E., et al.: A role of cell-mediated immunity in the pathogenesis of periodontal disease. J. Periodont. 45:351, 1974.

73. Horton, J.E., et al.: Elaboration of lymphotoxin by cultured human peripheral blood leukocytes stimulated with dental plaque-deposits, Clin. Exp. Immunol. 13:383, 1973.

74. Houston, F., et al.: Healing after root reimplantation in the monkey, J. Clin. Periodontol. 12:716, 1985.

75. Hove, K., and Stallard, R.: Diabetes and the periodontal patients, J. Periodont. 41:713, 1970.

76. Howard, J.G., et al.: Influence of molecular structure of the tolerogenicity of bacterial dextrans. III. Dissociation between tolerance and immunity to the alpha 1-6- and 1-3-linked epitopes of dextran B 1355, Immunology 29:611, 1975.

77. Hugoson, A.: Gingival inflammation and female sex hormones, J. Periodont. Res. (Suppl.) 5:1, 1970.

78. Isidor, F., et al.: New attachment formation on citric acid treated roots, J. Periodont. Res. 20:421, 1986.

79. Isidor, F., et al.: New attachment-reattachment following reconstructive periodontal surgery, J. Clin. Periodontol. 12:128, 1985.

80. Ivanyi, L, et al.: Cell-mediated immunity in periodontal disease. Cytotoxicity, migration, inhibition and lymphocyte transformation studies, Immunology 22:141, 1972.

81. Ivanyi, L., and Lehner, T.: Lymphocyte transformation by sonicates of dental plaque in human periodontal disease, Arch. Oral Biol. 9:1117, 1971.

82. Ivanyi, L., and Lehner, T.: Stimulation of lymphocyte transformation by bacterial antigens in patients with periodontal disease, Arch. Oral Biol. 15:1089, 1970.

83. Janoff, A., and Carp, H.: Proteases, antiproteases and oxidants. In Pathways of Tissue Injury During Inflammation, ed. G. Majno, R.S. Cotran, and W. Kaufman. Baltimore: Williams and Wilkins, 1982.

84. Janossy, G., et al.: Rheumatoid arthritis: A disease of lymphocyte macrophage immunoregulation, Lancet 11:527, 1981.

85. Jaun, H.: Mechanism of action of bradykinin-induced release of prostaglandin E, Arch. Pharmacol. 300:77, 1977.

86. Johnson, A.G., et al.: Studies on the O antigen of Salmonella typhosa. V. Enchancement of antibody response to protein antigens by purified lipopolysaccharide, J. Exp. Med. 103:225, 1956.

87. Johnson, B.D., and Engel, D.: Acute necrotizing ulcerative gingivitis—a review of diagnosis, etiology and treatment, J. Periodontol. 57:141, 1986.

88. Johnson, D.A., et al.: Role of bacterial products in periodontitis. I. Endotoxin content and immunogenicity of human plaque, J. Periodont. Res. 11:349, 1976.

89. Kaley, G., and Weiner, R.: Prostaglandin E.: A potential mediator of the inflammatory response. Ann. N.Y. Acad. Sci. 180:338, 1971.

90. Karring, T., et al.: Potentials for root resorption during periodontal wound healing, J. Clin. Periodontol. 11:41, 1984.

91. Keys, J.M., et al.: Mucosal induction of systemic T cell tolerance by Fusobacterium nucleatum, J. Periodontol. 57:441, 1986.

92. Khan, A., and Hill, N.O., eds. Human Lymphokines. New York: Academic Press, 1982.

93. Klebanoff, A., et al.: Myeloperoxidase-mediated antimicrobial systems and their role in leukocyte function. Biochemistry of the Phagocytic Process, ed. J.T. Schultz. Amsterdam: North Holland Publishing Co., 1970.

94. Klein, D.C., and Raisz, L.G.: Prostaglandins: Stimulation of bone resorption in tissue culture, Endocrinology 86:1436, 1970.

95. Kohler, C.A., and Ramfjord, S.P.: Healing of gingival mucoperiosteal flaps, Oral Surg. 13:89, 1960.

96. Kraal, J.H.: An analysis and clarification of status of periodontosis as a disease entity, J. Periodontol. 51:235, 1980.

97. Lally, E.T., et al.: Biosynthesis of complement components in chronically inflamed gingiva, J. Periodont. Res. 17:257, 1982.

98. Lavine, W., et al.: Impaired neutrophil chemotaxis in patients with juvenile and rapidly progessing periodontitis, J. Periodont. Res. 14:10, 1979.

99. Lederman, D., et al.: Gingival hyperplasia associated with nifedipine therapy, Oral Surg. 57:620, 1984.

100. Leggott, P.J., et al.: The effect of controlled ascorbic acid depletion and supplementation on periodontal health, J. Periodontol. 57:480, 1986.

101. Lehner, T.: Cellular immunity in periodontal disease: an overview. In Host-Parasite Interactions in Periodontal Diseases, ed. R.J. Genco and S.E. Mergenhagen. Washington, D.C.: American Society for Microbiology, 1982.

102. Lehner, T., et al.: Immunopotentiation by dental microbial plaque and its relationship to oral disease in man, Arch. Oral Biol. 21:749, 1976.

103. Lehner, T., et al.: Sequential cell-mediated immune responses in experimental gingivitis in man, Clin. Exp. Immunol. 16:481, 1974.

104. Lindhe, J., et al.: Connective tissue reattachment as related to presence or absence of alveolar bone, J. Clin. Periodontol. 11:33, 1984.

105. Lindhe, J., and Branemark, P.: Experimental studies on the etiology of pregnancy gingivitis, Periodont. Abstr. 50, 1968.

106. Listgarten, M.A.: Electron microscopic observations in the bacterial flora of acute necrotizing ulcerative gingivitis, J. Periodontol. 36:328, 1965.

107. Listgarten, M.A.: Normal development, structure, physiology and repair of gingival epithelium, Oral Sci. Rev. 1:3, 1972.

108. Listgarten, M.A.: Pathogenesis of periodontitis, J. Clin. Periodontol. 13:418, 1986.

109. Löe, H., and Holm-Pedersen, P.: Absence and presence of fluid from normal and inflamed gingivae, Periodontics 3:171, 1965.

110. Lucas, R.M., et al.: Nifedipine-induced gingival hyperplasia, J. Periodontol. 56:211, 1985.

111. Lynch, M.: Burket's Oral Medicine. 8th ed. Philadelphia:

J.B. Lippencott, 1984.

112. Mackler, B.F., et al.: Immunoglobulin-bearing lymphocytes and plasma cells in human periodontal disease, J. Periodont. Res. 12:37, 1977.

113. Mackler, B.F., et al.: Blastogenesis and lymphokine synthesis by T and B lymphocytes from patients with periodontal disease, Infect. Immun. 10:844, 1974.

114. Magnusson, I., et al.: Connective tissue attachment formation following exclusion of gingival connective tissue and epithelium during healing, J. Period. Res. 20:201, 1981.

115. Manor, A., et al.: Bacterial invasion of periodontal tissues in advanced periodontitis in humans, J. Periodontol. 55:567, 1984.

116. Marx, J.L.: Prostaglandins: Mediators of Inflammation, Science, 177:780, 1971.

117. Mashimo, P.A., et al.: The periodontal flora of juvenile diabetics: culture, immunofluorescence, and serum antibody studies, J. Periodontol. 54:420, 1983.

118. Melcher, A.H.: On the repair potential of periodontal tissues, J. Periodontol. 47:256, 1976.

119. Melcher, A.H.: Cells of the periodontium—Role in healing wounds, Ann. R. Coll. Surg. Engl. 67:130, 1985.

120. Mergenhagen, S.E., et al.: The role of lymphocytes and macrophages in the destruction of bone and collagen, Ann. N.Y. Acad. Sci. 256:132, 1975.

121. Mergenhagen, S.E., et al.: Immunologic reactions and periodontal inflammation, J. Dent. Res. 49:256, 1970.

122. Mergenhagen, S.E.: Thymocyte activating factors in human gingival fluids, J. Dent. Res. 63:461, 1984.

123. Mergenhagen, S.E.: Endotoxic properties of oral bacteria as revealed by the local Schwartzman reaction, J. Dent. Res. 39:267, 1960.

124. Miller, D.R., et al.: Role of the polymorphonuclear leukocyte in periodontal disease and health, J. Clin. Periodontol. 11:1, 1984.

125. Miranda, J.J., et al.: Studies on immunological paralyses. X. Cellular characteristics of the induction and loss of tolerance to levan (polyfructose), Immunology 23:843, 1972.

126. Mizel, S.B., and Farrar, J.J.: Revised nomenclature for antigen non-specific T cell proliferation and helper factors, Cell Immunol. 48:433, 1979.

127. Mohammed, A., et al.: The microvasculature of the rabbit gingiva as affected by progesterone and estrogen treated rats, J. Periodont. 45:50, 1974.

128. Montgomery, E.H., and White, R.R.: Kinin generation in the gingival inflammatory response to topically applied bacterial lipopolysaccharides, J. Dent. Res. 65:113, 1986.

129. Morley, H.: Prostaglandins and lymphokines in arthritis, Prostaglandins 8:315, 1974.

130. Morris, M.L.: The inductive properties of human dentin and cementum, J. Periodontol. 56:699, 1985.

131. Morrison, D.C., and Cochrane, C.G.: Direct evidence for Hageman factor (Factor XII) activation by bacterial lipopolysaccharides (Endotoxins), J. Exp. Med. 140:797, 1974.

132. Morrison, D.C., and Kline, L.F.: Activation of the classical and properdin pathways of complement by bacterial lipopolysaccharides (LPS), J. Immunol. 118:362, 1977.

133. Mouton, C., et al.: Serum antibodies to Oral Bacteroides asaccharolyticus (Bacteroides gingivalis): Relationship to age and periodontal disease, Infect. Immun. 31:182, 1981.

134. Mowat, A.M.I., and Parret, D.M.U.: Immunological response to fed protein antigens in mice. IV. Effects of stimulating the reticulo-endothelial system on oral tolerance and intestinal immunity to ovalbumin, Immunology 50:547, 1983.

135. Myrvik, Q.N., and Weiser, R.S.: Fundamentals of Immunology. 2nd ed. Philadelphia: Lea and Febinger, 1984.

136. Naik, D., et al.: Papillon-Lefevre syndrome, Oral Surg.

25:19, 1968.

137. Narayanan, A.S., and Page, R.C.: Connective tissues of the periodontium: A summary of current work, Collagen and Related Research 3:33, 1983.

138. Nisengard, R.J.: The role of immunology in periodontal disease, J. Periodont. 48:505, 1977.

139. Newman, H.N., and Addison, I.E.: Gingival crevice neutrophil function in periodontal lesions, J. Periodontol. 53:578, 1982.

140. Newman, M.G.: Current concepts of the pathogenesis of periodontal disease: Microbial emphasis, J. Periodontol. 56:734, 1985.

141. Nyman, S., et al.: Healing following reimplantation of teeth subjected to root planing and citric acid treatment, J. Clin. Periodontol. 12:294, 1985.

142. Nyman, S., and Karring, T.: Regeneration of surgically removed buccal alveolar bone in dogs, J. Periodont. Res. 14:86, 1979.

143. Nyman, S., et al.: New attachment following surgical treatment of human periodontal disease, J. Clin. Periodontol. 9:290, 1982.

144. Page, R.C.: Lymphoid cell responsiveness and human periodontitis. (Eds.): In Host-Parasite Interactions in Periodontal Diseases, ed. R.J. Genco and S.E. Mergenhagen, Washington, D.C.: American Society for Microbiology, 1982.

145. Page, R.C.: Gingivitis, J. Clin. Periodontol. 13:349, 1986.

146. Page, R.C., and Schroeder, H.E.: Periodontitis in Man and Other Animals: A Comparative Review, Basel: S. Karger, 1982.

147. Page, R.C., and Baab, D.A.: A new look at the etiology and pathogenesis of early-onset periodontitis. Cementopathia revisited, J. Periodontol. 56:748, 1985.

148. Page, R.C., and Schroeder, H.E.: Current status of the host response in chronic marginal periodontitis, J. Periodontol. 52:477, 1981.

149. Page, R.C., and Schroeder, H.E.: Pathogenesis of inflammatory periodontal disease. A summary of current work, Lab. Invest. 33:235, 1976.

150. Patters, M.R., et al.: Blastogenic response of human lymphocytes to oral bacterial antigens; comparison of individuals with periodontal disease to normal edentulous subjects, Infect. Immun. 14:1213, 1976.

151. Payne, W.A., et al.: Histologic features of the initial and early stages of experimental gingivitis in man. J. Periodont. Res. 10:51, 1975.

152. Pekovic, D.D., and Fillery, E.D.: Identification of bacteria in immunopathological mechanisms of human periodontal disease, J. Periodont. Res. 19:329, 1984.

153. Pinto, A.: Effect of hypothyroidism obtained experimentally on the periodontium of rat, J. Periodont. 45:217, 1974.

154. Polson, A.M.: The root surface and regeneration; present therapeutic limitations and future biologic potentials, J. Clin. Periodontol. 10:995, 1986.

155. Poli, G., et al.: Mononuclear and polymorphonuclear phagocyte functions in AIDS and prodromal syndrome. Paper presented at Int. Conf. on AIDS, Paris, June 23-25, 1986.

156. Quie, P.G., and Cates, K.L.: Clinical conditions associated with defective polymorphonuclear leukocyte chemotasis, Am. J. Pathol. 88:711, 1977.

157. Quie, P.G.: Neutrophil dysfunction and infection. In Advances in Host Defense Mechanisms, ed. J.I. Gallin and A.S. Fauci. New York: Raven Press, 1982.

158. Raisz, L., et al.: Complement dependent stimulation of prostaglandin synthesis and bone resorption, Science 185:789, 1974.

159. Ralls, S.A., and Cohen, M.E.: Problems of identifying "bursts" of periodontal attachment loss, J. Periodontol.

57:746, 1986.

160. Ranney, R.R., et al.: Relationship between attachment loss and precipitating serum antibody to actinobacillus actinomycetemcomitans in adolescents and young adults having severe periodontal destruction, J. Periodontol. 53:1, 1982.

161. Renggli, H.H.: Phagocytosis and killing by crevicular neutrophils. The Borderland Between Caries and Periodontal Disease, ed. T. Lehner, London: Academic Press, 1977.

162. Reuland-Bosma, U., and van Dijk, J.: Periodontal disease in Down's syndrome: A review, J. Clin. Periodontol. 13:64, 1986.

163. Rifkin, B.R., and Tai, H.H.: Elevated thromboxane B_2 levels in periodontal disease, J. Periodont. Res. 16:194, 1981.

164. Riott, I.M., Brostoff, J., and Male, D.K.: Immunology. St. Louis: C.V. Mosby Co., 1985.

165. Root, R.K., and Cohen, M.S.: Microbicidal mechanisms of phagocytic cells, Rev. Infect. Dis. 3:565, 1981.

166. Rostock, M.H., et al.: Severe gingival overgrowth associated with Cyclosporine therapy, J. Periodontol. 57:294, 1986.

167. Saglie, F.R.: A scanning electron microscope study of the relationship between the most apically located subgingival plaque and epithelial attachment, J. Periodontol. 48:105, 1977.

168. Saglie, F.R., et al.: The presence of bacteria in periodontal disease—1. A scanning and transmission electron microscopic study, J. Periodontol. 56:618, 1985.

169. Saglie, F.R., and Elbaz, J.J.: Bacterial penetration into the gingival tissue in periodontal disease, J. West. Soc. Periodont. 31:85, 1983.

170. Sanavi, F., et al.: The colonization and establishment of invading bacteria in periodontium of ligature -treated immunosuppressed rats, J. Periodontol. 56:273, 1985.

171. Sandholm, L: The cellular host response in juvenile periodontitis, J. Periodontol. 56:359, 1985.

172. Sanz, M., et al.: Invasion of junctional epithelium in human periodontitis by microorganisms, J. Dent. Res. 63:250, 1984.

173. Saxen, L., and Nevanlinna, H.R.: Autosomal recessive inheritance of juvenile periodontitis: Test of a hypothesis, Clin. Genet. 2:332, 1984.

174. Schenkein, H.A., and Genco, R.J.: Gingival fluid and serum in periodontal diseases. II. Evidence for cleavage of complement components C3, C3 proactivator (Factor B) and C4 in gingival fluid, J. Periodont. 48:778, 1977.

175. Schroeder, H.E.: Quantitative parameters of early human gingival inflammation, Arch. Oral Biol. 15:383, 1970.

176. Schroeder, H.E., et al: Correlated morphometric and biochemical analysis of early chronic gingivitis in man, Arch. Oral Biol. 18:899, 1973.

177. Schroeder, H.E.: Histopathology of the gingival sulcus. In The Borderland Between Caries and Periodontal Disease, ed. T. Lehner. London: Academic Press, 1977.

178. Schroeder, H.E., and Lindhe, J.: Conversion of established gingivitis in the dog into destructive periodontitis, Arch. Oral Biol. 20:775, 1975.

179. Schroeder, H.E.: Discussion: Pathogenesis of periodontitis, J. Clin. Periodontol. 13:426, 1986.

180. Sehgal, P.B., et al.: Human B_2 interferon and B-cell differentiating factor BSF-2 are identical, Science 235:731, 1987.

181. Seow, W.K., et al.: Modulatory effects of periodontopathic bacteria on polymorphonuclear leukocyte adherence, J. Dent. Res. 65:476 (abst.), 1986.

182. Seow, W.K., and Thong, Y.H.: Augmentation of human polymorphonuclear leukocyte adherence by interferon, Int. Arch. Allerg. Appl. Immunol. 79:305, 1986.

183. Seymour, G.J.: Possible mechanisms involved in the immuno-regulation of chronic inflammatory disease, J. Dent. Res. 66:2, 1987.

184. Seymour, G.J., and Mestecky, J.F.: The periodontium as a watershed between mucosal and systemic immunology, J. Dent. Res. 63:474, 1984.

185. Seymour, G.J., et al.: Conversion of a stable T-cell lesion to a progressive B-cell lesion in the pathogenesis of chronic inflammatory periodontal disease: An hypothesis, J. Clin. Periodontol. 6:267, 1979.

186. Shenker, B.J., and Dirienzo, J.M.: Suppression of human peripheral blood lymphocytes by Fusobacterium nucleatum, J. Immunol. 132:2357, 1984.

187. Slots, J., and Gibbons, R.J.: Attachment of Bacteroides melaninogenicus subsp. assaccharolyticus to oral surfaces and its possible role in colonization of the mouth and of periodontal pockets, Infection and Immunity, 19:254, 1978.

188. Slots, J., and Genco, R.J.: Black-pigmented Bacteroides species, Copnocytophagia species, and actinobacillus actinomycetemcomitans in human periodontal disease, J. Dent. Res. 63:412, 1984.

189. Slots, J.: Bacterial specificity in adult periodontitis—A summary of recent work, J. Clin. Periodontol. 13:912, 1986.

190. Smith, B.A., et al.: Increased concentrations of Fibronectin on healing after periodontal surgery, J. Dent. Res. 66 (Special Issue):150, abstr. no. 345, 1987.

191. Socransky, S.S., et al.: New concepts of destructive periodontal disease, J. Clin. Periodontol. 11:21, 1984.

192. Socransky, S.S.: Criteria for infectious agents in caries and periodontal disease, J. Clin. Periodontol. 6:16, 1979.

193. Spindler, S.J., et al.: Juvenile periodontitis. 1. Demonstration of local immunoglobulin synthesis, J. Periodontol. 57:300, 1986.

194. Stahl, S.S.: Repair potential of the soft tissue root interface, J. Periodontol. 48:545, 1977.

195. Stahl, S.S., et al.: Speculations about gingival repair, J. Periodontol. 43:395, 1972.

196. Stashenko, P.P., et al.: T cell responses of periodontal disease patients and healthy subjects to oral microorganisms, J. Periodont. Res. 18:587, 1983.

197. Stingl, G., et al.: The functional role of Langerhans cells, J. Invest. Dermatol. 74:315, 1980.

198. Stone, S., et al.: Scaling and gingival curettage. A radiographic study, J. Periodontol. 37:415, 1966.

199. Stossel, T.P.: Phagocytosis, Am. J. Pathol. 88:741, 1977.

200. Sutcliffe, P: A longitudinal study of gingivitis and puberty, J. Periodont. Res. 7:52, 1972.

201. Suzuki, J.B., et al.: Local and systemic production of immunoglobulins to periodopathogens in periodontal disease, J. Periodont. Res. 19:599, 1984.

202. Suzuki, J.B., et al.: Immunologic profile of juvenile periodontitis. II. Neutropphil chemotaxis, phagocytosis, and spore germination, J. Periodontol. 55:461, 1984.

203. Syrjanen, S., and Syrjanen, K.: Hyperplastic gingivitis in a child receiving sodium valporate treatment, Proc. Finn. Dent. Soc. 75:95, 1979.

204. Taichman, N.S., et al.: Neutrophil interactions with oral bacteria as a pathogenic mechanism in periodontal diseases, Advances in Inflammation Research 8:113, 1984.

205. Takeuchi, H., et al.: Oral microorganisms in the gingiva of individuals with periodontal disease, J. Dent. Res. 53:132, 1974.

206. Taubman, M.A., et al.: Association between systemic and local antibody and periodontal diseases. In Host Parasite Interactions in Periodontal Diseases, ed. R.J. Genco and S.E. Mergenhagen. Washington, D.C.: American Society for Microbiology, 1982.

207. Taubman, M.A., et al.: Periodontal bone loss in ovalbumin sensitized germfree rats fed antigen-free diet with ovalbumin, J. Periodont. Res. 18:292, 1983.

208. Taubman, M.A., et al.: Host response in experimental periodontal disease, J. Dent. Res. 63:455, 1984.
209. Tempel, T.: Host factors in periodontal disease. Periodontal manifestations of Chediak-Higashi syndrome, J. Periodont. Res. (Suppl.) 10:26, 1972.
210. Thielade, E.: The non specific theory in microbial etiology in inflammatory periodontal diseases, J. Clin. Periodontol. 13:905, 1986.
211. Thompson, R.A.: Familial defect of polymorph neutrophil phagocytosis associated with surface glycoprotein antigen (OKMI), Clin. Exp. Immunol. 58:229, 1984.
212. Tolo, K., and Brandtzaeg, P.: Relation between periodontal disease activity and serum antibody titers to oral bacteria. In Host-Parasite Interactions in Periodontal Diseases, ed. R.J. Genco and S.E. Mergenhagen. Washington, D.C.: American Society for Microbiology, 1982.
213. Van Dyke, T.E., et al.: The Papillon-LeFevre Syndrome: Neutrophil dysfunction with severe periodontal disease, Clin. Immunol. Immunopathol. 31:419, 1984.
214. Van Dyke, T.E., et al.:Neutrophil function and oral disease, J. Oral Pathol. 14:95, 1985.
215. Van Dyke, T.E., et al.: Neutrophil function in localized juvenile periodontitis phagocytosis, superoxide production and specific granule release, J. Periodontol. 57:703, 1986.
216. Van Dyke, T.E., et al.:Periodontal diseases and impaired neutrophil function, J. Periodont. Res. 17:492, 1982.
217. Van Dyke, T.E., et al.: Juvenile periodontitis as a model for neutrophil function: Reduced binding of complement chemotactic fragment, C5a, J. Dent. Res. 62:870, 1983.
218. Van Dyke, T.E., et al.: Periodontal diseases and neutrophil abnormalities. In Host-Parasite Interactions in Periodontal Diseases, ed. R.J. Genco and S.E. Mergenhagen. Washington, D.C.: American Society for Microbiology, 1982.
219. Van Dyke, T.E. et al.: Neutrophil chemotaxis dysfunction in human periodontitis. Infect. Immunity 27:124, 1980.
220. Walsh, L.J., et al.: Interleukin-1 modulates T6 expression on a putative intraepithelial Langerhans cell precursor population, J. Dent. Res. 65:1424, 1986.
221. Weinman, J.P., and Orban, B.: Diffuse atrophy of alveolar bone (periodontosis), J. Periodontol. 13:31, 1942.
222. Wilde, G., et al.: Host tissue response in chronic periodontal disease. VI. The role of cell-mediated hypersensitivity, J. Periodont. Res. 12:179, 1977.
223. Wilhelm, D.L.: Chemical mediators. In The Inflammatory Process, ed. B.W. Zweifach, et al. 2nd ed., Vol. II. New York: Academic Press, 1973.
224. Wilton, J.M.A.: The function of complement in crevicular fluid: In The Borderland Between Caries and Periodontal Disease, ed. T. Lehner. London: Academic Press, 1977.
225. Wilton, J.M.A.: Polymorphonuclear leukocytes of the human gingival crevice: Clinical and experimental studies and cellular function in humans and animals. In Host-Parasite Interactions in Periodontal Diseases, ed. R.J. Genco and S.F. Mergenhagen. Washington, D.C.: American Society for Microbiology, 1982.
226. Winkler, J.R., et al.: AIDS virus associated periodontal disease, J. Dent. Res. 65:741, abst. no. 139, 1986.
227. Wirthlin, M.R.: Current status of new attachment therapy, J. Periodontol. 52:529, 1981.
228. Wolbach, S.B., and Bessey, O.H., Tissue changes in vitamin deficiencies, Physiol. Rev. 22:233, 1942.
229. Wolff, L.F., et al.: Microbial interpretation of plaque relative to the diagnosis and treatment of periodontal disease, J. Periodontol. 56:281, 1985.
230. Wynn, S.E., et al.: In situ demonstration of natural killer (NK) cells in human gingival tissue, J. Periodontol. 57:699, 1986.
231. Yoshie, H., et al.: Periodontal bone loss and immune characteristics of congenitally athymic and thymic cell-reconstituted athymic rats, Infect. Immun. 50:403, 1985.
232. Yukna, R.A., et al.: A clinical study of healing in humans following the excisional new attachment procedure, J. Periodont. 47:696, 1976.
233. Zweifach, B.W.: Microvascular aspects of tissue injury. In The Inflammatory Process, ed. B.W. Zweifach et al. 2nd ed., Vol. II. New York: Academic Press, 1973.

10

THE ROLE OF OCCLUSION IN THE ETIOLOGY OF PERIODONTAL DISEASE

Faulty occlusal relationships of the teeth and abnormal occlusal forces may cause injury to the surface of the gingival tissues and/or induce traumatic lesions in the supporting periodontal structures. Occlusion may also indirectly affect the status (health or disease) of the periodontal tissues by interfering with plaque elimination and by influencing periodontal defense mechanisms. That influence may be expressed in reactions ranging from compensatory hypertrophy to disuse atrophy.

MALOCCLUSION AND PERIODONTAL DISEASE

Angle's classification of malocclusion is the most commonly used parameter for evaluating normal or abnormal occlusion.[4] Angle's assumption that malocclusion represented a periodontal handicap has since been questioned.[17] Most epidemiological studies on malocclusion and periodontal disease have been concerned with separate or combined effects of various specific occlusal features. An occlusion feature index for epidemiological assessment of specific aspects of abnormal occlusal relationships was developed at the National Institute of Dental Research. The following four occlusal features were included in the index:[45] (1) Mandibular crowding from cuspid to cuspid; (2) cusp-fossa relationships of the posterior teeth; (3) vertical overbite, measured by the portion of the mandibular incisors covered by the maxillary central incisors with the mandible in centric occlusion; and (4) horizontal overjet, measured from the incisal edge of the maxillary incisors to the labial surface of the mandibular incisors with the mandible in centric occlusion.

The PI index[51] was used to assess periodontal disease and the occlusal feature index to survey occlusion in 908 males between the ages of 17 and 26 years.[45] A positive correlation was found between the severity of periodontal disease and the extent of vertical overbite, abnormal posterior cuspal relationships, lower

anterior crowding, and horizontal overjet. Although some investigations have supported the concept of a weak correlation between features of malocclusion and severity of periodontal disease,[7,13,27,40] some have found no such correlation.[15,16,37,50]

It has been claimed that lower anterior crowding may enhance plaque retention and thus predispose to gingivitis, and that marked protrusion of maxillary anterior teeth will interfere with the normal lip seal, lead to mouthbreathing, and predispose to gingivitis.[14] The results of some surveys tend to confirm these assumptions,[37] while others refute them.[15,16] It appears that the important factor in the etiology of gingivitis for these patients is not the malocclusion itself but whether or not mouth-breathing occurs with the malocclusion.[32]

Recent studies indicate that malalignment of teeth decreases the effectiveness of the average type of oral hygiene and thus contributes to plaque retention and calculus formation and enhances severity of gingivitis. However, in persons with good oral hygiene, malposition of teeth is of no periodontal significance.[1,2]

Other occlusal abnormalities, such as crossbite[15,16] or extreme malposition or tipping of teeth, have been claimed to predispose to periodontal disease.[15,16,29,30,31,38] It appears, from studies of skulls[29] and from clinical observations, that prominent labial or lingual position of a tooth predisposes to both bony and gingival dehiscence, which may extend through the attached gingiva and into the alveolar mucosa.

Old observations[31] of unfavorable periodontal sequelae following loss of teeth and tipping often seem to be true,[15,16] but no correlation has been found between tooth irregularities and severity of periodontal disease in young patients on the basis of changes in axial inclination, displacement, or rotation of teeth.[6]

Malocclusion and periodontal disease cannot be studied in a meaningful way without an objective evaluation of the plaque and calculus present on the teeth. The main reason for the contradictory findings is probably related to differences in methods of evaluating the presence of local irritants and the severity of malocclusion.

TRAUMA FROM OCCLUSION AND PERIODONTAL DISEASE

Trauma from occlusion, by definition, is an injury to any part of the masticatory system resulting from abnormal occlusal contact relationships and/or from abnormal function or dysfunction of the masticatory system.[23,46] Trauma from occlusion thus may be manifest in the periodontium, hard structures of the teeth, pulp, temporomandibular joints, soft tissues of the mouth, and neuromuscular system.

However, in the context of periodontics, the term *trauma from occlusion* is usually applied to an occlusal periodontal relationship with evidence of traumatic periodontal injury. Trauma from occlusion refers to the effect of abnormal occlusal forces acting upon basically normal periodontal structures, while secondary trauma from occlusion refers to the effect of normal or abnormal occlusal forces on weakened periodontal structures. The term *traumatic occlusion* is used to characterize the specific occlusal features that lead to the trauma from occlusion.[23]

Historically, a number of reports have stated, on the basis of clinical observations, that trauma from occlusion is a significant causative factor in the etiology of periodontal disease.[33,39,56] However, epidemiological surveys utilizing scientifically sound scoring systems during the 1950s and 1960s established an overwhelmingly strong association between the presence of bacterial plaque or accretions on the teeth and incidence of periodontal disease.[48,52] Unfortunately, similar clinical scoring systems or indices for trauma from occlusion have not been developed. Thus, no epidemiological survey is available concerning the association or correlation between trauma from occlusion and periodontal disease. A study of vertical osseous defects showed no correlation with any occlusal factors; the only consistent correlation was with subgingival calculus.[19]

Present knowledge on the role of trauma from occlusion in the etiology of periodontal disease is only circumstantial and what it is based on is limited to clinical observations in humans and some experimental studies in animals. Admittedly, one study on humans reported increased tooth mobility, bone loss, and increased pocket depth associated with the presence of balancing interferences.[62] However, the alleged interferences were diagnosed from wear facets identified on casts, which cannot be accepted as documentation of occlusal interferences. In another study, no relationship between centric relation contacts and contacts in working, balancing, and protrusive mandibular movements related to severity of periodontal disease was found.[35]

A reduction in tooth mobility following occlusal adjustment has been reported,[41] indicating that occlusal interferences may influence tooth mobility. Increased tooth mobility, however, does not necessarily indicate the presence of trauma from occlusion[61] or relate directly to the severity of the periodontal disease.[42] The significance of tooth mobility in the diagnosis of trauma from occlusion will be discussed later in this chapter.

In appraising the significance to the peridontium of trauma from occlusion, it should be acknowledged that occlusal contacts registered as facet patterns on the teeth, and even occlusal interferences, do not necessarily mean trauma from occlusion, inasmuch as facets of wear may be produced by normal functional contacts, and occlusal interferences may be bypassed by the patient's neuromuscular mechanisms without trauma to any part of the masticatory system.

Because trauma from occlusion involves a harmful effect (an injury), it can, for ethical reasons, be studied experimentally only in animals and observed clinically in humans only as it may occur naturally or as a nonstandardized, iatrogenic side-effect of dental treatment.

PERIODONTAL DISEASE AND EXPERIMENTALLY INDUCED TRAUMA FROM OCCLUSION

A large number of animal studies and some human biopsy and autopsy studies have established in detail the histological features of trauma from occlusion in the periodontal tissues. In only a few exceptional cases of experimental trauma from occlusion has apical movement of the junctional epithelium been related to the trauma from occlusion.[9,36,57,60] In the overwhelming majority of well controlled experimental studies, gingival inflammation or pocket formation has not developed from traumatic occlusion.[12,59,61] Perhaps the supracrestal gingival fibers (Fig. 10-1) constitute a barrier against spread of inflammation and downgrowth of the junctional epithelium.[12] It is further assumed that the abundant gingival blood supply is unaffected by traumatic injury.[11] It has been reported that the connective tissue underlying the junctional epithelium gets its blood supply through the periodontal membrane and thus could be affected by periodontal trauma.[43]

A concept that trauma from occlusion is a "co-destructive" factor in periodontitis suggests that occlusal forces alter the alignment of transceptal and alveolar crest fibers so that the pathway of the gingival inflammation extends directly into the periodontal ligament.[20,21] Thus, excessive occlusal forces would produce periodontal membrane damage and bone resorption and so aggravate the tissue destruction caused

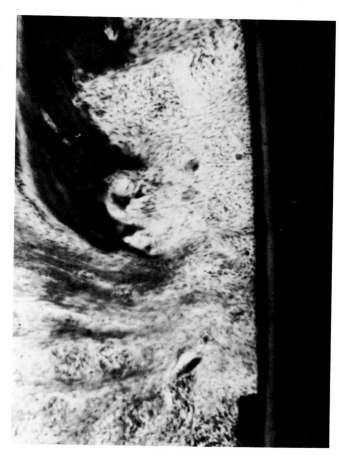

Fig. 10-1. Experimental trauma from occlusion. Maxillary central incisor in rhesus monkey. Note intact supracrestal fibers between the alveolar crest and the junctional epithelium.

by the inflammation. According to this concept, trauma from occlusion, combined with inflammation, would produce intrabony pockets, angular and crater-like osseous defects, and excessive tooth mobility.

Some investigators have failed to produce periodontal pockets by combining gingival irritation and trauma from occlusion,[12] and the spread of gingival inflammation into the periodontal membrane that is alleged to be associated with trauma from occlusion has not been consistently observed in animals[34] or in human biopsy[54] and autopsy material.[24] In a study, deepening of experimentally induced periodontal pockets and bone resorption were accelerated by progressive traumatic occlusion over a period of 6 months.[36]

Experimental studies in animals have established that transient periodontal trauma from occlusion and increased tooth mobility associated with jiggling of teeth may result in a widening of the periodontal space, eventually allowing the experimentally induced movements of the teeth to take place without any evidence of traumatic injury to the periodontium.[12,22,58,61] Thus, the initial increase in tooth mobility

was the result of repeated traumatic injuries to the periodontal structures, but, as repair took place and the movement pattern was repeated within limited or self-limiting boundaries, the mobility of the teeth was maintained without any evidence of sustained traumatic lesions in the periodontium. The role of trauma from occlusion in the pathogenesis of periodontal disease in humans certainly cannot be assessed on the basis of animal studies; however, such studies do provide important information regarding similar basic biologic reactions.

CLINICAL OBSERVATIONS AND CONCEPTS

The prevailing confusion regarding the role of trauma from occlusion in the etiology of periodontal disease stems basically from a lack of established diagnostic criteria for what constitutes periodontal trauma from occlusion on a clinical level. A common mistake in diagnosis is to equate increase in tooth mobility with trauma from occlusion. In order to make a diagnosis of trauma from occlusion, there has to be evidence of recognizable injury at the time of the examination. Such evidence is difficult to obtain, since most instances of traumatic occlusion are transient in nature.

Tooth movements, repair, and compensatory changes in the periodontal structures will usually eliminate clinical evidence of trauma from occlusion. Without periodontal or pulpal pain or tenderness, or roentgenographic evidence of active bone resorption, the occlusion cannot be diagnosed as traumatic occlusion. Such is the case even though histologic evidence of previous resorption and repair (partial or complete) may persist.

The presence or absence of increased vascular permeability may, as suggested many years ago,[26] be useful as a basis for diagnosing active trauma from occlusion in experimental animals.[58] Intially, as a result of trauma, there may be changes both in position and mobility patterns of the teeth, but after completion of a reparative phase following this initial trauma, an adaptive phase, with increased mobility, may persist indefinitely without evidence of new trauma.[58] The increased mobility, however, indicates hyperfunction related to the available support of the tooth, and a return to a normal mobility would indicate a more desirable balance in the dynamic interplay between occlusal forces and periodontal support.

The supporting periodontal structures may undergo a series of reversible changes in response to variations in occlusal load on the teeth or to altered quantity and quality of support. Such changes are clinically manifested in altered tooth mobility according to the following principles (Fig. 10-2).

hypofunction→disuse atrophy→low mobility

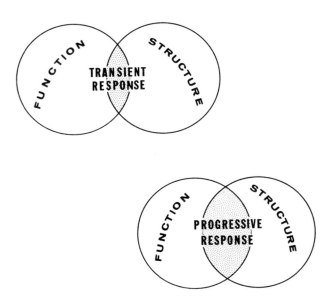

Fig. 10-2. The response of the supporting structures to function may be small and transient, as required for homeostasis, and be reflected in tooth mobility. Responses that reflect a continuous exceeding of homeostasis are progressive, nonadapting, and destructive. The state rather than the degree of mobility is then the primary concern in trauma from occlusion.

normal function→normal structure→normal mobility

hyperfunction→hypertrophy→increased mobility

As indicated by the arrows, adaptive or pathological periodontal changes may develop as the functional status is altered, but not necessarily in the order listed above, since trauma may, for example, be inflicted through adaptive steps of function and hyperfunction. The most confusing aspect clinically is that both hyperfunction within the adaptive physiological limits and traumatic occlusion are expressed as increased mobility. This means that other signs and symptoms beyond mobility are needed by the dentist to establish the diagnosis of trauma from occlusion. Such evidence might be soreness to pressure and/or roentgenographic evidence of active bone resorption (Fig. 10-3).

Self-limited mobility is a greater than normal, but constant, tooth mobility based on a physiological balance between the occlusal forces and the adaptive capacity of the periodontium. "Self-limited" implies that the progression of tooth movement has been stopped without splinting or other mechanical stabilization of the teeth. In persons with bruxism and normal periodontal support, one may find an increased widening of the periodontal space and a normal lamina dura, but no evidence of active trauma from occlusion (Fig. 10-4). The increased mobility apparently reaches a self-limited stage through periodontal adaptation to the abnormal occlusal forces.

Another example of self-limited mobility is often seen in the mandibular incisor region following periodontal treatment of teeth with advanced bone loss. Lingual movement of the teeth is usually limited or stopped as the impact of occlusal forces is dissipated to the adjacent teeth through interproximal contacts. When the teeth are apart, there is a tendency for the tongue to impose a labially directed force, which may be great enough to move teeth that have minimal support labially. Because the tongue force is constant and the periodontal support level is kept constant following the periodontal therapy, a nontraumatic balance between force and periodontal adaptation may develop, while in lingual and interproximal directions the movement patterns associated with the occlusal forces are self-limited by the contact relations of the teeth.

Abnormal mobility of this constant and limited type is compatible with periodontal health and normal function, and such teeth have excellent long-term prognoses despite the increased mobility and the widened periodontal space seen in the roentgenograms (Fig. 10-5).

Self-limited mobility without trauma from occlusion may also be established following periodontal treatment and occlusal adjustment for teeth with functional interproximal contacts but with anatomical possibility for buccolingual movement. When such teeth are

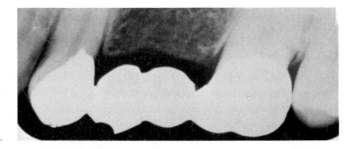

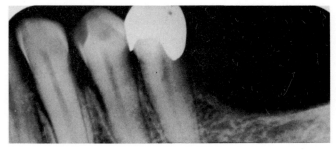

Fig. 10-3. Lamina dura at the mesial surface of the mandibular first bicuspid is well defined in spite of the widened periodontal space. The tooth has increased mobility but no signs of trauma from occlusion. The lamina dura at the mesial aspect of the second bicuspid is poorly defined, indicating resorption and repair. This tooth also has increased mobility caused by clasp arrangements on a free end saddle partial denture. This tooth also is sore to occlusal pressure and thus shows both roentgenologic and clinical signs of trauma from occlusion.

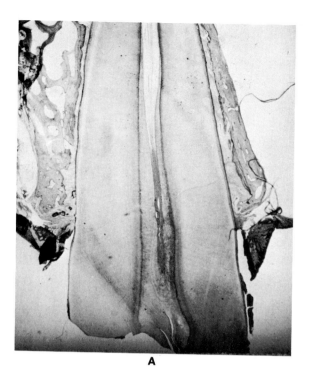

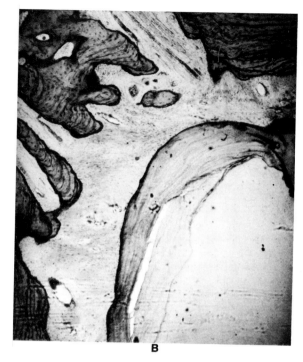

A

B

Fig. 10-4. *A,* Autopsy specimen of maxillary cuspid with extensive occlusal wear extending into secondary dentin in the previous pulp chamber. The periodontal space is two to three times wider at the alveolar crest as at the apical third of the root. The alveolar bone is very heavy, but there are no signs of active trauma from occlusion. *B,* Higher magnification of the apical area of the same tooth as in *A.* Note lamellated bone at the apical fundus of the alveolus and deposition lines in the apical cementum. Both these phenomena indicate compensatory eruption but not trauma in response to the severe occlusal attrition.

ground out of contact in lateral and protrusive excursions, the possibility of buccolingual mobility caused by bruxism is practically eliminated, and the eccentric forces from mastication (without actual tooth contact in these excursions) may be reduced to the tolerance level of the adaptive capacity of the periodontium. Following adequate periodontal therapy, such teeth often settle down to a constant mobility level, with a well defined lamina dura and a healthy periodontium. Grinding the teeth out of eccentric contacts thus may change progressive traumatic injury with increasing mobility to a nontraumatic, self-limited mobility, so long as there is no further progression of the periodontitis.

It has long been established that transient trauma from occlusion associated with orthodontic tooth movement, or from premature occlusal contacts from which teeth can move away, does not significantly alter gingival inflammation or the position of the epithelial attachment relative to the cementoenamel junction. It also appears that jiggling of teeth, both in humans[47] and in animals,[59] within a defined, limited range of movement, does not have any significant effect on the health status of the gingival tissues or pocket formation so long as the mobility is self-limiting.

However, selective indicants of destructive periodontal disease have been observed along teeth with

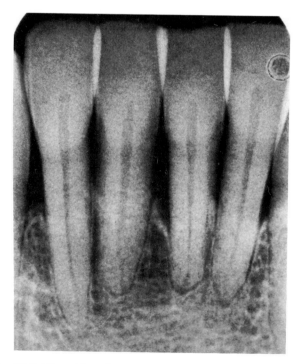

Fig. 10-5. The widened periodontal space bordered by a well-defined lamina dura in this mandibular incisor has been observed in an unaltered state over 15 years. The tooth has greater than normal mobility, but the mobility has not increased during the 15 years of observation.

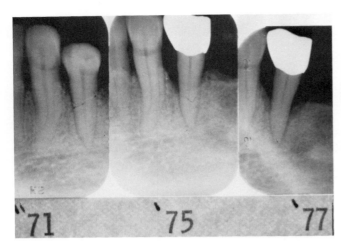

Fig. 10-6. Mandibular first bicuspid used as abutment for free-end saddle partial denture in 1971. Progressive bone loss was noted in 1975 and 1977. The mobility of this tooth also became gradually more severe and periodontal pockets developed, while the adjacent nontraumatized cuspid did not lose any bone.

progressive trauma from occlusion over several months or years. A typical example (Fig. 10-6) of such situations occurs with abutment teeth for free-end saddle partial dentures, where continuous ridge resorption in the saddle areas produces progressive trauma to the abutment teeth. With teeth subject to marginal irritation from plaque retention, clasps, and faulty framework connection with the teeth, there is, in addition to the trauma, a tendency for more rapid periodontal destruction to occur than for the other teeth in the same mouth.

Another example of continuous trauma from occlusion and accelerated periodontal breakdown occurs with teeth undergoing progressive tipping, in which the traumatic effect tends to increase with the increasing degree of tipping (Fig. 10-7). Unbalanced cantilevers on bridges may also lead to a progressively increasing traumatic effect as supporting structures for the tooth or teeth are lost, with gradually decreasing periodontal structures available to withstand the impact of the traumatizing forces. An unstable malocclusion, in which occlusal forces and lip and tongue pressure move the teeth in opposite directions, may also create progressive trauma from occlusion and lead to accelerated periodontal destruction.[49] Another example of periodontal breakdown associated with excessive occlusal forces is sometimes seen when the occlusal vertical dimension is being maintained by only one or two occlusal units, due to either loss of teeth or extreme malocclusion. It is an old observation that habit patterns such as biting on pencils or fingernails also may result in localized periodontal breakdown.[53]

Whether severely altered or grossly inadequate occlusion will lead to progressive periodontal breakdown depends to a great extent on the presence or absence of bruxism (Fig. 10-8), and on the amount of remaining support for the teeth, as well as on the individual biological potential for favorable periodontal response to the abnormal forces. It may also be assumed that the severity of the marginal gingival irritation at the onset of the trauma from occlusion will greatly influence the role of the trauma from occlusion in the progression of the periodontal destruction.[23]

The role of trauma from occlusion in destructive periodontal disease appears to increase with decrease in remaining support for the teeth, especially when the loss of support is associated with untreated periodontal pockets. The severity of the trauma is apt to increase with decreased support, while the retention of irritants in the periodontal pockets also increases with increase in pocket depth, thus aggravating both the trauma and the inflammation. In this context, it may be noted that inducing trauma from occlusion in dogs that already had periodontal pockets merely accelerated periodontal destruction, while in dogs without periodontal pockets, no pockets developed in association with the trauma.[59] However, it should not be overlooked that continued trauma from occlusion was maintained during the entire experimental period, as was evident in the steadily increasing mobility and capillary permeability for the dogs that showed deepening of the pockets. The dogs without pockets underwent only a transient period of 2 months of trauma from occlusion, because after that time the widened periodontal space and the healed periodontal tissues allowed for the self-limited jiggling of the teeth without further trauma from the occlusion or increase in tooth mobility. Thus, it cannot be concluded from this study that long-term trauma from occlusion will not induce pocket formation, since progressive trauma from occlusion was not maintained beyond 2 months.

CURRENT CONCEPTS OF TRAUMA FROM OCCLUSION

On the basis of experimental evidence and clinical observation, the following tentative statements may be made regarding the role of trauma from occlusion in the pathogenesis of periodontal disease. Some of these statements may have to be revised as more scientific knowledge becomes available

1. Transient trauma from occlusion will not initiate nor aggravate marginal gingivitis, nor will it initiate formation of periodontal pockets.

2. Trauma from occlusion will contribute to increased tooth mobility; however, greater-than-normal tooth mobility is not necessarily diagnostic of trauma from occlusion, since compensatory widening of the periodontal space may have taken place before the assessment of the mobility.

3. Progressive trauma from occlusion without self-

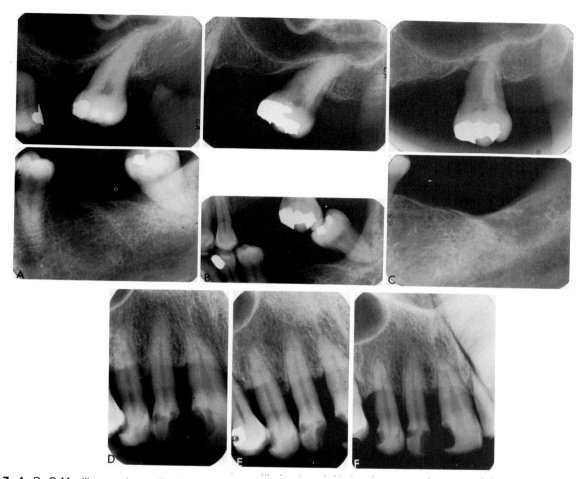

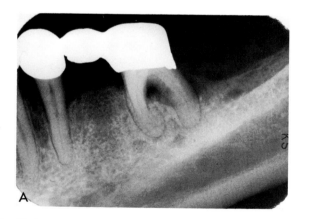

Fig. 10-7. *A, B, C* Maxillary and mandibular tipped third molars over a time span of 3 years. Note the progressive loss on bone especially at the mesial side and the final loss of the mandibular third molar as they tipped more and more. These teeth became increasingly more mobile despite periodontal therapy and recall for prophylaxis every 3 months. *D, E, F,* Roentgenograms of anterior teeth from the same patient and treated in the same way and over the same period of time as the molars. There was no indication of progressive trauma from occlusion on the anterior teeth and no noticeable loss of periodontal support.

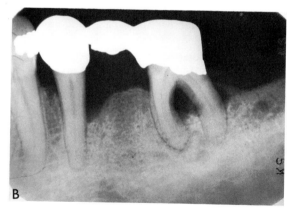

Fig. 10-8. *A, B,* Rapid periodontal breakdown associated with bruxism in an almost plaque-free mouth. Only 1 year separates the 2 roentgenograms.

limiting features tends to accelerate pocket formation and bone loss. This type of trauma from occlusion may be seen associated with unstable malocclusion and faulty dental restorations or appliances, and in cases of advanced periodontal disease with secondary trauma from occlusion. The modes of interaction between the trauma and the deepening of the pockets are not known.

4. Both primary and secondary types of trauma from occlusion are often related to bruxism, which becomes an especially significant factor in perpetuating the trauma in patients with advanced loss of periodontal support.

5. The periodontal significance of trauma from occlusion in patients with periodontitis also depends on the magnitude of the irritants in the periodontal pockets.

6. Trauma from occlusion probably plays a very minor role, if any, in the pathogenesis of early to moderate periodontitis.

Orthodontic movement of teeth with periodontal pockets will often result in periodontal abscesses if the teeth have not been scaled, while orthodontic treatment following scaling and root planing can usually be carried out without any detrimental periodontal effect. Thus, even transient trauma from occlusion may contribute to the progress of periodontitis, especially in teeth with intrabony pockets or furcation involvements, where there is no supracrestal "buffer zone" of transseptal or gingival fibers (Fig. 10-1) between the junctional epithelium and the traumatic periodontal injury. However, the hypothesis that intrabony pockets are usually the result of the pathway of the inflammation having been changed by trauma from occlusions has not been confirmed.[19]

Very few patients have evidence of progressive trauma from occlusion. The role of progressive trauma from occlusion both in the pathogenesis of pockets and in treatment may be considerably greater, however, for patients with advanced loss of periodontal support.

GINGIVAL TRAUMA FROM OCCLUSION

Although gingival lesions resulting from impinging overbite or shearing occlusion are not traditionally included in the concept of trauma from occlusion, they do represent periodontal injury caused by abnormal occlusion and should be considered as an occlusal factor in the etiology of periodontal disease. Such lesions have more inflammatory manifestations that do the traumatic lesions in the periodontal membrane, and the inflammatory response involves tissues at the dentogingival junction, where inflammation may lead to apically directed migration of the junctional epithelium. Trauma to the gingiva thus may induce and aggravate both gingivitis and periodontitis. Impinging overbite, with the mandibular incisors biting into the palatal mucosa and the maxillary incisors striking the labial mandibular gingiva, will rarely result in significant loss of periodontal support as long as all posterior teeth are present to maintain occlusal vertical dimension and the anterior teeth are kept scrupulously clean. The potential for wedging of hard food particles

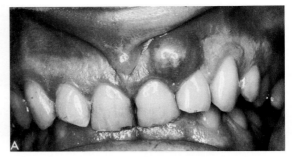

Fig. 10-9. Periodontal abscess caused by a cornhusk shred wedged into the palatal gingival sulcus of the central incisor.

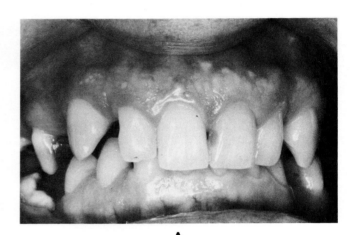

A

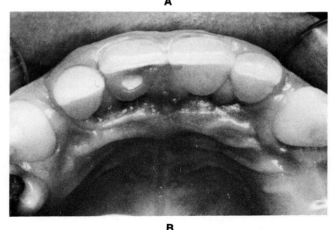

B

Fig. 10-10. *A, B,* Palatal gingival trauma associated with impinging overbite.

or other foreign bodies into the gingival crevice with subsequent inflammation or even abscess is of course much higher for impinging overbite than for normal occlusion (Fig. 10-9). The clinical significance of such malocclusion increases markedly with the loss of posterior teeth and the lowering of vertical dimension (Fig. 10-10).

A detrimental periodontal effect of faulty interprox-

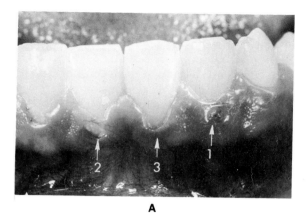

A

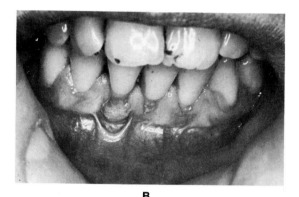

B

Fig. 10-11. *A,* Stages in gingival fenestration in a 14 year old. *1,* Early passage from crevice to gingival surface; *2,* almost complete loss of tissue; *3,* recession of gingiva via fenestration. *B,* Advanced recession with heavy deposits of calculus.

imal contacts and food impaction was described as early as 1930.[30] Food impaction may result from open contacts, faulty contacts with inadequate marginal ridges, plunger cusp effects, and occlusal interferences moving teeth during function.[54] The specific significance of food impaction in the etiology of periodontal disease has not been established on a scientific basis. A "mild correlation" between food impaction and attachment loss was reported in one epidemiological survey,[18] while another survey found no significant relationship between open contacts and bone loss.[35] It is often impossible to assess whether the contact was open initially and induced the food impaction, or whether the contact became open as a result of the periodontal disease. Open contacts without food impaction are generally considered to be of no periodontal significance. In spite of conflicting statements in the literature, clinical observations tend to support the concept that food impaction is a contributory factor in the etiology of periodontal disease.

Fractures of teeth, especially longitudinal hairline

fractures of molars associated with bruxism, may induce combined pulpal and periodontal lesions affecting the periodontal attachment.[28]

Claims that trauma from occlusion may lead to thickening of the free gingival margin[55] (McCall's festoons), gingival dehiscence (Stillman's clefts), or gingival recession have not been supported by research findings. Such concepts seem to lack scientific rationales based on current knowledge of periodontal physiology and pathology. Clefts are usually the result of calculus or faulty tooth-brushing (Fig. 10-11).

PERIODONTAL SIGNIFICANCE OF NONFUCTIONING OCCLUSION

The common sequela of nonfuction is atrophy of the periodontal structures and the supporting bone, accompanied by a tendency toward extrusion, especially of the maxillary posterior teeth. The periodontal effect of nonfunction versus function was studied in rhesus monkeys following extraction of all mandibular teeth on one side.[44] Observations over periods of up to 3 years indicated that gingival inflammation, plaque, and calculus formation all were more severe associated with the maxillary nonfunctioning than with the functioning teeth. As the nonfunctioning teeth erupted, bone was deposited on the alveolar process, but not fast enough to keep up with the eruption. The distance between the cementoenamel junction and the alveolar crest therefore increased more on the nonfunctioning than on the functioning side, meaning that the nonfunctioning teeth ended up with less bony support. The distance between the cementoenamel junction and the bottom of the epithelial attachment also become greater on the nonfunctioning than on the functioning side. However, this greater loss of attachment may have been related to the increased plaque and calculus formation rather than a direct effect of nonfunction. A marked decrease in width and alteration in structure of the periodontal membrane developed on the nonfunctioning side (Fig. 10-12). The findings of enhanced plaque retention and gingival inflammation related to nonfunction in monkeys have also been confirmed in humans.[2] Good oral hygiene can compensate for the natural tendency toward more severe gingivitis on the nonfunctioning than on the functioning side. The possible relationship between degree of inflammation and rate of eruption, as well as the failure to maintain alveolar crest height in nonfunction, is unknown.

A beneficial periodontal effect of heavy function has been postulated for primitive people such as Eskimos and Australian aborigines. It appears that these people, who depend on heavy occlusal function for survival, have an unusually high resistance to pocket formation, despite extensive plaque and calculus accumulation on their teeth.[5] When individuals from those

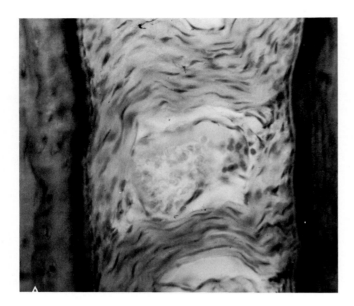

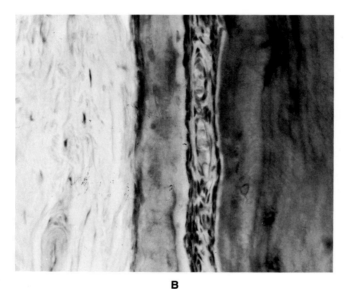

B

Fig. 10-12. *A,* Periodontium subjected to heavy occlusal function in a monkey. *B,* Periodontium after 3 years of nonfunction in the same monkey. The magnification is the same for both photographs. Note the narrow periodontal space, the thin alveolar process and thick cementum associated with nonfunction *(B).*

ethnic groups have changed to a softer diet requiring less occlusal function, their periodontal health has deteriorated.

It seems reasonable that the heavy collagenous fiber complex of a well-functioning periodontium would provide more resistance to penetration of inflammation than would the loose connective tissues making up the periodontium of nonfunctioning teeth. Functional movement of the teeth may also enhance the protective mechanisms of the gingival sulcus.

SUMMARY

Malocclusion may interfere with functional and artifical plaque removal and thus enhance the development of periodontal disease.

Only extreme degrees of malocclusion predispose to periodontal trauma from occlusion.

Progressive trauma from occlusion may reach a nontraumatic stage of periodontal adaptation related to limitations of the field of traumatic occlusal impact, and a constant, self-limited mobility pattern may ensue.

The role of trauma from occlusion in the pathogenesis of periodontal disease is still controversial, but experimental evidence and clinical observations indicate that periodontal pocket formation may be accelerated by progressive long-term trauma from occlusion.

Transient or short-term trauma from occlusion has no significant effect upon the status of the gingiva.

Mechanical gingival trauma from impingement or food impaction may cause and aggravate periodontal disease.

Nonfunction will alter the periodontium structurally and enhance plaque retention. However, with good oral hygiene, loss of periodontal support is not directly related to nonfunction.

REFERENCES

1. Ainamo, J.: Relationship between malalignment of teeth and periodontal disease, Scand. J. Dent. Res. 80:104, 1972.
2. Alexander, A.H.: The effect of lack of function of teeth on gingival health, plaque and calculus accumulation, J. Periodont. 41:438, 1970.
3. Alexander, A.G., and Tipnis, A.K.: The effect of irregularity of teeth and the degree of overbite and overjet on the gingival health. A study of 400 subjects, Br. Dent. J. 128:539, 1970.
4. Angle, E.H.: Classification of malocclusion, Dent. Cosmos 41:248, 305, 1899.
5. Baarregaard, A.: Dental condition and nutrition among natives in Greenland, Oral Surg. 2:995, 1949.
6. Beagrie, G.S., and James, G.A.: The association of posterior tooth irregularity and periodontal disease, Br. Dent. J. 113:239, 1962.
7. Bilimoria, K.F.: Malocclusion—its role in the causation of periodontal disease, J. All-India Dent. Ass. 35:293, 1963.
8. Box, H.K.: Treatment of the Periodontal Pocket, Toronto: University of Toronto Press, 1928.
9. Box, H.R.: Experimental traumatogenic occlusion in sheep, Oral Health 25:9, 1935.
10. Buckley, L.A.: The relationship between malocclusion and periodontal disease, J. Periodont. 43:415, 1972.
11. Cohen, D.W., et al.: Effects of excessive occlusal forces on the gingival blood supply, J. Dent. Res. 39:677, 1960.
12. Comar, M.D., Kollar, J.A., and Gargulo, A.W.: Local irritation and occlusal trauma as co-factors in the periodontal disease process, J. Periodont. 40:193, 1969.
13. Ditto, W.M., and Hall, D.C.: The survey of 143 periodontal cases in terms of age and malocclusion, Am. J. Ortho. 40:234, 1954.
14. Emslie, R.: The incisal relationship and periodontal disease, Parodontologie 12:15, 1958.
15. Geiger, A.M.: Occlusal studies in 188 consecutive cases of

periodontal disease, Am. J. Ortho. 48:330, 1962.

16. Geiger, A.M.: Occlusion in periodontal disease, J. Periodont. 36:378, 1965.

17. Geiger, A.M., Wassermann, B.H., Thompson, R.H., and Turgeon, L.R.: Relationship of occlusion and periodontal disease. V. Relation of classification of occlusion to periodontal status and gingival inflammation, J. Periodont. 43:554, 1972.

18. Gilmore, N.D.: An epidemiological investigation of vertical osseous defects in periodontal disease, Thesis, The University of Michigan, 1970.

19. Gilmore, N.D., and Russell, A.L.: A clinical epidemiological study of vertical osseous defects of the periodontium, J. Periodont. Res. (Suppl.) 10:17, 1972.

20. Glickman, I., and Smulow, J.B.: Alterations in the pathway of gingival inflammation into the underlying tissues induced by excessive occlusal forces, J. Periodont. 33:7, 1962.

21. Glickman, I.: Inflammation and trauma from occlusion co-destructive factors in chronic periodontal disease, J. Periodont. 34:5, 1963.

22. Glickman, I., and Smulow, J.B.: Adaptive alterations in the periodontium of the Rhesus monkey in chronic trauma from occlusion, J. Periodont. 39:101, 1968.

23. Glickman, I., and Smulow, J.B.: The combined effects of inflammation and trauma from occlusion in periodontitis, Int. Dent. J. 19:393, 1969.

24. Goldman, H.M.: Extension of exudate into supporting structures of teeth in marginal periodontitis, J. Periodont. 28:175, 1957.

25. Gottlieb, B., and Orban, B.: Die Veränderungen der Gewebe in übermässiger Beanspruchung der Zähne, Leipzig: G. Thieme, 1931.

26. Häuple, K: Über die feingeweblichen Veränderungen bei funktionell bedingtem Knochenumbau, Odont. Tidskr. 60:209, 1952.

27. Hellgren, A.L.: The association between crowding of the teeth and gingivitis. Report of the 32nd Congress of European orthodontic Society, The Hague, Netherlands, Albani, 1956, pp. 134-140.

28. Hiatt, W.H.: Incomplete crown-root fractures in pulpal-periodontal disease, J. Periodont. 44:369, 1973.

29. Hirschfeld, I.: A study of skulls in the American Museum of Natural History in relation to periodontal disease, J. Dent. Res. 5:241, 1923.

30. Hirschfeld, I.: Food impaction, J. A. D. A. 17:1504, 1930.

31. Hirschfeld, I.: The individual missing tooth: A factor in dental and periodontal disease, J. A. D. A. 24:67, 1937.

32. Jacobson, L., and Linder-Aronson, S.: Crowding and gingivitis: A comparison between mouthbreathers and nosebreathers, Scand. J. Dent. Res. 80:500, 1972.

33. Karolyi, M.: Beobachtungen über Pyorrhea alveolaris, Oest.-Ung. Vierteljahrschr. Zahnheilkd. 17:279, 1901.

34. Kenney, E.B.: A histologic study of incisal dysfunction and gingival inflammation in the rhesus monkey, J. Periodont. 42:3, 1971.

35. Knowles, J.W.: Occlusal interferences and periodontal disease, Thesis, The University of Michigan, 1966.

36. Lindhe, J., and Svanberg, G.: Influence of trauma from occlusion on progression of experimental periodontitis in the beagle dog, J. Clin. Periodontol. 1:3, 1974.

37. Massler, M., and Savara, B.S.: Relation of gingivitis to dental caries and malocclusion in children 14 to 17 years of age, J. Periodont. 22:87, 1951.

38. McCall, J.O.: Tooth malposition as a factor in periodontal disease, N. Y. J. Dent. 1:23, 1931.

39. McCall, J.O.: Traumatic occlusion, J. A. D. A. 26:519, 1939.

40. McCombie, F., and Stothard, O.L.: Relationship between gingivitis and other dental conditions, Can. Dent. Ass. J. 30:506, 1964.

41. Mühlemann, H.R., Herzog, H., and Rateitschak, K.H.: Quantitative evaluation of the therapeutic effect of selective grinding, J. Periodont. 22:11, 1957.

42. Mühlemann, H.R., Savdir, S., and Rateitschak, K.H.: Tooth mobility—its causes and significance, J. Periodont. 36:148, 1965.

43. Nuki, K., and Hock, J.: The organization of the gingival vasculature, J. Periodont. Res. 9:305, 1974.

44. Philstrom, B.L., and Ramfjord, S.P.: Periodontal effect of nonfunction in monkeys, J. Periodont. 42:748, 1971.

45. Poulton, D.R., and Aaronson, S.A.: The relationship between occlusion and periodontal status, Am. J. Ortho. 47:690, 1961.

46. Ramfjord, S.P., Kerr, D.A., and Ash, M.M., eds.: Proceedings of the World Workshop in Periodontics, 1966, Ann Arbor, Michigan: The University of Michigan, 1966.

47. Ramfjord, S.P., et al.: Subgingival curettage versus surgical elimination of periodontal pockets, J. Periodont. 39:167, 1968.

48. Ramfjord, S.P., et al.: Epidemiological studies of periodontal diseases, Am. J. Public Health 58:1713, 1968.

49. Ramfjord, S.P., and Ash, M.M., Jr.: Occlusion, 3rd ed. Philadelphia: W.B. Saunders Co., 1982.

50. Razdan, D.P., and Chawla, T.M.: Malocclusion—its association with periodontal disease, J. Indian Dent. Assoc. 42:39, 1970.

51. Russell, A.L.: A system of classification and scoring for prevalence surveys of periodontal disease, J. Dent. Res. 35:350, 1956.

52. Russell, A.L.: International nutrition surveys: A summary of preliminary dental findings, J. Dent. Res. 42:233, 1963.

53. Sorrin, S.: Habit, an etiologic factor of periodontal disease, Dent. Dig. 41:290, 1935.

54. Stahl, S.S.: The response of the periodontium to combined gingival inflammation and occluso-functional stress in four human surgical specimens, Periodontics 6:14, 1968.

55. Stillman, P.R., and McCall, J.O.: Textbook of Clinical Periodontia. New York: Macmillan Co., 1937.

56. Stillman, P.R.: The management of pyorrhea, Dent. Cosmos 59:405, 1917.

57. Stones, H.H.: An experimental investigation into the association of traumatic occlusion with periodontal disease, P. Roy. S. Med. 31:479, 1938.

58. Svanberg, G., and Lindhe, J.: Vascular reactions in the periodontal ligament incident to trauma from occlusion, J. Clin. Periodontol. 1:58, 1974.

59. Svanberg, G.: Influence of trauma from occlusion on the periodontium of dogs with normal or inflamed gingiva, Odontol. Revy 25:165, 1974.

60. Waerhaug, J., and Hansen, E.R.: Periodontal changes incidental to prolonged occlusal overload in monkeys, Acta Odont. Scand. 24:91, 1966.

61. Wentz, F.M., Jarabak, J., and Orban, B.: Experimental occlusal trauma initiating cuspal interferences, J. Periodont. 29:117, 1958.

62. Youdelis, R.A., and Mann, W.V.: The prevalence and possible role of nonworking contacts in periodontal disease, Periodontics 3:219, 1965.

11

EXAMINATION AND DIAGNOSIS

The basis for an accurate diagnosis and treatment plan is the systematic collection of data about the patient that are relevant to the prevention or treatment of periodontal disease. The subjective examination (interview) provides the examiner with an opportunity to obtain the patient's chief concern or reason for seeking treatment, his or her past history of dental treatment, and his or her past medical history. The physical examination consists of an evaluation of the oral structures, especially the periodontium, and the paraoral structures for signs of disease.

EXAMINATION

A comprehensive examination should include (1) the case history, (2) the clinical examination, (3) the diagnosis, and (4) the treatment plan. For obvious reasons, the clinical examination must largely be limited to the periodontium; however, it is expected that in clinical practice all the elements of the clinical examination will be covered in the oral examination.

CASE HISTORY

The case history provides the clinician with the opportunity to obtain the patient's chief complaint (if any), a review of the present illness and past dental and medical history, and a review of the systems (e.g., the cardiovascular system). The objectives of the case history are directed toward forming a tentative diagnosis and determining any systemic factors that might affect the diagnosis or influence the treatment plan.

The *chief complaint* is a description by the patient of the symptoms related to the disease for which treatment is being sought. From the standpoint of periodontal disease, the chief complaint does not usually relate to a symptom, except in the presence of acute necrotizing gingivitis or a periodontal abscess.

The *present illness* is a chronological account of the problem indicated by the chief complaint. Previous diagnoses and treatments rendered, as well as the effectiveness of those treatments, should be noted at this point in the case history. This part of the examination is often facilitated if the patient has completed a health questionnaire, such as a modified Cornell Medical Index Health Questionnaire. However, such a questionnaire is not a substitute for a comprehensive history.

The *past history* consists of the patient's previous experience of oral diseases and systemic diseases, and his treatment for those diseases. The past dental history should acquaint the dentist with the patient's previous dental treatment, professional and home-care procedures, frequency and nature of professional care, reasons for prior extractions of teeth, history of prior dental and periodontal disease, and bleeding and anesthetic problems in previous dental procedures. All these data aid in the development of the diagnosis and prognosis, and may have a significant influence on the plan of treatment.

The past medical history includes the patient's past systemic diseases, injuries and operations, and childhood diseases and sequelae. Of particular importance is a history of rheumatic fever or valvular defects of the heart for which premedication is required.

The objectives of the medical history are (1) to provide information about the whole patient that will aid in forming the diagnosis; (2) to determine systemic factors or disease that will require special considerations prior to, during, and after periodontal therapy; and (3) to alert the clinician to any past or present disease processes that may present a hazard to the dentist and dental assistants in relation to treatment, or that might place the patient at risk because of treatment or drug therapy.

CLINICAL EXAMINATION—GENERAL

The clinical or physical examination is carried out

using the principles of inspection, palpation, and probing, examining to the extent necessary those oral and paraoral structures of professional concern to the dentist. Specific techniques of inspection and bimanual or bidigital palpation of paraoral structures can be reviewed elsewhere.[25]

Paraoral Structures

A complete examination of the paraoral structures should include an evaluation of the head and skull, eyes, nose, skin, neck, and jaws. The extent to which these structures need to be evaluated will in large measure depend upon the chief and associated complaints.

The examination of the head is intended for the recognition of abnormalities in the facies, facial form and symmetry, the eyes and nose, the skin, the neck region, and the jaws, including the temporomandibular joints. Facial asymmetry is commonly seen in the presence of regional lymphadenopathy, periodontal and alveolar abscesses, neoplasia, and salivary gland disease.

The inspection of the eyes must be limited to detecting external departures from normal. The pinpoint pupil of the narcotic addict, the scleras in jaundice (icterus), and herpetic lesions are perhaps the signs most likely to be of direct value.

The examination of the nose is by visual inspection in conjunction with questions regarding obstruction and associated mouthbreathing. The gingivitis associated with chronic mouthbreathing cannot be treated effectively until the breathing has been controlled by elimination of the obstruction.

The status of the skin may reflect manifestations of systemic disease, but is most helpful in the differential diagnosis of dermatological lesions that appear simultaneously in the oral cavity.

The examination of the neck should be done on every patient by visual inspection and by palpation. The floor of the mouth, the base of the mandible, the submandibular salivary glands, and the lymph nodes in neck triangles, including the cervical nodes, should be routinely examined for enlargement, tenderness, or fixation. The most common causes of so-called occult lymph node adenopathy are acute and chronic infections of regional or systemic origin, leukemias, lymphomas, primary lymph node diseases, and metastases from malignant neoplasia.

A complete examination of the joints and mandibular movements is beyond the scope of this presentation, and the reader is referred to other sources.[25,53] However, the mandible, joints, and the masseter and temporalis muscles should be palpated for swelling and tenderness and inspected visually for asymmetry, and the joints should be checked for smooth gliding movements and the absence of noises and grating sensations (tactile fermitus). The movement of the mandible should be observed during opening and closing for deviations from a straight closing path, and for restrictions on the degree of opening. The normal opening range in adult males is 50-to-60 mm.[52] The lateral movements should be smooth, without interruption, and extend to the left and right without restriction for about 10 mm each way. Restrictions on such movements, and on opening, lateral, and protrusive excursions with the teeth out of contact, may be indicative of past or presently active joint or muscle dysfunction.

CLINICAL EXAMINATION—ORAL

The clinical or physical examination of the oral structures should begin with a general appraisal of the patient's oral hygiene, the extent of carious lesions, occlusal function, stability, tooth mobility, and status of the periodontium. The general appraisal should be brief but should provide the examiner with an idea how extensive the examination will be, what instruments may be needed, whether or not a referral may be needed immediately, and what areas may require special consideration.

Instruments and materials

Aside from instruments for special methods to be discussed later, only a few instruments and materials are necessary to carry out the examination of the oral structures. These are a mouth mirror, cotton rolls, cotton, thumb forceps, thin 2 × 2 sponges, finger cots, tongue depressor, chip-syringe or air-jet, dental floss, water syringe, articulating paper, and a periodontal probe.

Soft tissues

This part of the oral examination consists of a brief review of the lips, labial and buccal mucosa, palate, oropharynx, floor of the mouth, and tongue. The examination should be systematic, and all areas should be visually inspected for changes in color, form, and texture. All tissues should be palpated for underlying induration, swelling, and discomfort. Where possible, the palpation should be bimanual or bidigital.

Examination of Periodontium

The examination of the periodontium includes a visual inspection of the gingiva, probing of the gingival sulci for pathological deepening, and an evaluation of periapical and posterior bite-wing radiographs for alterations in the lamina dura and the height of the alveolar crest bone. The findings of the clinical examination are recorded on a periodontal chart. Also included on the chart are tooth mobility, the level of the free gingival margin, the level of the attachment, the approximate bone level, and missing teeth.

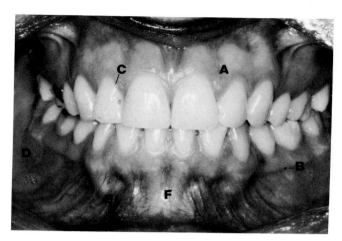

Fig. 11-1. Gingiva. *A,* Attached gingiva. *B,* Mucogingival line. *C,* Free gingival margin. *D,* Posterior vestibular fornix. *F,* Frenum area.

Gingiva

The gingiva (Fig. 11-1) is examined for aberrations from normal in color, form, consistency, adaptation to the teeth, the level of the free gingival margin in relation to the cementoenamel junction, the level of the attachment in relation to the cementoenamel junction, the zone of the attached gingiva, and bleeding or exudation. In some instances, a plaque score is obtained for all the teeth and recorded on a specific oral hygiene chart.

The term *normal* is used here to mean healthy as well as meeting certain anatomical criteria—color, form, consistency, crevice depth, bleeding, and level of attachment. *Healthy* here means free of disease at the time, but does not exclude evidence of prior disease. The surface of the attached gingiva is stippled, as occasionally is the free gingival margin. The zone of the attached gingiva is important for periodontal health, but the width may be difficult to determine in relation to the mucogingival junction, which is often indistinct.

The *normal color* of the gingiva is coral pink, but physiological pigmentation such as melanosis gingiva may alter this color generally or locally (Fig. 11-1, A). The intensity of the color in normal gingiva is related to the degree of keratinization (Fig. 11-1, B), thickness of tissue, and the subpapillary venous plexus. In gingivitis (Fig. 11-2, C,D), the color of the gingiva tends to be darker (red hue), with loss of keratinization or ulceration, and to have a faint blue hue if some keratinization remains.

The *form* of the gingiva is related to the teeth, the underlying bone, and the presence or absence of disease. In a normal gingiva the tissue just fills the interdental space and the gingival margin ends in a knifelike edge, is coronal to the cementoenamel junc-

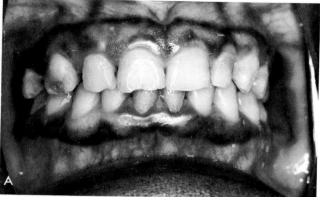

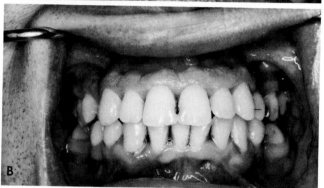

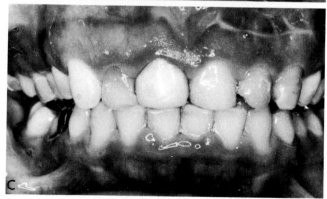

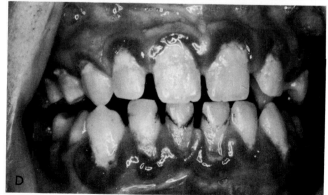

Fig. 11-2. Gingiva. *A,* Melanosis gingiva. *B,* Marked stippling. *C,* Soft, spongy tissue. Note scar above left maxillary lateral incisor. *D,* Marked gingivitis, with alteration of color, form, and density.

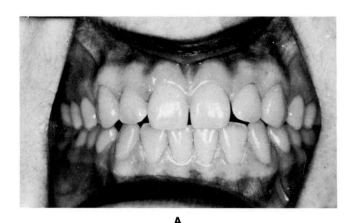

A

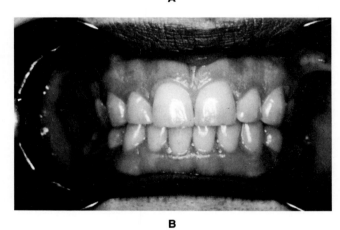

B

Fig. 11-3. Gingiva. *A,* Normal gingiva in young adult. *B,* Normal gingiva in older adult.

tion, and is closely adapted to the surface of the teeth (Fig. 11-3). Inasmuch as spacing between the teeth may occur, and the area below the contact area may vary even with a normal arrangement of teeth, the form and contour of the interdental tissues or papilla will vary with many factors, including type of adjacent teeth, facial-lingual position, mesialdistal position, spacing of teeth, carious lesions, and periodontal disease.

The consistency of the normal and healthy gingiva is firm and resilient. The consistency depends on the density of the tissues. In the presence of dense fibrous connective tissue that is firmly attached to the bone and teeth, the gingiva will feel firm and unyielding on palpation with the finger or side of an explorer blade. In the presence of active chronic inflammation with edema, passive congestion, granulation tissues, minimal keratinization of the surface epithelium, and loss of attachment and alveolar bone, the gingiva will feel soft and spongy on palpation. In the presence of suppuration and abscess formation (Fig. 11-4) the tissue may seem fluctuant and unsupported.

Normal healthy gingiva does not bleed on gentle probing. When the gingiva is correctly examined with a probe, there should be no bleeding from the gingival sulcus.[39] Even in normal tissues, slight bleeding may occur if probing is not done carefully, but the tendency for bleeding is very great in the presence of gingivitis or periodontitis because of the ulceration of the crevice and granulation tissue present in the crevicular wall. Gingival bleeding is used as an index of initial gingivitis.[7,39]

Periodontal probing

The periodontal probe with grooved markings at 3, 6, and 8 mm (Fig. 11-5), or at other distances from the tip, is used to clinically measure the depth of the gingival crevice and the level of the attachment relative to the cementoenamel junction. With careful and systematic use of the probe, the clinical measurements will be quite consistent; at least, the variation or error will not detract from the measurements' clinical diagnostic value.

Errors of measurement in clinical probing will occur because of (1) excessive probing force, (2) incorrect placement and angulation of probe, and (3) failure to systematically probe all areas. An excessively large probe, indistinct millimeter marking grooves or bands, incorrectly placed millimeter markings, and needle-tip probes may all be factors in probing errors. However, assuming the clinician has selected the correct probe, the development of consistent skill in using the probe is the best method of preventing errors. Even so, probing will not provide an accurate picture of the topography of the alveolar process, nor of the activity of the periodontal disease. It does provide information on a past history of periodontal disease, but not a complete one.

Exploration. Exploration of the root surfaces (Fig. 11-6) for evaluating the margins of restorations, detecting calculus, evaluating furcation involvement due

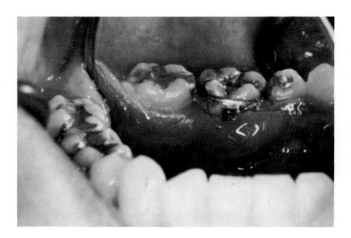

Fig. 11-4. Periodontal abscess. Acute abscess related to excess cement and orthodontic band.

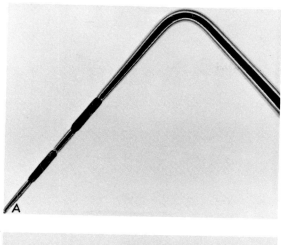

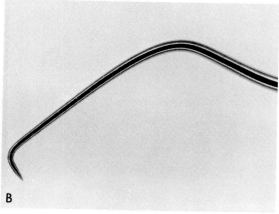

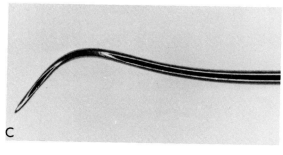

Fig. 11-5. Instruments. *A*, Periodontal probe. *B*, Shepherd's hook explorer. *C*, Cowhorn explorer.

to periodontal disease, and determining the effectiveness of instrumentation in preparing a biologically acceptable root surface, is carried out with a periodontal probe (Fig. 11-5A), shepherd's hook explorer (Fig. 11-5B), cowhorn explorer (Fig. 11-5C), and a mouth mirror. Exploration for furcation involvement of mandibular molars is done with a cowhorn type of explorer and with a shepherd's hook explorer with the tip ground down for the maxillary teeth. The furcation morphology or furcation entrance architecture varies considerably. The furcation entrance diameter of maxillary and mandibular teeth is 1.0 mm or less in a large percentage of the teeth[6] and requires an explorer with

a fine tip. However, the entrance diameter is only one consideration in establishing the prognosis and treatment. Also to be considered are the occluso-apical level of the furcation, remaining bone support, access for instrumentation, and root divergence.[16,19,55]

Depth of crevice. The probing depth of the gingival crevice varies according to location, state of eruption, and presence or absence of disease. The physiological

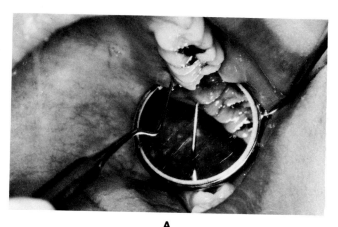

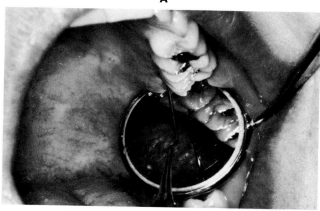

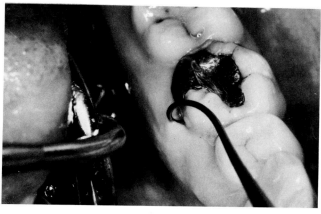

Fig. 11-6. Exploration. *A*, Entry of shepherd's hook explorer into furcation. *B*, Upward and distal movement to enter furcation. *C*, Use of cowhorn explorer to enter furcation of mandibular molar.

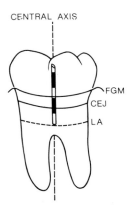

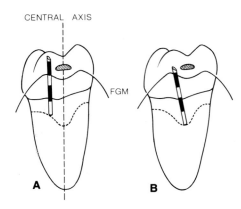

Fig. 11-7. Periodontal probing. Probe is held in the same plane as the central axis of the tooth. In the position indicated the probe must be placed at an angle (buccally) to reach the level of attachment, but remain in the plane of the central axis.

Fig. 11-9. Periodontal probing. *A,* Probing of distal or mesial pocket with probe in upright position in contact with adjacent molars. *B,* Probe placed at angle to reach depth of pocket.

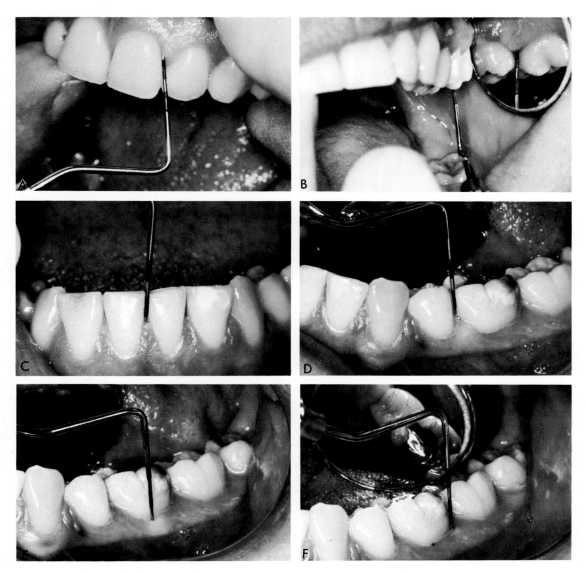

Fig. 11-8. Periodontal probing. *A,* Distal crevice of central incisor; *B,* distal pocket on maxillary molar; *C,* mesial surface of central incisor; *D,* mesial surface of mandibular molar; *E,* buccal surface of mandibular molar; *F,* distal line angle of molar.

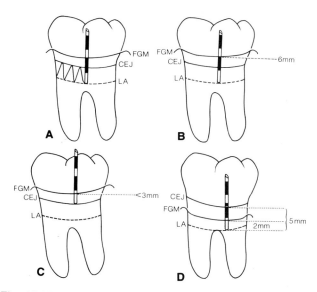

Fig. 11-10. Periodontal probing. *A,* Stepping of probe from cementoenamel junction to level of attachment. *B,* Measurement of depth of crevice. *C,* Measurement of free gingival margin to cementoenamel junction. *D,* In gingival recession, measurement to cementoenamel junction to free gingival margin to the level of attachment.

basis for establishing a depth for a normal gingiva has not been determined. However, on the basis of clinical trials and epidemiological surveys, it appears that the average depth of the normal gingiva is less than 3 mm, and usually the depth at the facial and lingual surfaces is less than that at the interproximal surfaces of the teeth. However, the crevice should not be considered abnormal simply if greater than 2 or 3 mm.

The depth of the gingival crevice may be markedly increased because of inflammatory gingival enlargement, which is referred to as hyperplastic gingivitis. The diagnosis can be accurate only if the attachment is not apical to the cementoenamel junction. If the

attachment were apical to the cementoenamel junction, the primary diagnosis in this case would be periodontitis. In the first instance, the deep sulcus has been called a pseudo- or gingival pocket; in the latter instance, it is a true periodontal pocket.

Level of attachment. The technique of probing re-

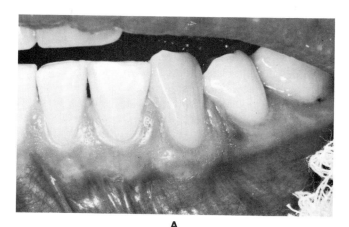

A

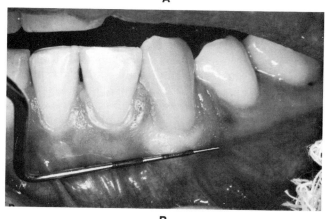

B

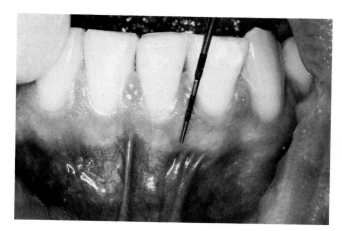

Fig. 11-11. Measurement of attached gingiva, from mucogingival line to level of attachment, using measurement of free gingival margin to level of attachment.

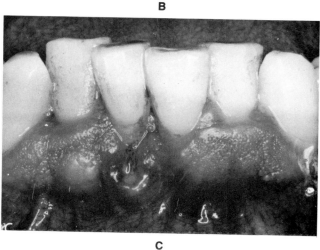

C

Fig. 11-12. Attached gingiva. *A,* Note mucogingival line at mandibular cuspid. *B,* Rolling the tissue at the mucogingival line to identify attached gingiva. *C,* Loss of attachment and cleft extending apically to the mucogingival line and attached gingiva.

quires that the examiner concentrate on one goal at a time. The first goal in probing is to determine the location of the attachment. The tip of the probe should always be held in contact with the tooth and the blade parallel with the central long axis of the tooth in one plane (Fig. 11-7). Probing is commenced at the most distal molar and carried around the upper arch tooth by tooth, testing the facial, then the lingual surfaces, or vice versa, and then the mandibular arch (Fig. 11-8). The probe is moved within the crevice in very short steps of approximately 1 mm from the distal to the mesial contact area. At the contact area of adjacentteeth, the probe must be angled in some instances in which the pocket extends more apically just beneath the contact area, where the probe cannot be positioned parallel to the long axis of the tooth (Fig. 11-9).

As the probe is stepped (Fig. 11-10) along the base of the crevice, the depth of the crevice is determined by the position of the free gingival margin on the probe (Fig. 11-10, B). However, the level of attachment or base of the crevice or periodontal pocket must be related to another landmark, the cementoenamel junction. Thus, the second goal in probing is to locate the cementoenamel junction. During the stepping procedure, the probe is lifted coronally to the cementoenamel junction and the distance from the free gingival margin to the cementoenamel junction is measured (Fig. 11-12, C). The difference between these two measurements is then the distance at which the attachment is apical to the cementoenamel junction. The difference is zero if the attachment is at the cementoenamel junction. If there is gingival recession so that the free gingival margin is apical to the ce-

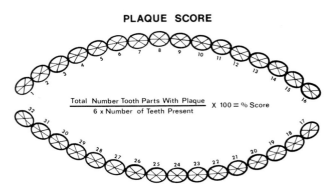

PLAQUE SCORE

$$\frac{\text{Total Number Tooth Parts With Plaque}}{6 \times \text{Number of Teeth Present}} \times 100 = \% \text{ Score}$$

Fig. 11-14. Plaque score chart. Chart used to record plaque present on 6 portions of each tooth. Score is derived as indicated. (Modified from O'Leary.)

mentoenamel junction, the depth of the crevice is read directly on the probe at the free gingival margin as before, and the level of the attachment relative to the cementoenamel junction is read directly on the probe at the cementoenamel junction (Fig. 11-10, D).

Attached gingiva. The width of the attached gingiva should be determined, because an adequate zone of attached gingiva is necessary for periodontal health (Fig. 11-11). The apical border of the mucogingival junction is often indistinct and difficult to detect, but the assessment may be aided by observing the movement of the alveolar mucosa.[63] The side of a periodontal probe is used to roll up the alveolar mucosa (Fig. 11-12, B). The site where such rolling does not occur is the clinically determined apical zone of the attached gingiva. Less than 1 mm. of attached gingiva may indicate chronic inflammation[30] or require meticulous care to prevent inflammation.[5] Inadequate width of the attached gingiva is a significant factor in prognosis (Fig. 11-12, C) and in determining surgical correction procedures.

Charting. The free gingival margin relative to the cementoenamel junction is usually drawn on the periodontal chart. In many dental offices, the level of the attachment is drawn on the chart as well. In Figure 11-13, the area between the free gingival margin and the level of attachment is shaded to demonstrate the crevice area. Also included is an estimate of the bone level taken from radiographs. The routine determination of alveolar crestal bone height by penetrating the soft tissue with a periodontal probe[13,34,35] is not advocated.

The extent of furcation involvement is also indicated on the chart, either by classification or by symbols. Many periodontal charts are available for individual use and have places for noting abnormal tooth mobility, overhanging margins of restorations, food impaction, and missing, impacted, and drifted teeth.

Dental plaque is scored after all mucosal tissues have been evaluated, as the color of the tissue may

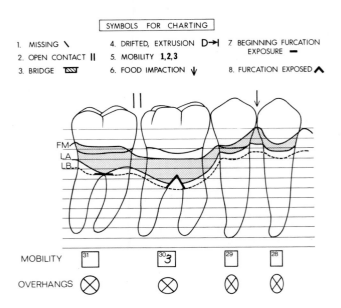

SYMBOLS FOR CHARTING

1. MISSING \
2. OPEN CONTACT ||
3. BRIDGE ⟐
4. DRIFTED, EXTRUSION D→|
5. MOBILITY 1,2,3
6. FOOD IMPACTION ↓
7. BEGINNING FURCATION EXPOSURE ━
8. FURCATION EXPOSED ⋀

MOBILITY 31 30 3 29 28

OVERHANGS ⊗ ⊗ ⊗ ⊗

Fig. 11-13. Charting. Basic parts of a periodontal chart. *FM,* free gingival margin; *LA,* level of attachment; *LB,* estimated level of bone from radiograph.

be altered by the plaque-disclosing solution. Repeated periodic scoring of plaque is indicated to demonstrate to both patient and dentist the patient's plaque control effectiveness. After all the teeth have been thoroughly disclosed, the amount of plaque is estimated using an index such as the plaque index score. The plaque at the free gingival margin is scored at present on the facial, lingual, and interdental tooth surfaces, and recorded on a plaque chart having schematic representations of each of 32 teeth divided into 6 areas (Fig. 11-14). The plaque control score is computed as a percentage of the total number of areas for the number of teeth present. It appears that patients are more highly motivated when plaque score percentages for the initial and subsequent examinations are recorded on a plaque index chart (Fig. 11-15) that visually demonstrates progress to the patient.[1,19]

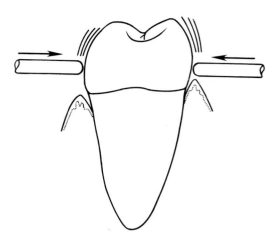

Fig. 11-16. Mobility test. A clinical test of mobility is carried out using the handles of two instruments. Mobility is graded on the basis of 1 to 3.

Tooth Mobility

Tooth mobility is tested at this time for recording on the periodontal chart. It is related at the time of the occlusal examination to other aspects of occlusion. Several sophisticated methods for measuring tooth mobility have been developed[27,37,44,47,50] for use in clinical studies,[26,31,38,51] but the methods are not suitable for the routine assessment of tooth mobility. Less objective methods have been utilized,[18,33,35] but the Miller index,[35] when modified, has been found to be a highly accurate, clinically acceptable method of assessing horizontal tooth mobility on an averaged basis.[31] In effect, the modified Miller index is a useful technique for epidemiological studies involving large populations,[31] and may be valid for use in some clinical studies if a significant number of evaluations are made, mouth scores are averaged per patient, and the examiner's results are calibrated. However, although the use of an index such as the Miller index is generally considered to be useful for diagnosis and treatment

planning for the individual practitioner,[42] this endorsement is not made without reservations.

The clinical assessment of mobility based on Miller's mobility index[35] uses the following measurement system: Mobility 1 = the first distinguishable sign of movement greater than normal; Mobility 2 = movement of 1 mm from normal position in any direction; Mobility 3 = movement of more than 1 mm in any direction. Rotation or depression is classified as Mobility 3. In a later modification, Miller made some changes, but still considered Mobility 1 as slight, Mobility 2 as moderate, and Mobility 3 as movement of more than 1 mm in any direction, including rotation or depression. Actual testing should be done with the handles of 2 instruments (Fig. 11-16).

A modification of the mobility index[34,36] using half scores 0, ½, 1, 1½, 2, 2½, and 3 appears to be valid.[31] Whether specific units are necessary in an index for use in a clinical practice or for clinical research has not been established. However, although many indices used at present in clinical practice are based on scores of 1, 2, and 3, and sometimes 1 to 4, specific units need not be used.[25,33] For clinical practice, the mobility scores of 1 to 3 suggested by Miller, or others modified with numerical criteria, appear to be acceptable. An example of such modification follows:

1 = First perception of movement greater than normal

2 = Moderate movement (~0.5 mm)

3 = Marked movement (~0.75 mm) in any direction

The use of 0.5 mm and 0.75 mm criteria[31] may be added to Miller's system[34] (above), or the specific units may be eliminated entirely if it seems that measurements obtained with them are no more objective than those obtained without them.

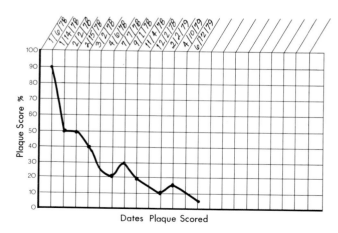

Fig. 11-15. Plaque record. Sequential plaque record showing a decrease in plaque score.

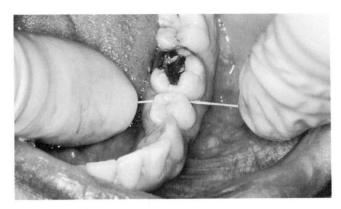

Fig. 11-17. Contact testing. Interproximal contacts are tested using dental floss. Contacts should be tight so that tape will snap in and out of the interproximal position.

Contacts

An evaluation of proximal contacts for tightness is an essential part of the periodontal examination, inasmuch as food impaction can be a significant factor in the cause and continuation of periodontal disease. Proper interproximal contacts may be lost because of faulty occlusal contact relations from restorations. This loss may cause distal movement of distal molars, improper marginal ridges, and increased mobility associated with occlusal trauma or periodontal disease. A diastema, or space between 2 adjacent teeth, may not lead to food impaction. However, in the presence of increased mobility, plunger cusps, and inadequate marginal ridges, food impaction involving the posterior teeth is a distinct possibility where there are only light contacts. The danger is even greater with open contacts. Contacts should be tested with dental floss (Fig. 11-17) and related to the patient's history of food being wedged between the teeth.

EXAMINATION OF TEETH

The examination of the teeth includes an assessment of number, contact relations, and missing, impacted, or unerupted teeth. The results of indicated vitality tests are also included on a dental chart.

Occlusion

The general appraisal of the occlusion is principally concerned with the influence of occlusal morphology on finding contact movements in protrusive and lateral movements, on closure patterns into centric relation, and on patterns of swallowing. The principal reason for evaluating these contact relations is the high correlation between the elimination of TMJ-muscle-pain dysfunction and the removal of (1) occlusal interferences to smooth gliding movements (balancing and protrusive); (2) interferences to closure in centric relation; and (3) interferences contributing to strained mandibular positions during swallowing and bruxism.

Other reasons relate to the establishment of occlusal stability, the pressure of secondary occlusal trauma, and the control of bruxism, all of which are important in the treatment of tooth mobility and advanced periodontal disease.

Other important aspects of the occlusion that should be evaluated are tooth mobility, contact relations of teeth, marginal ridge relations (Fig. 11-18), plunger cusps and food impaction, soft tissue trauma such as cheek biting, impinging overbite (Fig. 11-19), atypical facets of wear and extensive wear associated with bruxism (Fig. 11-20), and evidence of clenching and other habits that may influence the stability of the occlusion, such as pipe smoking, fingernail biting, and biting foreign objects. All these aspects of occlusion may influence the diagnosis, prognosis, and treatment of periodontal disease. A premature contact in centric relation is an occlusal interference to maximum intercuspal contact relations in the centric relation contact position (Fig. 11-21).

Balancing interferences are those on the nonfunctional or balancing side that interfere with working side contacts. Balancing side interferences may cause disclusion of working side contacts at some position

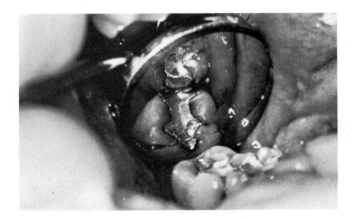

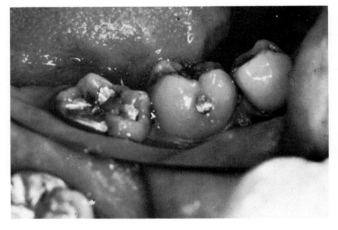

Fig. 11-18. Uneven marginal ridges. Uneven marginal ridges contribute to food impaction and are often occlusal interferences in centric.

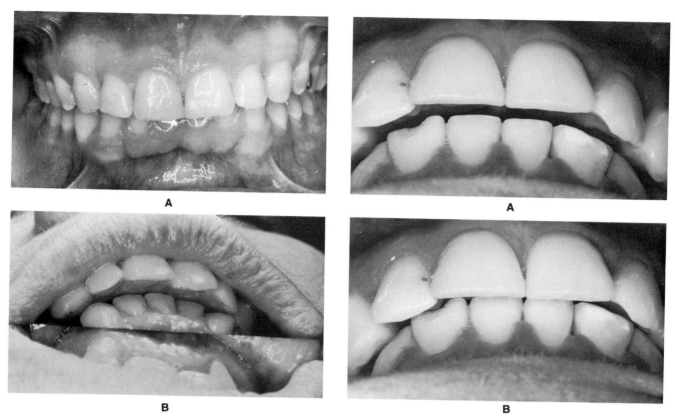

Fig. 11-19. Impinging overbite. *A,* Inflammation of lower labial gingiva because of vertical overlap and trauma related to incising foodstuffs. *B,* Impingement of mandibular incisors on maxillary gingiva.

Fig. 11-21. Jaw positions. *A,* Mandible in centric relation. *B,* Mandible in centric occlusion.

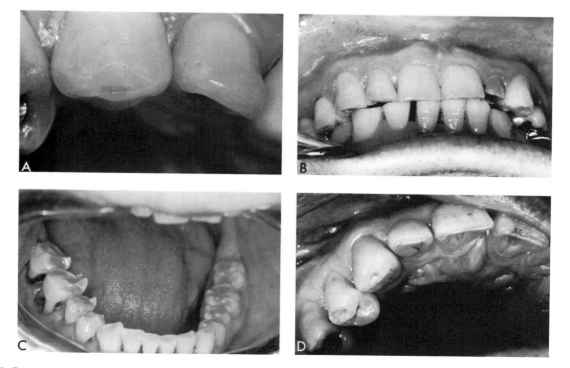

Fig. 11-20. Bruxism. *A,* Atypical facet of wear. *B,* Anterior wear and fracturing of teeth. *C,* Extensive wear from grinding at night. *D,* Fracturing of cusp tip of maxillary first premolar.

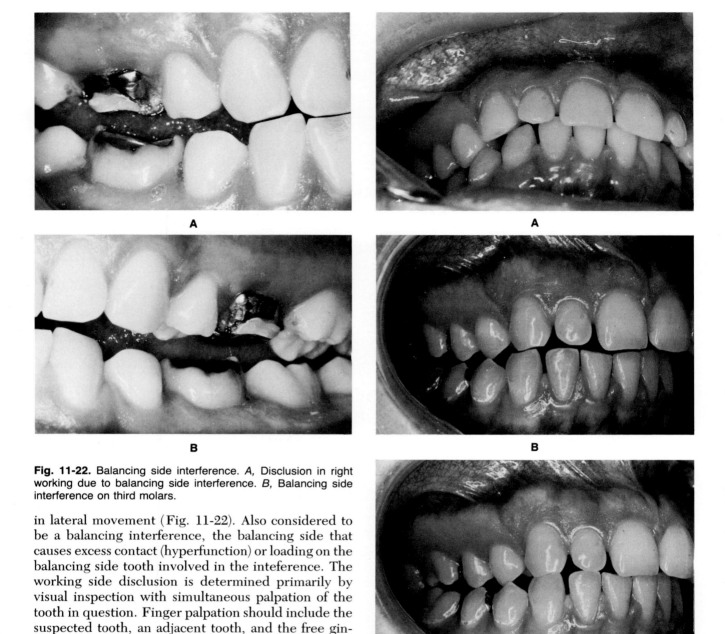

Fig. 11-22. Balancing side interference. *A,* Disclusion in right working due to balancing side interference. *B,* Balancing side interference on third molars.

in lateral movement (Fig. 11-22). Also considered to be a balancing interference, the balancing side that causes excess contact (hyperfunction) or loading on the balancing side tooth involved in the inteference. The working side disclusion is determined primarily by visual inspection with simultaneous palpation of the tooth in question. Finger palpation should include the suspected tooth, an adjacent tooth, and the free gingival margin. The presence of excess tooth mobility with a balancing contact is therefore considered to be a balancing side interference.

Working side interferences are those that interfere with smooth gliding movements on the function (working) side. Such interferences (Fig. 11-23) are detected by observing movements in gliding contacts and by palpating the working side teeth for heavy contacts and/or excess mobility.

Protrusive and lateral protrusive interferences are those contact relations that prevent smooth anterior gliding movements, cause disclusion of anterior teeth (Fig. 11-24), or, as a result of restorations, orthodontic movement of teeth, and occlusal instability, cause disclusion of teeth that are usually in contact in function

Fig. 11-23. Working side interference. *A,* Centric occlusion. *B,* Cuspid disclusion due to interferences on the first premolars. *C,* Contact between cuspids in right working and slight lateral protrusive interference.

or parafunction (Fig. 11-25). Such interferences may be detected by finger palpation and observation during directed gliding contact movements, and may be marked with articulating paper or sheet wax. When there is pain associated with traumatic occlusion or pulpitis, the movements necessary to detect the interferences may not be possible.

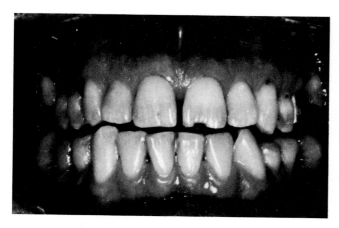

Fig. 11-24. Protrusive interference. Disclusion of anterior teeth due to posterior contacts.

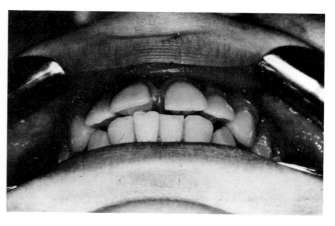

Fig. 11-25. Occlusal instability. Displacement of maxillary incisors related to discrepancy between centric occlusion and position of the teeth in malocclusion.

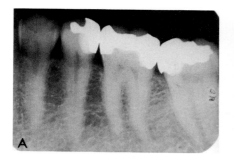
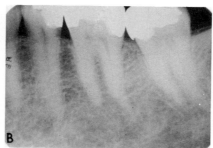
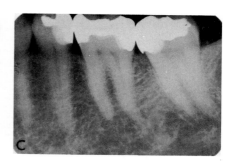
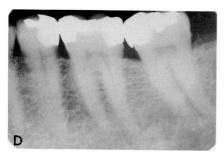
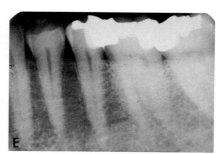

Fig. 11-26. Roentgenographic errors. *A,* Vertical error resulting in appearance of alveolar crest being above level of cementoenamel junction. Error in positioning also resulted in the missing of a portion of molar. *B,* Vertical error plus overexposure. *C,* Vertical angulation error, normal exposure. *D,* Normal angulation, normal exposure. *E,* Horizontal angulation error with overlapping of crowns.

ROENTGENOGRAPHIC EXAMINATION

The roentgenographic survey of the supporting structures is an essential part of the diagnostic procedure. However, it is necessary that the limitations of the roentgenogram in periodontal diagnosis be considered. A diagnosis should be made not on the basis of roentgenographic data alone, but in conjunction with a complete examination, including clinical probing.

Roentgenographic principles

The possibility of using roentgenograms fully in a diagnosis requires that films be correctly positioned (Fig. 11-26), exposed (Fig. 11-27), developed, and evaluated. Details of the technical procedures should be reviewed elsewhere.[65]

Positioning of the roentgenographic film depends upon the roentgenographic technique used and the anatomical features that may put restraints on such positioning. Proper positioning is necessary to avoid radiographic illusions (Fig. 11-28) due to faulty angulations.[29,61]

Roentgenographic survey

The roentgenographic periodontal survey should include an evaluation of the following: (1) presence or absence of lamina dura; (2) width of the periodontal membrane space; (3) height and form of the interdental alveolar bone crest; (4) root length and form; (5) periapical bone and root relationship; (6) overhanging margins of restorations; and (7) the status of interradicular areas (Fig. 11-29). When roentgenograms are being reviewed for potential disturbances, it is necessary constantly to factor into the analysis illusions

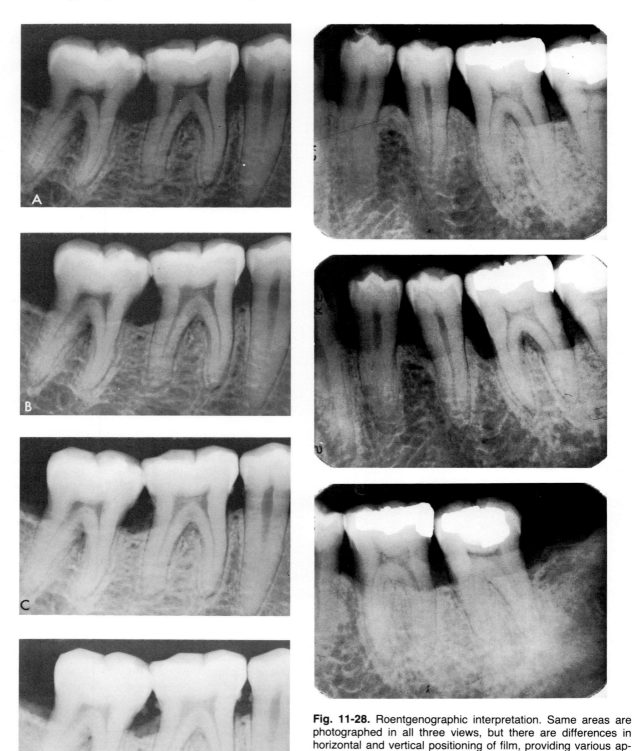

Fig. 11-27. Radiographs taken at the same angulation but at different levels of x-ray exposure from *A* through *D*. Photographic prints were made at the same level of light exposure for all. Note the increase in visualization of crestal bone and calculus as exposure was increased.

Fig. 11-28. Roentgenographic interpretation. Same areas are photographed in all three views, but there are differences in horizontal and vertical positioning of film, providing various appearances to alveolar bone.

due to faulty horizontal and vertical angulations, data from the clinical examination (probing exploration, symptoms, etc.), and limitations of the roentgenograms in periodontal diagnosis.

Without considering the effect of disease on the alveolar bone, those factors that influence the presence or absence and the appearance (thickness and

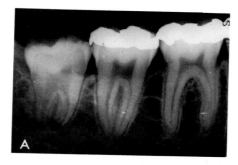

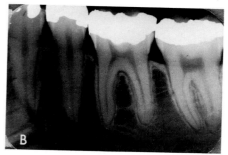

Fig. 11-29. Normal appearing alveolar bone. Note relationship of alveolar bone crest to cementoenamel junction, tooth position, and crown shape. Lamina dura is present in all areas. No clinical evidence of periodontal disease. *A,* Right side; *B,* Left side.

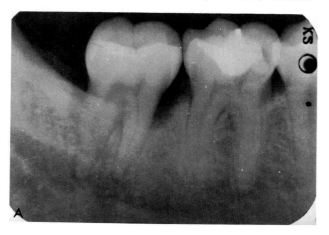

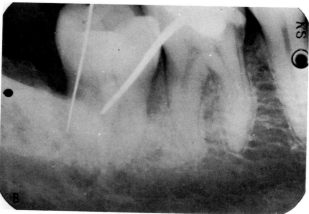

Fig. 11-30. Supplemental aid. Use of silver paint to demonstrate loss of attachment level on roentgenograms. *A,* Extent of bone loss not clearly seen, as demonstrated by *B.*

clarity) of the lamina dura include the following: (1) variation in vertical and horizontal angulation of the x-ray beam; (2) concavity and convexity of root surfaces; (3) curvature of roots; (4) level of the cementoenamel junction; and (5) thickness of the alveolar bone.

The most common observable loss of continuity of lamina dura is related to the presence of bone loss associated with periodontal disease. However, roentgenograms alone cannot indicate (1) the presence or absence of periodontal pockets; (2) early bone loss in periodontal disease; (3) early furcation involvement; (4) the location of the epithelial attachment; and (5) the status of the alveolar crest and process on facial and lingual surfaces of the teeth.

When a periodontal pocket is present, as indicated by probing, a loss of bone at mesial, distal, or interradicular areas can be visualized on the roentgenograms, provided that enough bone resorption has taken place. In general, the area of bone loss must be larger than the roentgenographic image. In one study,[49] septal defects less than 3 mm could not be visualized on the roentgenograms. The loss of bone at the alveolar crest is usually underestimated on roentgenograms because of inadequate visualization of the buccal or lingual aspects of the interdental septum.[60] Thus, observation of the extension of bone loss to the buccal or lingual is not generally possible because the teeth obscure the view, but interproximal infrabony pockets can be visualized.[48]

Adjunctive devices, such as a calibrated or endodontic silver point (Fig. 11-30) to assess the base of a periodontal pocket on the roentgenogram, or an Everett-Fixott grid attached to the film to superimpose 1 mm. squares on the film in assessing bone changes, are sometimes used to facilitate the roentgenographic diagnosis. The use of barium, Lipiodol, or lead-containing materials is not recommended, because of the hazards involved, for introduction into periodontal pockets to assess bony topography.

The width of the periodontal membrane space (radiolucent line around the teeth) may also vary considerably because of the same factors enumerated with the lamina dura (Fig. 11-31). The width of the roentgenographic periodontal membrane space must be related to clinical mobility, to function, and to the widths of the spaces of other teeth when an increase in the width of a periodontal space of a particular tooth is in question. The width of the periodontal membrane varies with function, occlusal stress, occlusal trauma, and orthodontics. The same amount of width can be interpreted as being different on the basis of a change in exposure time or a change in kilovoltage. Differences in widths of the periodontal membrane space on a tooth must be related automatically to what the visual impression of the space would be if the horizontal or vertical angulation were to be changed (Fig.

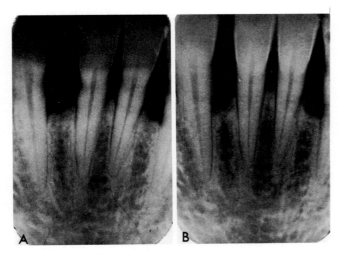

Fig. 11-31. Periodontal membrane space. *A,* Periodontal membrane space not clearly demonstrated on mesial aspect of incisor. *B,* With horizontal position and vertical angulation changed, the periodontal membrane space is seen clearly. This demonstrates the difficulty of evaluating the width of the periodontal membrane space.

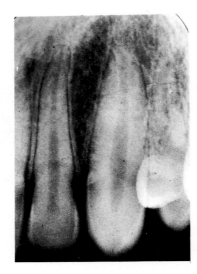

Fig. 11-32. Lamina dura and periodontal membrane space. The lamina dura and periodontal membrane space are clearly seen around the lateral incisor, but there was no clinical evidence of hypermobility, facets of wear, or symptoms of trauma.

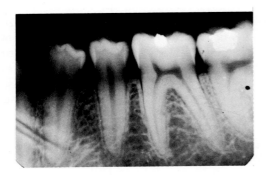

Fig. 11-33. Normal alveolar bone. Roentgenogram of young adult with no clinical evidence of gingivitis.

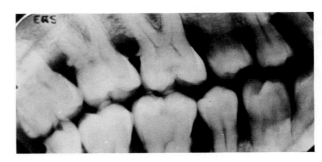

Fig. 11-34. Posterior bite-wing roentgenograms. Overlapping of maxillary teeth obscures contact areas for caries and septal bone for earliest signs of loss. Overlapping is less for mandibular teeth, and proximal caries and septal bone are clearly seen. Note crestal bone form and curve of Spee.

11-32). Also, a given horizontal angulation may produce 1 or more periodontal membrane spaces or lines about the root of a molar tooth.[62]

Without consideration of destructive changes of disease, the height and form of the interproximal alveolar bone on roentgenograms should be related to (1) vertical and horizontal angulation of the x-ray beam; (2) the contour of approximating teeth; (3) position of the cementoenamel junction; (4) eruption level of the teeth; and (5) angulation of the teeth. If the angulation of the x-ray beam is optimal, all the other variations can be related to the principle that bone and enamel (or CEJ) are usually separated by about 1 to 1.5 mm of radiolucency (soft tissue) in the absence of destructive disease (Fig. 11-33). In the anterior part of the mouth, the interproximal septa are thin and tend to form a peak, whereas on the posterior aspects the alveolar bone crest tends to be broad and flat because of the convexity of the proximal curvatures of the mo-

lar teeth. Uneven height of the teeth to the occlusal plane, or malposed teeth, as seen with stepping of the marginal ridges, produce a slope to the alveolar crest (Fig. 11-34). These aspects of radiographic interpretation are important in avoiding misinterpretation about bone loss. Prior surgery should also be considered (Fig. 11-35, A,B), as should periodontal-pulpal problems (Fig. 11-35, C).

The evaluation of roentgenograms for the presence or absence of calculus on the facial and lingual surfaces of the teeth is not possible. Because calculus may not be sufficiently large or calcified to be seen on the mesial and distal aspects of a tooth,[20] the use of roentgenograms can only be considered as an adjunct to clinical exploration for calculus (Fig. 11-36).

The possibility of detecting open margins or small overhanging margins on restorations (Fig. 11-37) is very much dependent on the coincidence of the position of marginal defect and the vertical or horizontal

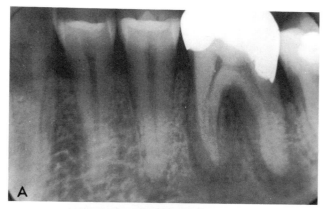

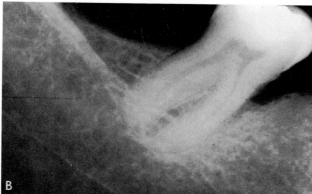

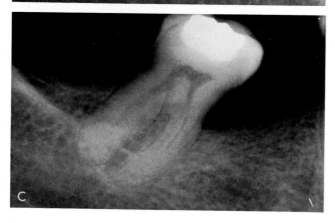

Fig. 11-35. Roentgenographic aids. *A*, Connection between periodontal pocket and periapical lesion. Sequential roentgenograms demonstrating bone level before *(B)* and after *(C)* surgery.

angulation of the x-ray beam. Thus, a precise paralleling technique may preclude by chance the detection of a defective margin on the mesial or distal aspect of a restoration. Therefore, use of radiographs for a systematic evaluation of margins is not possible and cannot take the place of clinical exploration.

The use of radiographs to detect vertical fractures is generally of low yield, except in gross fractures (Fig. 11-38). Estimates of the coronal extent of the pulp and the extent of caries may be highly misleading because of incorrect angulation of film (Fig. 11-38, B).

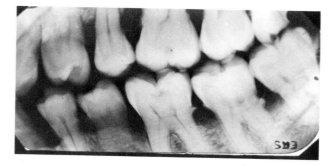

Fig. 11-36. Calculus. The detection of calculus on roentgenograms is incidental. The evaluation of calculus removal must be done clinically.

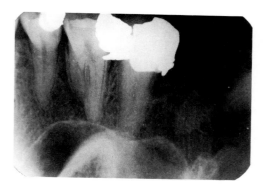

Fig. 11-37. Overhanging margin. Presence of gross overhanging margin and associated bone loss.

TRAUMATIC OCCLUSION

The assessment of injury to the supporting structures of the teeth in relation to disturbances in the masticatory system, either directly from the occlusion or secondarily to trauma from occlusion in other areas of the masticatory system, must be based on clinical evidence supported by radiographic data (Fig. 11-39). Often, trauma from occlusion is present without radiographic signs of injury to the supporting structures. The mechanism of the neuromuscular response and atypical facial pain is not clear. Conversely, major changes in the supporting structures may be seen without overt clinical symptoms. The mere widening of the periodontal membrane space in conjunction with jiggling of a tooth may represent adaptation and not injury.

In the presence of neuromuscular disturbances, pain, or soreness of teeth, and on the detection of significant alterations in the lamina dura, periodontal membrane space, and root form, a diagnosis of traumatic occlusion should be considered. Confirmation may be accomplished if the symptoms subside with direct treatment of the cause, such as elimination of occlusal interferences (Fig. 11-40). Root fractures, root resorption, hypercementosis, and pulpitis may

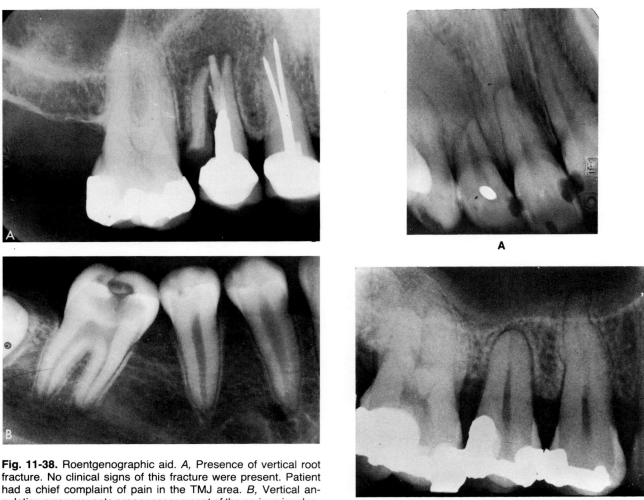

Fig. 11-38. Roentgenographic aid. *A,* Presence of vertical root fracture. No clinical signs of this fracture were present. Patient had a chief complaint of pain in the TMJ area. *B,* Vertical angulation error prevents proper assessment of the carious involvement of the molar in relation to pulp.

Fig. 11-39. Root resorption. *A,* No clinical symptoms indicating activity. *B,* Hypermobility and chronic sore tooth.

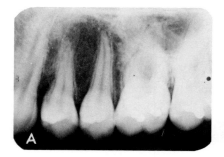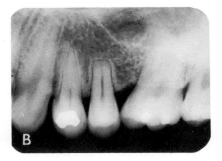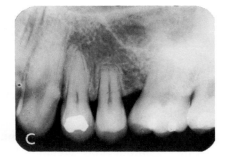

Fig. 11-40. Traumatic occlusion. *A,* Initial roentgenogram taken for complaint of pain. *B,* Restoration placed in first premolar prior to roentgenogram. First indication of root resorption with increased mobility. Occlusal adjustment done at this time. *C,* Several months after adjustment. No further resorption or clinical evidence of trauma.

result from occlusal dysfunction. Although root resorption, clinical hypermobility and increased width of the periodontal membrane space without discomfort, or other evidence of injury may be thought of as adaptation, the limitations of roentgenographs as well

as clinical observations have to be considered in the diagnosis. The cause of adaptation, or even injury without radiographic evidence, may be very difficult to locate, inasmuch as the response may be due to dysfunction distant to the mobile tooth. Thus, the diagnosis of trauma from occlusion cannot be based solely on radiographic evidence, but must be related to a complete examination.

OTHER DIAGNOSTIC METHODS

In addition to traditional diagnostic methods used in the dental office, other aids are likely to become available from laboratory research methods. These aids will be able to detect minute changes in the periodontium that are not now detectable with probing, palpation, inspection, and radiographic assessment. The traditional methods provide historical data, but they offer little information about the acitivity of the disease at the time of the examination, and virtually nothing about the susceptibility of an ostensibly well patient to factors predisposing to active periodontal disease. Such information would be extremely beneficial in the prevention and treatment of periodontal disease.

Some of the methods to be discussed are currently available for differential diagnosis, some have not reached the point of being practical for routine laboratory or clinical diagnosis, and one or two can be considered to be useful diagnostic procedures. None is useful at present for predicting the onset of periodontal disease, and the use of all these in clinical practice to make a diagnosis of a clinical entity is questionable. One or two may be useful for objectively monitoring goals of minimal inflammation in periodontal therapy.

GINGIVAL CREVICULAR FLUID (GCF)

The presence of fluid in the gingival crevice has been described for several decades, and the relationship of its flow and composition to gingival health has been studies extensively.[9,10] Gingival crevicular flow has been monitored to assess the severity of gingival disease and the response to therapy, to measure the effectiveness of oral hygiene, to determine the effectiveness of periodontal therapy, to evaluate the rate of local destruction, and to assess the relationship between GCF and systemic disease.

Although there is no particular advantage in the analysis of multiple components of the gingival fluid with present techniques of analysis, the gingival fluid does offer an easily obtainable body fluid with numerous tissue markers not yet evaluated. The opportunities for detecting disease profiles are enormous and several models to approach the problem are evident.

MICROBIOLOGICAL METHODS

The development of potentially useful microbiotic methods for routine laboratory or clinical diagnosis would appear to follow logically from research demonstrating basic mechanisms involved in the pathogenesis of periodontal disease. Research has been directed toward (1) detection of bacteria that predominate in periodontal lesions; (2) detection of bacteriological products that appear to mediate periodontal tissue responses; (3) detection of human isolates known to induce lesions in experimental animals; (4) evaluation of immune response to bacterial plaque; (5) development of selective media for the easy cultivation of suspected pathogens; and (6) the enumeration of predominant microflora on the basis of disease categories or development. The development of routine laboratory diagnostic methods of microbiological assay would appear to rest on the solution to several problems.

The analysis of bacterial products, such as endotoxins, hydrogen sulfide, polyamines, enzymes, and bacterial collagenase, as well as others, has provided promise that they can be assessed in terms of multiple components and related to clinical correlates of disease.[17] Such profiling might also be useful if coupled with products of host cells, including lysozyme, phosphatases, neutrophil products, and many others.

The use of sophisticated methods to evaluate bacteria and their products includes probes to simplify the identification of specific bacteria by enzyme-linked immunoassay (LISA),[12] immunofluorescence,[17] flow cytometry,[28] and DNA analysis.[58] The diagnosis of juvenile periodontitis is primarily based on clinical probing, radiographs, and history. If further assistance is necessary, serum antibody titers to *A.a.* may be useful. However, disease activity is not determined by these means, only by history. The use of dark-field microscopy does not appear to be a diagnostic test of destructive periodontal disease. The use of microbial methods of identification to provide measures of disease activity appears to be limited. The use of sophisticated probes such as DNA analysis may offer the most sensitive tests for microbes.

It is expected that in the future there will be tests to accurately measure susceptibility to periodontal disease, but none have yet been reported.[15] Susceptibility tests would identify patients likely to develop or to experience further periodontal breakdown. Microbiological assays would involve the detection and enumeration of potential pathogens. At present, the cause-and-effect relationship between bacterial and periodontal disease has not been established,[56] but microorganisms can be considered to be suspect if known to (1) predominate at disease sites in humans; (2) induce lesions under specific laboratory conditions in animals; or (3) produce metabolic products considered to mediate inflammation.[15] Additional data are necessary before the routine diagnosis and prediction of periodontal disease can be based on the analysis of the flora of the gingival crevice or periodontal pocket.

IMMUNE RESPONSES

Although the immune systems mediate some of the responses of the tissue to plaque, it does not appear that presently used serological or hypersensitivity procedures can be used to detect the susceptibility of patients to periodontitis. Immunological methods show considerable promise, but at present there are no practical predictive diagnostic tests for use in clinical practice.

Clinical correlates of disease and elevated antibody titers to periodontopathic bacteria suspected of causing periodontitis have been considered to be of possible diagnostic value. However, the relationships of LJP/antibody to *A.a.* ANUG/antibody to *B. intermedius* and intermediate-size spirochetes; and AP/antibody to *B. gingivalis* remain to be clarified.

OTHER TESTS

Aside from the differential white cell count made from peripheral blood in evaluating leukemic gingivitis, recent studies have demonstrated a polymorphonuclear leukocyte dysfunction in juvenile periodontitis;[8,32] that is to say, a reduction in phagocytosis and a decreased response of neutrophils to chemotactic stimuli. Neutrophil dysfunction also occurs in cyclic neutropenia,[11] agranulocytosis,[2] and Chèdiak-Higashi disease.[59] The detection of chemotactic defects in peripheral polymorphonuclear leukocytes could be a useful diagnostic aid in the differential diagnosis of certain types of periodontal disease. Further work may demonstrate its value in relation to specific bacteria.[40]

A fluorescein test has been advocated for evaluating the clinical severity of gingivitis,[36] but its value has not been documented by other investigators, except in relation to the sulcus bleeding index.[36,39] The test is based on the swallowing of capsules of sodium fluorescein and recovery of fluorescein with mouthwashing procedures.

SUMMARY

Traditional clinical and laboratory diagnostic aids have provided a historical evaluation of the periodontium on an anatomical basis. However, recent trends in diagnostic methods are directed toward the need to assess the susceptibility to and progression of periodontal disease. Such methods which are in the process of development, parallel the recognition of a need for objective criteria in laboratory studies that consider the mechanisms involved in the pathogenesis of periodontal disease. Such recognition has also risen out of awareness of the use of laboratory methods in areas other than periodontics, the use of indexing methods by clinicians, and the renewed interest in nonparametric statistical methods. In addition, there has been an increased awareness that prevention of periodontal disease requires more information about the intensity of predisposing factors that must be present before clinical lesions become obvious.

Traditional diagnostic methods do not measure (1) the presence or absence of active disease, especially low levels of periodontal disease at the time of the examination; (2) periodontal disease susceptibility; and (3) the rate of destruction of the supporting structures. It is hoped that future methods will determine these parameters of disease in such a way as to be practical at the level of clinical and laboratory practice.

Several diagnostic methods for determining the numbers of potentially pathogenic bacteria in plaque samples, and for measuring immune response to plaque or bacteria, are in the process of development. However, there are no microbiological assays of practical diagnostic value available, whereby susceptibility to periodontal disease can be evaluated, for use in clinical practice. Some possibilities exist in the institutional setting for evaluating the bacterial flora associated with juvenile periodontitis; however, how the flora may be related to tests of dysfunction of polymorpholeukocyte, or to susceptibility, is not known. The basic diagnostic problem for the clinician is usually not recognition of juvenile periodontitis, but the prevention of the periodontal destruction and information on the activity of the process.

Monitoring the flow of gingival crevicular fluid has become simplified to the point that the process can be accomplished with a meter in a matter of minutes in the dental office. GCF-flow measurements are used in clinical trials to assess (1) the severity of gingival inflammation; (2) effectiveness of periodontal therapy; and (3) response of tissues to the placement of restorations and prosthetic applicances. GCF could be used to demonstrate the effect of plaque control to patients. The significance of GCF measurements in a periodontal practice has not been determined.

Roentgenograms are an essential adjunct to a complete examination of the oral health of the patient. Irrespective of their limitations, they do not detract from a diagnosis if interpreted correctly and in light of findings from probing. Data from roentgenograms do not provide evidence of early bone change of periodontal disease or of more advanced destruction on the facial and lingual surfaces. Roentgenograms cannot be used effectively to determine the activity of periodontal disease, but do provide evidence of bone loss in the past. A loss of interproximal septal bone is most likely to be seen, but seeing it will depend upon the extent of involvement of the facial and lingual plates of bone, area of mouth, amount and density of bone covering the teeth, angulation of the x-ray beam, and morphology and position of the roots of the teeth.

Roentgenograms made with standardized methods of producing "identical" radiographs are useful adjuncts to periodontal probing in evaluating the progress of periodontal disease and treatment in clinical trials. There may be no advantage in using the more sophisticated but complex procedural systems over the less precise, but more practical, systems in clinical practice.

Roentgenograms are necessary adjuncts for evaluating traumatic occlusion and play a primary role in the detection of osseous lesions due to pulp disease, neoplasia, and systemic diseases.

REFERENCES

1. Barrickman, R.W.: Graphing indexes reduces plaque, J.A.D.A. 87:1404, 1973.
2. Bauer, W.H.: The supporting tissues of the tooth in acute secondary agranulocytosis (arsphenamin neutropenia), J. Dent. Res. 25:501, 1946.
3. Brasher, W.J., and Rees, T.D.: Systemic conditions in the management of periodontal patients, J. Periodont. 41:349, 1970.
4. Brill, N., and Bjorn, H.: Passage of tissue fluid into human gingival pockets, Acta Odont. Scand. 17:11, 1959.
5. Bowers, G.M.: A study of the width of the attached gingiva, J. Periodont. 34:201, 1963.
6. Bower, R.C.: Furcation morphology relative to periodontal treatment: furcation entrance architecture, J. Peridont. Res. 18:412, 1983.
7. Carter, H.G., and Barnes, G.P.: The gingival bleeding index, J. Periodont. 45:801, 1974.
8. Cianciola, L.J., Genco, R.J., Patters, M.R., McKenna, J., and van Oss, C.J.: Defective polymorphonuclear leukocyte functions in a human periodontal disease, Nature 265:445, 1977.
9. Cimasoni, G.: The crevicular fluid, Monographs in Oral Science. Vol. 3. New York: S. Karger, 1974.
10. Cimasoni, G.: Crevicular fluid updated. Basel: S. Karger, 1983.
11. Cohen, M.M., and Morris, A.L.: Periodontal manifestations of cyclic neutropenia, J. Periodont. 32:159, 1961.
12. Dzink, J.L., et al.: ELISA and conventional techniques for identification of black-pigmented Bacteriodes isolated from periodontal pockets, J. Periodont. Res. 18:369, 1983.
13. Easley, J.R.: Methods of determining alveolar osseous form, J. Periodont. 38:112, 1967.
14. Egelberg, J.: Gingival exudate measurements for evaluation of inflammatory changes of the gingivae, Odont. Revy 15:381, 1964.
15. Ellen, R.P.: Microbiological assays for dental caries and periodontal disease susceptibility, Oral Sci. Rev. 8:3, 1976.
16. Everett, F.G.: Birfurcation involvement, Oregon Dent. J. 28:2, 1959.
17. Fine, D.H., and Mandel, I.D.: Indicators of periodontal disease activity: An evaluation, J. Clin. Periodontol. 13:533, 1986.
18. Forsberg, A., and Hagglund, G.: Mobility of the teeth as a check of periodontal therapy, Acta Odont. Scand. 15:305, 1958.
19. Garnick, J.J.: Use of indexes for plaque control, J.A.D.A. 86:1325, 1973.
20. Gettleman, L., et al.: Preliminary evaluation of the hisotoxicity and radiopacity of lead-containing elastic impression materials, J.A.D.A. 96:987, 1978.
21. Glickman, I.: Bifurcation involvement in periodontal disease, J.A.D.A. 40:528, 1950.
22. Golub, L.M., Borden, S.M., and Kleinberg, I.: Area content of gingival crevicular fluid and its relation to periodontal disease in humans, J. Periodont. Res. 6:243, 1971.
23. Greenberg, J., Laster, L., and Listgarten, M.A.: Transgingival probing as a potential estimator of alveolar bone level, J. Periodont. 47:514, 1976.
24. Hassell, T.M., Gormann, M.A., and Saxer, U.P.: Periodontal probing: Interinvestigator discrepancies and correlations between probing force and recorded depth, Helv. Odont. Acta 17:38, 1973.
25. Kerr, D.A., Ash, M.M., and Millard, H.D.: Oral Diagnosis. 6th ed. St. Louis: C.V. Mosby Co., 1982.
26. Korber, K.H.: Periodontal pulsation, J. Periodont. 41:382, 1970.
27. Korber, K.H., and Korber, E.: Untersuchungen uber die kaufunktionale Beanspruchung des Zahnes, Dtsch. Zahnaerztl. Z. 18:576, 1963.
28. Kornman, K.S., et al.: Detection and quantification of Bacteroides gingivalis in bacterial mixtures by means of flow cytometry, J. Periodont. Res. 19:570, 1984.
29. Lang, N.P., and Hill, R.W.: Radiographs in periodontics, J. Clin. Periodontol. 4:16, 1977.
30. Lang, N.P., and Löe, H.: Relationship between the width of keratinized gingiva and gingival health, J. Periodont. 43:623, 1972.
31. Laster, L., Laudenback, K.W., and Stoller, N.H.: An evaluation of clinical tooth mobility, J. Periodont. 46:603, 1975.
32. Lavine, N., Stolman, J., Maderazo, E., Ward, P., and Cozen, R.: Defective neutrophil chemotaxis in patients with early onset periodontitis, J. Dent. Res. 55 (Special Issue B), I.A.D.R. Abstract No. 603, 1976.
33. Lovdal, A., et al.: Tooth mobility and alveolar bone resorption as a function of occlusal stress and oral hygiene, Acta Odont. Scand. 17:61, 1959.
34. Mann, W.V.: The correlation of gingivitis, pocket depth and exudate from the gingival crevice, J. Periodont. 34:379, 1963.
35. Miller, S.C.: Textbook of Periodontia. Philadelphia: Blakiston, 1936.
36. Mormann, W., Regolati, B., Lutz, F., and Saxer, V.P.: Gingivitis fluorescein test in recruits, Helv. Odont. Acta 19:27, 1975.
37. Mühlemann, H.R.: Periodontometry, a method for measuring tooth mobility, Oral Surg. 4:1220, 1951.
38. Mühlemann, H.R.: Tooth mobility, a review of clinical aspects and research finds, J. Periodont. 38:686, 1967.
39. Mühlemann, H.R., and Sons, S.: Gingival sulcus bleeding— a leading symptom in initial gingivitis, Helv. Odont. Acta 15:107, 1971.
40. Nisengard, R.J.: The role of immunity in periodontal disease, J. Periodont. 48:505, 1977.
41. O'Leary, T.J., et al.: Severe periodontal destruction following impression procedures, J. Periodont. 44:43, 1973.
42. O'Leary, T.J.: Indices for measurement of tooth mobility and clinical studies, J. Periodont. Res. 9 (Suppl. 14):94, 1974.
43. O'Leary, T.J., et al.: Factors affecting tooth mobility, Periodontics 4:309, 1966.
44. O'Leary, T.J., and Rudd, K.D.: An instrument for measuring horizontal tooth mobility, Periodontics 1:249, 1963.
45. O'Leary, T.J., et al.: The plaque control record, J. Periodontol. 43:39, 1972.
46. Oliver, R.C., Holm-Pedersen, P., and Löe, H.: The correlation between clinical scoring, exudate measurements and microscopic evaluation of inflammation in the gingiva, J. Periodont. Res. 40:201, 1969.
47. Parfitt, G.J.: Measurement of the physiological mobility of individual teeth in an axial direction, J. Dent. Res. 39:608, 1960.
48. Patur, B., and Glickman, I.: Clinical and roentgenographic evaluation of the post-treatment healing of infrabony pockets, J. Periodont. 33:164, 1962.
49. Pauls, V., and Trott, J.R.: A radiological study of experimentally produced lesions in bone, Dent. Pract. 16:254, 1966.

50. Picton, D.C.A.: A method of measuring physiologic tooth movements in man, J. Dent. Res. 36:814, 1957.

51. Picton, D.C.A.: A study of normal tooth mobility and the changes with periodontal disease, Dent. Pract. 12:167, 1962.

52. Poissant, C.: Clinical evaluation of the treatment of functional temporomandibular joint disturbances, Thesis, The University of Michigan, 1973.

53. Ramfjord, S.P., and Ash, M.M.; Occlusion. 3rd ed. Philadelphia: W.B. Saunders Co., 1982.

54. Rudin, H.J., et al.: Correlation between sulcus fluid rate and clinical and histological inflammation of the marginal gingiva, Helv. Odont. Acta 14:21, 1970.

55. Saxe, S.R., and Carman, D.K.: Removal or retention of molar teeth: The problem of the furcation, Dent. Clin. North Am. 13:783, 1969.

56. Socransky, S.S.: Relationship of bacteria to the etiology of periodontal disease, J. Dent. Res. 49:203, 1970.

57. Spray, J.R., and Garnick, J.J., Doles, L.R., and Klaivitter, J.G.: Microscopic demonstration of the position of periodontal probes, J. Periodont. 49:148, 1978.

58. Strzempko, M.N., et al: Moles percent G and C DNA-DNA hybridization and ultrastructure of "fusiform" Bacteroides, J. Dent. Res. (Special Issue A) 64, abst. nos. 1129,300, 1985.

59. Temple, T.R., Kimball, H.R., Kakehashi, S., and Amen, C.R.: Host factors in periodontal disease: periodontal manifestations of Chediak-Higashi syndrome, J. Periodont. Res. (Suppl.) 10:26, 1973.

60. Theilade, J.: An evaluation of the reliability of radiographs in the measurement of bone loss in periodontal disease, J. Periodont. 31:143, 1960.

61. Thunthy, K.H.: Radiographic illusions due to faulty angulations, Dent. Radiogr. Photogr. 51:1, 1978.

62. Van der Linden, L.W.J., and Van Aken, J.: The periodontal ligament in the roentgenogram, J. Periodont. 41:243, 1970.

63. Vincent, J.W., Machen, J.B., and Levin, M.P.: Assessment of attached gingiva using the tension test and clinical measurements, J. Periodont. 47:412, 1976.

64. Wege, W.R.: A technique for sequentially reproducing intraoral film, Oral Surg. 23:454, 1967.

65. Wuehrmann, A.H., and Monson, L.R.: Dental Radiography. 2nd ed. St. Louis: C.V. Mosby Co., 1969.

12

GINGIVITIS, GINGIVOSTOMATITIS, AND GINGIVAL ATROPHY

Gingivitis is an inflammatory process that usually originates at the dentogingival junction and affects the functional gingival component of the periodontium. It is primarily a disease of the gingiva, but may spread secondarily to the alveolar or oral mucosa. Inflammatory disease originating in the oral mucosa independent of the teeth, with or without involvement of the gingiva, is called *stomatitis*.

The term *gingivostomatitis* is used to designate a combined inflammatory manifestation in the gingiva and the alveolar mucosa when the inflammation is of nondental origin or significance. Gingivitis is thus a true periodontal disease. However, gingivostomatitis or other manifestations of stomatitis should not be considered periodontal disease, and will therefore be discussed here from a differential diagnostic and management standpoint.

Gingival atrophy and recession may or may not be related to gingival inflammation, but because loss of tissues affects the gingiva as a functional unit, they have to be considered part of gingivo-periodontal disease.

The classification of gingivitis, gingivostomatitis, and gingival atrophy shown in Table 12-1 takes into consideration these concepts of gingivo-periodontal disease.

CLINICAL FEATURES OF GINGIVITIS

The clinical features of importance for diagnosis and assessment of the results of therapy include alterations in gingival color, form, density, gingival crevice depth, position of epithelial attachment, bleeding tendency, and crevicular fluid.

The normal *gingival color* (Fig. 12-1, A) ranges from pale pink to darker shades because of various degrees of melanin pigmentation. The color may vary further

Table 12-1. Classification of Gingivitis, Gingivostomatitis, and Gingival Atrophy

SIMPLE GINGIVITIS
Ordinary acute or chronic inflammatory response to plaque, calculus, and iatrogenic irritants on the surfaces of the teeth
COMPLEX GINGIVITIS
Gingival inflammatory response modified by local or systemic factors
Gingival hyperphasia (or Enlargement)
Mouthbreather's gingivitis
Hereditary gingival fibromatosis
Dilantin gingivitis
Pregnancy gingivitis
Leukemic gingivitis
Acute and Recurrent Necrotizing Gingival Lesions
Necrotizing ulcerative gingivitis (NUG)
GINGIVOSTOMATITIS
Desquamative Gingivostomatitis
Chronic desquamative gingivitis
Benign mucous membrane pemphigoid
Erosive lichen planus
Allergic gingivostomatitis
Thermal electrical and chemical gingivostomatitis
Dermatological diseases with gingival manifestations
Infective Gingivostomatitis
Herpetic gingivostomatitis
Other acute oral infection
Infective granulomas
TRAUMATIC GINGIVITIS
Impingement from occlusion, food impaction, or dental appliances
Trauma from faulty oral hygiene practices or other habits
GINGIVAL ATROPHY OR RECESSION
Systemic Origin
Senile atrophic gingivitis
Local Causes
Faulty oral hygiene practices
Malposition of the teeth
Sequelae or periodontal disease and therapy

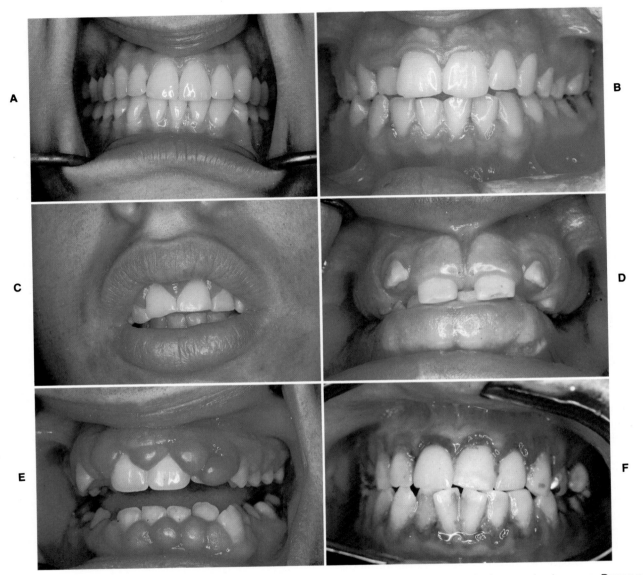

Fig. 12-1. *A,* Normal gingiva. Uniform pale pink color. Knife-edged margins and papillae filling the interproximal spaces. Dense and resilient to palpation. Shallow crevice with probing ending at or coronal to the cementoenamel junction. No tendency for bleeding and no tenderness associated with routine probing.

B, Simple gingivitis. Uneven red color. Thickened margins and blunted, swollen papillae. Soft and "boggy" or edematous to palpation. Crevice depth may be increased due to the swelling, but the level of attachment is at the cementoenamel junction. There is marked tendency for bleeding upon slight provocation, but minimal tenderness to touch.

C, Mouthbreather's gingivitis. Lack of lip seal with exposed, glossy red and bulbous gingival papillae.

D, Hereditary gingival fibromatosis. Marked hyperplasia of both free and attached gingiva in 12-year-old girl, with only minor signs of inflammation. Note malposition of the teeth related to the fibrotic hyperplastic tissues.

E, Dilantin gingivitis. Seventeen-year-old male on Dilantin therapy for 3 years. Characteristic increase in size of the interdental papillae, which with time will create gingival clefts. The swollen papillae may later become confluent and cover the entire tooth. The swelling may secondarily involve the attached gingiva. In this instance, the swelling is also aggravated by mouthbreathing.

F, Leukemic gingivitis. Male, 27 years old, with acute myelogeneous leukemia. Red or bluish-red gingival margins. Swollen and soft. Marked increase in bleeding tendency, but minimal tenderness to touch. Severity related to amount of plaque.

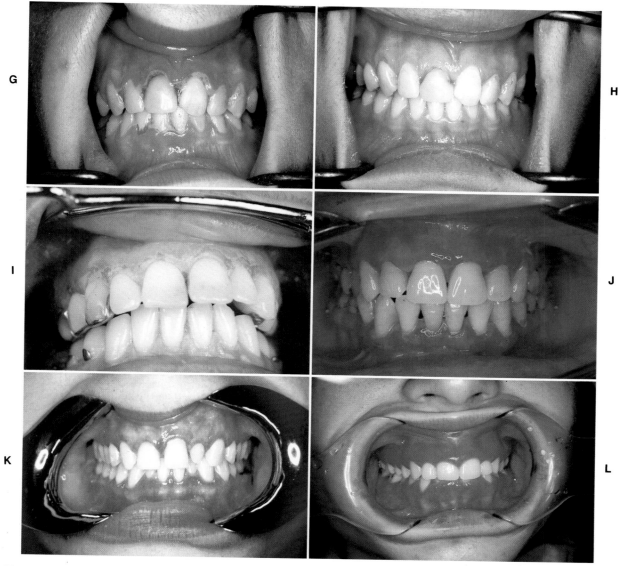

Fig. 12-1. *G,* Necrotizing ulcerative gingivitis in 22-year-old female. Necrosis of papillae and free gingival margins, most severe around poorly fitting acrylic crown. Gray pseudomembrane over necrotizing lesions. Marked redness, increased bleeding tendency, and soreness to touch.

H, After treatment, including removal of subgingival margins of the acrylic crown. Normal gingival color, form, density, and crevice depth without bleeding tendency or soreness to touch.

I, Allergic desquamative gingivitis. Patchy desquamation of gingival epithelium in the maxilla, leaving a red, tender surface. This was an acute allergic response to a sulfa drug (Gantrisin) used in the treatment of cystitis in a female 29 years old. The patient had both gingival and genitalial lesions, which abated after withdrawal of the drug.

J, Benign mucous membrane pemphigoid. Female, 34 years old. Ruptured vesicles with redness, tenderness, and desquamation. No ocular or genitalial lesions.

K, Erosive lichen planus. Female, 30 years old. Gingival lesions characterized by redness, tenderness, and increased bleeding tendency. Often discrete signs of keratinized striation may be observed associated with the lesions. At the time the photograph was taken there was no evidence of lichen planus in the buccal mucosa or elsewhere on the body.

L, Allergic gingivostomatitis related to chewing gum. Severe redness, desquamation, and soreness of the gingiva. The patient also had angular cheilitis and tongue lesions. All lesions subsided after the use of chewing gum was stopped.

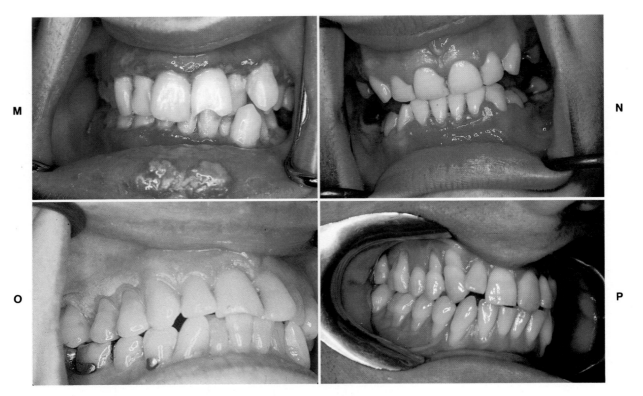

Fig. 12-1. *M,* Herpetic gingivostomatitis. Female, 29 years old. High fever, severe pain, and tenderness to touch, superficial ulceration and desquamation of the gingiva. Note also herpetic ulcer on lower lip.

N, Traumatic gingivitis in mandibular anterior region from impingement of maxillary anterior teeth as a result of deep overbite and loss of posterior teeth. Also poor oral hygiene. Female, 47 years old.

O, Senile atrophic gingivitis. Female, 67 years old. Atrophy and hyperkeratosis of gingival mucosa.

P, Gingival recession. Male, 41 years old. Horizontal toothbrushing with hard brush over many years. Note how the recession is most pronounced over the teeth that are in buccal version, while the second bicuspid, which is positioned further palatally, is not affected. Also evidence of root surface abrasion from the faulty brushing.

as a result of inflammation. The pink gingival color is a reflection of the blood in the subepithelial plexus of blood vessels and the translucency of the gingival mucosa.

For the diagnosis of gingivitis, emphasis should be placed on variations in color in the marginal or papillary gingiva compared to the rest of the gingiva, rather than on the overall color hue.

Alterations in *gingival form* in gingivitis are related to swelling, which is a cardinal sign of inflammation. Thus, a thickening of the free gingival margin and a blunting of the interdental papillae are common clinical features of gingivitis. Deviations from the usual thin marginal gingiva to a thick one, without any other signs of inflammation, are not diagnostic of gingivitis.

Surface stippling will be lost because of the edema in acute gingivitis. However, with low-grade chronic gingivitis, there may be stippling in spite of crevicular inflammation if the gingiva is stimulated by surface massage.

Decreased density of the gingiva related to inflammation is accompanied by edema and destruction of collagen. Thus, in simple gingivitis, the gingiva is usually softer and less resilient than normal. While decreased density is a sign of gingivitis, gingivitis cannot be excluded because of the presence of a firm and dense gingiva.

The *gingival crevice* may be of increased depth in gingivitis due to swelling of the gingiva; however, normal crevice depth does not rule out gingivitis, so measurements of crevice depth are of limited value in the diagnosis of gingivitis.

The position of the *epithelial attachment* in relation to the bottom of the gingival crevice (located by a thin probe) and the cementoenamel junction is important in differentiating between gingivitis and periodontitis and in determining the type of treatment and prognosis.

In recent years, an increasing significance has been given to a *bleeding tendency* associated with gentle probing of the gingival crevice.[94] Such bleeding does not occur when the gingival crevice is normal or healthy. In patients with good oral hygiene and slight subgingival calculus, bleeding upon probing may be the only clinical sign of gingivitis. This is true because in such patients color, form, density, depth of crevice, and attachment level may all be normal and the crevicular inflammation may be detectable only from the increased bleeding tendency from this nonvisible part of the gingiva. Therefore, gingivitis cannot be ruled out by normal color, form, and density without systematic probing of the gingival crevices around all the teeth. For laboratory diagnosis of gingivitis, *gingival fluid tests* have a demonstrated value.

SIMPLE GINGIVITIS

Simple gingivitis is plaque-induced and starts at the surface of the dentogingival junction. It may be found somewhere in the mouth in nearly every adult person, and is the most common of all oral diseases (Fig. 12-1, *B*). If not treated, it may spread to the deeper gingival structures and eventually develop into periodontitis.

The greatest clinical significance of simple gingivitis is that it may develop into periodontitis, and a main objective in its treatment is to prevent such progression. Fortunately, there are indications that this goal may be achieved without complete cure of the gingivitis.[4]

Therapy

Because bacterial plaque is the direct cause of simple gingivitis, therapy must be aimed at total elimination of plaque or reduction to a tolerable level in terms of total mass and numbers of pathogenic organisms.

The procedures recommended for elimination of plaque and plaque-retaining surface features of the teeth are discussed in chapters 17 and 18. In some situations, such as with subgingival margins of dental restorations, it may not be possible to achieve a complete cure of simple gingivitis and still maintain subgingival margins.[120] From a practical standpoint, it is seldom possible to maintain plaque control over several months to such an extent that there are absolutely no signs of gingivitis anywhere in the mouth. Fortunately, if the patient has his teeth cleaned professionally at regular intervals not exceeding every 3 months, mild marginal gingivitis without such serious sources of crevicular plaque retention as subgingival calculus and iatrogenic restorations seemingly does not jeopardize the attachment apparatus of the teeth to any significant degree.[118]

No numerical levels for "permissible," nonsignificant plaque and gingivitis scores have been established. A stage of diminishing returns from efforts on plaque control will often be reached at an individual level of performance.[66] Clinical judgment supplemented by repeated plaque scores is needed to determine if or when that level has been reached.

Bleeding associated with oral hygiene procedures, or appearance of exudate when pressure is applied upon the gingiva, are certainly indications of active periodontal disease beyond the compromise stage. Such findings indicate a definite need for professional care, while transient marginal gingival color changes may be of lesser clinical significance.

Thus, although the optimal goal for treatment of simple gingivitis is to restore gingival health completely (Fig. 12-2, *A, B*), an acceptable compromise may be to reduce the disease to such an extent that it no longer represents a threat to the maintenance of the dentition for the lifetime of the individual.

Restoration of normal gingival form and crevice depth beyond what occurs during elimination of inflammation has been recommended in the form of surgical recontouring (gingivoplasty). Surgery is usually of more esthetic than hygienic value, although surgical reduction of the third molar gum flaps may be needed to cure the gingivitis. Similarly, with lack

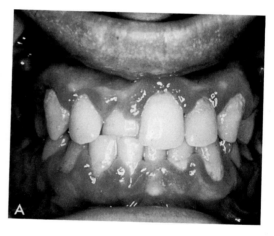

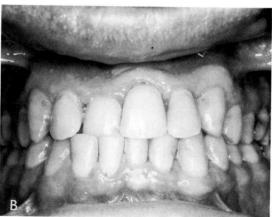

Fig. 12-2. *A,* Chronic simple gingivitis with changes in color, form, density, and increased crevice depth associated with swelling of the gingiva. Bleeding wtih slight provocation. Male, 47 years old. *B,* After scaling and instruction in oral hygiene, there was great improvement, but there is still some plaque on the teeth and mild marginal gingivitis.

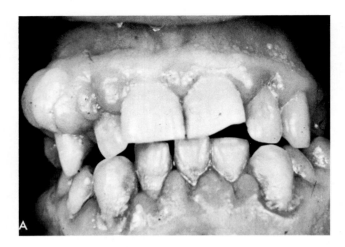

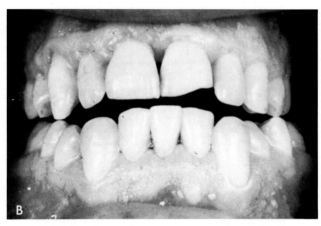

Fig. 12-3. *A,* Extensive gingival hyperplasia associated with chronic simple gingivitis. Male, 55 years old, no oral hygiene. *B,* After scaling, home care and gingivoplasty. Improvement has occurred, but there is still chronic gingivitis.

of attached gingiva, mucogingival surgery may be needed to cure the gingivitis (see chapter 25). Severe gingival hyperplasia as a result of long-standing chronic gingivitis may be very fibrotic and may affect esthetic appearance and interfere with normal masticatory function. Such gingival enlargement should be removed surgically (Fig. 12-3, A, B). The indications and the required surgical procedures are discussed in chapter 22.

COMPLEX GINGIVITIS

In complex gingivitis, the gingival response to plaque and other irritants has been altered by either local or systemic influences not ordinarily present. On the basis of clinical appearance, one diversified group of such manifestations is often termed gingival hyperplasia or gingival enlargement, although gingival hyperplasia may also occur in simple gingivitis of both the acute and chronic types.

Gingival Hyperplasia

Gingival hyperplasia includes an increase in the size of the gingiva due to a reactive increase in tissue cells, fluid, and the presence of inflammatory cells. Included in this category are mouthbreather's gingivitis, hereditary gingival fibromatosis, Dilantin gingivitis, pregnancy gingivitis, and leukemic gingivitis.

Mouthbreather's gingivitis

The alternating drying and wetting of the gingival mucosa in mouthbreathers may alter the appearance of the part of the gingiva that is not covered by the resting lips (Fig. 12-1, C). The uncovered mucosa may become glossy red and enlarged to various degrees.[53,76] The pathogenesis of these mucosal changes is not known. The gingival changes are most often observed on the labial gingiva related to protruded maxillary anterior teeth, and the uncovered part of the gingiva may be demarcated from the part covered by the lip by a distinct border or "lip line" (Fig. 12-4, A, B, C). The disturbance may appear as an intensive redness of the palatal gingiva bordering the maxillary anterior teeth.

The alternating drying and wetting of the teeth by saliva will result in rapid accumulation of a thick salivary pellicle on the teeth, but does not seem to increase the amount of plaque.[53] Whether this coating of the teeth predisposes to more and different types of plaque formation with altered irritation potentials compared to persons with normal lip seal is not known. Nor is it known if mouthbreather's gingivitis predisposes to periodontitis to a greater extent than does simple gingivitis, although calculus has been found to be more prevalent in mouthbreathers than in persons with nasal respiration.[3]

Diagnosis. The collapsed inactive nostrils and protruding maxillary front teeth in persons with a lack of lip seal often suggest the diagnosis of mouthbreathing before oral examination (Fig. 12-1, C). The characteristic gingival manifestation of mouthbreathing is glossy, red, and enlarged interdental papillae and thick gingival margins on the labial aspect of the maxillary anterior and biscuspid teeth. On the palatal aspect, the demarcation between the affected and unaffected mucosa is not as well defined as on the labial side, but there is often a red gingival margin close to the teeth, with tenderness and a tendency for bleeding upon slight provocation.

Therapy. Anything that can be done to facilitate normal nasal breathing should be encouraged. Consultation with a physician to assure that the nasal passages are fully patent should be recommended. Orthodontic treatment to gain lip seal may be indicated, and deliberate practice in nasal breathing should be encouraged. However, changing the habit of mouth-

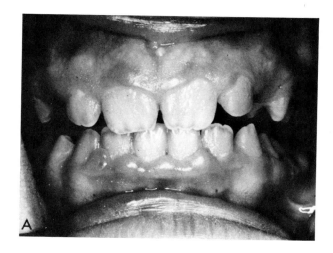

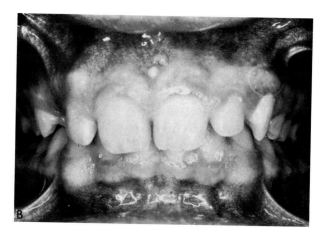

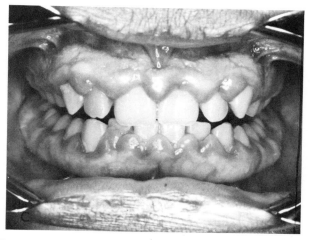

breathing to nasal breathing is very dfficult, and attempts are often unsuccessful. A number of patients also have unavoidable periodic nasal obstruction with allergic rhinitis. Mouthbreathing is such cases will continue in spite of attempts at treatment. For these individuals, meticulous and frequent oral hygiene (at least 2 times a day) should be instituted. Some benefit with regard to decreased gingival reaction has been claimed from covering the affected parts of the gingiva with Vaseline or Orabase before going to sleep.[76] However, no studies under controlled conditions have established the long-term benefit of such practice.

Hereditary gingival fibromatosis

Hereditary gingival fibromatosis or hyperplasia (Fig. 12-1, D) is a rare gingival disease with many names (elephantiasis of the gingiva, giantism of the gingiva, fibromatosis gingivae, multiple epulides, hypertrophic gingivitis).[10,108,125,128] In many instances, there are convincing family histories of the disease being associated with a hereditary developmental anomaly apparently transmitted by a dominant autosomal gene.[24,125] Other cases deviate from that pattern,[14] and in some instances, a family history of inheritance cannot be established.

Gradual enlargement of the entire gingiva is usually noticed during and after eruption of the permanent dentition, but occasionally it has also been observed to start during eruption of the deciduous teeth[24,90] (Fig. 12-5). The greatest enlargement often occurs on the palatal aspects of the maxillary molars (Fig. 12-6). There is no pain and no increased bleeding tendency, except sometimes upon crevicular probing. The gingival tissues are normal in color, and firm, often with pronounced stippling. Histologically, the hyperplastic

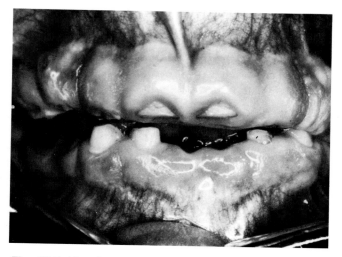

Fig. 12-4. *A,* Mouthbreather's gingivitis in 11-year-old boy. Note hyperplasia of mandibular anterior gingiva above demarcation for the "lip line" from contact with the resting lip. *B,* Same patient as in *A* after hygienic therapy and use of Vaseline to cover the gingiva at night. There is noticeable reduction in swelling. *C,* Severe gingival hyperplasia associated with mouthbreathing in 18-year-old male. Both maxillary and mandibular labial and buccal gingiva are uncovered by the lips during rest. The hyperplasia extends to the posterior parts of the mouth.

Fig. 12-5. Hereditary gingival fibromatosis around deciduous teeth in 5-year-old male child. His mother and two brothers also had the same condition. Note how both free and attached gingiva are affected.

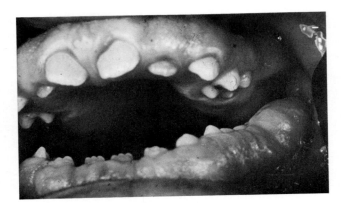

Fig. 12-6. Palatal and buccal hyperplasia in 33-year-old male with hereditary gingival fibromatosis.

gingival tissues are made up of fibrous connective tissue with coarse collagenous fiber bundles. The only evidence of inflammation is immediately under the crevicular lining.[103] The histological features may be indistinguishable from advanced Dilantin hyperplasia or fibroid epulis. Hypertrichosis of varied severity has been reported to accompany the gingival enlargement in some cases.[108]

Diagnosis. The diagnosis should be based on the clinical findings and a positive family history of a similar condition. If such a history is not available, Dilantin hyperplasia may be excluded if the patient does not use the drug.

Treatment. The hyperplastic gingival tissues should be removed surgically for esthetic and functional reasons. This may be accomplished either by gingivectomy or by undermining reverse bevel flap procedures (see chapters 22 and 23). The surgery is often postponed until after the eruption of the second molars, but in severe cases partial removal of hyperplastic tissues may be done at an earlier age. The rate of recurrence of the hyperplasia is to a great extent dependent on the patient's oral hygiene. With meticulous oral hygiene, the regrowth may be very slow, and the surgery may not have to be repeated for 10 to 20 years. Slight orthodontic treatment may be indicated following removal of the hyperplastic tissues, which have a tendency to wedge the teeth apart, especially in the maxillary anterior region. Whether hyperplasia will develop under complete dentures if the teeth are extracted is controversial. One case has been reported in which this did not occur,[90,128] but we have seen hyperplasia recur under a complete maxillary denture in a mother of three children, all of whom had hereditary gingival fibromatosis (Fig. 12-7). Because this is not a true neoplasm, and the condition may be controlled by periodic surgical interventions and good oral hygiene, extraction of the teeth because of the hyperplasia is not indicated.

Dilantin gingivitis

After the introduction of phenytoin (diphenylhydantoin) for treatment of seizures (epilepsy),[1] a number of cases regarding hyperplastic gingival changes have been reported.[32,61]

It soon became apparent that only about 40 to 50% of individuals taking Dilantin developed hyperplastic gingival changes.[1,78,117] A significant correlation has been documented between the degree of gingival hyperplasia and the dosage and duration of the medication.[1] The rate of hyperplastic growth appears to be greatest during the 1st year on the drug, and greater in younger than older individuals. A statistically significant correlation has been reported between the degree of hyperplasia and the level of oral hygiene.[1]

The gingival hyperplasia may start 1 to 6 months after the drug therapy is initiated. It usually starts as inflammatory overgrowth of the interdental papillae and, in the early stages, is confined to the interdental papillae, but may later involve the free gingiva (Fig. 12-1, E).

The papillae initially appear red, swollen, and soft (Fig. 12-8, A, B). Later the edematous, swollen tissues undergo fibrosis, become denser and less red in color, and the bleeding tendency upon provocation decreases until in long-standing lesions the surface texture of the gingiva is almost normal, although there is always evidence of inflammation where the gingiva contacts the tooth.

Histologically, early gingival hyperplasia is charac-

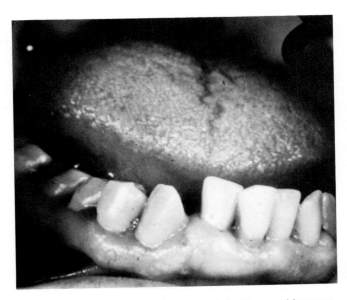

Fig. 12-7. Hereditary gingival fibromatosis in 42-year-old woman. She has had gingivoplasty three times since she was a young girl. For esthetic reasons her maxillary teeth were extracted the time she had the first mandibular gingivoplasty. She experienced hyperplasia under the maxillary dentures and she has had surgical removal of hyperplastic maxillary tissues twice. She has 3 sons, all of whom have hereditary gingival fibromatosis.

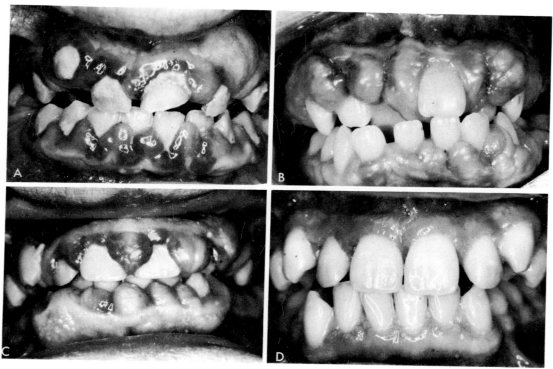

Fig. 12-8. *A,* Dilantin gingivitis in 11-year-old girl with complete lack of oral hygiene. Soft, red and swollen papillae with abundant accumulation of plaque on the teeth. *B,* Dilantin gingivitis in 28-year-old female. Dense, fibrotic gingival hyperplasia, which has displaced several of the teeth and resulted in malocclusion. *C,* Dilantin gingivitis in 20-year old male. *D,* Same patient as in *C.* One year after gingivoplasty and institution of good oral hygiene.

terized by severe and diffuse inflammation. In long-standing hyperplasia, the inflammatory changes are often confirmed close to the gingival crevice, while the rest of the fibrotic gingiva is indistinguishable from hereditary gingival fibromatosis or fibroid epulides.

In spite of extensive research and numerous theories, the mechanism whereby Dilantin induces gingival hyperplasia is not entirely clear. It was suggested 25 years ago that the hyperplasia is an aggregated connective tissue response to local irritation in patients in whom Dilantin has affected adrenocortical function,[116] but this has not been substantiated scientifically.

Diagnosis. Positive history of the use of Dilantin and presence of gingival hyperplasia are the fundamental prerequisites for the diagnosis of Dilantin gingivitis. Dilantin is still the best drug available for control of grand mal seizures, and it is not necessary to interfere with this drug therapy in order to treat the gingival hyperplasia successfully. However, the patient should take the minimal effective dosage of Dilantin for control of epilepsy in order to prevent gingival hyperplasia. Another drug that predisposes to gingival hyperplasia is cyclosporin, which is used primarily in organ transplant patient to prevent graft rejection.[104]

Treatment. It has been shown that the hyperplasia can be prevented by good oral hygiene.[1,41] If the hyperplastic tissues are removed surgically by gingivectomy or flap procedures and the patient maintains good oral hygiene, the hyperplasia will not return[1,41] (Fig. 12-8, *C, D*). The problem is the management of good oral hygiene, especially in mentally retarded persons. It has been recommended that chlorhexidine gluconate be used to supplement plaque control for patients on Dilantin therapy who are not mentally or physically able to maintain adequate oral hygiene. Mild Dilantin hyperplasia in early inflammatory stages may regress almost completely by prophylaxis and good oral hygiene, and does not require surgical removal of the hyperplastic tissues.

Pregnancy gingivitis

That gingivitis may be aggravated during pregnancy has been known for over a century.[44] Most commonly, it has been assumed that this increase in gingival inflammation is caused by an altered metabolic response to bacterial plaque on the teeth,[17,51,82] rather than being a specific pathological entity of periodontal disease caused by systemic changes and primarily due to the pregnancy itself.[130] During pregnancy, there is a marked increase in the blood levels of estrogen and

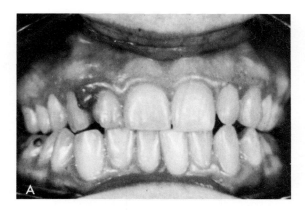

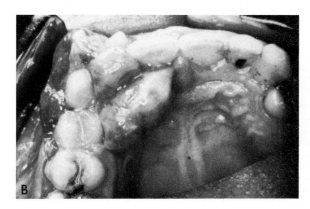

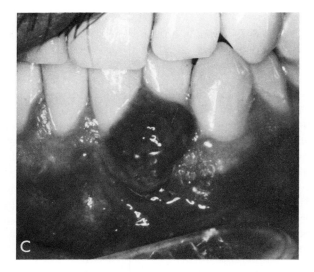

Fig. 12-9. *A,* Pregnancy gingivitis with small pregnancy tumor between right maxillary cuspid and lateral incisor. Twenty-seven-year-old female, seventh month of pregnancy. A similar tumor was present but subsided after previous pregnancy. Generalized gingivitis and poor plaque control. *B,* Large pregnancy tumor. Twenty-six-year-old woman, eighth month of pregnancy. The tumor has displaced teeth and interferes with masticatory function. Severe bleeding tendency upon minor provocation. *C,* Recurrent pyogenic granuloma in 21-year-old male. After two unsuccessful tries at removal, periosteum and some alveolar bone with periodontal membrane had to be removed, after which the tumor did not recur.

progesterone. Parturition is followed by a marked fall in those levels. Since the increase in gingivitis occurs at about the same time as the rise in the blood levels of these sex hormones, it has been suggested that the altered behavior of the gingival tissues during pregnancy may be due to the increased hormonal levels.[79] It has been reported that *B. intermedius* is associated with the appearance and severity of pregnancy gingivitis and that proportional bacterial counts correlated with levels of plasma estrogen and progesterone which may act as nutrients for these organisms.[67]

In a well-controlled longitudinal study,[51] it was demonstrated that gingivitis became more severe during pregnancy, but without any corresponding concomitant change in amount of bacterial plaque on the teeth, thus confirming a relationship between the increase in gingivitis and some metabolic change related to pregnancy.[79,114] It may be that progesterone, by acting on the gingival microcirculation, is more responsible for the increased inflammatory response than is estrogen.[50,71,73]

No notable changes occur in the gingiva during pregnancy in the absence of local irritants, and there is no evidence to indicate that pregnancy itself causes gingivitis.

Hormonal contraceptives may also induce gingival manifestations indistinguishable from pregnancy gingivitis.[23,72,98] However, such gingival manifestations are very rare, considering the common use of oral contraceptives, and do not occur at all in patients with good plaque control.[98] Crevicular fluid exudate may be increased during menstruation in patients with gingivitis, whereas patients with gingival health are not affected.[49]

Clinical and histological features. Nonspecific enlarged red gingival papillae that bleed upon slight provocation are seen in pregnancy gingivitis. Sometimes, one papilla may grow out like a tumor (Fig. 12-9, *A*), but such lesions are not neoplastic.[59] In severe cases, both the marginal and the papillary gingivae are shiny red or bluish-red, soft, and usually smooth, while the "granulomas" may have a pebbled, raspberry-like appearance.[32] The crevicular depth may increase, as a result of gingival swelling rather than of loss of attachment. There is no pain associated with the gingivitis unless there is impingement upon the swollen tissues by the occlusion (Fig. 12-9, *B*). There is also a significant increase in horizontal tooth mobility during pregnancy.[17]

The typical clinical appearance of pregnancy gingivitis is seen only in a small percentage of pregnant women with gingivitis.[80] It starts as an apparent activation of chronic gingivitis to a more acute type during the 2nd or 3rd month of pregnancy, with increase in gingival bulk through the 8th month, when it starts to regress. Without treatment, the gingiva returns over some months to the same chronic gingivitis that the patient had before the pregnancy.[17]

The histopathological appearance of pregnancy gingivitis is that of a nonspecific, highly vascular inflammation[31,82] with heavy cellular infiltration. Newly formed capillaries predominate in the inflamed tissues. Surface ulceration may occasionally be observed. Pregnancy tumors, clinically and histologically,[59] are the same as pyogenic granulomas seen in nonpregnant persons (Fig. 12-9, C).

Diagnosis. A positive history of pregnancy or use of contraceptive pills is a prerequisite for the diagnosis of pregnancy gingivitis. The clinical and histopathological features are not in themselves diagnostic, although the clinical appearance of swelling and marked color changes with pronounced bleeding tendencies may be highly suggestive of pregnancy gingivitis.

Treatment. Pregnancy gingivitis responds well to regular hygienic therapy, including removal of local irritants and institution of good oral hygiene (chapters 16 and 17), and should be treated as simple gingivitis. Severe gingival hemorrhage or sensitivity may interfere with regular scaling and root planing. Local anesthetics should then be used, but with the limitations on systemic aspects of periodontal care discussed in chapter 15. With pregnancy tumors, surgical removal may be needed. This preferably should be done during the 2nd trimester, and the lesions have to be excised to the bone, with the periosteum included. With subsequent good oral hygiene, the tendency for recurrence is small.[98]

Leukemic gingivitis

Gingival enlargement with increased bleeding tendency may be found in patients with acute leukemias,[11,124] mainly the monocytic and the acute myelogenous leukemias (Fig. 12-1, F).

The leukemia does not cause the gingivitis,[69] but the lowered resistance to infection due to lack of normal functional leukocytes tends to aggravate already present gingivitis, and the increased bleeding tendency with these diseases often discourages vigorous oral hygiene. The result is an increase in plaque harboring infective organisms. It has also been claimed that the large immature cells in acute monocytic leukemia may act as emboli in the fine gingival capillary loops and create stasis.[124]

Clinical and histopathological features. The gingival tissues are soft, swollen, and appear bluish-red. The bulbous interdental papillae may exhibit surface necrosis, with a pseudomembrane resembling necrotizing ulcerative gingivitis (NUG), but the inflammation is usually not as well delineated as in ordinary NUG. In severe cases, the hyperplastic gingiva may almost cover the crowns of the teeth. The marked increase in bleeding tendency is often a major complaint.

Histologically, there is a dense diffuse infiltration of predominantly immature leukocytes both in the free and in the attached gingiva.[31] Surface ulcerations with a fibrinous pseudomembrane are not uncommon, and the underlying leukemia may easily be overlooked as a faulty diagnosis of NUG is made.

Diagnosis. The diagnosis of leukemia gingivitis is made from blood studies and history of leukemia. Histopathological features are diagnostic of leukemia, but if leukemia is suspected on the basis of the clinical appearance or poor response to local therapy, blood studies rather than biopsy are recommended, as the bleeding response and the healing process following the biopsy may be complicated by the leukemia, and the evidence of leukemia may be missed in the biopsy specimens. No biopsy should be performed if it is known that the patient has leukemia.

Treatment. If the patient is being treated for the leukemia, the most favorable time for the periodontal treatment should be determined in conference with the patient's physician. If local irritants are eliminated, the leukemic gingivitis will subside to a great extent. It is advisable to do a superficial debridement first and to instruct the patient to use a soft toothbrush. If deep scaling is needed for removal of calculus, antibiotic coverage and local anesthetics may be recommended. Then cover the instrumented area with 3% acromycin ointment and a periodontal dressing, and limit the scaling to one quadrant at each session. No periodontal surgery is indicated for patients with leukemic gingivitis. Because these patients have very poor response to dental plaque and other irritants, it is mandatory that the teeth be kept as clean as possible and that all irritating dental appliances be corrected or eliminated.

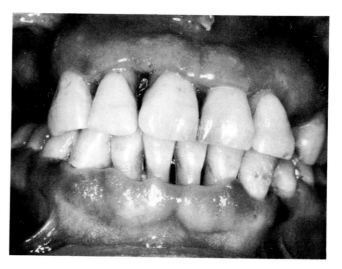

Fig. 12-10. Recurrent necrotizing ulcerative gingivitis following several unsuccessful episodes of treatment with chromic acid. Male, 27 years old. Note loss of interproximal tissues.

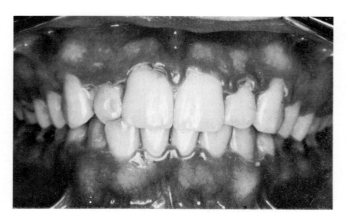

Fig. 12-11. Necrotizing ulcerative gingivitis. Female, 23 years old, who had had a sore mouth for 3 to 4 days. Necrosis with loss of interdental papillae related to right maxillary lateral incisor. Gray pseudomembrane-covered necrotic lesions. Beginning involvement also of free gingival margins in the maxilla.

Acute and Recurrent Necrotizing Gingival Lesions

Various forms of acute or chronic, progressive, or self-limiting necrotizing lesions may involve the gingiva, periodontium, and adjacent structures as a reuslt of physical or chemical agents, irradiation, infections, and unknown factors. The most common lesion is acute necrotizing ulcerative gingivitis (NUG), or Vincent's infection. Rare necrotizing processes such as exanthematous necrosis, Takahara's disease (acatalasia), gangrenous stomatitis (noma), and mercury poisoning may involve the periodontium, but are not considered to be periodontal diseases.

Necrotizing ulcerative gingivitis (NUG)

Painful ulceration of the gingiva has been described since far back in historical times. Xenophon reported in 401 B.C. that many of the soldiers retreating from the Persian wars were affected with sore, foul-smelling mouths.[48] Hunter, in 1778, clearly differentiated this painful disease from periodontitis,[31] and the classic description of the disease dates back to Plaut[101] and Vincent.[121] In the 1890s, these investigators implicated fusiform and spirochetal bacteria in the etiology of the disease, which since that time has often been referred to as Vincent's infection (Fig. 12-1, *G, H*). Other names for the disease are *ulceromembraneous gingivitis, gingivitis ulcerosa, necrotizing gingivitis, fusospirochetal gingivitis, pseudomembranous ulcerative necrotizing gingivitis,* and *trench mouth* (because of its frequent occurrence among soldiers in the frontline trenches during World War I).[109] The descriptive term *necrotizing ulcerative gingivitis* (NUG) is preferred over *acute necrotizing ulcerative gingivitis* (ANUG), because a necrotizing and ulcerative lesion has to be assumed to be acute, and the terms *subacute* and *chronic necrotizing ulcerative gingivitis* are con-

fusing misnomers for recurrent or residual acute necrotizing ulcerative lesions (Fig. 12-10).

Clinical features of NUG. NUG starts as an acute painful swelling and redness, usually at the tips of the interdental papillae in areas of previous gingivitis associated with plaque, calculus, and poor dental restorations. It may also start in 3rd molar gum flaps or at poorly fitting crown margins. These locations were called "incubation zones" by Box 50 years ago.[9] Spirochetes and fusiform bacteria are commonly found in these locations, even without NUG (Fig. 12-11).

Within hours or a very few days after the patient experiences the initial burning painful sensation, ulceration and bleeding upon the slightest provocation appear. The ulcers become covered by a gray-yellow fibrinous exudate constituting a pseudomembrane (Fig. 12-1, *G,* 12-1, *I*), which is easily removed to reveal a raw, bleeding, and very tender surface.[5,35] Sloughing of the progressively necrotic interdental papillae creates craterlike lesions surrounded by an intensive red halo at the swollen borders of the ulceration. The lesions may spread from the papillae along the gingival margins, creating crater-like depressions. In severe cases, there may be spontaneous bleeding, and the lesions may occasionally spread even to the adjacent alveolar mucosa. Lesions not connected with the gingival ulcers may, in a few instances, develop in locations with lymphoid tissues, such as the tonsillar regions and the residual Waldeyer's ring in the soft palate (Fig. 12-12). These mucosal lesions are called *Vincent's angina,* and have the same punched-out, necrotic, crater-like ulcers as the gingival manifestations of the disease.

In patients with extremely poor resistance associ-

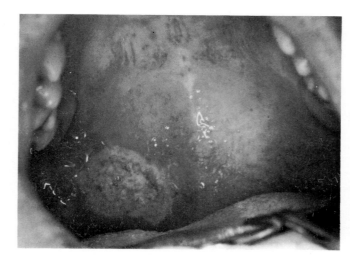

Fig. 12-12. Vincent's angina in 19-year-old female with necrotizing ulcerative gingivitis. The palatal lesion has a necrotic, punched-out base surrounded by a red halo. It healed promptly following penicillin therapy.

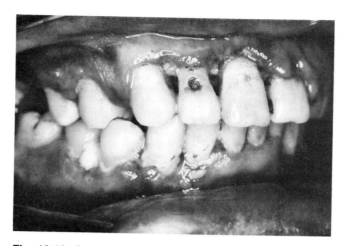

Fig. 12-13. Cancrum oris with bare necrotic bone in male 19 years old. General malaise and high fever. Responded to prolonged high dosage of penicillin therapy and oral hygiene.

ated with severe malnutrition, the gingival necrosis may progress to and expose the alveolar process. These severe lesions are called *cancrum oris*,[25] and have been described in children from areas where there is extreme malnutrition.[26,83] With even more severe facial necrosis, the lesions are called *noma*. Such cases are extremely rare in the western world. Cancrum oris indicates that, besides gingival lesions, the patient has osteomyelitis and may develop fever, with temperatures of up to 103° F (Fig. 12-13).

The patients with NUG often complain of a foul taste and a wedging sensation between the teeth. A peculiar pungent halitosis of decay, distinctly different from the common halitosis of an unclean mouth, may be observed in severe cases. There is often lymphadenopathy in the regional neck glands. A slight increase in body temperature is only rarely present,[40] although the patients may complain of mild malaise, anorexia, and dysphagia. Blood counts may show a slight leukocytosis.

According to a survey[5] of 218 patients with NUG, the most common signs and symptoms of the disease were (1) gingival bleeding (95%); (2) blunting of the interdental papillae (94%); (3) fetid odor (84%); (4) pseudomembrane (73%); (5) pain (86%); and (6) bad taste in the mouth (40%). Of great diagnostic significance is the presence of a painful, bleeding, necrotizing ulcer, which better than anything else characterizes the disease.

Epidemiology. Since ancient times, NUG has occurred in individuals or groups of people living in stressful situations.[31] Therefore, prevalance figures from general population samples would be meaningless. The highest incidence has been reported for young males (18 to 20 years of age) in wartime[109] or during college examination.[27,58] Common denominators are stress[84] and heavy smoking.[100] In the United

States, the disease very seldom occurs in children, but severe manifestation of NUG has been observed in poorly nourished children in other parts of the world.[83] It is also very unusual to find NUG in persons over 40 years of age.

It has been well established that the disease is not communicable.[109] Experimental transfer of organisms from active lesions of 1 person to another will not initiate the disease, even if the gingival tissues are traumatized beforehand,[64,110] and so-called epidemics of NUG can always be traced to group exposure to stress, such as the trench mouth phenomenon in World War I.[109]

As with other forms of periodontal disease, NUG seems to have a higher incidence in the lower than in the higher socioeconomic groups.[31] In these populations, plaque scores are also high. It appears, however, that the disease rarely, if ever, starts in a clean, healthy mouth.[58] From clinical observations, it appears that the incidence of NUG in an average American population is very low at the present time.

Histopathology. The histological appearance of NUG is a fairly well demarcated necrotic ulcer covered by a fibrinous membrane incorporating dead cells, nuclear cell debris, numerous dead, dying, and living polymorphonuclear cells, plus a large number of bacteria, with a preponderance of fusiforms and spirochetes.[13]

In contrast to simple gingivitis and periodontitis, bacteria have been observed within the tissues in the NUG lesions by both light[13] and electron microscopy.[43,74,75] The surface of the wound is covered by a variety of organisms, but the penetration into the inflamed tissues is by spirochetes and fusiform bacilli only. The deepest penetration, extending for several cell layers into living connective tissue and epithelium, is by spirochetes.[75] However, this penetration does not necessarily indicate that the spirochetes are the cause of the lesion.

Etiology. The term *Vincent's infection* is an expression of the old belief that NUG is caused by an infection of Vincent's[121] organisms (fusiform bacilli and spirochetes). There is no question about the preponderance of these organisms in the active disease.[107] The fact that the symptoms of the disease abate remarkably in less than 24 hours following antibiotic drug therapy also tends to support the infection theory.[122] However, it becomes more difficult to sustain the theory of a specific infection when it is considered that these organisms are also present in simple chronic gingivitis, and that all attempts to produce NUG lesions by transfer of fuso-spirochetal organisms have failed.[110] Establishment of necrotizing lesions in guinea pigs following injection of infectious material[42,107] is meaningless, since similar reactions may also be produced by injection of plaque from patients with simple gingivitis and even from patients with no clinical evidence of any periodontal disease.[110] Similar lesions may also be induced by other organisms, such as *Bacteroides melaninogenicus*, without the concomitant presence of spirochetes and fusiforms.[89]

The strongest support for the theory of a specific infection as the cause of NUG has been the demonstration of spirochetes and fusiform organisms penetrating the tissues at the base of the NUG lesions.[74,75] A major limitation in the study of the spirochetal effect in NUG is the present inability to culture most oral spirochetes. Thus experimental investigations of these organisms are seriously hampered, and no definite evidence is available at present to establish that any specific organism or group of organisms is the initial cause of NUG.

One of the most consistent observations in studies of NUG patients is the history of recent stress, as is evident from the disease's association with wartime experiences[109] and students during examination periods.[27] Corticosteroid release is increased under emotional stress.[86] This may alter connective tissue turnover and increase tissue permeability and vasomotor tonicity.[28]

Another hypothetical explanation of the relationship between stress and NUG is that increased epinephrine output during stress[112] may lead to constriction of the capillary loops of the end circulation in the gingival papillae,[62,63] and thus adversely affect gingival resistance.[56] The often-claimed association between heavy smoking and NUG[100] could also be explained by the release of epinephrine that occurs with smoking,[12,123] with resultant vasoconstriction and relative anoxia in the papillary areas. Smoking may also produce a transient lowering of the oxidation-reduction potential in the mouth. However, this does not seem to favor the anaerobic fractions of the bacterial flora in dental plaque.[57] Another interesting observation is that smoking may impair leukocytic function.[22] The 3 chief interrelated factors predisposing to NUG seem to be sepsis, stress, and smoking, and all of these factors will influence gingival circulation.[56]

Another predisposing factor may be the lowered gamma globulin level that has been noted in patients with NUG.[68,127] However, a possible effect of an altered immune reaction in the pathogenic complex of NUG has not been demonstrated. Certain systemic diseases,[31] such as infectious mononucleosis, acute leukemia, cyclic neutropenia, Down's syndrome,[18] metallic poisoning and severe malnutrition,[26] and debilitating diseases,[20] seem to predispose to NUG, which may indicate that lowered resistance is a predisposing etiological factor.

In summary, the interplay between potentially pathogenic organisms and altered defense mechanisms in the host that leads to NUG has not been fully elucidated at the present time, and NUG generally is considered to be an opportunistic infection.

Diagnosis. The diagnosis of NUG is made on the basis of the history of the symptoms and clinical signs of the disease.[5] The two most common and characteristic symptoms are pain and severe bleeding tendency; foul taste, malaise, and occasional slight fever are less common symptoms. The most important signs are necrotic lesions with blunting of the gingival papillae, severe pain, and bleeding upon slight provocation; less diagnostic signs are the presence of a pseudomembrane over the lesion, fetid odor, and regional lymphadenopathy.

Bacteriological or cytological smears are not useful in establishing the diagnosis of NUG; neither are biopsies,[13] as the histopathological appearance of NUG is similar to that from trauma and chemical burns.

In differential diagnosis, the following lesions should be ruled out: herpetic gingivostomatitis (no necrotic tissue loss but high fever), leukemia and neutropenia (blood studies), and candidiasis (clinical appearance and culture of organisms). Other diseases may also have some of the signs and symptoms of NUG, but their history is different: gonorrhea, syphilis, heavy metal poison, tularemia, cat scratch disease, erythema multiform, and histoplasmosis.[8]

Treatment. After World War I, treatment of NUG was usually based on the hypothesis that the disease was a contagious fusospirochetal infection. Because the suspected organisms were anaerobic, and the spirochetes were susceptible to arsenicals, oxidizing agents and arsenicals were used for the treatment of the disease. Later it was observed that topical applications of escharotics alleviated the pain, and during World War II, chromic acid, silver nitrate, and phenol were commonly used in treatment of NUG, combined with aniline dyes for antibacterial effect.

Since Lyons (1948) stated the NUG could be cured by hygienic procedures only,[81] and it was pointed out that escharotic drugs only eliminated the pain by necrosis of nerve endings and other tissues in the wound,[33] arsenicals and escharotics have not been commonly used.

Antibiotics[30,122] or oxidizing agents have been more popular. They may alleviate the symptoms and lead to partial regression of the lesions, but they will not effect a cure unless a meticulous hygienic regime is implemented in addition to the drugs. A drug that has been suggested recently for treatment of NUG is metronidazole.[29,122] Although this drug may not be as immediately effective in elimination of symptoms as penicillin, it has been claimed to be relatively free from side effects. However, none of these drugs has any advantages over hygienic therapy alone, except possibly in the cases with systemic symptoms of the disease. The fact that the disease is noncontagious also negates the need for antibiotics in uncomplicated cases, since equally fast and lasting relief of pain may

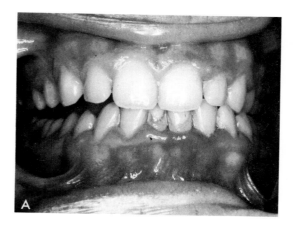 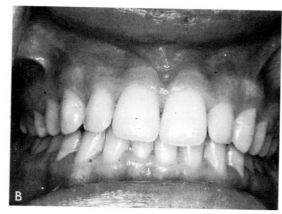

Fig. 12-14. *A,* Necrotizing ulcerative gingivitis in mandibular anterior region. Interproximal necrosis with swollen gingival margins and pseudopapillae. Female, 20 years old. *B,* After repeated scaling, polishing, and instruction in oral hygiene. Note normal gingival form.

be achieved by hygienic therapy alone. Furthermore, even with antibiotics, satisfactory hygienic therapy is needed to cure the disease.

The recommended treatment is debridement of the teeth, which involves polishing the teeth carefully with a rubber cap and pumice. Then apply topical Xylocaine and remove all accessible calculus. If removal of calculus is painful in spite of the topical anesthetics, anesthetize the site by injection. The sooner calculus removal and root planing is accomplished, the sooner will the lesions heal. If time is not available at the initial appointment for complete prophylaxis, at least polish the teeth and remove gross calculus. Instruct the patient in circular scrub toothbrushing and in the use of dental floss, which he should start to practice 12 to 24 hours after the initial appointment. Use 1½% hydrogen peroxide mouthrinse every 2 hours.

The next visit to the dentist should be 1 to 3 days later, depending on how thorough the initial debridement was. At the second appointment, scaling, root planing, removal of overhangs, and polishing should be completed. Instruction in oral hygiene with emphasis on the use of dental floss should be repeated, and the use of hydrogen peroxide rinses discontinued. Subsequent weekly appointments with instruction in oral hygiene and complete polishing of the teeth should be repeated until the gingiva has regenerated to an acceptable form (Fig. 12-14, A, B).

If there is considerable gingival deformity with pseudopapillae from recurrent attacks of NUG, the access for cleaning of the interproximal tooth surfaces is poor. In such cases, a gingivoplasty after the initial debridement (see Fig. 22-6, A, B) will shorten the time needed for complete cure of the disease.[31] Such cases with pseudopapillae and active necrosis in the interproximal spaces are often designated *subacute Vincent's infection.* The patients have usually been treated repeatedly with antibiotics without adequate

debridement and have a history of remissions and exacerbations of symptoms. From a pathological standpoint, the inflammatory manifestations during the periods of recurrent necrosis must still be considered acute, and we prefer the term *recurrent NUG* rather than *subacute NUG.*

During the time when NUG was treated with repeated application of demineralizing caustics such as chromic acid, it was common to find deep interproximal craters involving loss of bone (Fig. 12-10). These cases were called *chronic Vincent's infection.* The exposed root surfaces were soft from the demineralization caused by the acid, and very sensitive because of accumulation and penetration of bacteria and bacterial products.

If the NUG has developed into osteomyelitis, cancrum oris, or noma, the patients should be treated with large doses of penicillin over at least 2 to 3 weeks, in addition to debridement of the local lesions. Any patient with NUG and body temperature over 100° F may be treated with penicillin in addition to the routine oral debridement.

The treatment of NUG is not complete until a gingival architecture that allows efficient oral hygiene is established.[85] There is a tendency for the patients to reject further treatment when the initial symptoms have abated, and then to return for further treatment when the pain recurs, as it often does if the treatment has not been carried through to complete resolution of the lesions.

Summary. NUG is a unique acute tissue-destroying gingival disease with poorly understood etiology and pathogenesis. The clinical signs and symptoms are distinct and diagnostic. Treatment by debridement and efficient oral hygiene is usually followed by a dramatically favorable response. The disease may recur if the treatment is not carried to complete resolution of the lesions and restitution of normal gingival architecture.

GINGIVOSTOMATITIS
Desquamative

Several types of lesions are characterized primarily by extensive desquamation of the gingiva or mucosa. Included in this classification are chronic desquamative gingivitis, benign mucous membrane pemphigus (pemphigoid), and erosive lichen planus. Other lesions, related to allergens, thermal and electrical injury, and specific dermatological disease, may also exhibit desquamative characteristics.

Chronic desquamative gingivitis

The descriptive term *chronic desquamative gingivitis* was first suggested by Merrit in 1933,[92] but the disease had been described much earlier under different names.[102,119] It was said to occur most often in females after the age of 30,[31] but may in fact appear any time after puberty and may also affect males. It has been reported in dentate as well as in nondentate persons.[97,111] The gingival mucosa is glistening red, with small, dull, grayish patches involving both the free and the attached gingiva (Fig. 12-1, I). The surface epithelium may be rubbed or peeled off, leaving a red, tender surface. There is a dry, burning sensation in the mouth, and sensitivity to thermal changes. Highly spiced food cannot be tolerated, and toothbrushing is painful. Histologically, there is severe, immediate subepithelial inflammation and a tendency to separation between the epithelium and the connective tissues. The histological findings are not diagnostic, however, because similar pathological changes have been observed by both light[34] and electron microscopy[55,95] for benign mucous membrane pemphigoid and erosive lichen planus, and there are growing indications that the chronic desquamative gingivitis is not a disease entity but a variant of vesicular dermatological disorders,[87,88] such as lichen planus and mucous membrane pemphigoid[106] or immunopathological[105] and allergic responses.

The tenderness of the gingiva hinders plaque control, and patients often develop secondary acute marginal gingivitis in response to plaque retained on the teeth.

Diagnosis. The preliminary diagnosis of desquamative gingivitis is made on the basis of the gingiva and the absence of established signs and symptoms of definable dermatological or allergic reactions. By careful examination and observation, which may have to be extended over several years,[106] it will usually be found that the desquamation is due to dermatological or allergic disorders rather than representing an entity of chronic desquamative gingivitis. Chronic desquamative gingivitis is considered to be a term to describe a gingival manifestation of a variety of diseases, most frequently dermatoses such as benign mucous membrane pemphigoid, pemphigus, and erosive lichen planus.

Treatment. Because the etiology is unknown, there is no rational therapy. Experimental therapy with estrogen or other hormones is discouraged. Supportive therapy should consist of careful oral hygiene with soft toothbrushes and dental floss. Fortunately, the desquamative gingival lesions usually have remissions and sometimes disappear without returning.

Mucous membrane pemphigoid

Mucous membrane pemphigoid (Fig. 12-1, J) is basically characterized by bullous gingival lesions, sometimes containing a clear and at other times a red serosanguineous fluid. These bullae break open after a short time—usually before the patient comes to the doctor's office—and the lesion is then covered by a desquamating gray epithelial coating from the outer wall of the bulla. Most often, the gingival mucosa on the labial aspect appears red and glistening, without any evidence of bullous lesions, and the patient may have to be observed over some time before a definite diagnosis can be made.[106] Biopsy will not establish the diagnosis, as other desquamative lesions have similar histopathological features.[88,126] However, pemphigus can be ruled out by histological examination. Recent attempts at immunopathological diagnosis appear promising.[105,106]

Treatment. With the etiology unknown, there is no rational therapy for this disease. Supportive therapy with meticulous oral hygiene, using a soft toothbrush and dental floss, is helpful for the secondary gingivitis and may be supplemented by topical application of hydrocortisone or other topically acting fluorinated corticosteroid ointments[129] before the patient retires at night. This may reduce the inflammation when used for over 2 to 4 weeks, but provides no cure for the disease. We have seen a few cases of spontaneous remission of this disease after 2 to 4 years' duration.

Erosive lichen planus

The most frequent source of desquamative gingival lesions is lichen planus.[54] The gingival manifestations may be bullous, but more often they are glistening gray patches that, when examined carefully, may have lacelike elevations. Sometimes the manifestations appear as a shiny red mucosal surface with some gray papules or erosive lesions (Fig. 12-1, K). The lesions are usually not painful, except for areas of ruptured bullae that may be irritated by hot or spicy food.

The most common location for oral lichen planus is in the buccal mucosa in the line of occlusion,[113] but it may also occur on the tongue and lips. The buccal lesions usually have the typical lacelike pattern of glistening Wickham's striae. The presence of such lesions makes the diagnosis of the gingival involvement easy. Histopathological examination will show edema and degeneration of the basal portion of the epithelium, with heavy leukocytic infiltration close to the degenerated basement lamina, but these findings are not in themselves diagnostic of lichen planus.[55,58]

Treatment. There is no satisfactory treatment for lichen planus. Only the supportive treatment of nontraumatic oral hygiene can be recommended. The duration of the disease may vary from a few months to many years, and seems to be related to psychic stress in the patient's life.

Allergic gingivostomatitis and other drug reactions

Gingival desquamation may occur as a result of ingested or parenterally administered drugs. Such stomatitis medicamentosa, caused by, for example, sulfa drugs or antibiotics,[31] is usually widespread in the oral cavity, but may start as a burning sensation and desquamation in the gingival region. The stomatitis may also develop with contact sensitivity (stomatitis venenata) to drugs that have been used topically, such as eugenol in periodontal dressings or topical antibiotics. Allergy to certain types of chewing gum (Fig. 12-1, L) is a classic example of severe gingivitis with an allergic basis, which usually also involves the lingual mucosa and the corners of the mouth.[60]

Thermal, electrical, and chemical gingivostomatitis

Topical application of aspirin, phenol, alcohol, and ethyl chloride may induce gingival inflammation with a tendency to surface desquamation (Fig. 12-15). A similar but more widespread mucosal inflammation may be seen from irritating substances such as chloroform and from substances used in toothpastes to prevent breath odors. Thermal burns from food or

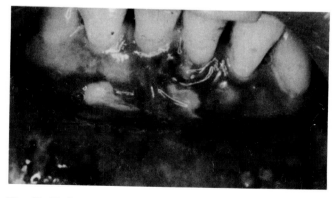

Fig. 12-15. Aspirin burn. Male, 45 years old. One aspirin tablet had been applied topically over a periodontal abscess on tooth #24. Superficial mucosal burn with gray membrane on gingiva and inside of lip.

other hot substances brought into contact with the gingiva will also appear as desquamating lesions. The diagnosis of such lesions must be based on the history of exposure to the irritant, rather than on the specific clinical and histological appearance of the lesions. The treatment is palliative until natural healing occurs.

Erosive gingival lesions have been observed following insertion of dissimilar metal alloys in restorations (which are affected by electrolytic activity of saliva) or removable dental appliances. Ulcerations may develop at the gingival margin contacting the restorations, and occasionally in the adjacent buccal and tongue mucosa. Hyperkeratosis, and even polypoid hyperplasia of the gingiva, may be other manifestations of galvanic irritation.[6] The saliva is an excellent electrolyte, and it has been demonstrated that gold, copper, and zinc ions from gold inlays will penetrate adjacent hard and soft tissues. Such copper and zinc ions deposited in the mucosa, as well as electrical irritation from galvanic current, may induce a severe gingivostomatitis. The rational therapy is to replace the offending restorations with cement or plastic material, to be followed by metals that are not dissimilar to the other restorations in the dentition.

Dermatologic diseases with gingival manifestations

A number of dermatological diseases may cause desquamative oral lesions[31] such as pemphigus, erythema multiforme, lupus erythematosus, psoriasis,[21] and others. Most of these diseases leave a much more widespread and severe involvement than do the lesions of desquamative gingivostomatitis. The management of these diseases is not part of dental practice, and any time such diseases are suspected, the patient should be referred for medical care.

Infective Gingivostomatitis

In addition to NUG, which is considered to be periodontal disease, other infective diseases may also involve the gingiva and mucosa. Included in this category are herpetic gingivostomatitis, gonorrhea, candidiasis, and lesions of the chronic infective granulomas such as tuberculosis, syphilis, and histoplasmosis.

Herpes

A primary infection with the herpes simplex virus (HV1) may lead to a disease called acute herpetic gingivostomatitis.[131] The disease usually occurs in children before 2 years of age, but has been seen in persons up to 50 years of age (Fig. 12-1, M).

The onset is very sudden, with high fever (103° to 104° F), and the oral lesions are apt to break out about 24 hours after the fever began.[15,91] The entire gingival

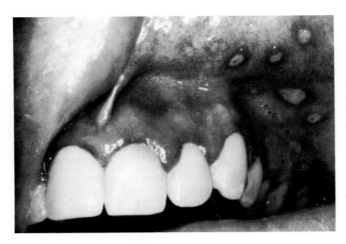

Fig. 12-16. Herpetic gingivostomatitis. Female, 25 years old. Fever, malaise, and extremely sore mouth. Bluish, swollen, and very tender gingival mucosa. Note discrete herpetic lesions (ruptured vesicles) in buccal mucosa. Well-demarcated red halo around the ruptured vesicles.

surface becomes red and extremely sore to the touch; then vesicles and bullae form. However, since these break easily, what is seen is a shallow ulceration, covered by a grayish membrane and surrounded by a distinct red halo (Fig. 12-16). Sometimes there may be no overt vesiculation, but a bluish-red shiny discoloration of the very tender gingiva is seen. The symptom of high, sudden fever should make one suspect herpetic gingivostomatitis in patients with very sore gingiva. The patient often develops vesicles elsewhere on the oral mucosa 2 to 3 days later. The disease is sometimes misdiagnosed as NUG, but the high fever, severe malaise, and the different location from that of NUG, and the lack of necrosis of the gingival lesions of herpetic gingivostomatitis, should make the differential diagnosis clear.

The acute phase of herpetic gingivostomatitis with the high fever will usually subside in a week to 10 days, but it may take another week for the lesions to heal completely. The disease is self-limiting and heals without therapy and without any residual scars.

There is no effective treatment for the herpetic infection. Mild soothing mouthwashes, Phenergan (syrup) or Xylocaine Viscous may be used prior to meals, as the pain makes it difficult to eat.

Acute herpetic gingivostomatitis is contagious,[15] but most adults have developed immunity in childhood. However, because dentists have occasionally developed severe paronychia from working on patients with acute herpetic lesions, the use of gloves is recommended. Only seldom, if ever, will a person develop a recurrence of the disease.[39]

Other acute infections

Other acute oral infections, such as gonorrhea and

candidiasis,[31] may cause development of gingivostomatitis, but in these infections there is usually widespread involvement of the oral mucosal membranes, and the gingival mucosa is not involved to any greater extent than the rest of the oral mucosa. Those lesions are usually classified as stomatitis rather than as gingivostomatitis.

Infective granulomas

A number of chronic infective granulomas (tuberculosis, syphilis, histoplasmosis) may produce gingival lesions that may pose problems in differential diagnosis of gingival disease.[8,31] However, they cannot be characterized as gingivostomatitis, and the granulomatous thick and firm borders of the lesions should alert the clinician to this type of disease (Fig. 12-17).

AIDS

The incidence of acquired immunodeficiency syndrome (AIDS) is increasing rapidly. It may provide some problems in differential diagnosis with other mucosal oral lesions,[99] since the appearance at early stages may be just red spots or asymptomatic plaques that later may develop into Kaposi's sarcoma. If this disease is suspected, refer the patient for medical care.

TRAUMATIC GINGIVITIS

Impingement from occlusion, food impaction, or dental appliances Gingival injury from severe malocclusion is discussed in detail in Chapters 10 and 19.

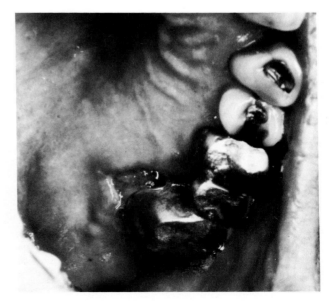

Fig. 12-17. Oral histoplasmosis. Male, 57 years old. General malaise. Painful necrotic lesion with exposed bone at the base of the lesion. Note thick, rolled borders with a granulomatous appearance. Had not responded to penicillin therapy. The patient also had two other similar gingival lesions. The diagnosis was made from biopsy and cultures from the lesion. All lesions healed following prolonged treatment with amphotericin B in a hospital.

Whenever occlusal function causes gingival lesions, occlusal therapy is required (Fig. 12-1, N). Meticulous oral hygiene will help to reduce gingival swelling and thus decrease the potential for occlusal gingival trauma.

Food impaction[46] is also discussed in Chapter 10. It is important to recognize that food impaction with subsequent gingival irritation may occur between teeth that apparently have close contact relations when tested in nonfunction. The food impaction may be related to plunger cusp effects of occlusal interferences, with opening of contacts during masticatory function.

Dental appliances, such as impinging partial denture clasps or indirect retainers, may cause severe gingivitis and gingival recession in spite of good oral hygiene. It is generally assumed that the gingivitis associated with faulty margins of restorations is not the direct result of mechanical trauma from these margins, but is caused by plaque retention favored by the faulty margins. Similarly, faulty pontic design of bridgework may enhance plaque retention rather than directly cause traumatic gingivitis. Toothpicks and interdental stimulators used in a faulty manner may cause gingival irritation. Gingival lesions caused by mechanical injury are usually erosive and superficial in nature and will heal readily when the source of irritation is detected and eliminated (Fig. 12-18, A, B). Faulty toothbrushing over a long time is more apt to produce atrophy than gingival inflammation.[47]

Traumatic gingival lesions may also be caused by self-mutilation of the gingiva with fingernails or various mechanical objects.[52,115] This is often done without conscious recognition, and it may be difficult to establish the true diagnosis. Gingival lesions from long-standing poor habits may be deep and almost granulomatous in nature. Severe gingival recession may be caused by such oral habits.

The diagnosis of traumatic gingivitis has to rely heavily on the history of trauma, whereas in simple plaque-induced gingivitis there is no such history. The differential diagnosis is not a great problem. Treatment of traumatic gingivitis is always aimed at elimination of the source of the trauma.

GINGIVAL ATROPHY OR RECESSION SYSTEMIC IN ORIGIN

The concept of passive eruption of teeth with gradual physiological gingival recession with age[37,38] has not been substantiated. With adequate and nontraumatic oral hygiene, the boundary between the epithelial and connective tissue attachment to the teeth can be maintained at the cementoenamel junction with age. However, due to the common presence of gingival inflammation and the tendency to faulty toothbrushing,[96] no group has been able to demon-

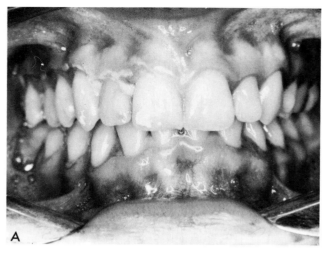
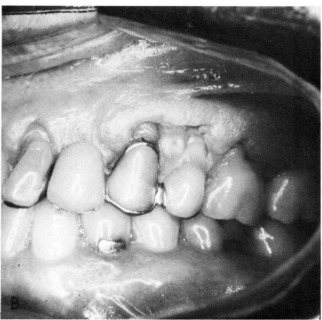

Fig. 12-18. *A,* Erosive, traumatic lesions on the gingiva and in the mucobuccal fold, right side, following faulty use of new, stiff toothbrush. Some superficial sloughing of traumatized mucosa. *B,* Gingival recession and dental abrasion from long-time faulty horizontal brushing with hard toothbrushes.

strate under controlled conditions the maintenance of this ideal relationship longitudinally in population groups.[118] Gingival recession is found in nearly 50% of young adults and in up to 100% of persons over the age of 45 years.[36]

Senile atrophic gingivitis

A uniform generalized atrophy of skin and mucous membranes usually occurs after the age of 60 years. Decreased output of sex hormones seems to affect the mucosal linings of the genitalia to a greater extent than it does the oral and gingival mucosa.[77]

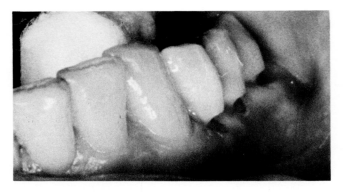

Fig. 12-19. Wedge-shaped defects caused by horizontal toothbrushing with hard brush and abrasive toothpowder.

In a few postmenopausal women with kraurosis vulvae, pronounced atrophic and hyperkeratotic changes of the gingiva may occur. Atrophy may develop, with a grayish surface of the gingiva resembling early leukoplakia (Fig. 12-1, O, and the patient may have a sensation of dryness and mild burning in the mouth when exposed to spicy, hot, or cold foods. This condition has been called *senile atrophic gingivitis*, although there is not necessarily any evidence of inflammation. The hyperkeratotic gingival changes have not been reported to have such a potential for cancerous development as is seen in kraurosis vulvae, and the gingival atrophy is of no significance to maintenance of periodontal support. There is no acceptable therapy for these oral changes. Because kraurosis vulvae is precancerous, patients with senile atrophic gingivitis should always be referred for gynecological examination.

Local Causes
Faulty oral hygiene practices

Gingival recession (Fig. 12-1, P) occurs most often on the buccal surfaces of the maxillary cuspids, bicuspids,[36,65] and first molars.[96] The most common cause of the gingival atrophy or recession is faulty use of toothbrushes or other devices for oral hygiene. The recession is often accompanied by V-shaped abrasion (Fig. 12-19) of tooth substance.[36] The gingival and dental changes caused by faulty toothbrushing were described in great detail by Hirschfeld.[47] Decreased incidence of gingival recession with improvement in oral hygiene has been confirmed in longitudinal studies.[70,96] Gingival recession is of significance mainly because it causes poor esthetic appearance and root sensitivity. Caries is seldom found in areas of gingival recession from faulty oral hygiene.

Treatment. The patient should be instructed in toothbrushing with a soft brush and a minimal amount of a nonabrasive dentifrice (see Chapter 18). If there are any indications of interdental recession from faulty use of interdental cleaning and stimulating devices, use of these devices should be discontinued in favor of dental floss, or, if their use is desired, instruction in correct use should be given in front of a mirror. Change of toothbrushing habits may lead to partial gingival regeneration (creeping reattachment), as is shown in Fig. 12-20, A, B.

With esthetically objectionable recession, or recession involving frenum attachments or complete loss of attached gingiva, reparative peridontal surgery may be indicated (see Chapter 25). Dental restorations may be needed if the abrasions extend close to the pulp.

Malposition of teeth

Another significant cause of gingival recession is malposed teeth.[36,45] Teeth in marked buccal or lingual position relative to the alveolar process are covered by thin bone or no bone, and usually by a very thin gingiva.[31] In extreme malposition, there often develop gingival clefts denuding the labial or lingual surfaces of the teeth. Depending on the state of oral hygiene

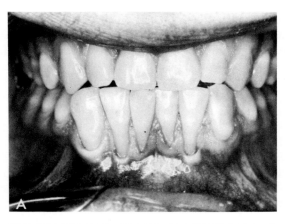

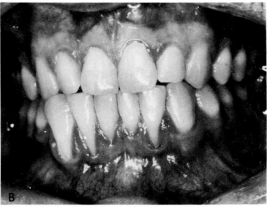

Fig. 12-20. *A,* Gingival recession caused by extremely vigorous brushing five to six times a day with hard brushes. Male 21 years old. Was instructed in the use of soft toothbrush. No surgical therapy. *B,* Same patient 3 years later. Note partial regeneration of gingiva, and no more pull on the free gingiva associated with lip pull.

and presence or absence of attached gingiva, there may or may not be inflammation associated with the recession.[36] The assumption that gingival recession is caused by trauma from occlusion[93] has not been substantiated and appears to be unlikely. Although disuse atrophy of the periodontal membrane will result, this does not seem to have any significant effect on the gingival tissues if the oral hygiene is good.[2]

Treatment for malposition should include orthodontic correction of the malocclusion, careful oral hygiene with a soft brush, and surgical procedures if "creeping reattachment" does not occur following the orthodontic and hygienic phase of the treatment.

Sequelae of periodontal disease and therapy

Gingival recession may be caused by traumatic gingivitis and by periodontitis. It may be localized to areas of traumatic impacts from dental appliances, occlusal impingement, and food impaction. Calculus on labial or lingual surfaces may cause gingival clefts, and general gingival recession may result from periodontitis associated with calculus and faulty margins of restorations. However, all of these developments are inflammatory in nature and do not have the appearance usually associated with atrophy or gingival recession.

Recession caused by faulty oral hygiene practice or by malposition of the teeth is usually located on the labial and occasionally on the lingual surfaces of the teeth, with the interdental tissues in a normal position. On the other hand, recession as a result of periodontal disease and treatment tends to be generalized as horizontal alveolar atrophy, lowering the gingival level on the proximal as well as on the buccal and lingual surfaces of the teeth.

It has been recommended that acrylic shields or stents be used as a substitute for the lost gingival tissues. However, this is not very satisfactory from either an esthetic or a hygienic standpoint.[52]

REFERENCES

1. Aas, E.: Hyperplasia gingivae diphenyl-hydantoinea, Acta Odont. Scand. Suppl. 34, 1963.
2. Alexander, A.G.: The effect of lack of function of teeth on gingival health, plaque, and calculus accumulation, J. Periodont. 41:438, 1970.
3. Alexander, AG: Habitual mouthbreathing and its effects on gingival health, Parodontologie 24:49, 1970.
4. Axelsson, P., and Lindhe, J.: The effect of a preventive programme on dental plaque, gingivitis and caries in school children. Results after one and two years, J. Clin. Periodontol. I:126, 1974.
5. Barnes, G.P., Bowles, S.F., and Carter, H.G.: Acute necrotizing ulcerative gingivitis; a survey of 218 cases, J. Periodont. 44:35, 1973.
6. Bergenholtz, A.: Multiple polypous hyperplasias of the oral mucosa with regression after removal of amalgam fillings, Acta Odont. Scand. 23:111, 1965.
7. Bergenholtz, A., Hedegaard, B., and Söremark, R.: Studies of the transport of metal ions from gold inlays into environmental tissues, Acta Odont. Scand. 23:135, 1965.
8. Broome, W.C., Hutchinson, R.A., and Mays, E.E.: Histoplasmosis of the gingiva. Report of a case, J. Periodont. 47:95, 1976.
9. Box, H.K.: Necrotic Gingivitis, Toronto: University of Toronto Press, 1930.
10. Buckner, H.J.: Diffuse fibroma of the gums, J.A.D.A. 24:2003, 1937.
11. Burket, L.W.: A histopathologic explanation for oral lesions in acute leukemia, Am. J. Orth. Oral Surg. 30:516, 1944.
12. Brun, J.H.: The action of nicotine on the peripheral circulation, Ann. N.Y. Sci. 90:8, 1960.
13. Cahn, L.R.: The penetration of the tissue of Vincent's organisms, J. Dent. Res. 9:695, 1929.
14. Cernea, P., et al.: Les hyperplasies gingivales familiales, Rev. Stomatol. 56:620, 1955.
15. Chilton, N.W.: Herpetic stomatitis, Am. J. Orth. Oral Surg. 30:355, 1944.
16. Cimasone, G.: The Gingival Fluid. Basel: S. Karger, 1974.
17. Cohen, D.W., et al.: A longitudinal investigation of the periodontal changes during pregnancy and fifteen months postpartum. Part II. J. Periodont. 42:653, 1971.
18. Cohen, M.M., et al.: Oral aspects of mongolism, Oral Surg. 14:92, 1961.
19. Courant, P.R., Paunio, J., and Gibbons, R.J.: Infectivity and hyaluronidase activity of debris from health and diseased gingiva, Arch. Oral Biol. 10:119, 1965.
20. Courtley, R.L.: Vincent's infection, Br. Dent. J. 74:34, 1943.
21. Doben, D.T.: Psoriasis of the attached gingiva. Case report, J. Perriodont. 47:38, 1976.
22. Eichel, B., and Shahrich, H.A.: Tobacco smoke toxicity, loss of human oral leukocytic function and fluid cell metabolism, Science 166:1424, 1969.
23. El-Askiry, G.M., et al: Comparative study of the influence of pregnancy and oral contraceptives on the gingivae, Oral Surg 30:472, 1970.
24. Emerson, T.G.: Hereditary gingival hyperplasia. A family pedigree of four generations, Oral Surg. 19:1, 1965.
25. Emslie, R.D.: Cancrum oris, Dent. Pract. 13:481, 1963.
26. Enwonwu, C.O.: Epidemiological and biochemical studies of NUG and noma (cancrum oris) in Nigerian children, Arch. Oral Biol. 17:1357, 1972.
27. Giddon, D.B., Zackin, J.S., and Goldhaber, P.: Acute necrotizing ulcerative gingivitis in college students, J.A.D.A. 68:381, 1964.
28. Giddon, D.B., Clark, R.E., and Varni, J.G.: Apparent digital vasomotor hypotonicity in the remission stage of acute necrotizing ulcerative gingivitis, J. Dent. Res. 48:431, 1969.
29. Glenright, J.D., and Sideway, D.A.: The use of metronidazole in the treatment of acute ulcerative gingivitis, Br. Dent. J. 121:174, 1966.
30. Glickman, I.: The use of penicillin lozenges in the treatment of Vincent's infection and other acute gingival inflammations, J.A.D.A. 34:406, 1947.
31. Glickman, I.: Clinical Periodontology, 4th ed. Philadelphia, W.B. Saunders Co., 1972.
32. Glickman, I., and Lewitus, M.: Hyperplasia of the gingiva associated with Dilantin (sodium diphenylhydantoinate) therapy, J.A.D.A. 28:199, 1941.
33. Glickman, I., and Johannessen, L.B.: The effect of a six percent solution of chromic acid on the gingiva of the albino rat. A correlated gross biomicroscopic and histologic study, J.A.D.A. 41:674, 1950.
34. Glickman, I., and Smulow, J.B.: Histopathology and histochemistry of chronic desquamative gingivitis, Oral Surg. 21:325, 1966.
35. Goldhaber, P., and Giddon, D.B.: Present concepts concerning the etiology and treatment of acute necrotizing ul-

cerative gingivitis, Int. Dent. J. 14:468, 1964.

36. Gorman, N.J.: Prevalence and etiology of gingival recession, J. Periodont. 38:316, 1967.

37. Gottlieb, B.: Der Epithelansatz am Zahne, Deutsche Monatschr. Zahnheilkd. 39:142, 1921.

38. Gottlieb, B., and Orban, D.: Active and passive eruption of the teeth, J. Dent. Res. 13:214, 1933.

39. Griffin, J.W.: Recurrent intraoral herpes simplex virus infection, Oral Surg. 19:209, 1965.

40. Grupe, H.E., and Wilder, L.S.: Observations of necrotizing gingivitis in 870 military trainees, J. Periodont. 27:255, 1956.

41. Hall, W.B.: Dilantin hyperplasia, a preventable disease, J. Periodont. Res. (Suppl.) 4:36, 1969.

42. Hampp, E.G., and Mergenhagen, S.E.: Experimental infections with oral spirochetes, J. Infect Dis. 109:43, 1961.

43. Heylings, P.: Electron microscopy of acute ulcerative gingivitis (Vincent's type). Demonstration of the fusospirodental complex of bacteria within the pre-necrotic epithelium, Br. Dent. J. 122:51, 1967.

44. Hilming, F.: Gingivitis gravidarum-Undersögelser over klinik og aetiologi med aetiologi sligt henblik pa C-vitaminets betydning, Thesis, Copenhagen, 1950.

45. Hirschfeld, I.: A study of skulls in the American Museum of National History in relation to periodontal disease, J. Dent. Res 5:241, 1923.

46. Hirschfeld, I.: Food impaction, J.A.D.A. 17:1504, 1930.

47. Hirschfeld, I.: The Toothbrush: Its Use and Abuse, Brooklyn, Dental Items of Interest, 1939.

48. Hirschfeld, I., Beube, F., and Siegal, E.H.: The history of Vincent's infection, J. Periodont. 11:89, 1940.

49. Holm-Pedersen, P., and Löe, H.: Flow of gingival exudate as related to menstruation and pregnancy, J. Periodont. Res. 2:13, 1967.

50. Hugoson, A.: Gingival inflammation and female sex hormones, J. Periodont. Res. (Suppl. 5) 1970.

51. Hugoson, A.: Gingivitis in pregnant women. A longitudinal clinical study, Odont. Revy. 22:65, 1971.

52. Hurt, W.C.: Periodontics in General Practice, Springfield, Il., Charles C. Thomas, 1976.

53. Jacobson, L.: Mouthbreathing and gingivitis, J. Periodont. Res. 8:269, 1973.

54. Jandinski, J.J., and Shklar, G.: Lichen planus of the gingiva, J. Periodont. 47:724, 1976.

55. Johnson, F.R., and Fry, L.: Ultrastructural observation on lichen planus, Arch Derm 95:596, 1967.

56. Kardachi, B.J.R., and Clarke, M.G.: Aetiology of acute necrotizing ulcerative gingivitis: A hypothetical explanation, J. Periodont. 45:830, 1974.

57. Kenney, E.B., Saxe, S.R., and Bowles, R.D.: The effect of cigarette smoking on anaerobiosis in the oral cavity, J. Periodont. 46:82, 1976.

58. Kerr, D.A.: Gingival and periodontal disease, J.A.D.A. 32:31, 1945.

59. Kerr, D.A.: Granuloma pyogenicum, Oral Surg. 4:158, 1951.

60. Kerr, D.A., McClatchey, K.D., and Regezi, J.A.: Allergic gingivostomatitis (due to gum chewing), J. Periodont. 42:709, 1971.

61. Kimball, O.P.: The treatment of epilepsy with sodium diphenyl hydantoinate, J.A.D.A. 112:1244, 1939.

62. Kindlova, M.: Vascular supply of the periodontium in periodontitis, Int. Dent. J. 17:476, 1967.

63. Kindlova, M., and Scheinin, A.: The vascular supply of the gingiva and the alveolar mucosa in the rat. II. Spontaneous and experimentally induced changes of the microcirculation, Acta Odont. Scand. 26:629, 1968.

64. King, J.D.: Nutritional and other factors in trench mouth with special reference to the nicotinic acid component of Vitamin B complex, Br. Dent. J. 75:113, 1943.

65. Kitchin, P.C.: The prevalence of tooth root exposure and the relation of the extent of such exposure to the degree of abrasion in different age classes, J. Dent. Res. 20:565, 1941.

66. Knowles, J.W.: Oral hygiene related to the long term results of periodontal therapy, Mich. State Dent. J. 55:147, 1973.

67. Kornman, K.A., and Loesche, W.J.: The subgingival microflora during pregnancy, J. Periodont. Res. 15:11, 1980.

68. Lehner, T.: Immunoglobulin abnormalities in ulcerative gingivitis, Br. Dent. J. 127:165, 1969.

69. Levin, S.M., and Kennedy, J.E.: Relationship of plaque and gingivitis in patients with leukemia, Va. Dent. J. 50:22, 1973.

70. Lightner, L.M., et al: Preventive periodontic treatment procedures: Results over 46 months, J. Periodont. 42:555, 1971.

71. Lindhe, J., Attström, R., and Björn, A.L.: The influence of progesterone on gingival exudation during menstrual cycles, J. Periodont. Res. 4:97, 1969.

72. Lindhe, J., and Björn, A.L.: The influence of hormonal contraceptives on the gingiva of women, J. Periodont. Res 2:1, 1967.

73. Lindhe, J., and Branemark, P.I.: Changes in microcirculation after local application of sex hormones, J. Periodont. Res. 2:185, 1967.

74. Listgarten, M.A., and Lewis, D.W.: The distribution of spirochetes in the lesion of acute necrotizing ulcerative gingivitis: an electron microscopic and statistical survey, J. Periodont. 38:379, 1967.

75. Listgarten, M.A., and Lewis, D.W.: The distribution of spirochetes in the lesion of acute necrotizing ulcerative gingivitis: an electron microscopic and statistical survey, J. Periodont. 38:379, 1967.

76. Lite, T., Dimaio, D.J., and Burman, L.R.: Gingival patterns in mouthbreathers, Oral Surg. 8:382, 1955.

77. Litwack, D., Kennedy, J.E., and Zander, H.A.: Response of oral epithelia to ovariectomy and estrogen replacement, J. Periodont. Res. 5:263, 1970.

78. Livingston, S., and Livingston, H.L.: Diphenylhydantoin gingival hyperplasia, Amer. J. Dis. Child. 117:265, 1969.

79. Löe, H.: Periodontal changes in pregnancy, J. Periodont. 36:37, 1965.

80. Löe, H., and Silness, J.: Periodontal disease in pregnancy. I. Prevalence and Severity, Act. Odont. Sc. 21:533, 1963.

81. Lyons, H.: Acute necrotizing periodontal disease: An appraisal of therapy and a critical criterion, J.A.D.A. 37:271, 1948.

82. Maier, A.W., and Orban, B.: Gingivitis in pregnancy, Oral Surg. 2:334, 1949.

83. Malberger, E.: Acute infectious oral necrosis among children in the Gambia, West Africa, J. Periodont. Res. 2:154, 1967.

84. Manhold, J.H., Doyle, J.L., and Weisinger, E.H.: Effects of social stress on oral and other bodily tissues. II. Results offering substance to an hypothesis for the mechanism of formation of periodontal pathology, J. Periodont. 42:109, 1971.

85. Manson, J.: Recurrent Vincent's disease. A survey of 61 cases, Br. Dent. J. 110:386, 1961.

86. Maupin, C., and Bell, W.: The relationship of 17-hydroxycorticosteroids to ANUG, J. Periodont. 46:721, 1975.

87. McCarthy, F.P., McCarthy, P.L., and Shklar, G.: Chronic desquamative gingivitis: A reconsideration, Oral Surg. 13:1300, 1960.

88. McCarthy, P.L., and Shklar, G.: Diseases of the Oral Mucosa, New York, McGraw-Hill Book Co., 1964.

89. McDonald, J.B., et al.: The pathogenic concepts of an experimental fusospirochetal infection, J. Infect. Dis. 98:15, 1956.

90. McIndoe, A., and Smith, B.O.: Congenital familial fibromatosis of the gums with the teeth as a probable aetiologic factor, Brit. J. Plast. Surg 11:62, 1958.

91. McNair, S.T.: Herpetic stomatitis, J. Dent. Res. 29:647, 1950.

92. Merrit, A.H.: Chronic desquamative gingivitis, J. Periodont. 4:30, 1933.

93. Miller, S.C.: Textbook of Periodontia, 3rd ed., Philadelphia, The Blakiston Co., 1950.

94. Mühlemann, H.R., and Sons, S.: Gingival sulcus bleeding: A leading symptom in initial gingivitis, Helv. Odont. Acta 15:107, 1971.

95. Nikai, H., Rose, G.G., and Cattoni, M.: Electron microscopic study of chronic desquamative gingigivitis, J. Periodont. Res. (Suppl. 6), 1971.

96. O'Leary, T.J., et al.: The incidence of recession in young males: A further study, J. Periodont. 42:264, 1971.

97. Oles, R.: Chronic desquamative gingivitis, J. Periodont. 38:485, 1967.

98. Pearlman, B.A.: An oral contraceptive drug and gingival enlargement; the relationship between local and systemic factors, J. Clin. Periodontol. 1:47, 1974.

99. Petit, J.C., et al.: Progressive changes of Kaposi's sarcoma of the gingiva and palate. Case report on an AIDS patient, J. Periodont. 57:159, 1986.

100. Pindborg, J.J.: Gingivitis in military personnel with special reference ot ulceromembranous gingivitis, Odont. Tidskr. 59:407, 1951.

101. Plaut, H.C.: Studien zur bakteriellen Daignostik der Diphtherie und der Anginen, Deutsch. Med. Wochenschr. 20:920, 1894.

102. Prinz, H.: Chronic diffuse desquamative gingivitis, Dent. Cosmos 74:331, 1932.

103. Ramfjord, S.P.: The histopathology of inflammatory gingival enlargement, Oral Surg. 6:516, 1953.

104. Rateitschak-Plüiss, E.M., et al.: Gingival hyperplasia by cyclosporin—A medication, Schw. Zahnheilk 93:56, 1983.

105. Rogers, R.S., and Jordon, R.E.: The immunopathology of oral inflammatory diseases, J. Clin. Res. 34:396A, 1976.

106. Rogers, R.S., Sheridon, P.J., and Jordon, R.E.: Desquamative gingivitis, clinical, histopathologic and immunopathologic investigations, Oral Surg. 42:316, 1976.

107. Rosebury, T., McDonald, J.B., and Clark, A.: A bacteriologic survey of gingival scrapings from periodontal infections by direct examination, guinea pig inoculation, and anerobic cultivation, J. Dent. Res. 29:718, 1950.

108. Ruston, M.A.: Hereditary or idiopathic hyperplasia of the gums, Dent. Pract. 7:136, 1957.

109. Schluger, S.: Necrotizing ulcerative gingivitis in the army: Incidence, communicability, and treatment, J.A.D.A. 38:174, 1949.

110. Schwartzman, J., and Grossman, L.: Vincent's ulceromembranous gingivostomatitis, Arch. Pediat. 58:515, 1941.

111. Scopp, I.W., Desquamative gingivitis, J. Periodont. 35:149, 1964.

112. Shannon, I., Kilgore, W.G., and O'Leary, T.: Stress as a predisposing factor in ANUG, J. Periodont. 48:240, 1969.

113. Shklar, G., and McCarthy, P.L.: The oral lesions of lichen planus, Oral Surg. 14:164, 1961.

114. Silness, J., and Löe, H.: Periodontal disease in pregnancy. II. Correlation between oral hygiene and periodontal condition, Acta Odont. Scand. 22:121, 1964.

115. Sorrin, S.: Habit: An etiologic factor of periodontal disease, Dent. Dig. 41:290, 1935.

116. Staple, P.H.: Some tissue reactions associated with 5:5-diphenylhydantoin (Dilantin) sodium therapy, Br. Dent. J. 95:289, 1953.

117. Stern, L., Eisenbud, L., and Klattel, J.: Analysis of oral reactions to dilantin sodium, J. Dent. Res 22:157, 1943.

118. Suomi, J.D., et al.: The effect of controlled oral hygiene procedures on the progression of periodontal disease in adults: Results after third and final year, J. Periodont. 42:152, 1971.

119. Tomes, J.: A System of Dental Surgery. 4th ed., P. Blakiston Son and Co., 1897.

120. Valderhaug, J., and Bineland, J.M.: Peridontal conditions in patients 5 years following insertion of fixed prosthesis, J. Oral Rehabil. 3:237, 1976.

121. Vincent, H.: Sur l'etiologie et sur les lesions anatomopathologique de la pourriture d'hospital, Ann. Inst. Pasteur 10:448, 1896.

122. Wade, A.B., Blake, G., and Mirza, K.: Effectiveness of metronidazole in treating the acute phase of ulcerative gingivitis, Dent. Pract. Dent. Rec. 16:440, 1966.

123. Watts, D.T.: The effects of nicotine and smoking on the secretion of ephinephrine, Ann. N.Y. Acad. Sci. 90:74, 1960.

124. Wentz, F.M.: Oral manifestations of the blood diseases, J.A.D.A. 44:698, 1952.

125. Weski, H.: Elephantiasis gingivae hereditaria, Deutsch. Monatschr. Zahnheikd. 38:557, 1921.

126. Wilgram, G.F.: Pemphigus and bulbous pemphigoid. In Ultrastructure of Normal and Abnormal Skin, ed. A.S. Zelickson. Philadelphia, Lea & Febiger, 1967.

127. Wilton, J., et al.: Mediated immunity and humoral antibodies in acute ulcerative gingivitis, J. Periodont. Res. 6:9, 1971.

128. Zackin, S.J., and Weisberger, D.: Hereditary gingival fibromatosis, Oral Surg. 14:828, 1961.

129. Zegarelli, E.V., et al.: Triamcinolone in the treatment of acute and chronic lesions of the oral mucous membranes, Oral Surg. 13:170, 1960.

130. Ziskin, D.E., Blackberg, S.M., and Stout, A.P.: The gingivae during pregnancy. An experimental study and a histopathological interpretation, Surg. Gynecol. Obstet. 57:719, 1933.

131. Ziskin, D.E., and Holden, M.: Acute herpetic gingivostomatitis, J.A.D.A. 30:1697, 1943.

The term *periodontitis* refers to inflammation of the supporting structures of the teeth associated with loss of attachment and bone. Although there is no generally accepted classification of periodontitis, a "Glossary of Periodontic Terms," published as a supplement to the *Journal of Periodontology*,[43] does subdivide periodontitis into adult, juvenile, necrotizing ulcerative gingivo-periodontitis, prepubertal, and rapidly progressive periodontitis. These categories will be used here to discuss the nature of periodontitis.

If the emphasis were to be placed upon proved microbial specificity, the term *periodontitis* could represent a group of diseases that were etiologically specific infections.[71,78] However, "specificity" may no longer relate to single periodontal pathogens, but to any of a number of pathogens.[105,113] For example, *A. actinomycetimcomitans*, *B. gingivalis*, and *B. intermedius* are closely associated with active periodontitis in humans.[101] However, it should not be concluded that such associations represent actively progressing diseases,[6,8] even though these gram-negative rods have virulence factors that may give them special importance in the etiology of periodontitis.[102] The probability is not great for obtaining a representative sample of microorganisms[113] (or other diagnostic criteria) from an active site of a disease characterized by seemingly random onsets and sporadic exacerbations interspersed with long periods of remission.[45,53] (The phrase "seemingly random" is used because population studies have shown that not all subjects, teeth and surfaces are equally susceptible to disease.[65])

CLASSIFICATION OF PERIODONTITIS

Although it has been proposed that microbial infections are the most likely cause of periodontitis,[100,105] and that different forms of the disease suggest the possibility of different etiological syndromes,[99] it is not possible to classify periodontitis as a series of specific infections or to speak of different periodontal diseases that may have different specific etiologies.[113] There is no accepted classification of periodontitis based on microbiologic etiologic factors. Therefore, the classification of periodontitis suggested in Chapters 6 and 12 will be used. Those forms of periodontitis that do not have specific systemic and/or local modifying factors will be described as *simple* periodontitis, and those with significant modifying factors will be described as *complex* periodontitis.

The model we will use for simple periodontitis will be adult periodontitis (AP), and the model for complex periodontitis will be juvenile periodontitis (JP). Most cases of periodontal disease are difficult to classify clinically on the basis of different specific etiologies;[113] i.e., they may range gradually from gingivitis to more or less advanced destructive periodontitis, more or less rapidly advancing, and more or less prepubertal, adolescent, young adult, or "over-35-years-of-age" periodontitis.

At least five different forms of periodontitis are described. They are prepubertal, juvenile, rapidly progressive, adult periodontitis,[81] and necrotizing ulcerative gingivo-periodontitis.[43] As previously indicated, these may be difficult to identify retrospectively and prospectively, as well as at the time of examination.

Attempts to classify periodontitis on the basis of microbial infections by different specific groups of microorganisms have not been completely successful. Although it seems reasonable to differentiate between *Bacteroids* periodontitis (rapidly progressive periodontitis), *Actinobacillus/Capnocytophaga* periodontitis (juvenile periodontitis), and *Capnocytophaga* periodontitis (severe periodontitis in juvenile diabetes),[38] the flora in periodontal pockets are complex, and additional data are needed before the various forms of periodontitis can be classified on the basis of the potential pathogenicity of these microorganisms.

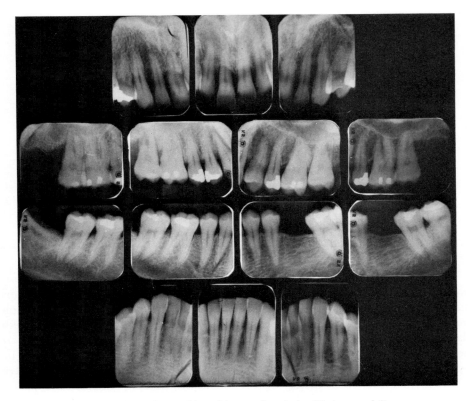

Fig. 13-1. Radiographic evidence of periodontitis in an adult.

Adult Periodontitis

Adult periodontitis (AP) is a common form of periodontitis considered to have an onset in the late teens or later, and to progress slowly throughout life.[65] AP is not continuous, inasmuch as periods of inactivity and regression have been suggested.[45] Peripheral environmental factors such as bacterial plaque are prominent, but other factors, such as neutrophil dysfunction and hormonal disturbances which modify the response of the tissues to microbial injury, are not considered to be present.[43]

Adult periodontitis is associated with varying degrees of gingivitis and loss of attachment and bone loss (Fig. 13-1). Gingivitis may not be a significant aspect of AP, and of course is frequently present in the absence of periodontitis. The diagnosis of AP is based upon periodontal probing aided by radiographs, as well as by the age of the patient. Loss of attachment and periodontal pockets cannot be detected radiographically in all cases without insertion of silver points at the time the radiographs are taken. The destruction seen at age 35 years could reflect the effects of early-onset periodontitis.

The diagnosis of adult periodontitis can be made on the basis of the loss of any attachment, or a specific amount of loss, as measured by a periodontal probe. If AP is determined on the basis of any attachment loss greater than zero, the prevalence of this form of periodontitis is much greater than if the diagnosis of AP is based on the criterion of 3 mm. loss or greater. Although this value has been used in studying AP prevalence,[81] it is not generally used in clinical practice.

The prevalence of adult periodontitis has been discussed in Chapter 6 and will not be reviewed here; however, some of the distributive aspects of attachment loss will be considered. The pattern of tissue loss tends to be bilaterally symmetrical in the dentition of affected populations,[70] but symmetry may not be

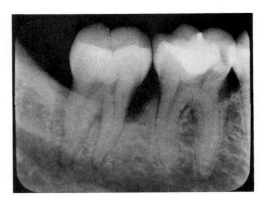

Fig. 13-2. Radiographic view of bone loss in periodontitis most severely involving the second molar.

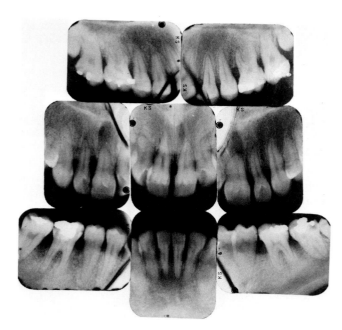

Fig. 13-3. Radiographs of young adult with history of treatment for juvenile periodontitis.

the case in every individual. Some teeth and surfaces are not at equal risk for the development of periodontal lesions (Fig. 13-2). Also, some individuals are more susceptible to periodontitis than others.

The microbiological profile of adult periodontitis is not consistent, but *Bacteroides intermedius, B. gingivalis, Actinobacillus actinomycetemcomitans, Wolinella recta,* and spirochetes are strongly associated with advanced periodontitis.[109,110] Twenty-seven species have been implicated as common etiologic agents in moderate adult periodontitis.[72] However, there is insufficient consistency in the microbial flora to implicate any of these bacteria singly or in combination as primary etiologic agents in adult periodontitis.[65,102]

The immunologic profile of individuals with adult periodontitis does not provide a consistent indication of a particular microorganism, or even of several, as being the cause of AP.[27,111,112] Correlations between AP and elevated antibody titers to *B. gingivalis* have been reported,[39] but this microorganism has not been implicated as the major cause of AP. The absence of a specific antibody titer increase in adult periodontitis may relate to polyclonal activation.[9,104]

In adults 35 years of age or older who have not had early-onset forms of gingivitis and who have not had repeated long-term episodes of acute necrotizing ulcerative gingivitis, the general features of periodontitis are those of a chronic inflammatory process in which the severity of the response is consistent with the degree of plaque accumulation. There are no known serum neutrophil or monocyte abnormalities; there is no evidence of rapid progression, although 1

or several sites may convert to rapidly progressive periodontitis; there may be both vertical and horizontal patterns of bone loss; and loss of attachment may be generalized, although the process may more commonly and severely affect the molars and incisors.

Adult periodontitis does not respond to antibiotics in the same way as does periodontitis that is secondary to neutrophil defects. It requires persistent professional care for control of subgingival plaque.

Complex periodontitis

Here we will consider forms of periodontitis that reflect the influence of factors modifying the host's resistance to bacteria or their products. Many patients with early-onset periodontitis have abnormalities of polymorphonuclear leukocytes. In addition, several systemic diseases may predispose the patient to periodontitis,[81] including some that appear to predispose the patient to rapidly progressive periodontitis.[86]

Juvenile periodontitis Juvenile periodontitis (JP) is a form of periodontitis that has its onset about the time of puberty and is localized predominantly in the first molars and/or incisors (Fig. 13-3 and 13-4). The term *periodontosis*[119] is a reflection of earlier concepts of noninflammatory degenerative disease of systemic origin.[46,47,118] The supposed absence of an inflammatory component was never generally accepted,[7,92] although the recognition of periodontosis as a clinical entity has been proposed.[3] The term *localized juvenile periodontitis* is widely used and does not presuppose a degenerative pathologic process. The prevalence of this disease in teenagers is probably less than 0.1%.

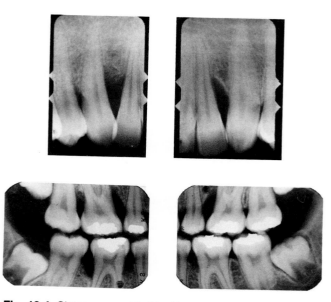

Fig. 13-4. Sixteen-year-old girl with provisional diagnosis of juvenile periodontitis. Only maxillary lateral incisors affected. Microbiologic, hematologic, and neutrophil chemotactic examinations, as well as family and dental histories, were negative.

Most patients with JP have neutrophil chemotactic dysfunction, and in some cases abnormalities of monocyte chemotaxis as well.[40,84,117] Evidence for a genetic basis for JP has been presented,[106,114] including an autosomal mode of inheritance with full penetrance[95] and an X-linked dominant mode.[115] Although *Actinobacillus actinomycetemcomitans (A.a.)* and *Capnocytophaga* species[103,126] have been implicated in the etiology of JP, and elicit a humoral immune response as reflected by serum antibodies,[34,66] the susceptibility to injury by these microbes is very probably genetic.

It has not been shown that there is an association between JP and histocompatibility leukocyte antigen (HLA); in other words, that the inheritance is linked with major histocompatibility antigen (MHA). Thus, the possibility of an immunogenetic basis for the disease has not been supported in respect to an association between JP and MHA.

Because *A.a.* may not be present in the plaque, the microbial etiology of JP is more complex than implicating an association only with *A.a.* and *Capnocytophaga*.[114] Furthermore, antibodies may not reflect the composition of the pocket flora. Antibodies against putative periodontopathic bacteria not found in periodontal pockets may also be found.[83]

The absence of specific serum antibodies for the microflora present in periodontal pockets, and the presence of serum antibodies for *A.a.* when these microorganisms are not detected in pocket microflora, are inconsistencies that have generated a number of hypotheses to explain JP as an infection primarily by *A.a.* and to a lesser extent by *Capnocytophaga* species. Because of the problems in making a retrospective diagnosis of JP on the parents of patients with JP, and in making a prospective diagnosis on normal siblings who have not reached circumpubertal age, it is difficult to reconstruct the familial distribution of this relatively rare disease which has an equivocal genetic mode of transmission.

The tendency for LJP to manifest itself at puberty and "burn out" in the late twenties has focused attention on potential changes in the microbial flora in children of circumpubertal age. The reasons for such a "window" of destruction or lowered defenses during this period of time do not seem to be explained simply on the basis of "opportunistic" microorganisms.

There is some evidence of a difference between the subgingival flora of children and adults,[4] and there may be an increased level of black pigmented *Bacteroides* during puberty.[26] However, the prevalence of this periodontal disease-associated organism (specifically, *B. intermedius*) is very low in prepubescent children and predominates only in circumpubertal plaques.[123] These changes at puberty have suggested that, as in pregnancy,[55] there is a relationship between levels of hormones and levels of black-pigmented *Bacteroides* in subgingival plaque.

The diagnosis of juvenile periodontitis as a distinct clinical entity of a degenerative process[3] has been questioned.[7,92] Attempts to characterize a number of forms of periodontitis that may begin before, during, or after puberty suggest the need for diagnostic criteria that reflect the cause of the disease, rather than the symptoms.

Most of the individuals manifesting early-onset aggressive forms of periodontitis have abnormalities of

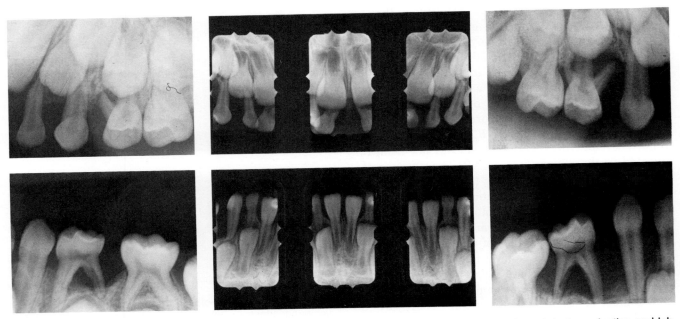

Fig. 13-5. Severe periodontitis involving primary dentition. Chemotatic examination, family history, hematologic evaluation and laboratory tests were negative. The microbial flora largely anaerobes. Inconsistent for prepubertal, as well as juvenile, periodontitis.

peripheral blood phagocytes that can be detected as abnormal cell motility or adherence.[80] Therefore, the need is evident for unique criteria for the prospective diagnosis of juvenile periodontitis, as well as of other forms of early-onset periodontitis (Fig. 13-5).

The features of localized juvenile periodontitis periodontosis) include circumpubertal age of onset; 3:1 females to males affected; familial tendency; lack of relationship between local etiologic factors and presence of deep periodontal pockets; rapid loss of alveolar bone; vertical loss of bone about the 1st molars and 1 or more incisor teeth in an otherwise healthy adolescent; and primary teeth not affected.[3] The question of "burnt-out" lesions may reflect the predominant tendency for LJP to be limited to molars and incisors. When these teeth are lost, the disease is perceived as "burnt out." However, after its onset at puberty, the destructive process may slow down or spontaneously cease.

For the treatment of juvenile periodontitis, the antibiotic choice appears to be tetracycline. Traditional initial therapies such as scaling, root planing, oral hygiene instruction, or occlusal adjustment, followed by surgical therapy in the form of open curettage, have been suggested to provide consistent success.[25]

Prepubertal periodontitis Prepubertal periodontitis (PP) affects deciduous teeth in young children and has been suggested to be a clinical disease entity.[85] PP occurs in a localized and a generalized form, and like JP is a relatively rare form of early-onset periodontitis. The disease begins about the age of 4 years or before, during or immediately after eruption of the primary teeth, but may affect the permanent dentition.

In PP, there is an abnormality in chemotaxis of either blood neutrophils or monocytes or both, resulting from an inability of these cells to adhere to surfaces. The defect in adherence relates to the absence of a membrane glycoprotein. The defect has been found in a cell surface determinant designated as 60.3 and another designated as LFA-1, and is not found in JP and rapidly progressive periodontitis (RP).[82]

The features of generalized PP include the early onset of the disease during or after the eruption of the primary teeth; rapid destruction of bone; severe inflammation of gingiva accompanied by gingival proliferation; involvement of all primary teeth, although permanent dentition may or may not be affected; a tendency for the disease to be refractory to antibiotic therapy; defects in neutrophils and monocytes; frequent respiratory infections (respiratory, otitis, etc.); cleft formation or recession; and sometimes destruction of tooth roots.[81,85]

Histologic features of generalized PP show an absence of neutrophils from the gingiva, but a dense lymphoid cell infiltrate consisting of plasma cells is present in the connective tissue.[81] Thus, extensive bone loss may occur in the absence of neutrophils.

The features of localized PP include minimal or no gingival inflammation; a few teeth affected but no apparent pattern present; either neutrophils or monocytes but not both affected; no apparent history of frequent infections, although patients may have otitis media; destruction not as rapid as in generalized form; and affected areas treatable by root scaling and planing, along with antibiotic therapy.

Rapidly progressive periodontitis Rapidly progressive periodontitis (RP) has been defined as a form of periodontitis that usually begins between puberty and 35 years of age or later.[43] It may be associated with systemic disease and be refractory to all forms of therapy. Most patients with RP demonstrate abnormalities in peripheral blood neutrophil function that are manifested in an impaired chemotactic ability.[117] RP has been described as a distinct clinical condition.[86]

The features of RP include an active phase of severe, rapid bone destruction involving most of the teeth; spontaneous or rapid slow-down of the process; proliferation and severe inflammatory response during active phase; functional defects in neutrophils or monocytes in the majority of affected patients; the possibility of previous juvenile periodontitis; and systemic disturbances that may include weight loss, mental depression and general malaise.[86,87] Treatment consisting of root planing and antibiotic therapy is generally effective.

Many patients with RP have serum antibodies specific for various species of *Bacteroides*, *Actinobacillus*, or both. These gram-negative, anaerobic, assacharolytic rods, and possibly *Capnocytophaga*, have been implicated as important pathogens.[86] The cyclic nature of the disease has suggested the possibility that serum antibody is protective and may be the basis for arresting the disease. In this respect, there appears to be a relationship between RP and serum antibodies and defects in host defense mechanisms.

SYSTEMIC DISEASE AND PERIODONTITIS

A number of diseases appear to make individuals prone to periodontitis. Hereditary or genetic factors may be involved.

Systemic diseases that may modify the response of the host to bacteria and predispose it to periodontitis include Papillon-LeFèvre syndrome, hypophosphatasia, Chédiak-Higashi syndrome, chronic granulomatous disease, Down's syndrome, diabetes mellitus, neutropenia, hypergammoglobulinemia-E,[23,88] ichthyosis,[88] and Crohn's disease.[28,60,98]

Papillon-LeFèvre syndrome

Papillon-LeFèvre syndrome (hyperkeratosis palmoplantaris) is a rare genetic disease (possibly a recessive genetic trait) in which there is severe and premature destruction of the periodontal supporting structures.[19,50,75] Less than 75 cases have been reported. The skin manifestations of the disease are hyperkeratosis of the palms and the hands and soles of the feet, dry skin, and spare, fine body hair. Periodontitis begins in some cases at less than 3 years of age and progresses rapidly to loss of all the deciduous teeth. The disease may continue through puberty and affect all the permanent dentition.[37] However, the periodontitis beginning in puberty may involve only the first molars and incisors,[54] as in localized juvenile periodontitis (see Fig. 16-4). Histologically, the lesions demonstrate a heavy plasma cell infiltrate.[81] Removal of local irritants does little to prevent the disease and the resulting loss of teeth.

Hypophosphatasia

Hyphosphosphatasia is a rare genetic disease that results in the premature loss of the deciduous dentition.[8,13] Mild forms of the disease may exhibit only oral clinical and radiographic evidence. The term *odontohyphophosphatasis* has been suggested where the dental findings are the predominant manifestations.[13] Laboratory tests may be necessary to make a differential diagnosis from Papillon-LèFevre syndrome, cyclic diseases, and noncyclic neutropenia.

The disease may appear clinically in infants, young children, and adults. The infantile form is generally lethal. Hypophosphatasia in childhood is characterized by premature exfoliation of deciduous teeth (chiefly the incisors), retarded growth, and rachitis-like deformities. The exfoliation of teeth appears to be related to disturbed cementogenesis.

On the basis of pedigree, biochemical abnormalities (deficiency of the enzyme alkaline phosphatase and excretion of phosphoethanolamine in the urine), and the clinical phenotype of premature tooth loss, hypophosphatasia in mild cases has been considered a dominant trait affecting both osteogenesis and cementogenesis, with mild clinical expression in the heterozygote.[29] Adult forms without apparent skeletal disease may occur, and an autosomal dominant inheritance has also been suggested.[30]

Chédiak-Higashi syndrome (CHS)

Tooth loss at a young age due to severe periodontitis occurs in humans and animals with Chédiak-Higashi syndrome. The teeth are usually lost before adulthood. Neutrophil and monocyte chemotaxis is defective in this hereditary disease.[120] There is a reduced ability of the lysosomes to fuse with phagosomes. The defect may involve the cell's cytoskeletal elements. In this respect, macrophages and neutrophils are weakly active.

Chronic granulomatous disease

Chronic granulomatous disease (CGD) of childhood is a rare inherited disturbance in which patients are susceptible to infection because their neutrophils and monocytes lack enzymes necessary to kill many species of bacteria and fungi. CGD patients develop severe infections of the skin, lymph nodes, liver, and other tissues.[57] Neutrophils and monocytes from these patients do not make oxygen reduction products.[22]

The oral manifestations of CGD include gingivitis, localized early periodontitis, and generalized early-to-moderate periodontitis, but no evidence of juvenile, severe, or rapidly progressing disease, in spite of leukocyte defects.[22] Periodontal disease may or may not be present. Routine antibiotic prophylaxis given to patients with CGD may explain the absence of the disease in the presence of the neutrophil defect.

Down's syndrome (DS)

Down's syndrome (trisomy-21, mongolism) is an inherited disturbance caused by an autosomal abnormality (additional autosome 47, +21). The major clinical findings are mental retardation, characteristic facies, and marked hypotonia. The prevalence of periodontitis in adult Down's syndrome patients appears to be greater than in normal subjects of the same age and sex.[5]

Although it has been suggested that bone loss occurs only rarely in young Down's syndrome patients, several studies have reported advanced periodontal disease in young DS patients,[14,108] and periodontal disease resembling acute necrotizing ulcerative gingivitis has been reported.[14,15,56]

The increased susceptibility of persons with DS to periodontitis and NUG-like gingivitis may be related to the reported impaired neutrophil function[59,91] and the high prevalence of *Bacteroides melaninogenicus* in the gingival crevice of institutionalized trisomy 21 patients.[69]

The pattern of periodontitis in Down's syndrome first involves the mandibular incisors and then extends to the maxillary incisors and molars of the permanent dentition.[58] The pattern is similar for the primary dentition.[96]

Diabetes mellitus

Diabetes mellitus is a diagnostic term for a constellation of anatomic and biochemical abnormalities secondary to a disorder of carbohydrate metabolism involving glucose homeostasis. One of the protean manifestations commonly cited is an increased susceptibility to periodontal disease. The definitive etiology of diabetes mellitus continues to be enigmatic, and prevention and cure remain in the realm of clinical management.[74]

The prevalence of periodontitis in populations of insulin-dependent diabetes mellitus (IDDM) may differ. Generalizations are inappropriate because, while

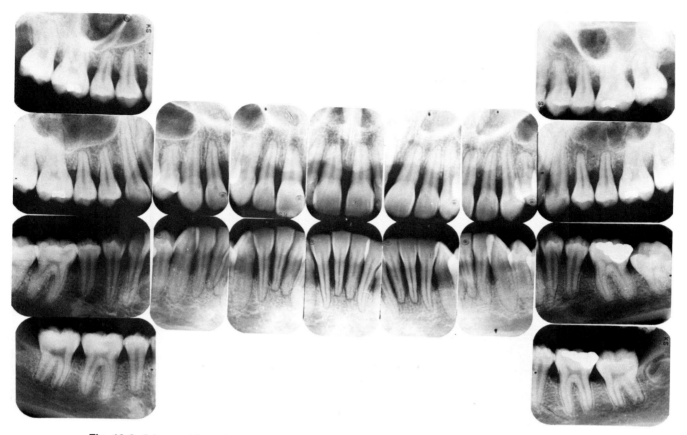

Fig. 13-6. Advanced bone loss associated with periodontitis in a young girl with cyclic neutropenia.

some populations may not exhibit signs of periodontitis,[6] reports of other populations suggest that IDDM patients have a higher frequency of periodontal disease sites with attachment loss.[17,94]

The level of periodontal disease in diabetic patients in general does not appear to differ from that in non-diabetic patients,[51,67,79] but an increase has been reported for diabetics 30 to 40 years of age,[42] and for insulin dependent diabetics 40 to 60 years of age.[124] From the standpoint of juvenile diabetes versus adult diabetics, and controlled versus poorly controlled diabetes, the reports provide conflicting conclusions, especially in relation to periodontitis.

Defects in neutrophil chemotaxis, which tend to be associated with severe forms of periodontitis, have been reported in IDDM.[67,68] Thus, the high susceptibility of periodontitis in juvenile diabetics 5 to 20 years of age[17] is most likely to be due to defective neutrophil function when present. Suppressed polymorphonuclear leukocyte chemotaxis is a major diabetic complication.[52]

Neutropenia/agranulocytosis

Neutropenia, as a benign, quantitative defect in the pool of circulating neutrophils, is diagnosed on the basis of the number of polymorphonuclear leukocytes, but a specific diagnosis is based on the cause of the depressed number of neutrophils. Neutropenia is diagnosed on the basis of less than 1500 polymorphonuclear leukocytes per μl. The cause of the depression may be inherent or acquired.

Cyclic neutropenia, chronic benign neutropenia of childhood, and Chèdiak-Higashi syndrome occur with an identifiable local agent. Acquired forms of neutropenia include those due to drugs and to infection. Chronic benign neutropenia of childhood,[2] agranulocytosis,[24] congenital familial neutropenia,[64] and familial benign chronic neutropenia[25] are profound noncyclical depressions in the number of polymorphonuclear leukocytes in the circulating blood. The oral manifestations of cyclic neutropenia may reflect advanced periodontitis (Fig. 13-6) affecting both the deciduous and permanent dentitions,[21,62,90,97] some manifestations of chronic benign neutropenia are persistent gingivitis and periodontitis.[25,93] Effective treatment of periodontal disease associated with neutropenia and agranulocytosis may be related more to control of systemic infections with antibiotics than simply to control of plaque.[107] All teeth do not appear to be equally involved with periodontitis, and periodontal therapy and restorative treatment may have added significance in the maintenance of less affected teeth.

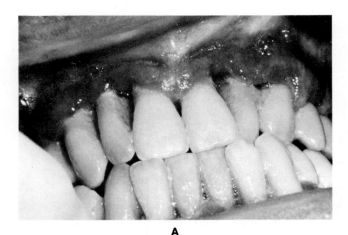

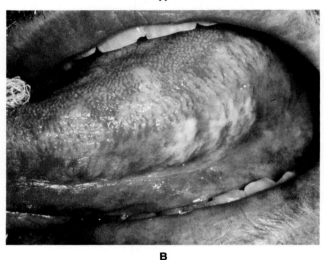

Fig. 13-7. *A,* Periodontitis associated with AIDS. *B,* White leukoplakic patches on lateral border of tongue. No symptoms are produced and unlike Candida, do not rub off.

AIDS

A rapidly progressive periodontitis has been observed in patients with AIDS. The periodontitis has-been potentially related to HIV virus and has been referred to as *AVAP* (AIDS-virus-associated periodontitis).[121] No cause-and-effect relationship between HIV and the periodontitis has been assumed. Documented cases of this potentially related intraoral expression of HIV virus infection include at least eight HIV-seropositive, nine ARC (AID-related-complex), and twenty-one AIDS patients.[122]

The clinical features of AVIP resemble those observed in acute necrotizing ulcerative gingivitis (ANUG), superimposed on rapidly progressive periodontitis (Fig. 13-7A). Severe pain, bleeding, and an intense erythema of the attached gingiva and alveolar mucosa are characteristics of this form of periodontal disease. Leukoplakia-like white patches on the tongue (Fig. 13-7B) are common. The rapid loss of bone, and

perhaps the generalized erythema of the alveolar mucosa, have been considered to differentiate this rapidly progressing form of periodontitis from ANUG, which, on the basis of recurrent episodes, causes bone loss.

DIAGNOSIS OF PERIODONTITIS

The diagnosis of periodontitis may be based upon clinical probing for loss of attachment and the presence of periodontal pockets. Dental radiographs are used for assessing the status of interdental alveolar bone in relation to periodontitis. Except on the basis of repeated measurements, these diagnostic procedures provide no information on disease activity or rate of progression of the disease. Thus, on the basis of periodontal probing and radiographs, it is possible to determine historically the effect of periodontal disease, but it is not possible to determine anything about disease activity or to make predictions about episodes of attachment loss prior to its occurrence.[131]

The diagnosis of periodontitis without further qualification can be made with a periodontal probe, but qualification to specify prepubertal, juvenile, rapidly progressive, and adult periodontitis requires additional information. The criteria for these forms of periodontitis have been discussed, and the overlapping of signs and symptoms is apparent.

In several respects, the age of onset is important in differentiating the various forms of early-onset periodontitis, and knowledge of an underlying systemic disease and/or neutrophil defect may be necessary in determining the nature of the periodontitis. Thus, assays of the function of polymorphonuclear leukocytes may be of diagnostic value in a small percentage of cases exhibiting rapidly destructive juvenile and adult periodontitis.[89] Not all patients with juvenile periodontitis (LJP) have been shown to have depressed neutrophil chemotaxis.[116]

Diagnostic Methods

Several tests for periodontitis are in the process of development, and their effectiveness has been reviewed.[36,77,89] A diagnosis of periodontitis can be made with a periodontal probe, and interproximal bone loss can be evaluated using traditional radiographs. However, an evaluation of disease activity, susceptibility to disease, and response to therapy is not possible with these methods, and sophisticated analytic techniques for measuring several potential indicators of disease activity in saliva, blood, crevicular fluid, and dental plaque are being developed. Putative indicators may relate to host cells (responsiveness, products and surface markers), products of tissue injury, and specific bacteria and their products.[36,49,89]

Host cells, products and responses

Considerable emphasis has been placed on the functional assessment of polymorphonuclear leukocytes (PNNs) or neutrophils, including the in vitro and in vivo determination of their chemotactic activity. Although neutrophil chemotaxis has been routinely assayed by in vitro techniques,[10,76] and in vivo techniques have been developed using a skin window,[1] a less traumatic technique has been developed that monitors reduced PMNL migration in the gingival sulcus using chemotactic agents, such as casein, N-formylmethionylleucyl-phenylalanine (N-fMLP), placed into the gingival crevice.[44,52] The effectiveness of the method in identifying individuals who may be susceptible to severe forms of periodontal disease has yet to be determined.

The detection of isotype-specific antibodies has been facilitated by the development of enzyme-linked immunosorbent assay procedures (ELISA),[31] which may also offer the potential for rapid and simplified identification of organisms commonly associated with periodontitis, such as localized juvenile periodontitis (antibody to *A.a*),[66] acute necrotizing ulcerative gingivitis (antibody to *Bacteroides intermedius* and intermediate size spirochetes),[16] and severe adult periodontitis (antibody to *Bacteroides gingivalis*).[73] Sera and saliva from patients with LJP may have elevated antibody levels to *A.a.*,[33] and the predictive value of a positive serum test (significantly elevated anti-*A.a.*-IgG) has been found to be 86% and the specificity 89%.[41] The value of ELISA antibody determination remains to be determined on the basis of correlations, established by prospective longitudinal studies, between *A. actinomycetemcomitans* antibody titers and consequent development of periodontal disease.

Antibody levels to putative infecting periodontopathic microorganisms may be elevated locally and detectable in the gingival fluid.[111] A number of potential indicators of periodontal disease are present in the fluid obtained from gingival crevices, including leukocytes and ionic species,[18] serum proteins,[12] immunoglobulin (Ig),[11] and Ig with antibody activity.[32] The detection, using static crevicular fluid (SGF), of IgG antibody to homologous organisms demonstrated a proportion of agreement of 54% to 78% for elevated SCF antibody and the presence of corresponding microorganisms at the same site.[35] Evidence suggests that gingival plasma cells have antibody specificity and that GCF Ig is synthesized locally. The use of SCF antibody for detecting microorganisms and as an indicator of disease activity has yet to be determined. The composition of gingival crevicular fluid seems to be a promising source of information for the detection of disease activity.

The development of a biochemical profile of GCF constituents would provide an opportunity to monitor a large number of factors associated with the inflammatory response and breakdown of connective tissue, including bone resorption.[61] The composition of GCF includes a number of bacterial products (e.g., endotoxins, enzymes) and host cell products, including a number of enzymes from host cells, as well as from neutrophils. The simultaneous examination of a number of these enzymes to provide a profile of active disease could lead to extensive combinations and to research to clarify meaningful markers of disease activity. The products of tissue injury present in the GCF are potential indicators of periodontal disease.

The rapid identification of bacteria implicated in various forms of periodontal disease has been considered as a method useful for clinical diagnosis. More specifically, indirect immunofluorescence microscopy using specific serodiagnostic reagents for the clinical detection of *B. gingivalis* has been suggested to be useful for the diagnosis of adult periodontitis.[125] However, although specific species of bacteria have been identified as prominent in chronic periodontal disease, no specific organisms or groups of organisms have yet been directly implicated as causal agents for any periodontal disease.[89]

Microscopic assessment "at chairside" of pathogens associated with periodontal disease provides rapid bacterial evaluation by morphotypes, but the limitations include inability to speciate or study individual microbes or to determine susceptibility to antibiotic therapies. As yet, the method has not been shown to predictably detect levels of pathogenic morphotypes associated with periodontal disease.[48]

SUMMARY

Periodontitis has been identified as inflammation of the supporting structures of the teeth that involves a loss of connective tissue attachment and alveolar bone. Manifestations of periodontitis occur at different ages, although such expressions in variations in the disease appear to be more related to host defenses (e.g., neutrophil function) than to any specific function of aging. Even so, the provisional clinical diagnosis of early-onset forms of periodontitis is made on the basis of periodontal probing and the dental-medical history of the patient, including the age of onset.

A definitive diagnosis of some forms of periodontitis may require the identification of disturbances of neutrophil function, including chemotaxis and cell adherence. In such instances, a clinical diagnosis of a specific form of periodontitis may not be possible, and reliance on laboratory studies may be necessary. An example of such a study is the use of a unique marker to differentiate prepubertal gingivitis from juvenile periodontitis and rapidly progressive periodontitis.

The use of a biochemical profile to identify specific forms of disease and to specify disease activity has yet to be accomplished. The development of simple methods of evaluating enzymatic activity of dental plaque appears to be a particularly attractive area of research into test systems meant to differentiate active from inactive sites of disease activity.

REFERENCES

1. Addison, I.E., et al: A human skin window technique using micropore membranes, J. Immunol. Methods 54:129, 1982.
2. Andrews, R.G., et al: Chronic benign neutropenia of childhood associated with oral manifestations, Oral Surg. 20:719, 1965.
3. Baer, P.N.: The case for periodontosis as a clinical entity. J. Periodontol. 42:516, 1971.
4. Balit, H.L., et al.: The increasing prevalence of gingival *Bacteroides melaninogenicus* with age in children, Arch Oral Biol. 9:435, 1964.
5. Barnett, M.L., et al.: The prevalence of periodontitis and dental caries in a Down's syndrome population, J. Periodontol. 57:288, 1986.
6. Barnett, M.L., et al.: Absence of periodontitis in a population of insulin-dependent diabetes mellitus (IDDM) patients, J. Periodontol. 55:402, 1984.
7. Bernier, J.L.: The role of inflammation in periodontal disease, Oral Surg. 2:583, 1949.
8. Beumer, J., et al.: Childhood hypophosphatasia and the premature loss of teeth, Oral Surg. 35:63, 1973.
9. Bick, P.H., et al.: Polyclonal B-cell activation induced by extracts of Gram-negative bacteria isolated from periodontal disease sites, Infect. Immun. 34:43, 1981.
10. Boyden, S.: Chemotactic effect of mixtures of antibody and antigen on polymorphonuclear leukocytes, J. Exp. Med 115:453, 1962.
11. Brandtzaeg, P.: Immunochemical comparison of proteins in human gingival pocket fluid serum and saliva, Arch Oral Biol. 10:795, 1965.
12. Brill, N., and Bronnestrom, R.: Immunoelectrophoretic study of tissue fluid from gingival pockets, Acta Odont. Scand. 18:95, 1960.
13. Brittain, J.M., et al: Odontohypophosphatasia: A report of two cases, J. Deut. Child. 43:106, 1976.
14. Brown, R.H.: Longitudinal study of periodontal disease in Down's syndrome, N. Z. Dent. J. 74:137, 1978.
15. Brown, R.H.: Necrotizing ulcerative gingivitis in mongoloid and nonmongoloid retarded individuals, J. Periodont. Res. 8:290, 1973.
16. Chung, C.P., et al.: Bacterial IgG and IgM antibody titers in acute necrotizing ulcerative gingivitis, J. Periodontol. 54:557, 1983.
17. Cianciola, L.J., et al.: Prevalence of periodontal disease in insulin dependent diabetes mellitus (juvenile diabetes), J.A.D.A. 104:653, 1982.
18. Cimasoni, G.: Crevicular Fluid Updated, Monographs in Oral Science, Ed. H.M. Meyers. Basel: S. Karger, 1983.
19. Coccia, C.T., et al.: Papillon-LeFevre Syndrome: precocious periodontosis with palmar-plantar hyperkeratosis, J. Periodontol. 37:408, 1966.
20. Cogen, R.B., et al.: Host factors in juvenile periodontitis, J. Dent. Res. 65:394, 1986.
21. Cohen, D.W., and Morris, A.L.: Periodontal manifestations of cyclic neutropenia, J. Periodontol. 32:159, 1961.
22. Cohen, M.S., et al.: Phagocytic cells in periodontal defense. Periodontal status of patients with chronic granulomatous disease of childhood, J. Periodontol. 56:611, 1986.
23. Dahl, M.V., et al.: Infection, dermatitis, increased IgE and impaired neutrophil chemotaxis, Arch Derm. 112:1387, 1976.
24. Davey, K.W., and Konchak, P.A.: Agranulocytosis. Dental care report, Oral Surg. 28:116, 1969.
25. Deasy, M.J., et al: Familial benign chronic neutropenia associated with periodontal disease—a case report, J. Periodontol. 51:206, 1980.
26. Delaney, J.E., and Kornman, K.S.: Subgingival microflora associated with puberty, J. Dent. Res. (abst.) 63:263, 1984.
27. Doty, S.L., et al.: Humoral immune response to oral microorganisms in periodontitis, Infect. Immun. 37:499, 1982.
28. Dudney, T.P., and Todd, I.P.: Crohn's disease of the mouth, P. Roy. S. Med. 62:1237, 1969.
29. Eastman, J., and Bixler, D.: Lethal and mild hypophosphatasia in half-sibs, J. Craniofac. Genet. Dev. Biol. 2:35, 1982.
30. Eberle, F., et al.: Adult hypophosphatasia without apparent skeletal disease: "Odontohyphosphatasia" in four heterozygote members of a family, Klen-Wochenschr. 62:371, 1984.
31. Ebersole, J.L.: An ELISA for measuring serum antibody to *Actinobacillus actinomycetemcomitans*, J. Periodont. Res. 15:621, 1980.
32. Ebersole, J.L., et al.: Gingival crevicular fluid antibody to oral microorganisms. I. Method of collection and analysis of antibody, J. Periodont. Res. 19:124, 1984.
33. Ebersole, J.L., et al.: Human immune responses to oral microorganisms. I. Association of localyzed juvenile periodontitis (LJP) with serum antibody responses to *Actinobacillus actinomycetemcomitans*, Clin. Exp. Immunol. 46:856, 1981.
34. Ebersole, J.L., et al.: Human immune response to oral microorganisms. I. Association of localized juvenile periodontitis (LJP) with serum antibody responses to *Actinomycetes actinomycetemcomitans*, Clin Exp. Immunol. 47:43, 1982.
35. Ebersole, J.L., et al.: Local antibody responses in periodontal diseases. In New Approaches to the diagnosis and chemotherapeutic management of the periodontal diseases, J. Periodontol. (Special Issue) 56:51, 1985.
36. Fine, D.H., and Mandel, I.D.: Indicators of periodontal disease activity: An evaluation, J. Clin. Periodontol. 13:533, 1986.
37. Galatin, D.R., and Bradford, S.: Hyperkeratosis palmoplantaris and periodontosis: The Papillon-LeFevre syndrome, J. Periodontol. 40:40, 1969.
38. Genco, R.J.: Progress in periodontal research. Findings from the Periodontal Disease Clinical Research Center, State University of New York at Buffalo, Northeast Soc. Periodontist Bull. 11:5-14, 1981.
39. Genco, R.J., and Slots, J.: Host responses in periodontal diseases, J. Dent. Res. 63:441, 1984.
40. Genco, R.J., et al.: Neutrophil chemotaxis impairment in juvenile periodontitis: Evaluation of specificity, adherence, deformability, and serum factors, J. Reticuloendothel. Soc. 28:81s, 1980.
41. Genco, R.J., et al.: Serum and gingival fluid antibodies as adjuncts in the diagnosis of *Actinobacillus actinomycetemcomitans*-associated periodontal disease, J. Periodontol. (Special Issue) 56:41, 1985.
42. Glavind, L., et al.: The relationship between periodontal state and diabetes duration, insulin storage, and retinal changes, J. Periodontol. 39:341, 1968.
43. Glossary of Periodontic Terms, J. Periodontol. (Supplement), November, 1986.
44. Golub, L.M., et al.: The response of human sulcular leucocytes to a chemotactic challenge. A new in vivo assay, J. Periodont. Res. 16:171, 1981.
45. Goodson, J.M., et al.: Patterns of progression and regression of advanced destructive periodontal disease, J. Clin Periodontol. 9:472, 1982.
46. Gottlieb, B.: Etiology and therapy of alveolar pyorrhea, Z. Stomatol. 18:59, 1920.
47. Gottlieb, B.: The new concept of periodontoclasia, J. Periodontol. 17:7, 1944.
48. Greenstein, G., and Polson, A.: Microscopic monitoring of pathogens associated with periodontal diseases. A review, J.

Periodontol. 56:740, 1985.

49. Gusberti, F.A., et al.: Diagnostic methods for the assessment of potential periodontal disease activity: Enzymatic activities of bacterial plaque and their relationship to clinical parameters. In Borderland Between Caries and Periodontal Disease III, ed. T. Lehner and G. Cimasoni. Basel: S. Karger, 1987.

50. Haneke, E., et al.: Increased susceptibility to infections in the Papillon-LeFevre syndrome, Dermatologica 150:283, 1975.

51. Hove, K.A., and Stallard, R.E.: Diabetes and the periodontal patient, J. Periodontol. 41:713, 1970.

52. Iacono, V.J., et al.: In vivo assay of crevicular leukocyte migration. In New Approaches to the diagnosis and therapeutic management of the periodontal diseases, J. Periodontol. (Special Issue), 1985.

53. Imrey, P.B.: Considerations in the statistical analysis of clinical trials in periodontitis, J. Clin. Periodontol. 13:517, 1986.

54. Ingle, J.E.: Papillon-LeFevre syndrome: Precocious periodontosis with associated epidermal lesions, J. Periodontol. 30:230, 1959.

55. Jensen, J., et al.: The effect of female sex hormones on subgingival plaque, J. Periodontol. 52:599, 1981.

56. Johnson, N.P., and Young, M.A.: Periodontal disease in mongols, J. Periodontol. 34:41, 1963.

57. Johnston, R.B., Jr., and Newman, S.L.: Chronic granulomatous disease, Pediatr. Clin. North Am. 24:365, 1977.

58. Kisling, E., and Krebs, G.: Periodontal conditions in adult patients with mongolism (Down's syndrome), Act. Odont. Scand. 21:391, 1963.

59. Kretschmer, R.R., et al.: Leukocyte function in Down's syndrome quantitative NBI reduction and bacteriodal capacity, Clin Immunol. Immunopathol. 2:449, 1974.

60. Lamster, I., et al.: An association between Crohn's disease, periodontal disease and enhanced neutrophil function, J. Periodontol. 49:475, 1978.

61. Lamster, I.B., et al.: Development of a biochemical profile for gingival crevicular fluid, J. Periodontol. (Special Issue) 56:13, 1985.

62. Lamster, I.B., et al.: Infantile agranulocytosis with survival into adolescence: Periodontal manifestations and laboratory findings, J. Periodontol. 58:34, 1987.

63. Lang, N.K., et al.: Bleeding on Probing. A Predictor for the progression of periodontal disease? J. Clin. Periodontol. 13:590, 1986.

64. Levine, S.: Chronic familial neutropenia with marked periodontal lesions: Report of a case, Oral Surg. 12:310, 1959.

65. Listgarten, M.A.: Pathogenesis of periodontitis, J. Clin. Periodontol. 13:418, 1956.

66. Listgarten, M.A., et al.: Comparative antibody titers to *Actinobacillus actinomycetemcomitans* in juvenile periodontitis, chronic periodontitis, and periodontally healthy subjects, J. Clin. Periodontol. 8:155, 1981.

67. Manouchehr-Pour, M., et al: Impaired neutrophil chemotaxis in diabetic patients with severe periodontitis, J. Dent. Res. 60:729, 1981.

68. McMullen, J.A., et al.: Neutrophil chemotaxis in individuals with advanced periodontal disease and a genetic predisposition to diabetes mellitus, J. Periodontol. 52:167, 1981.

69. Meskin, L.H., et al.: Prevalence of *Bacteriodes melaninogenicus* in the gingival crevice are of institutionalized trisomy 21 and cerebral palsy patients and normal children, J. Periodontol. 39:326, 1968.

70. Miller, S.C., and Seidler, B.B.: Relative alveoloclastic experience of the various teeth, J. Dent. Res. 21:365, 1942.

71. Miller, W.D.: The Micro-organisms of the Human Mouth (1890). Reprinted Basel: S. Karger, 1973, p. 321.

72. Moore, W.E.C., et al.: Bacteriology of moderate (chronic) periodontitis in mature adult humans, Infect. Immun. 42:510, 1983.

73. Mouton, C., et al.: Serum antibodies to oral *Bacteroides asaccharolyticus (Bacteroides gingivalis)*. Relationship to age and periodontal disease, Infect. Immun. 31:182, 1981.

74. Murrah, V.A.: Diabetes mellitus and associated oral manifestations: A review, J. Oral Pathol. 14:271, 1985.

75. Naik, D., et al.: Papillon-LeFevre syndrome, Oral Surg. 25:19, 1968.

76. Nelson, R.D., et al.: Chemotaxis under agarose: A new and simple method for measuring chemotaxis and spontaneous migration of human polymorphonuclear leukocytes and monocytes, J. Immunol. 115:1650, 1975.

77. New approaches to the diagnosis and chemotherapeutic management of the periodontal diseases, J. Periodontol. 56: (Special Issue), 1985.

78. Newman, M.G.: Current concepts of the pathogenesis of periodontal disease, J. Periodontol. 56:734, 1985.

79. Nichols, C., et al.: Diabetes mellitus and periodontal disease, J. Periodontol. 49:85, 1978.

80. Page, R.C., and Baab, D.A.: A new look at the etiology and pathogenesis of early-onset periodontitis, J. Periodontol. 56:748, 1985.

81. Page, R.C., and Schroeder, H.: Periodontitis in man and other animals. A comparative review. Basel: S. Karger, 1982.

82. Page, R.C., et al.: Characteristics of early-onset periodontitis and identification of the molecular abnormality in one form. 7th International Conference on Periodontal Research, Ittingen, Switzerland, Sept. 8-11, 1986.

83. Page, R.C., et al.: Clinical and laboratory studies of a family with a high prevalence of juvenile periodontitis, J. Periodontol. 56:602, 1985.

84. Page, R.C., et al.: Defective neutrophil and monocyte mobility in patients with early-onset periodontitis, Infect. Immun. 47:169, 1985.

85. Page, R.C., et al.: Prepubertal periodontitis. I. Definition of a clinical entity, J. Periodontol. 54:257, 1983.

86. Page, R.C., et al.: Rapidly progressive periodontitis, J. Periodontol. 54:197, 1983.

87. Palcanis, K.G., et al.: Rapidly progressive periodontitis, J. Periodontol. 57:378, 1986.

88. Pincus, S.H., et al.: Defeceive neutrophil chemotaxis with varient ichthyosis, hyper-immunoglobulinemia E and recurrent infection, J. Pediatr. 87:908, 1975.

89. Polson, A.M., and Goodson, J.M.: Periodontal diagnosis. Current states and future needs, J. Periodontol. 56:25, 1985.

90. Prichard, J.F., et al.: Prepubertal periodontitis affecting the deciduous and permanent dentition of a patient with cyclic neutropenia. A case report and discussion, J. Periodontol. 55:114, 1984.

91. Quie, P.G., and Cates, K.L.: Clinical conditions associated with defective polymorphonuclear leukocyte chemotaxis, Am. J. Pathol. 88:711, 1977.

92. Ramfjord, S.P., Kerr, D.A., and Ash, M.M., eds. World Workshop on Periodontics, June 6-9, 1966. Ann Arbor, Michigan, University of Michigan, 1966.

93. Reichart, P.A., and Dornow, H.: Gingivo-periodontal manifestations in chronic benign neutropenia, J. Clin Periodontol. 5:74, 1978.

94. Rylander, H., et al.: Prevalence of periodontal disease in young diabetics, J. Clin. Periodontol. 14:38, 1987.

95. Saxen, L.: Hereditary juvenile periodontitis, J. Clin. Periodontol. 7:276, 1980.

96. Saxen, L., et al: Periodontal disease associated with Down's syndrrome: An orthopantomographic evaluation, J. Periodontol. 48:337, 1977.

97. Scully, C., et al.: Oral manifestations in cyclic neutropenia, Br. J. Oral Surg. 20:96, 1982.

98. Segal, A.W., and Lowei, G.: Neutrophil dysfunction in

Crohn's disease, Lancet ii:219, 1976.

99. Seymour, G.T.: Possible mechanisms involved in the immunoregulation of chronic inflammatory periodontal diseases, J. Dent. Res. 66:2, 1987.

100. Slots, J.: The predominant cultivable microflora of advanced periodontitis, Scand. J. Dent. Res. 85:114, 1977.

101. Slots, J.: Bacterial specificity in adult periodontitis, J. Clin. Periodontol. 13:912, 1986.

102. Slots, J., and Gevco, R.J.: Black-pigmented *Bacteroides* species, *Capnocytophagia* species, and *Actinobacillus actinomycetemcomitans* in human periodontal disease: Virulence factors in colonization, survival and tissue destruction, J. Dent. Res. 63:412, 1984.

103. Slots, J.: The predominant cultivable organisms in juvenile periodontitis, Scand. J. Dent. Res. 84:1, 1976.

104. Smith, S., et al.: Polyclonal B-cell activation, severe periodontal disease in young adults, Immunology and Immunopathology 16:354, 1980.

105. Socransky, S.S.: Microbiology of periodontal disease—present status and future considerations, J. Periodontol. 48:497, 1977.

106. Spektor, M.D., et al.: Clinical studies of one family manifesting rapidly progressive juvenile and prepubertal periodontitis, J. Periodontol. 56:93, 1984.

107. Spencer, P., and Fleming, J.E.: Cyclic neutropenia: A literature review and report of a case, J. Dent. Child. 52:108, 1985.

108. Sznajder, N., et al.: Clinical periodontal findings in trisomy 21 (mongolism), J. Periodont. Res. 3:1, 1968.

109. Tanner, A.C.R., et al.: A study of the bacteria associated with advancing periodontitis in man, J. Clin Periodontol. 6:278, 1979.

110. Tanner, A.C.R., et al.: Microbiota of periodontal pockets losing crestal alveolar bone, J. Periodont. Res. 19:279, 1984.

111. Taubman, M.A., et al.: Association between systemic and local antibody in periodontal disease. In Host-Parasite Interactions in Periodontal Diseases, ed. R.J. Genco and S.E. Mergenhagen. Washington, D.C.: American Society for Microbiology, 1982.

112. Tew, J.G., et al.: Immunological studies of young adults with severe periodontitis, J. Periodont. Res. 16:403, 1981.

113. Theilade, E.: The non-specific theory in microbial etiology of inflammatory periodontal diseases, J. Clin. Periodontol. 13:905, 1986.

114. Vandesteen, G.E., et al.: Clinical, microbial and immunologic studies of a family with a high prevalence of early-onset periodontitis, J. Periodontol. 55:159, 1984.

115. Vandesteen, G.E., et al.: Leukocyte function, microflora and antibody studies of four families with periodontitis, J. Periodont. Res. 17:498, 1982.

116. Van Dyke, T.E., et al.: Periodontal diseases and neutrophil abnormalities. In Host-Parasite Interactions in Periodontal Disease, ed. R.J. Genco and S.E. Mergenhagen. Washington, D.C.: American Society for Microbiology, 1982.

117. Van Dyke, T.E., et al.: The polymorphonuclear leukocyte (PMNL) locomotor defect in juvenile periodontitis. Study of random migration, chemokinesis, and chemotaxis, J. Periodontol. 53:682, 1982.

118. Wannenmacher, E.: Umschau auf dem Gebiet der Paradentose, Zentralbl Gesamte Zahn-Mund-Kieferheilkd. 3:81, 1938.

119. Weinman, J.P., and Orban, B.: Diffuse atrophy of alveolar bone (Periodontosis), J. Periodontol. 13:31, 1942.

120. White, J.G., and Clawson, C.C.: The Chediak-Higashi syndrome: The nature of the giant neutrophil granules and their interactions with cytoplasms and foreign particulates, Am J. Pathol. 98:151, 1980.

121. Winkler, J.R., et al.: AIDS virus associated with periodontal disease, J. Dent. Res. (Spec. Iss.) 65:741, 1986.

122. Winkler, J.R., and Murray, P.A.: Periodontal disease. A potential intraoral expression of AIDS may be rapidly progressive periodontitis, CDA Journal, January, 1987.

123. Wojcicki, C.J., et al.: Differences in periodontal disease-associated microorganisms of subgingival plaque in prepubertal, pubertal and postpubertal children, J. Periodontol. 58:219, 1987.

124. Wolf, J.: Dental and periodontal conditions in diabetes mellitus. A clinical and radiographic study, Proc. Finn. Dent. Soc. (Suppl. VI) 73:26, 1977.

125. Zambon, J.J., et al.: Rapid identification of periodontal pathogens in subgingival dental plaque. Comparison of indirect immunofluorescence microscopy with bacterial culture for detection of *Bacteroides gingivalis*, J. Periodontol. (Special Issue) 56:32, 1985.

126. Zambon, J.J., et al.: *Actinobacillus actinomycetemcomitans* in human periodontal disease. Prevalence in patient groups and distribution of biotypes and serotypes within families, J. Periodontol. 54:707, 1983.

14

TREATMENT PLANNING IN PERIODONTICS

The goal of all dental and periodontal therapy is to establish and maintain oral health, comfortable function, and optimal esthetics. To what extent these objectives may be achieved depends on the status of the patient's dentition at the time of admission, and the patient's desire and ability to cooperate with the dentist. The ability of the dentist and his dental health team may also have a bearing on the plans and results. Since there is no one-time cure for most periodontal diseases, long-term favorable results are determined by mutual cooperation between patients and professional personnel that goes beyond mere technical skill. Thus, the treatment plan should have both a technical-mechanical or drug aspect and a psychological-educational and motivational direction, focused on plaque control and maintenance care for the indefinite future.

Treatment Rationale

The most common cause of periodontal disease is an opportunistic bacterial infection,[9] which has to be contained in order for the disease to be cured. Any systemic or local disorder that may impair normal body responses to irritants should also be recognized and corrected, if possible. Fortunately, with rigid control of bacterial irritation, periodontal disease can be treated successfully even if unfavorable systemic factors persist.[26]

Although many aspects of periodontal inflammation appear to be self-destructive, characterized by collagenolysis and fiber degeneration, the inflammatory process is protective in an attempt to contain the injurious agents, and the inflamed tissues do not have to be surgically removed for improved healing.[11] Most of the pathogenic organisms live on the tooth surface and in the crevice or pocket, but some may also be present within the tissues of the pocket wall.[27] How-

ever, there is ample evidence that elimination of the surface organisms, without any specific antimicrobial therapy,[28] will lead to healing of the periodontal lesion.[29]

The great challenge in periodontal therapy is to eliminate the surface irritants and to correct the conditioning factors that may allow the opportunistic infection to return. The aim of periodontal therapy is to make the teeth biologically acceptable to the surrounding periodontal tissues.

Goals for Periodontal Therapy

In the report from a recent workshop, it was stated that "the goal of periodontal therapy is to restore health and function to the periodontium and to preserve the teeth for a lifetime."[7] More specifically, successful therapy is characterized by (1) a clinically healthy gingiva that is uniformly pink in color, firm, and dense, with the gingival sulcus attached firmly to the teeth, so that one may probe gently with a thin probe without causing bleeding or secretion; (2) a clinical attachment level that is maintainable with probing over time; (3) comfortably functioning stable occlusion; (4) acceptable esthetics to the patient; and (5) roentgenologic evidence of an even and well-defined lamina dura over the alveolar crest (Fig. 14-1). Although these optimal goals may not always be achieved for every tooth in the dentition, very few patients will end up edentulous if proper periodontal care has been applied.[8]

Treatable and Nontreatable Patients

Following a thorough appraisal of the patient and the dentition, it has to be decided whether all or some teeth with advanced periodontal disease can be successfully treated, and, furthermore, whether these

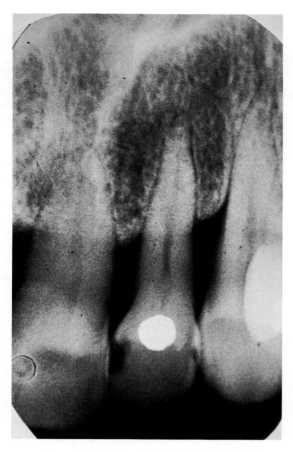

Fig. 14-1. Well-defined lamina dura over the alveolar crest 6 months after periodontal treatment.

teeth are a health hazard to the patient, in which case they should be removed and replaced with prosthetic appliances. Between the extremes of treating all or extracting all of the remaining teeth, there are usually a large number of potential solutions to the patient's periodontal and dental problems.[7]

A defeatist attitude has often prevailed among dentists and patients regarding the management of teeth with advanced periodontal bone loss.[22] In cases of advanced disease, the majority of dental practitioners used to consider periodontal therapy a delaying maneuver followed sooner or later by the loss of teeth and a poor denture base. Well-controlled clinical trials have now documented that the progress of even advanced periodontitis can be stopped and the teeth maintained over a long period of time.[8,10] It has also been documented that under complete dentures there is a continuous loss of alveolar ridge bone;[30] therefore, whenever it is possible, at least a few teeth are maintained to allow for overlay dentures rather than extracting all teeth.[12]

In borderline cases, the functional demands upon the dentition have to be considered. Bruxism will have a detrimental effect on the prognosis of poorly sup-

ported teeth. It has become increasingly evident that improved periodontal, restorative, and occlusal therapy make it possible to establish long-lasting comfortable dentitions with fewer remaining teeth and much less periodontal support than was previously necessary.[15] The possibility of orthodontically moving displaced teeth into a useful position, regardless of age and periodontal status, also makes it feasible to use abutment teeth that previously would have been considered hopeless. Treatment planning ultimately requires an up-to-date overview of what the various branches of modern dentistry can offer.

The initial step in all periodontal treatment planning is a careful evaluation of each tooth in an attempt to determine if a feasible response to treatment can be expected; however, every tooth given a dubious prognosis should not necessarily be scheduled for extraction. It has often been reported that teeth that were considered hopeless have continued to function satisfactorily over many years;[5] therefore, palliative periodontal treatment may be considered for some patients.

Indications for Palliative Treatment

Unfortunately, palliative periodontal treatment is often equated with superficial, mostly supragingival tooth cleaning, which in advanced periodontal disease is a complete waste of time. Nothing in periodontal therapy is more demanding than palliative treatment of inaccessible furcations and lesions extending close to the apex of the teeth, and in order to be better than no treatment, it has to be taken seriously.

Candidates for palliative treatment should have normal resistance to bacterial infection, and include (1) patients with short life expectancy due either to advanced age or systemic disease with poor survival prognosis, (2) patients with severe mental and physical handicaps, (3) patients with severe furcation involvement and generalized advanced periodontitis (Fig. 14-2), and (4) patients with limited financial resources for extensive restorative dentistry.

Palliative treatment should not be prescribed for patients with valvular heart defects, poorly controlled diabetes, or other diseases in which periodontal pockets may act as a serious focus of infection, thus threatening the patients' health.

Obstacles to Success of Periodontal Therapy

A few potentially negative factors should be considered in the treatment planning:

1. Lack of patient interest. Patients who have advanced periodontitis and are unreliable with their commitments have a poor prognosis.

2. Furcation involvement with poor access (Fig. 14-3).

3. Extensive root caries. Fluorides and adjustment

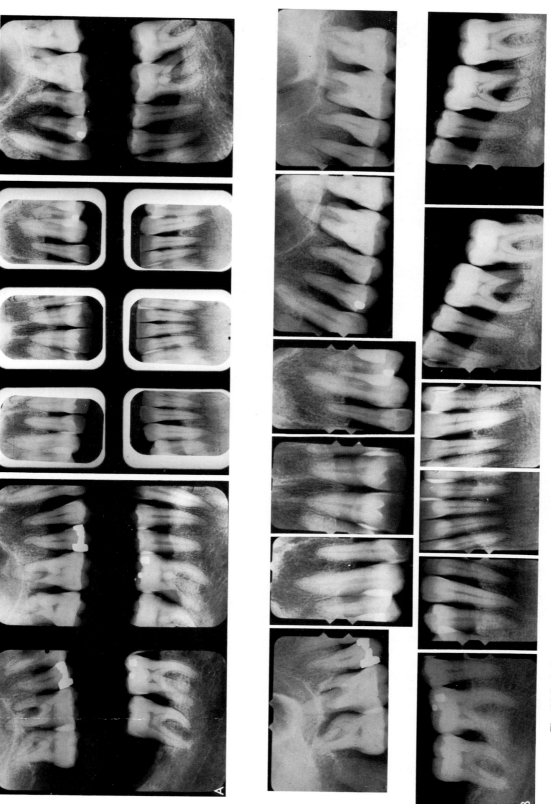

Fig. 14-2. *A,* Roentgenogram showing advanced periodontitis prior to treatment in a 42-year-old patient. Extensive furcation involvements of all maxillary molars and of one mandibular molar. *B,* Same patient 13 years later. The patient had maintenance prophylaxis every 3 months. Two maxillary molars developed retrograde pulpitis and all maxillary molars were extracted.

continued

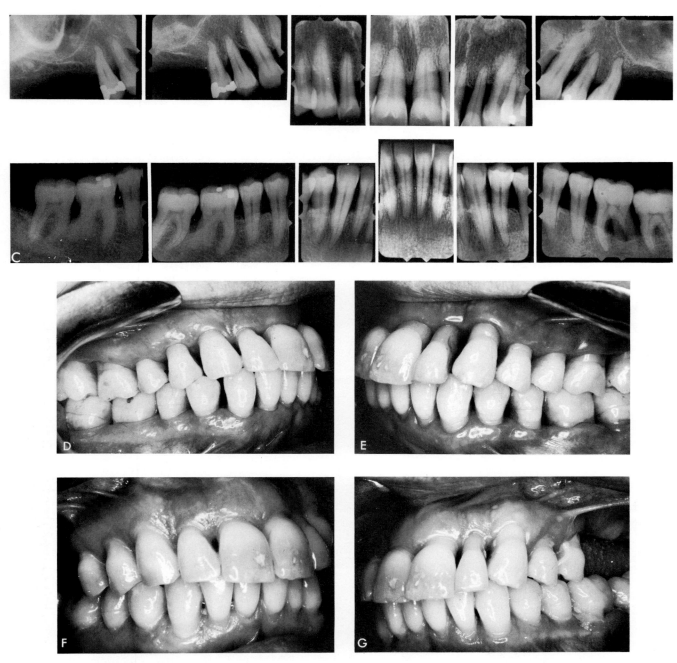

Fig. 14-2 continued. *C,* Roentgenograms taken 16 years after initial treatment, in which no splinting of the teeth was done. Although the teeth have more than normal mobility, they function comfortably, and the periodontal status is stable except for continuous bone loss around the mandibular first molar, which has through-and-through furcation involvement. *D,E,* Clinical appearances of tissues prior to treatment. *F,G,* Sixteen years after initial treatment. The teeth on the right side were treated with subgingival curettage, while partial pocket elimination surgery was done on the left side. The patient also had occlusal adjustment, which may have contributed to the closure of the interdental contacts and lessened the mobility of the teeth. Deep, inactive periodontal pockets can still be probed along almost all of the remaining teeth, but no bleeding or exudate is seen on probing the gingival crevice or on palpating the gingiva.

of diet should be considered essential (Fig. 14-4).

4. Esthetic problems have to be solved to the satisfaction of the patient (Fig. 14-5).

5. Financial inability or unwillingness to replace all lost teeth is not necessarily an obstacle to succes of periodontal therapy (Fig. 14-6).[8]

Sequential Plan for Periodontal Therapy

The first consideration in all treatment is the safety of the patient. Any kind of treatment that is potentially harmful to the patient's systemic and oral health is contraindicated. The primary objective is to treat a

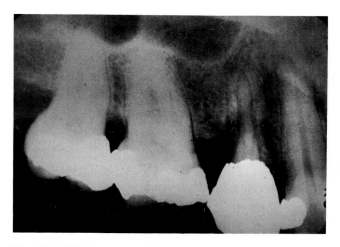

Fig. 14-3. Replacement of the maxillary bicuspid with a fixed bridge is preferable to periodontal treatment in the presence of such deep pockets and furcation involvement of the bicuspid.

patient with periodontal disease rather than merely to treat periodontal disease. Although each case of periodontal disease has to be analyzed and considered for individualized therapy, there is a logical sequential order of considerations and procedures that should be applied to every patient with periodontal disease.[17,25]

Systemic phase

All aspects of systemic health relevant to the etiology, treatment, and prevention of the patient's periodontal disease are evaluated.

Hygienic phase

All dental accretions and obstacles to effective oral hygiene have to be eliminated. The patient is then instructed and motivated to undertake effective plaque control. The optimal treatment plan for the patient is established.

Corrective phase

Occlusal aberrations of significance to periodontal health and function are eliminated, periodontal pockets and mucogingival deficiencies are evaluated, and restorative procedures indicated for the health, function, and esthetics of the dentition are carried out.

Maintenance phase

An individualized recall program is established to assure the maintenance of the patient's oral health.

The sequence of steps to be followed in the management of patients with periodontal disease is listed in the following outline.

Outline for Treatment Sequence

I. Systemic Phase
   1. Systemic health considerations.
   2. Premedication.

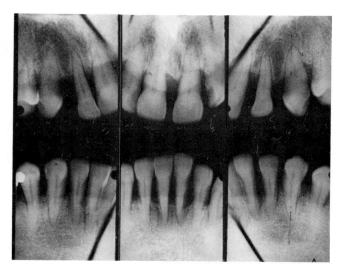

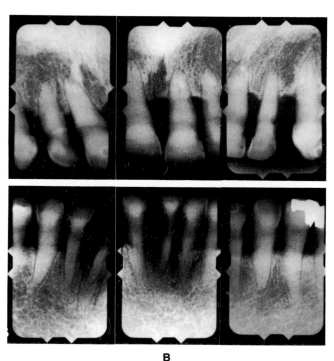

Fig. 14-4. *A,* Advanced periodontitis in a 43-year-old patient. *B,* Same patient 8 years later. Root caries with "softening" of the root surfaces make it difficult to maintain the teeth, although the periodontal status is stable.

   3. Referral to physician.
II. Hygienic Phase
   1. Patient education.
   2. Preliminary gross scaling.
   3. Excavation of deep caries, temporary restorations, endodontics.
   4. Instruction in oral hygiene.
   5. Extraction of hopeless teeth.
   6. Temporary splints, temporary replacement of lost teeth.

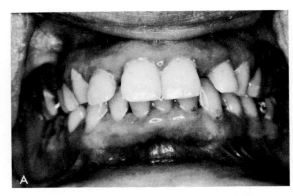

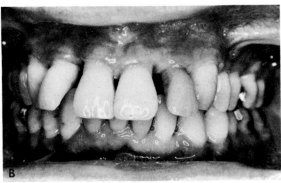

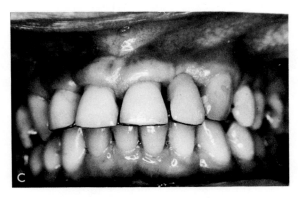

Fig. 14-5. *A,* Advanced periodontitis in a 25-year-old patient. *B,* After pocket elimination surgery. *C,* After orthodontic treatment and splinting of the anterior teeth.

7. Fine scaling and root planing.
8. Preliminary occlusal adjustment.
9. Evaluation of oral hygiene and tissue response.
10. Reassessment of entire treatment plan.

III. Corrective Phase
1. Maintenance of plaque control.
2. Orthodontic treatment.
3. Biteplanes.
4. Occlusal adjustment.
5. Hemisections with temporary splinting.
6. Periodontal surgery.
7. Treatment of hypersensitive teeth—topical fluoride.
8. Restorative dentistry.

9. Rechecking and refining of occlusion.

IV. Maintenance Phase
1. Reexamination for effectiveness of plaque control, recurrence of periodontal disease, caries, and occlusal problems. Reinforcement of oral hygiene instruction, performance of prophylaxis, including application of topical acidulated fluorophosphate.[6]
2. Roentgenographic survey or bitewings as needed. Comparing with prior roentgenographs.
3. Recementing and checking every 2 to 3 years of any fixed splints that are temporarily cemented.
4. Treatment of any active pockets.
5. Treatment of carious lesions.
6. Endodontic therapy if pulpal or periapical lesions have developed.
7. Replacement of dental restorations, bridges, and appliances that no longer satisfy health, function, or esthetic requirements.
8. Creation of new occlusal biteplanes when old ones are broken down, worn out, or lost.
9. Complete reevaluation of the entire periodontal and dental status of patients who return after having dropped out of the regular maintenance program for 1 or more years.

Obviously, very few patients need all of the procedures included in this comprehensive outline, and any step not needed should be bypassed until the next applicable procedure is reached. However, the sequence of procedures should be adhered to, both in planning and execution of periodontal therapy.

SPECIFIC CONSIDERATIONS FOR EACH STEP OF THE TREATMENT PLAN
Emergency treatment of acute pain

A differential diagnosis of the source of the pain may reveal that it is related to a periodontal abscess, pulpal disease, traumatic injury, necrotizing ulcerative gingivitis, painful mouth lesions not directly related to the periodontium, or occlusal dysfunction.

Before any emergency treatment is instituted, a brief medical history shold be obtained, in order to protect the patient and the operator against any health hazards or complications from infections, bleeding tendencies, or other conditions. The various emergency situations encountered in patients with periodontal disease are discussed in Chapter 15.

The systemic phase

The systemic phase of periodontal treatment should be concerned with the general implications of periodontal disease and periodontal treatment. The various considerations for and therapeutic aspects of the systemic phase are discussed in Chapter 16.

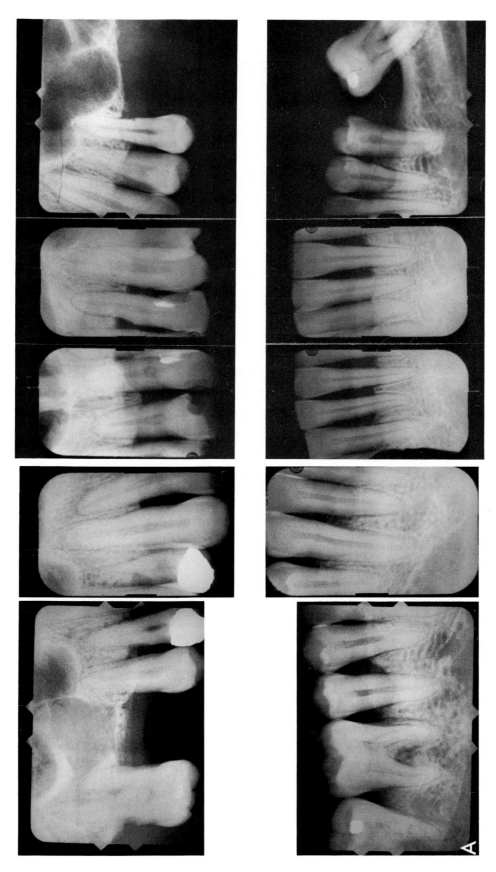

Fig. 14-6. A, Advanced periodontitis, trauma from occlusion, and partial edentulism in a 35-year-old patient. Treatment was scaling and root planing, occlusal adjustment, and subgingival curettage followed by recall for prophylaxis every 3 months. *continued*

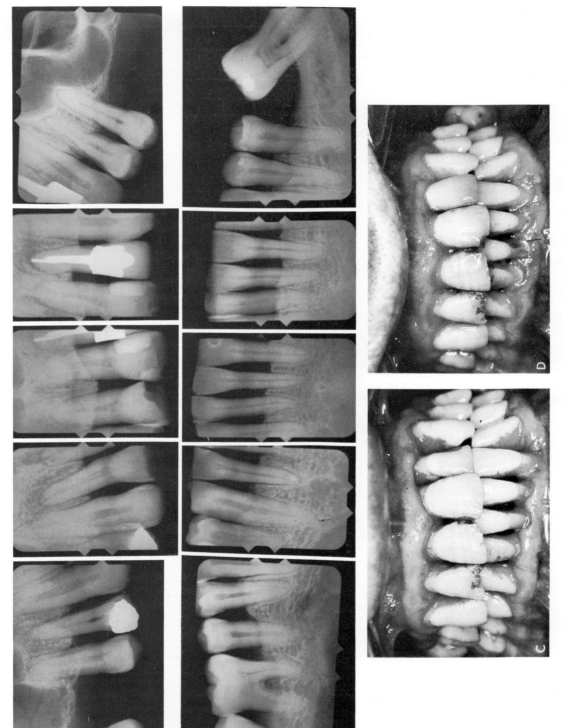

Fig. 14-6 continued. *B,* Twelve years later. There has been no noticeable progress in loss of bony support for the teeth, although more than normal mobility of several teeth persisted and the lost teeth were not replaced. *C,* Clinical appearance of tissues prior to treatment. *D,* Twelve years after initial treatment. Note poor oral hygiene in spite of frequent recalls and good patient education and motivation. However, the repeated professional cleaning of the teeth served to maintain the level of periodontal attachment.

The hygienic phase

It is evident from studying the localized inflammatory nature of gingival and destructive periodontal disease that active local therapy aimed at eliminating the causative irritants will constitute by far the most important part of the treatment. Among the local irritants that must be eliminated are bacterial plaque, calculus, chemicals, mouth-breathing, faulty dental appliances or restorations, food impactions, and faulty toothbrushing habits.

Patient education. Since dental plaque and calculus formation associated with inadequate oral hygiene are by far the most common causes of periodontal diseases, it seems natural to start the therapy by eliminating these active irritants. However, from the standpoint of patient management, it is advisable to initiate the treatment with a session of patient education. This provides an opportunity to demonstrate dramatically in the patient's own mouth the relationship between plaque and periodontal disease.

The concept of plaque control, as well as the rationale for the other aspects of the treatment plan, should be understood by the patient before the active treatment is initiated. For the treatment to be successful, it is important that time and effort for patient education be included in the treatment plan. Periodontal treatment without patient understanding and commitment is an exercise in futility.

Preliminary scaling. The next step should be preliminary gross scaling and superficial polishing of the teeth, followed by specific instruction in oral hygiene as described in Chapter 18.

Deep caries. Deep carious lesions should be excavated and temporary restorations placed. Any teeth needing endodontic therapy should be treated at this time, since further periodontal treatment will be useless if endodontic treatment cannot be completed successfully. It is assumed that any emergency endodontic problems were solve during the initial emergency treatment of the patient.

Oral hygiene instruction. The patient should be instructed in effective oral hygiene procedures as soon as gross obstacles to the safe and comfortable use of plaque control devices have been eliminated. Oral hygiene supervision and education should be included in every periodontal appointment, since adequate plaque control is essential for the success of the therapy.

Hopeless teeth. If some teeth have been diagnosed as hopeless and are not in a strategic position for the maintenance of occlusal relations, such teeth should be extracted at this time. Partially impacted third molars with communication to the oral cavity, or teeth with advanced periodontal disease, or caries without functional or esthetic value, should also be extracted.

Completely impacted third molars should not be extracted unless there is roentgenographic evidence of pathological processes around these teeth. The common assumption that eruptive pressures from impacted or crowded third molars will lead to anterior crowding has not been substantiated.[7]

Unfortunately, there are no generally accepted guidelines for what constitutes a tooth with a hopeless periodontal prognosis, and there are no definite guidelines for what constitutes a nonrestorable tooth or a tooth with a hopeless endodontic prognosis. Ultimately, these decisions are based on the clinical judgment of the therapist. There is a considerable difference of opinion among dentists regarding how far one should go in trying to save teeth with advanced periodontal lesions (Fig. 14-7), advanced carious lesions, advanced malposition, complicated root canal anatomy, unsatisfactory esthetic appearance, and so forth.

Temporary splinting. Temporary splinting of hypermobile teeth may expedite such treatment procedures as scaling, occlusal therapy, and surgical periodontal therapy. Temporary replacement of lost teeth

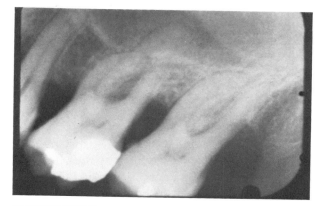

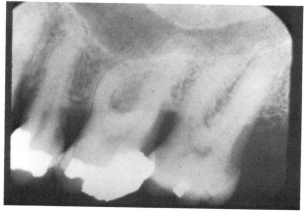

Fig. 14-7. Topical extraction of the first molar was contemplated because of advanced furcation involvement and risk for further periodontal loss for the adjacent second bicuspid and second molar. *Bottom,* Ten years after successful treatment.

may also be achieved through temporary splinting. Temporary appliances may be used to maintain an acceptable esthetic appearance and adequate function during the remainder of the periodontal therapy. For further discussion of temporary or provisional splinting, see Chapter 19.

Fine scaling and root planing. Three to 4 weeks after gross scaling and institution of oral hygiene, the inflammation has subsided, and the inflammatory infiltrate has been replaced to a considerable extent by collagenous connective tissue fibers. Fine scaling and root planing are needed to eliminate irritation from subgingival calculus and contaminated cementum. Clinically, this can now be done safely within defined boundaries of connective tissue attachment to the teeth. For details, see Chapter 17.

Occlusal adjustment. A preliminary occlusal adjustment should be done during the hygienic phase in cases of severe occlusal disharmony and in patients with complaints related to trauma from occlusion. However, for patients in need of comprehensive, complete occlusal adjustment, this adjustment is usually done in the corrective phase of periodontal therapy, after the teeth have settled into their normal position following the reduction of gingival inflammation.

Reassessment. Four to 6 weeks following the completion of the scaling and root planing, the patient's periodontal status should be reevaluated. For a large number of patients with gingivitis and incipient periodontitis due to poor oral hygiene, the hygienic or initial phase of the periodontal therapy will cure the disease; however, if residual active periodontal lesions persist, or if the patient is in need of other aspects of dental therapy, the treatment is extended into a corrective phase. It is important to reassess the entire periodontal and dental status of the patient at the end of the hygienic phase, then to make a definite decision concerning the need for further treatment.

Corrective phase of periodontal therapy

Plaque control. In order to ensure the success of the complete periodontal therapy, due attention must be paid to the patient's plaque control at every appointment during the corrective phase.

Orthodontic treatment. Indications for orthodontic treatment[14] in patients with periodontal disease are discussed in Chapter 19 and 27. If such treatment is indicated, it should be done at this stage of the periodontal treatment, prior to the comprehensive occlusal adjustment and the periodontal surgical therapy. Periodontal surgery should be postponed until the completion of orthodontic treatment for patients needing such treatment because 1) some pockets may be eliminated by such orthodontic treatment as the uprighting of tipped molars;[1] 2) intrabony pockets related to orthodontic intrusion of teeth may be treated by

surgical reattachment therapy following definitive positioning of the teeth;[21] and 3) retention following orthodontic therapy is enhanced by new fiber attachments that develop after periodontal surgery.[2]

Biteplanes. Biteplane splints are recommended for patients with neuromuscular problems and for stabilization of occlusion, as indicated in Chapter 19.

Occlusal adjustment. Occlusal adjustments should be completed at this stage in patients with signs and symptoms of trauma from occlusion who have tooth mobility or discomfort that can be alleviated by such adjustments. Of course, if the patient has no need of orthodontic treatment, biteplanes, or occlusal adjustments, the therapy can proceed to the next stage (hemisections, if needed, or surgical treatment of residual periodontal defects).

Hemisections. For molars with through-and-through furcation involvement, hemisection may be considered,[21] with the extraction of one of the involved roots and the application of a temporary splint to the remaining root and adjacent teeth until healing of the extraction site and pocket surgery have been completed and restorative dentistry can be done to well-established reference positions of the gingival margins.

Periodontal surgery. This phase should be postponed for 6 to 8 weeks following the completion of the hygienic phase of the therapy. One reason for this delay is that periodontal pockets or mucogingival defects that initially appeared to need surgical treatment will often abate following the hygienic phase of the therapy.[13] The changes are not confined only to the shrinkage of the gingiva; following the hygienic phase, even pockets that appeared to extend apically to the mucogingival line now often appear to end within the attached gingiva, thus modifying the need for surgical therapy. A second main reason for postponing the surgical procedures is that the increased density of the gingival tissues after healing allows optimal ease of manipulation and precision during surgery.

The selection of a surgical modality for the various teeth and areas in the mouth should be based on a thorough knowledge of indications and contraindications for surgical procedures,[3,4,16,18,19,20] outlined in Chapters 20 through 26.

Hypersensitive teeth. Hypersensitive teeth should be treated with fluoride application. Whenever the periodontal treatment has resulted in root exposure, the patient should be treated with acidulated fluorophosphate for caries prevention following the completion of the periodontal surgery.

Restorative procedures. For patients who have had extensive periodontal surgery, restorative procedures involving the gingival margins should be delayed until at least 2 months following the surgery. There is an unavoidable period of gingival recontouring and reshaping following periodontal surgery, which may continue for years following the periodontal treatment; however, the basic gingival-tooth relationships are usually established fairly well within 2 to 3 months after the surgery.

Occlusion. At the completion of the corrective phase, the occlusive relationships should be reexamined and refined. Usually only minor corrections are required.

The maintenance phase of periodontal therapy

The corrective phase is completed when healing after all therapeutic procedures is complete,[23] usually within 6 months of the treatment procedures[31] (see Chapter 28). For periodontitis patients, recall for evaluation and prophylaxis is usually scheduled every 3 months.[8] For gingivitis patients and for patients with very good oral hygiene, the recall may be every 6 or 12 months. Recall should also include retreatment of active lesions and application of fluorides. The entire dental status, including caries, restorations and occlusion, should be evaluated once every 6 or 12 months. Bitewing radiographs may be taken once a year.

Without a well-controlled maintenance program, the prognosis is guarded to poor for all periodontitis patients. This should be emphasized to the patients when treatment plans are presented.

REFERENCES

1. Brown, D.S.: The effect of orthodontic therapy on certain types of periodontal pockets. I. Clinical findings, J. Periodont. 44:742, 1973.
2. Crum, R.E., and Anderson, G.F.: The effect of gingival fiber surgery on the retention of rotated teeth, Am. J. Orthod. 65:626, 1974.
3. Ellegaard, B., and Löe, H.: New attachment of periodontal tissues after treatment of infrabony lesions, J. Periodont. 42:648, 1971.
4. Hiatt, W.H., and Schallhorn, R.G.: Intraoral transplants of cancellous bone and marrow in periodontal lesions, J. Periodont. 44:194, 1973.
5. Hirschfeld, L., and Wasserman, B.: A long term survey of tooth loss in 600 treated periodontal patients, J. Periodont. 49:225, 1980.
6. Horowitz, H.S., and Heifetz, S.B.: The current status of topical fluorides in preventive dentistry. In Fluorides and Dental Caries, ed. E. Newburn. Springfield, Il.: Charles C. Thomas, 1972.
7. Kakehashi, S., and Parakkal, P.F.: Proceedings from the State of the Art Workshop in Surgical Therapy for periodontitis, J. Periodont. 53:476, 1982.
8. Knowles, J.W., et al.: Results of periodontal treatment related to pocket depth and attachment level: Eight years, J. Periodont. 50:225, 1979.
9. Lang, N.P., Gusberti, F.A., and Siegrist, B.E.: Altiologie der Parodontal Erkrankeungen, Schw. Monets, Zahnmed. 95:59, 1985.
10. Lindhe, J., and Nyman, S.: Long-term maintenance of patients treated for advanced periodontal disease, J. Clin. Periodontol. 11:504, 1984.
11. Lindhe, J., and Nyman, S.: Scaling and granulation tissue removal in periodontal therapy, J. Clin Periodontol. 12:374, 1985.
12. Miller, P.A.: Complete dentures supported by natural teeth, J. Prosthet. Dent. 8:924, 1958.
13. Morrison, E.C., Ramfjord, S.P., and Hill, R.W.: Short-term effects of initial, non-surgical periodontal treatment (Hygienic phase), J. Clin Periodontol 7:199, 1980.
14. Moyers, R.E.: Handbook of Orthodontics. 3rd ed. Chicago: Yearbook Medical Publishers, 1973, p. 527.
15. Nyman, S., and Lindhe, J.: A longitudinal study of combined periodontal and prosthetic treatment of patient with advanced periodontal disease, J. Periodont. 50:163, 1979.
16. Prichard, J.F.: The infrabony technique as a predictable procedure, J. Periodont. 28:202, 1957.
17. Ramfjord, S.P.: Rational plan for periodontal therapy, J. Periodont. 24:88, 1953.
18. Ramfjord, S.P., et al.: Subgingival curettage versus surgical elimination of periodontal pockets, J. Periodont. 39:167, 1968.
19. Ramfjord, S.P.: How far should we go in trying to save the periodontally involved tooth? J. Alabama Dent. Assoc. 53:18, 1969.
20. Ramfjord, S.P., et al.: Longitudinal study of periodontal therapy, J. Periodont. 44:66, 1973.
21. Ramfjord, S.P.: Periodontal aspects of restorative dentistry, J. Oral Rehab. 1:107, 1974.
22. Ramfjord, S.P.: Changing concepts in periodontitis, J. Prosthet. Dent. 52:781, 1984.
23. Ramfjord, S.P.: Maintenance care for treated periodontitis patients, J. Clin. Periodontol. 14:433, 1987.
24. Renggli, H.H., and Schweizer, H.: Splinting of teeth with removable bridges. Biological effects, J. Clin. Periodontol. 1:43, 1974.
25. Robinson, H.B.G., and Kerr, D.A.: A postgraduate course in periodontal diseases. Sixth Annual Postgraduate Seminar. Nashville, Tennessee State Dental Association, June 28 -July 24, 1948.
26. Rylander, H., and Ericson, I.: Manifestations and treatment of periodontal disease in a patient suffering from cyclic neutropenia, J. Clin. Periodontol. 8:77, 1981.
27. Saglie, F.R., et al.: Identification of tissue invading bacteria in human periodontal disease, J. Periodont. Res. 17:452, 1982.
28. Saxen, L., et al.: Treatment of juvenile periodontitis without antibiotics. A follow-up study, J. Clin. Periodontol. 13:714, 1986.
29. Tagge, D.L., O'Leary, T.J., and Kafrawy, A.H.: The clinical and histological response of periodontal pockets to root planing and oral hygiene, J. Periodont. 46:527, 1975.
30. Tallgren, A.: The continuing reduction of the residual ridges in complete denture wearers: A mixed longitudinal study covering 25 years, J. Prosthet. Dent. 27:120, 1972.
31. Westfelt, E., et al.: Significance of frequency of professional toothcleaning for healing following periodontal surgery, J. Clin. Periodontol. 10:148, 1983.

15

EMERGENCY PERIODONTAL TREATMENT

Emergency treatment for periodontal problems is an important aspect of every practice. Complaints of severe bleeding, acute pain, traumatic injury, and serious oral discomfort or systemic distress should be given immediate attention, and measures to alleviate bleeding and pain should be instituted as soon as possible. However, no treatment should be rendered until the medical and dental history have been obtained and a diagnosis established. Failure to render prompt and appropriate treatment may lead to a patient's leaving a practice and to grounds for legal action against the practitioner. Problems related to hemorrhage are discussed in Chapter 20 ("Objectives and Principles of Periodontal Surgery"). All the precautions normally followed for patients at risk for AIDS and hepatitis should be followed.

PAIN OF PERIODONTAL AND PULPAL ORIGIN

Acute infections of periodontal origin are accompanied by swelling, pain, and sometimes elevation of body temperature, with malaise. The most common acute infections of periodontal significance are (1) acute necrotizing ulcerative gingivitis; (2) gingival and periodontal abscesses; (3) pulpal and periapical infections; and (4) infected gingival or periodontal cysts.

The diagnosis and management of acute necrotizing ulcerative gingivitis is discussed in Chapter 12. If the patient has no elevation in temperature, the emergency treatment should be debridement and instruction in oral hygiene. With symptoms of fever and malaise, the patient should also be given antibiotic treatment, preferably with penicillin if there is no history of sensitivity to this antibiotic. Instructions should be given to the patient as to what to do if a fever develops and/or there is an increase in severity of symptoms.

GINGIVAL AND PERIODONTAL ABSCESSES

An abscess is a suppurative inflammation usually associated with bacterial infection. A gingival or periodontal abscess is the result of pyogenic organisms having gained access and established foothold within the gingiva or in the deeper periodontal tissues (Fig. 15-1).

Pathogenesis

Bacteria usually are implanted through a traumatic interruption of the epithelial surface by toothbrush bristles, seeds, corn husks, dental procedures, or trauma from occlusion on teeth with intrabony pockets or with bifurcation and trifurcation involvement. The gaining of a foothold by the bacterial infection and the formation of an abscess also depend on the defense mechanisms in the infected tissues. With undiagnosed and poorly controlled diabetes or traumatic lesions associated with the infection, the changes for abscess formation are enhanced. Thus, an abscess may form following trauma to a gingival flap covering a partially erupted tooth (pericoronitis), when a tooth with an intrabony pocket is moved orthodontically against the bony wall of the pocket without preparatory periodontal treatment, or if a bridge or crown is placed on a molar with a bifurcation or trifurcation involvement, especially if such a tooth has been nonfunctional and has had atrophic periodontal structures prior to the dental restoration.

It has been suggested[11] that "hematogenous infection may become localized in an area of trauma from occlusion by the so-called "anachoretic" effect."[16] A periodontal abscess could then develop without extension from either gingival or pulpal infection.

Obstruction of the gingival opening of deep and tortuous pockets may lead to abscess formation. Trauma from subgingival scaling will introduce bacteria into the pocket wall[12] and sometimes, especially in patients with uncontrolled diabetes, initiate a periodontal abscess. Lateral perforation of the root during

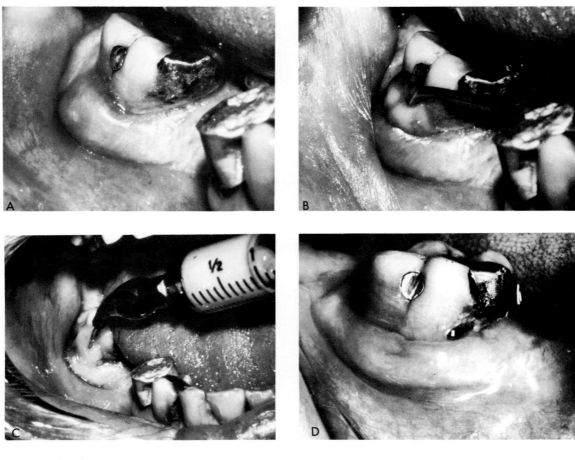

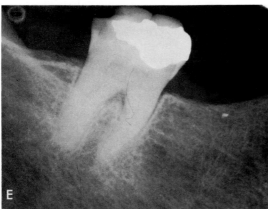

Fig. 15-1. *A,* Periodontal abscess with fluctuant swelling. *B,* Plastic instrument placed into the buccal pocket with pus. *C,* Pocket has been irrigated; ophthalmic achromycin ointment is placed into the pocket. *D,* One month after *C,* pocket has healed to the preabscess level. *E,* Roentgenogram 1 year after the abscess was treated. Note almost normal bone level.

root canal therapy or hairline longitudinal fracture of teeth also may induce periodontal abscesses.

Periapical or lateral abscesses associated with pulpal infection may drain along the root surface and appear as periodontal abscesses (Fig. 15-2).

Because a gingival or periodontal abscess starts from the gingival crevice or pocket, there is a connection between the site of the abscess and the gingival crevice. However, with deep pockets and a thin bone wall related to the abscess, the abscess may drain through the buccal or lingual alveolar process as well as along the root surface.

Diagnosis

A gingival or periodontal abscess is a painful lesion, and the involved tooth is usually very sore to biting or percussion. The abscess has a sudden onset, and there is usually swelling and tenderness of the gingival tissues, as well as leukocytosis and regional lymph-adenopathy, sometimes with fever and malaise. However, one may have gingival abscesses or pericoronitis without any soreness to percussion of the tooth. The tissue destruction can be very rapid, and new pockets 5 to 10 mm deep may form within a week. The extent of periodontal destruction associated with the abscess can be determined by careful probing along the tooth surface with a thin probe. Pulp vitality should always be tested; however, in multirooted teeth a periapical abscess may be present in one root and the other root may have vital pulp, and even in single-rooted teeth it is not uncommon to obtain a positive vitality response despite pulpal and periapical infection. Thus, the results of vitality testing may be inconclusive in a differential diagnosis between abscesses originating in the periodontal tissues and those originating in the pulp.

Roentgenograms are only moderately helpful in establishing a differential diagnosis between pulpal or periodontal origin of periodontal abscesses. An early periapical infection may show very little or no roentgenographic involvement of the bone, and abscesses with drainage on the buccal or lingual aspect of a tooth may be invisible on X-rays. The differential diagnosis between an abscess of periodontal and an abscess of pulpal origin is very important, since the prognosis for complete periodontal repair is much better for an abscess of pulpal origin than for one of periodontal origin.

Unquestionably, a number of apparently periodontal abscesses are of combined periodontal and pulpal origin, such as is seen associated with advanced periodontitis extending into the bifurcation or close to the apex of teeth, with accessory pulp canals. In this case, the pulp may be infected from the periodontal lesion, and the pulpal infection may subsequently lead to a periapical abscess, with periodontal drainage.

An important fact in the differential diagnosis between an abscess of periodontal origin and one of pulpal origin is that, in teeth with deep caries or extensive restoration, the abscesses are most often of pulpal origin, even with positive vitality response.

The elevation in temperature associated with periodontal abscess is usually very minimal. A significant elevation in temperature may be a warning of possible osteomyelitis. With acute osteomyelitis, several teeth are sore to percussion and there is severe throbbing pain involving an extended area. Osteomyelitis is an uncommon complication of a periodontal abscess; however, such cases have been observed and an illustration is given in Figure 15-3. Immediate diagnosis and treatment is extremely important in such cases.

Treatment of periodontal abscesses

A sterile instrument should be carefully introduced along the tooth surface into the area of the lesion, separating the soft tissues from the tooth in an attempt to establish drainage. It is appropriate to take a sample for culture, especially if an antibiotic is to be prescribed. While the soft tissues are being deflected from the tooth, the pocket should be irrigated with warm sterile saline. The gingival crevice should be searched for foreign objects, such as dislodged toothbrush bristles, corn husks, berry seeds, orthodontic ligatures, or any other foreign particles. Gross calculus should be removed. Then an ophthalmic antibiotic ointment should be introduced into the pocket. Use a glass syringe with a blunt, soft metal needle (Denitol syringe). Remove the glass plunger of the syringe and squeeze some of the ophthalmic antibiotic ointment, such as 3% Achromycin, from the tube into the syringe, partially replace the plunger, and hold the syringe under hot tap water until the antibiotic ointment is liquid and can be squeezed out through the needle. Hold the syringe with the needle along the tooth surface with the blunt tip moved into the area of the lesion, and inject the antibiotic ointment into the pocket or between the gum flap and the tooth with pericoronitis (not into the tissues) while withdrawing the syringe. If there is a definite fluctuant point to the abscess or the gingival surface, this can be penetrated by a sharp instrument; however, avoid making a large surgical incision or instituting drains in the area of the abscess, as this will only complicate the healing. Periodontal surgery is not recommended at this time. The swelling will regress quickly following drainage along the tooth surface and the application of the antibiotic. If the abscess is intercepted at an early stage of its development, it can usually be aborted by this therapy.

Systemic antibiotics are not usually necessary, but are indicated if the patient has a definite fever and there is danger that osteomyelitis may develop. Local

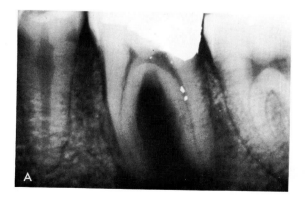 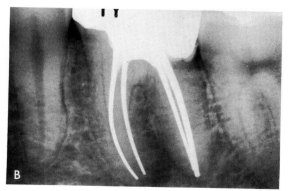

Fig. 15-2. *A,* Furcation involvement and extensive bone loss associated with periapical abscess. *B,* After successful endodontic therapy, complete healing.

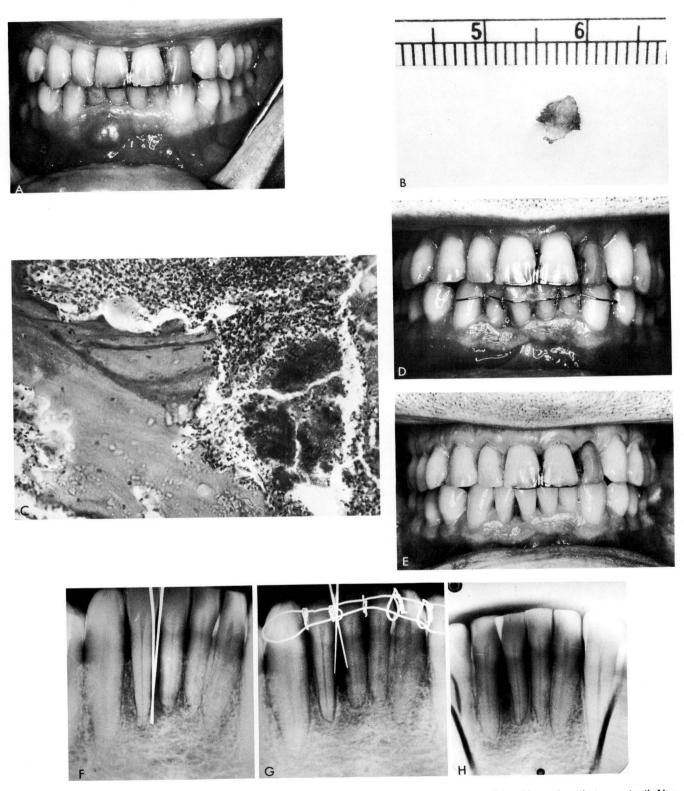

Fig. 15-3. *A*, Periodontal abscess with osteomyelitis in a 44-year-old patient. *B*, Sequestrum of dead bone from between teeth Nos. 25 and 26. *C*, Histologic section of the sequestrum. Note dead bone surrounded by pus and large bacterial colonies. *D*, The teeth have been splinted temporarily and the patient placed on systemic antibiotic therapy for 2 weeks. *E*, Clinical picture one year after the osteomyelitis. *F*, Roentgenogram after sequestrum was removed. *G*, Roentgenogram 5 months after the acute lesion occurred. There was healing of pockets and partial regeneration of alveolar bone. *H*, One year follow-up after initial treatment, showing well-defined alveolar bone and interdental septum, indicating complete healing.

lymphadenopathy of the neck glands will generally subside in a day or two following the use of topical antibiotic. Prescribe analgesics if the patient is in disturbing pain. Grinding the involved tooth at this time is not recommended, even if it feels high to the patient and a secondary TMJ/muscle pain dysfunction is present. Following the resolution of the infection, the tooth will move back to its normal position. Temporary splinting of the teeth is not indicated unless there is extensive mobility associated with trauma from occlusion.

The patient should be given an appointment to return within 24 hours. At this time, there is usually considerable relief from the pain and swelling. The soft tissue wall of the lesion should again be separated from the tooth with a periodontal file or plastic instrument, and the lesion irrigated with sterile saline. Scaling should be performed; however, the root surface should not be scraped apically to the subgingival calculus, since such scratching of the roof surface may interfere with subsequent healing.[13] Ophthalmic antibiotic ointment should again be placed in the pocket. Be sure to fill the entire pocket with the ointment. Again check the patient's temperature and the teeth adjacent to the involved area for possible sensitivity to percussion to assure that the patient is not developing osteomyelitis.

Later the patient should be seen for short periods once a week for 4 weeks. These appointments are for superficial scaling of the exposed tooth surfaces and for plaque control. Optimal plaque control during the time of healing is of great importance for the success of the treatment (Fig. 15-4).

If the abscess was a pericoronitis associated with a 3rd molar gingival flap, the flap should now be removed or the tooth extracted, if there is not sufficient space for it in the arch. In other cases, an appointment should be scheduled for 3 to 4 weeks after the initial treatment in order to undertake complete probing of the pocket area and to determine what further treatment may be needed.

Prognosis

After 3 to 4 months, the pockets created by the abscess have usually healed and have returned to the states of the initial pockets prior to abscess formation. Even furcation areas may heal if the furcation was not exposed in a periodontal pocket prior to the abscess. Such healing of furcation involvements resulting from an acute periodontal abscess has been described in the literature,[2,11] but it is rare, since most cases of periodontal abscesses and furcation involvements represent acute flare-ups of periodontal lesions already involving the furcation before the abscess formed.

Treatment and prognosis for the periodontal pockets present 3 to 4 months after the initial treatment of the

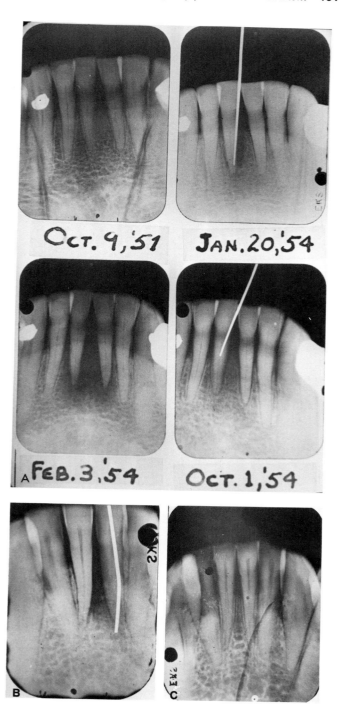

Fig. 15-4. *A,* Periodontal abscess treated with antibiotic ointment February 3, 1954, with complete healing by October 1, 1954. *B,* Periodontal abscess with pocket beyond apex. The pulp is vital. *C,* Complete healing 1 year later.

abscess are the same as for similar chronic periodontal pockets.[10]

Untreated or inadequately treated abscesses may develop into draining lesions, sometimes with chronic draining fistulas through the gingiva. Such lesions have been called chronic abscesses, which is a mis-

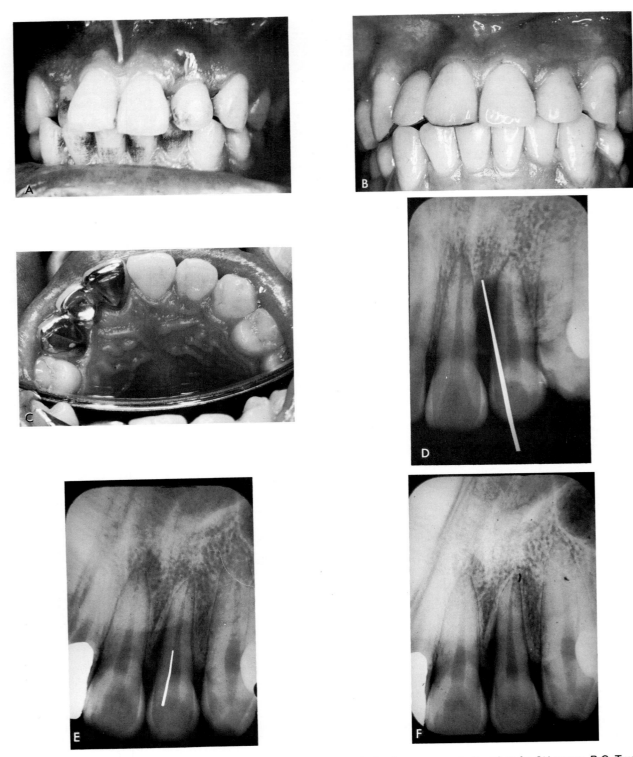

Fig. 15-5. *A,* Draining fistulous tract between teeth Nos. 9 and 10. This lesion has appeared off and on for 2½ years. *B,C,* Two years after treatment: no clinical pockets. *D,* Roentgenogram at admission. Silverpoint can be placed in the mesiopalatal pocket of tooth No. 10. *E,* One year after treatment the silverpoint cannot be placed into the previous pocket. Note well-defined lamina dura but widened periodontal space. *F,* Five years after the initial treatment, the bone defect still is present, but no pocket can be probed.

nomer, because an abscess is an acute suppurative inflammatory process. Chronic or recurrent abscesses with fistulous tracts are usually of pulpal origin; how-ever, they may be residual lesions following an acute periodontal abscess, as indicated in Figure 15-5. Such lesions should be treated in the same way as any other lesions of chronic periodontitis, usually with a modified Widman flap procedure (see Chapter 24).

If there is a history of recurrent periodontal abscesses, the possibility that the patient has diabetes should be carefully investigated.

PULPAL AND PERIAPICAL INFECTIONS

Pain from acute pulpitis associated with caries often may be alleviated temporarily by superficial excavation of the carious lesion with sharp curettes and placement of an antiseptic medication, such as chlorobutanol in oil of clove, covered by zinc oxide-eugenol cement.[19]

Chronic pulpitis or periapical inflammation can be eliminated only by extirpation of the pulp or through access for drainage from the periapical tissues; or both, if the infection has extended beyond the apex of the tooth.

Another source of pulp pain may be thermal and mechanical irritation associated with cervical abrasion of teeth. Temporary relief from such pain will usually follow topical application of fluoride preparations or combinations of fluorides and varnishes (Zarozen). However, lasting elimination of chronic root sensitivity may be difficult to attain, despite the dozens of procedures that have been recommended.

A periapical pulpal abscess with periodontal drainage should be treated endodontically after establishing drainage both through the crown and through the periodontal opening of the abscess.[5] Pulpal infections may also initiate abscesses in the furcation area[7,17] and on the lateral aspects of roots of teeth through accessory canals (Fig. 15-6). These lesions should be treated in the same way as a periapical abscess.[18] No surgical periodontal treatment should be undertaken at this time. Gross calculus should be removed and instruction given in home care. Three to 4 months after completion of the endodontic treatment, the periodontal status should be reevaluated and complete periodontal treatment instituted as needed. The reason for this delay of surgical procedures is that the prognosis for healing of the periodontal destruction caused by an acute periapical or lateral abscess of pulpal origin is excellent following adequate endodontic therapy. The ultimate prognosis for the tooth, however, depends on the extent of the periodontal lesion prior to the development of the abscess, since the most favorable result one can hope for is healing to the level of the pocket prior to the abscess. If the tooth had a through-and-through furcation involvement prior to the abscess, the long-term periodontal prognosis is guarded. Similarly, if single-rooted teeth had very extensive bone loss prior to the development of the abscess, the prognosis for such teeth is poor. Past clinical charts and x-rays should be consulted, if available; otherwise, the presence of calculus on the root surfaces or in the furcation area will indicate that, prior to the abscess, the pockets extended at least beyond the location of the calculus.

In cases in which the cause of the pain or abscess is obscure, the possibility of a longitudinal hairline tooth fracture should be considered.[6] Such a fracture may give rise to painful abscesses and has a poor prognosis.

INFECTED GINGIVAL OR PERIODONTAL CYSTS

Gingival[9] and periodontal cysts[8] are rare lesions, but, when present, may become infected through extension of periodontal or pulpal disease. A gingival cyst may appear as a bluish nodule on the gingiva. Although it does not represent periodontal disease, this type of cyst may become infected and drain through the gingiva. Such a cyst may not appear in a roentgenogram, and bone resorption may or may not be associated with the cyst. A lateral periodontal cyst will usually appear on the x-ray as a well-defined lesion on the side of the root, but it may also extend through the alveolar process and appear as a swelling on the gingiva. Most gingival and lateral periodontal cysts appear in the region of the mandibular cuspids and bicuspids. Occasionally, such cysts may become infected and form an abscess that may or may not have any communication with the periodontal pocket or the pulp. The treatment for such lesions is surgical enucleation of the cyst.

PAIN RELATED TO TRAUMA FROM OCCLUSION

Intrinsic trauma. Symptoms of pain may be related to trauma from occlusion and involve any part of the masticatory system, including the periodontium. The

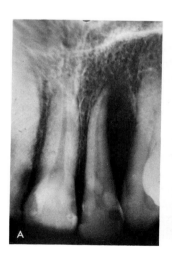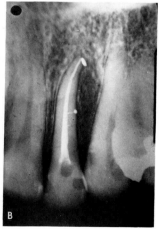

Fig. 15-6. *A,* Patient referred to periodontist with diagnosis of periodontal abscess on tooth No. 10. However, the tooth was devital and endodontic therapy was performed. *B,* Roentgenogram 6 months later shows complete regeneration of the periodontal lesion. Note distal accessory pulp canal at the middle of the root.

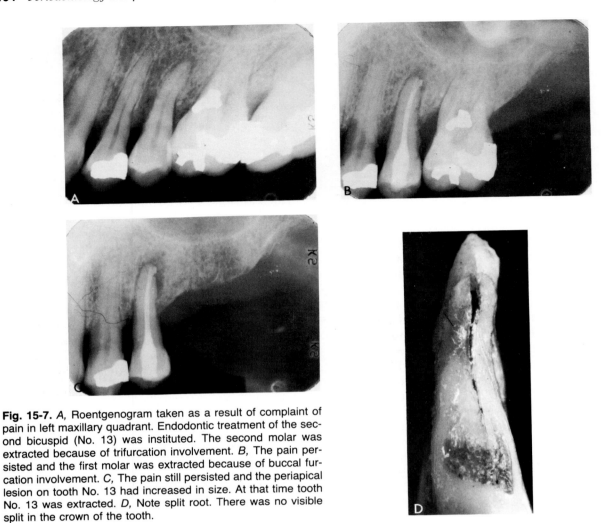

Fig. 15-7. *A*, Roentgenogram taken as a result of complaint of pain in left maxillary quadrant. Endodontic treatment of the second bicuspid (No. 13) was instituted. The second molar was extracted because of trifurcation involvement. *B*, The pain persisted and the first molar was extracted because of buccal furcation involvement. *C*, The pain still persisted and the periapical lesion on tooth No. 13 had increased in size. At that time tooth No. 13 was extracted. *D*, Note split root. There was no visible split in the crown of the tooth.

traumatic lesions may be surface injuries from occlusal impingement, faulty dental appliances, and food or other foreign body impactions, or the site of the injury may be in the subcrestal periodontal tissues associated with dysfunctional trauma from occlusion. In patients with advanced periodontitis and minimal residual support for the teeth, one may find acute painful trauma from occlusion and from accidental biting on hard objects.

For both gingival and deeper periodontal trauma, the sources of the trauma should be eliminated and an opportunity for rest of the involved tissues should be provided. Impacted food or foreign bodies should be removed, impinging clasps or other faulty appliances corrected, gross occlusal disharmony eliminated, and teeth with severe acute secondary trauma from occlusion given temporary stabilization, if needed. If the pain is of neuromuscular or tempormandibular joint origin, an occlusal splint or biteplane may be indicated.

One of the most difficult types of traumatic pain with regard to both diagnosis and treatment is pain associated with longitudinal hairline fractures of teeth. These fractures are most often seen in mandibular molars.[6] The pain may be related to pulpitis or a periodontal abscess, or both, and in serious cases may require removal of the pulp or extraction of the involved tooth (Fig. 15-7).

Extrinsic trauma. Teeth that have been displaced, fractured, or evulsed as a result of traumatic accidents require immediate treatment.

After diagnostic procedures, including roentgenograms, a decision on temporary splinting must be made. If the traumatized tooth is neither appreciably displaced nor fractured, no immediate treatment is indicated beyond attention to soft tissue injuries and a prescription of pain relieving drugs.

If the involved tooth is noticeably displaced in a horizontal or vertical direction, it must be repositioned. The use of fine wire ligatures applied to the cerivcal area of the tooth and then affixed to a Hawley retainer has been recommended for gradual repositioning of such a displaced tooth.[4] As soon as the tooth has been brought into the desired position, it should be immobilized with bonding procedures. Vitality tests are meaningless until several weeks have elapsed following the trauma.

Teeth with root fractures but some residual periodontal attachment of the crown extending subcrestally all around the fracture site should be immobilized temporarily with bonding.[14] The prognosis for such teeth is often surprisingly good. Coronal fractures may require pulpal treatment.

An evulsed tooth should be reimplanted, even if it has been out of the mouth for several hours.[1] The tooth should be cleaned in saline solution and a root canal filling placed if the tooth is fully developed. Do not remove the adherent remains of periodontal fibers and do not touch the root surface at all. If the apical foramen is wide open, use of calcium hydroxide[4] in the root canal (or not root canal filling at all) has been recommended.

Anesthetize the site, debride the vacant alveolus, and irrigate the area with sterile saline solution. Replace the tooth and immobilize it. Place the patient on antibiotic therapy for 1 to 2 weeks. Unfortunately, such reimplanted teeth have a tendency for root resorption and ankylosis. The average functional life expectancy for such a tooth is 4 to 5 years following the reimplantation.

PATIENTS IN DISTRESS

Patients may present signs and symptoms that they think require emergency attention, although they may not have bleeding or pain. Patients with psychoneurotic disorders may not be acceptable candidates for periodontal therapy. A few persons may be under psychic stress so severe that they need emergency psychiatric care, despite the fact that their subjective symptoms are dentally related.

It is important that the dentist's initial response to the patient's anxiety be empathy, understanding, and reassurance. If the dentist is successful in diminishing anxiety at the initial encounter with the distressed patient, the entire dental and periodontal therapy will be facilitated greatly. The dentist should strive for a therapeutic alliance with the stressed emergency patient.[3]

REFERENCES

1. Andreasen, J.O.: Traumatic Injuries to the Teeth. St. Louis: C.V. Mosby Co., 1972.
2. Bunting, R.W.: Oral Hygiene and the Treatment of Parodontal Diseases. Philadelphia: Lea and Febiger, 1936.
3. Dworkin, S.F.: Psychodynamics of dental emergencies, Dent. Clin. North Am. 17:403, 1973.
4. Hargis, H.W.: Trauma to permanent anterior teeth and alveolar processes, Dent. Clin. North Am. 17:505, 1973.
5. Hiatt, W.H.: Periodontal pocket elimination by combined endodontic-periodontic therapy, Periodontics 1:152, 1963.
6. Hiatt, W.H.: Incomplete crown-root fracture in pulpal-periodontal disease, J. Periodont. 44:369, 1973.
7. Johnson, H.B., and Orban, B.: The inter-radicular pathology as related to accessory root canals, J. Endodont. 3:21, 1948.
8. Moskow, B.S., et al: Gingival and lateral periodontal cysts, J. Periodont. 41:249, 1970.
9. Moskow, B.S., and Weinstein, M.M.: Further observations on the gingival cyst. Three case reports, J. Periodont. 46:178, 1975.
10. Nabers, J.M., Meador, H.L., and Nabers, C.L.: Chronology, an important factor in the repair of osseous defects, Periodontics 2:304, 1964.
11. Prichard, J.F.: Advanced Periodontal Disease: Surgical and Prosthetic Management. 2nd ed. Philadelphia: W.B. Saunders Co., 1972.
12. Ramfjord, S., and Kiester, G.: The gingival sulcus and the periodontal pocket immediately following scaling of teeth, J. Periodont. 25:167, 1954.
13. Ramfjord, S.P., and Costich, E.R.: Healing after simple gingivectomy, J. Periodont. 34:401, 1963.
14. Ramfjord, S.P., and Ash, M.M., Jr.: Occlusion. 3rd ed. Philadelphia: W.B. Saunders Co., 1983.
15. Ramfjord, S.P., and Nissle, R.R.: Modified Widman flap, J. Periodont. 45:601, 1974.
16. Robinson, H.B.G., and Boling, L.: The anachoretic effect in pulpitis. I. Bacteriological studies, J.A.D.A. 28:268, 1941.
17. Rubach, W.C., and Mitchell, D.F.: Periodontal disease, accessory canals and pulp pathosis, J. Periodont. 36:34, 1965.
18. Simring, M., and Goldberg, M.: The pulpal pocket approach: Retrograde periodontitis, J. Periodont. 35:22, 1964.
19. Sommer, R.F., Ostrander, F.D., and Crowley, M.C.: Clinical Endodontics. Philadelphia: W.B. Saunders Co., 1956.

16

SYSTEMIC PHASE OF PERIODONTAL THERAPY

Before the systemic phase of the patient's periodontal therapy is planned, the results of a health questionnaire,[21] the medical history, and any oral findings pertinent to the patient's systemic health should be available.

The systemic phase of the periodontal therapy is concerned with (1) precautions for protecting the health of the therapist, auxiliary personnel, and other patients against contagious diseases; (2) protection of the patient against potentially harmful systemic effects of the periodontal therapy; (3) making allowances for systemic diseases or disorders that may influence the etiology of the patient's periodontal disease, his healing potentials, and his systemic response to the therapy; (4) control of anxiety and low pain threshold; and (5) considerations of systemic supportive therapy.

PROTECTION AGAINST CONTAGIOUS DISEASES

As a rule, only emergency therapy should be considered for patients during the active contagious stage of a disease that can be transmitted by contact via the oral cavity. Routine periodontal treatment should be postponed until the patient has received medical treatment for an infectious disease. However, there are instances in which the patient may not be aware of his systemic disease, or in which all manifestations of disease may have abated but the patient is still a carrier of the infective agents. Or the patient may have an incurable disease such as AIDS.

Some of the most serious systemic conditions transmitted orally are venereal diseases and hepatitis. The infectious oral lesions of syphilis and AIDS are usually recognizable clinically,[6] but recent reports indicate numerous instances of oral and pharyngeal gonococcal infections, with no or very mild clinical manifestations, that were unknown to the patients.[8] Serious consequences of the spread of hepatitis virus associated with routine dental practice have been reported.[24] Herpes simplex and tuberculosis are other infectious diseases with a high transmission potential.

Guidelines have been suggested to protect dentists as well as office personnel, laboratory technicians, and patients from cross-infection by hepatitis B and AIDS.[27] There may be over 200 million carriers of the hepatitis virus worldwide, and the vast majority do not know they are carrying it. Because infection is associated with exposure to blood, dentists in the U.S. are 6 times more at risk than the public. All blood and saliva must be considered to be potentially infectious. Hepatitis B infection may be a greater risk to dentists than AIDS virus HTLV-III if the infectivity and transmission risk of the latter remains low.

There were at least 1.5 million, if not twice that number, Americans infected with the AIDS virus in 1986. AIDS is contagious, and every person who has the virus is capable of giving AIDS to someone else.

The projection of 270,000 accumulative cases of AIDS over the next 5 years does not include cases of ARC, AIDS-Related Complex, which is invariably a precursor of AIDS and is sometimes fatal in itself. There may be 10 times as many cases of ARC as there are cases of AIDS. The projected number of AIDS cases may be quite low, and some estimates suggest that by 1991 there will be 5 to 10 million Americans infected. It is thought that over 1/2 of the individuals with the virus in the blood will develop the disease and die. Control of the disease may be 5 to 10 years away. The main risk groups are male homosexuals and intravenous-drug users.

The following are recommendations for personnel dealing with patients suffering from hepatitis B and AIDS infection: wear gloves for all contact procedures; wear protective eye glasses and face masks;[27] use disposable hypodermic needles; and sterilize all instruments. All materials, impressions, and casts must be sterilized, disinfected, or disposed of in a manner to

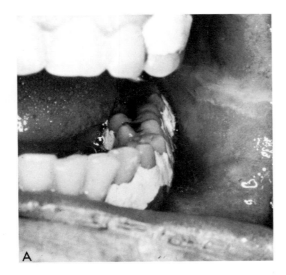

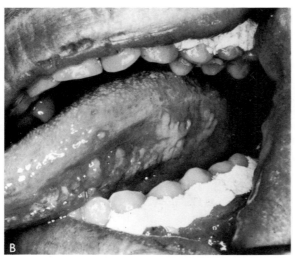

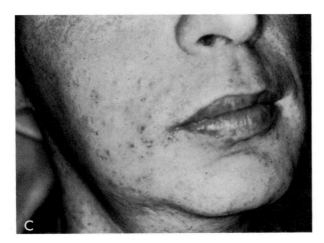

Fig. 16-1. Response of mucosa and skin to periodontal dressing. *A*, Erythema was present and there was a burning sensation in buccal mucosa after initial placement of dressing. The dressing was replaced, because the diagnosis of a sensitivity reaction was not made at that time. *B*, One day later, the patient had developed vesicular lesions on the surface of the tongue and the buccal mucosa. *C*, Sublingual swelling and allergic dermatitis also developed.

safeguard laboratory personnel, maintenance workers, and other patients. Dental assistants should follow the same precautions as the dentist.

A patient should always be referred for a medical examination prior to periodontal treatment if the medical history and the oral examination indicate that the patient may have an overt or a hidden systemic disease.

Unlike the evidence that herpes simplex virus type 2 (HSV-2) has an oncogenic potential, there is no evidence that the same potential exists for type 1 (HSV-1). Although HSV-2 almost invariably involves infections of the genitalia, the dentist must be aware of the close and potentially overlapping significance of these two types of herpes virus.

PROTECTION OF THE PATIENT'S HEALTH

A large number of systemic conditions may affect the treatment planning, although they may be of no direct importance in the pathogenesis and healing of the periodontal lesions. In a survey, it was found that over 50% of patients over 40 years of age had systemic conditions that might influence the periodontal therapy.[4] For patients with life-threatening systemic disorders, such as severe coronary insufficiency or hypertensive heart disease, the patient's physician should be consulted with regard to the management of the patient, who may require the facilities of a hospital rather than a private office. If such patients are to be treated in the dental office, it is advisable to plan short appointments and to use a local anesthetic without any or with minimal vasoconstrictive drugs.[1]

Allergies and drugs

Full knowledge of the patient's allergies is essential before any drugs can be prescribed or administered. Allergies to Novocain, penicillin and sulfa derivatives are some of the most common and serious hazards in dental practice. Allergies to iodine and to eugenol used in periodontal dressings (Fig. 16-1) should be identified so that the use of such products can be avoided. Other common drugs, such as aspirin,[4,18,38,46] may alter the clotting and the white cell count of the blood and thus affect the treatment of periodontal disease. The frequent use of anticoagulants is another important consideration in treatment planning.[44] Due consideration must also be given to secondary effects of other drugs, such as aspirin and tetracycline,[3] for patients on anticoagulant therapy. Consultation with the patient's physician (preferably in writing) is mandatory in such cases. The letter of referral should state the contemplated procedures and the timing of the periodontal procedures so that the physician can adjust the patient's intake of anticoagulants and determine the safety of other drugs that the dentist may want to use.

Drugs prescribed as part of the periodontal therapy

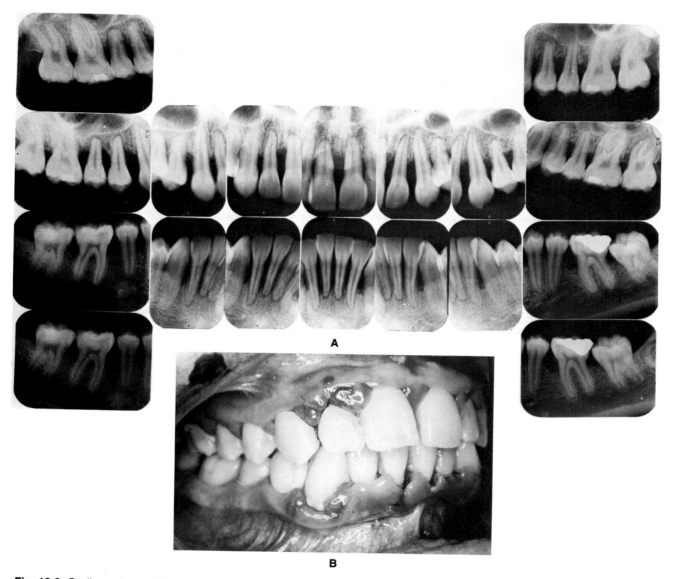

Fig. 16-2. Cyclic neutropenia in a 14-year-old girl. *A,* Advanced loss of bone. *B,* Soft tissue changes in advanced periodontitis.

may interfere with the effectiveness of drugs that the patient is already taking, or they may create a dangerous summation or synergistic action with these drugs; therefore, no new drugs should be prescribed without fully understanding the possible interaction with other drugs being used by the patient.[1] Systemic diseases such as ulcerative colitis may restrict the use of common drugs such as tetracyclines, which would be serious irritants to such patients. A dentist should never change a drug therapy that has been prescribed by a physician for a systemic disorder without the written consent of the physician.

Interaction of drugs is becoming a very important consideration in our "drug-oriented" society.[3] Many patients are on barbiturates or tranquilizers or both. These drugs are depressants and have the potential for summation or synergistic effects with drugs that may be used during periodontal therapy. The patient

should also be made aware of the interaction between such drugs and alcohol.

SYSTEMIC DISEASES OR DISORDERS REQUIRING PREMEDICATION

Patients with cardiac disease or disorders involving the endocardium are susceptible to endocarditis as a result of blood-borne infection.[13] The most common of such disorders are rheumatic heart disease, congenital valvular heart defects, syphilitic aortic valvular disease, and collagen diseases involving the endocardium; in addition, patients wearing prosthetic appliances in their hearts are included in this category. It is essential for the safety of such patients that they receive adequate premedication during periodontal treatment and that all periodontal sources of infection be eliminated.[12] The premedication should be in accordance with the recommendations of the American

Heart Association.[1]

There should be no compromising of complete pocket elimination for such patients, even if this elimination may necessitate the extraction of teeth that may have been retained in other patients; good oral hygiene with meticulous plaque control is a must as well. Oral irrigation devices should be avoided for such patients, owing to the inherent risk of bacteremias.[15]

Patients with an abnormally low number of polymorphonuclear cells (such as patients with neutropenia and some leukemias), as well as patients with inadequately controlled diabetes (manifested by repeated episodes of ketoacidosis), have a seriously lowered resistance to bacterial infection and should be scheduled for premedication associated with periodontal treatment (Fig. 16-2).

Patients with severe polymorphonuclear or monocyte deficiencies may also be subject to infections from oral organisms that are nonpathogenic in normal individuals; therefore, every effort must be made to establish perfect plaque control in these cases. Since these patients may develop life-threatening infections from a wider selection of organisms than the common antibiotics may deal with, every possible precaution should be taken to avoid tissue infection during periodontal therapy and to produce the fewest possible lesions during therapeutic procedures; such precautions necessitate minimal or no periodontal surgery.

OTHER CONDITIONS REQUIRING SPECIAL PRECAUTIONS

Patients with severe hypertension may need sedative drugs, and patients with hypertension may also need premedication to avoid syncope.

Individuals with known cirrhosis of the liver, or even patients without diagnosed cirrhosis who have had a high alcohol intake over many years, are potential risks for periodontal surgery, since their blood clotting mechanisms may be altered.[30] Medical consultation is advised prior to the periodontal treatment of such patients.

Patients with any kind of purpura or hemophilia (pseudophilia and true hemophilia) should only be treated following medical consultation. Extra precautions against bleeding should be included in the treatment of such patients. Such precautions may include the treatment of only a few teeth at each sitting and the placement of periodontal dressings over the treated area, even if the treatment procedure only included the scaling of teeth. Oral bleeding associated with blood diseases is a serious symptom that can often be eliminated by periodontal treatment and a strict but careful oral hygiene regime, regardless of the bleeding disorder.

Pregnancy is another systemic condition that should be considered in treatment planning. It is advisable to avoid systemic medication during at least the 1st trimester of the pregnancy. Recent studies have suggested an association between the ingestion of minor tranquilizers during pregnancy and the increased risk of congenital anomalies.[28,36,37] Because malformations have been induced experimentally in animals by the administration of cortisone during the early stage of pregnancy, increased cortisone output should be avoided. It may be advisable not to expose the patient to any stressful situation during this early stage of pregnancy. It is also best to avoid scheduling periodontal therapy around the time of the missed 2nd and 3rd menstrual periods in order to prevent any possible association with miscarriage, as well as during the last month of pregnancy, to avoid extra stress and bacteremia. Periodontal surgery should not be scheduled for the 1st or 2nd day of a menstrual period, because the clotting mechanism of the blood may be significantly altered at that time.[20] Patients with a history of total body or local irradiation involving oral structures should be carefully evaluated prior to periodontal treatment, and periodontal surgery should be kept to a minimum. Premedication with antibiotics may be considered.

In addition, avoid scheduling electrosurgery for patients with pacemakers, since the electrosurgery may affect the function of the pacemaker.

SYSTEMIC DISORDERS AND PERIODONTAL TREATMENT

The role of systemic conditions in the etiology of periodontal disease has been discussed in Chapter 9. Here will be considered only how such systemic disorders may relate to periodontal treatment.

Every possible attempt should be made to alleviate systemic diseases, such as blood disorders and diabetes, as much as possible before definitive periodontal treatment is initiated. However, hygienic aspects of periodontal therapy may be carried out with remarkable success even during active stages of these systemic diseases. Diabetes control may be facilitated by the successful treatment of periodontal disease.[48] Thus, the periodontal treatment may have a beneficial influence on the systemic health of the patient.

Nutritional Disturbances

The significance of the nutritional status of the patient in the etiology and treatment of periodontal disease has always been controversial.[17] It appears that unless the patient has nutritional deficiency disease (which should be treated by the patient's physician), there is no scientific evidence to support supplemental nutritional treatment as part of the periodontal therapy. Efforts to treat periodontal disease with vitamins or other dietary supplements have been unsuccess-

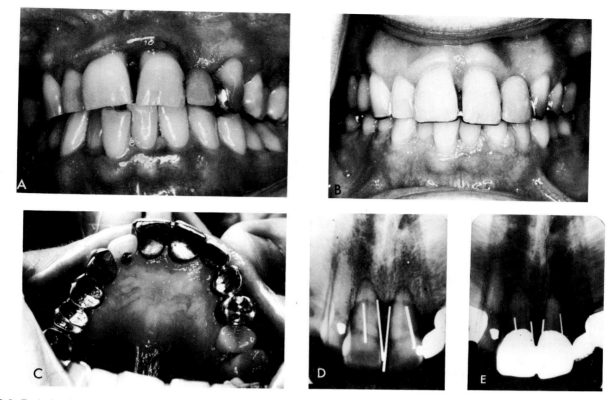

Fig. 16-3. Periodontitis in diabetic patient, aged 48 years. *A,* Prior to periodontal therapy. *B,C,* Clinical result of periodontal therapy 1 year later. Inflammation has been eliminated. *D,* Roentgenograms prior to the treatment. *E,* Roentgenograms 1 year after completion of the treatment. Note gain in support, as evidenced by the positions of the silver pins placed in the bottom of the pockets for contrast.

ful.[31] Routine administration of vitamins, proteins, or minerals for the purpose of enhancing a favorable periodontal response in patients who have no diagnosed nutritional disease has no valid basis.[11] An analysis of dietary intake records kept by the patient for a week or two is a totally useless means for appraising the patient's nutritional status. Various suggested biochemical tests of ascorbic acid levels, blood calcium levels, blood phosphorus levels, and so forth, are totally valueless in periodontal treatment planning. Deviations from the "normal" standard values for dietary composition are not very significant, and following adequate local periodontal therapy, no differences in response to therapy have been found to be attributable to variations in specific biochemical test values.

The fact that almost complete protein deprivation in rats[40] or scurvy in guinea pigs[35] may alter the connective tissue aspect of healing should not be interpreted to imply that periodontal healing will be disturbed unless a person has the ideal protein or vitamin C intake. The biological adaptability to variation in intake of vitamins and proteins, as well as minerals, has become more and more apparent in recent studies,[18] and the concept of "subclinical" nutritional deficiencies based on deviations from so-called "normal intake tables" has not found any scientific support.

Obviously, nutritional deficiency diseases should be treated because they represent a pathologic state; however, periodontal disease is not a nutritional deficiency disease and should be treated by eliminating the irritants that are the causes of the periodontal lesions. In the unlikely event that a periodontal patient has a nutritionally deficiency disease, the disease should usually be treated first, by placing the patient under the care of a physician prior to definitive periodontal therapy. However, local periodontal therapy may be entirely successful in the presence of a nutritional disorder. If so, hygienic therapy with plaque control should be initiated immediately, even if the patient has a nutritional deficiency disease.

Hormonal Factors

Clinical experience indicates that the response to periodontal treatment is as good in a diabetic as in a nondiabetic person, provided that the diabetes is fairly well controlled (Fig. 16-3). Juvenile or "brittle" diabetics have angiopathic changes and lowered resistance to infection; however, it appears that with proper antibiotic coverage, the periodontal healing following treatment progresses fairly well for such patients.

Routine premedication with antibiotics is not indicated for patients with controlled diabetes. Hypogly-

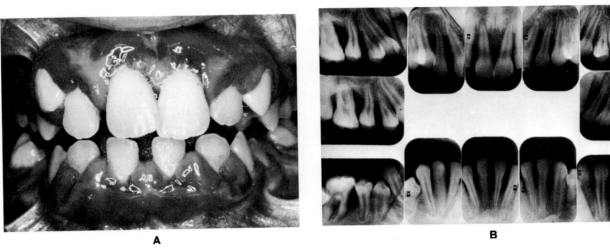

Fig. 16-4. *A,B,* Periodontal changes in an 11-year-old girl with hyperkeratosis of hands and feet (Papillon-LeFèvre's syndrome). Note severe inflammation and almost complete loss of periodontal support.

cemia may become aggravated by the stress of periodontal surgery, and for such patients precautions may be needed to help them avoid hypoglycemia reactions. Surgery should be postponed if there is any indication that the patient may have an exaggerated response at the time of surgery or if the patient normally eats a candy bar or sugar at that time of day.

It has been shown convincingly that the incidence of gingivitis may be increased during pregnancy[25] and possibly by the use of contraceptive pills,[14,32] which create the state of a pseudopregnancy. However, gingivitis in pregnant women can be treated and prevented in an entirely satisfactory manner by regular local therapy. The significant clinical implication is that pregnant women and women using contraceptive pills should be especially attentive to plaque control. Fortunately, pregnancy gingivitis does not seem to accelerate the loss of periodontal support for the teeth,[9] although a slight increase in tooth mobility has been observed during pregnancy.[24] There is no indication that humoral alterations during pregnancy interfere in any way with periodontal lesion healing.

Therapeutic doses of cortisone over a long period of time may have considerable metabolic effects, with systemic manifestations of a reduced rate of fibroblastic activity in wound healing and lowered resistance to infection. However, these hormonal effects do not seem to produce clinically recognizable periodontal alterations in patients on cortisone therapy,[23] and such patients can be treated successfully by regular local periodontal therapy with no significant delay in healing. Whether such patients should have premedication with antibiotics and additional corticosteroids[16] is controversial. Unless there is a serious infectious condition in the mouth, antibiotics are not recommended.

No relationship between osteoporosis and peri-odontal disease has been documented, so attempts to affect the periodontal healing response favorably with estrogen therapy or mineral supplementation[22] as part of the treatment of osteoporosis have no scientifically acceptable basis. Unquestionably, severe hormonal and metabolic disturbances, such as hyperparathyroidism of either the primary or secondary type, may alter the jaw bones and even the periodontal structures; however, such lesions should not be confused with common destructive periodontitis. There is no evidence to indicate that hyperparathyroidism or renal insufficiency with osteolytic lesions has any connection whatsoever with periodontal disease[39,41] or response to periodontal therapy. Hyperthyroidism, if severe, should be controlled prior to periodontal surgery in order to avoid thyrotoxic episodes.[16]

Blood Diseases

Neutropenia signifies a lowered periodontal resistance[43] and a guarded prognosis for periodontal disease (Fig. 16-2). Therapy should be palliative and directed at meticulous plaque control. Premedication with antibiotics is recommended for subgingival scaling. It is important to avoid gingival lacerations during the scaling.

Acute monocytic or acute myeloblastic leukemia often leads to gingival enlargement[47] and an increased gingival bleeding tendency in patients with inadequate oral hygiene. Such symptoms may interfere with the systemic care of the patient and should be treated immediately on a palliative hygienic basis, similar to patients with neutropenia.

Patients with various forms of purpura or hemophilia should always be referred for medical care, but the hygienic phase of periodontal therapy, if performed in a careful manner, may reduce greatly or even stop abnormal gingival bleeding.[33]

All systemic medications for bleeding disorders, including the administration of vitamin K, should be the responsibility of the patient's physician rather than the dentist.

Metabolic and Hereditary Disturbances

Periodontal lesions may accompany a few metabolic diseases, such as eosinophilic granuloma, Gaucher's disease,[45] and Letterer-Siwe's disease. These lesions are not manifestations of periodontitis or periodontosis and will not respond to regular periodontal therapy. Phenytoin (Dilantin) seemingly has a metabolic effect that predisposes patients to hyperplasia of the gingival tissues if their oral hygiene is inadequate. The chief concern in treatment planning for such patients is the need for meticulous plaque control. There is no need to consult with the patient's physician regarding a change in medication in order to facilitate the periodontal therapy.

Patients with Down's syndrome[10,42] often have more advanced periodontal lesions around the incisors and 1st molars than normal individuals of the same age. There are no indications that these patients have unusual or unfavorable responses to periodontal treatment. The periodontal prognosis appears to be hopeless for patients with Papillon-LeFèvre's syndrome (hyperkeratosis palmoplantaris with periodontosis),[7] probably owing to defects in the gingival epithelium (Fig. 16-4).

Severe hypophosphatasia seems to interfere with cementogenesis and thus signifies a very poor prognosis for the teeth.[5] Sturge-Weber's syndrome[2] may result in hemangiomatous gingival lesions that must be removed, preferably with electrosurgery, but the periodontal prognosis for the involved teeth is good (Fig. 16-5).

Control of Anxiety and Pain

Many individuals with a sincere desire for healthy teeth do not seek dental care because of anxiety and apprehension related to dental treatment. Modern dentistry offers a number of very effective means for controlling apprehension and pain. Judicial use of such means is highly recommended.[1] During both the initial interview with the patient and the oral examination procedures, the patient's anxiety profile and pain threshold should be observed closely. For apprehensive patients, it is advisable to prescribe Librium or Valium to be taken the night before the procedure, in the morning, and ½ hour before the treatment. For patients who apparently have a very low pain threshold during examination, routine administration of local anesthetics and drugs for the control of postoperative pain should be included in the treatment plan. In order to allow for good relations among the apprehensive patient, the dentist, and the office staff, more

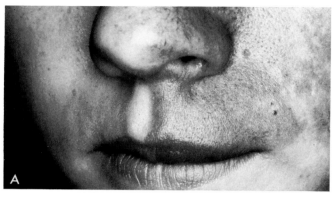
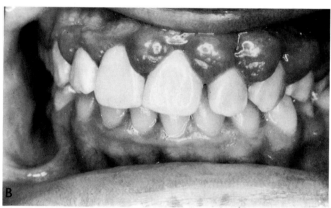
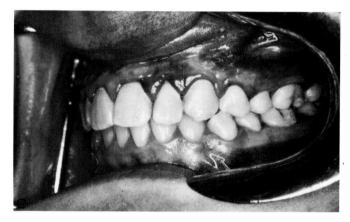

Fig. 16-5. Sturge-Weber's syndrome. *A,* Hemangioma in left half of face. *B,* Hemangioma of gingival tissues. *C,* Following gingivoplasty with electrosurgery.

than the routinely scheduled time and consideration than are usual with the average patient may need to be given.

Considerations for Systemic Supportive Therapy

So far, the search for systemic modalities of therapy that might support local tissue responses by improving healing potential and increasing resistence to local irritants has been futile. It is hoped that nutritional and hormonal supplements and immunity-controlling vaccines or agents might be developed. However, at present, no agents are available that will accelerate healing in the absence of nutritional deficiency disease, metabolically boost periodontal response, or increase periodontal resistance to bacterial plaque.

REFERENCES

1. American Dental Association—Council on Dental Therapeutics: Accepted Dental Therapeutics, 40th ed., Chicago: American Dental Association, 1984.
2. Baer, P.N., et al.: Gingival hemangioma associated with Sturge-Weber syndrome, Oral Surg. 14:1383, 1961.
3. Beckman, H.: Dilemmas in Drug Therapy, Philadelphia: W.B. Saunders Co., 1967.
4. Brasher, W.J., and Rees, T.D.: Systemic conditions in management of periodontal patients, J. Periodont. 41:349, 1970.
5. Bruckner, R.J., Rickles, N.H., and Porter, D.R.: Hypophosphatasia with premature budding teeth and aplasia of cementum, Oral Surg. 15:1351, 1962.
6. Burket's Oral Medicine: Diagnosis and Treatment. Ed. M.A. Lynch. Philadelphia: Lippincott, 1984.
7. Carvel, R.J.: Palmar-plantar hyperkeratosis and premature periodontal destruction, J. Oral Med. 24:73, 1969.
8. Chue, P.W.Y.: Gonorrhea—its natural history, oral manifestations, diagnosis, treatment and prevention, J.A.D.A. 90:1297, 1975.
9. Cohen, D.W., et al.: A longitudinal investigation of the periodontal changes during pregnancy and 15 months postpartum: Part II, J. Periodont. 42:653, 1971.
10. Cutress, T.W.: Periodontal disease and oral hygiene in trisomy 21, Arch. Oral Biol. 16:1345, 1971.
11. Dachi, S.F., Saxe, S.R., and Bohannan, H.M.: The failure of short term vitamin supplementation to reduce sulcus depth, J. Periodont. 37:221, 1966.
12. DeLeo, A.A., et al.: The incidence of bacteremia following oral prophylaxis on pediatric patients, Oral Surg. 37:36, 1974.
13. Eisenbud, L.: Subacute bacterial endocarditis precipitated by nonsurgical dental procedures, Oral Surg. 15:642, 1962.
14. El-Ashiry, G.M., et al.: Comparative study of the influence of pregnancy and oral contraceptives on the gingiva, Oral Surg. 30:472, 1970.
15. Felix, J.E., Rosen, S., and App, G.R.: Detection of bacteremia after the use of an oral irrigation device in subjects with periodontitis, J. Periodont. 42:785, 1971.
16. Glickman, I.: Clinical Periodontology, 4th ed. Philadelphia: W.B. Saunders Co., 1972.
17. Glickman, I.: Nutrition in the prevention and treatment of gingival and periodontal disease, J. Dent. Med. 19:179, 1964.
18. Hirsh, J., et al.: Relation between bleeding time and platelet connective tissue reaction after aspirin, Blood 41:369, 1973.
19. Hodges, R.E.: What's new about scurvy? Am. J. Clin. Nutr. 24:383, 1971.
20. Jacobs, H.G., and Selle, G.: Zur Frage der Blutungsneigung bei Zahnarztlich-chirurgischen Eingriffen während der Menstruation, Deutsche Zahnarztl. Ztschr. 29:1074, 1974.
21. Kerr, D.A., Ash, M.M., Jr., and Millard, H.D.: Oral Diagnosis, 5th ed. St. Louis: C.V. Mosby Co., 1978.
22. Kristoffersen, T., Bang, T., and Meijer, K.: Lack of effect of high doses of fluoride in prevention of alveolar bone loss in rats, J. Periodont. Res. 5:127, 1970.
23. Krohn, S.: Effect of the administration of steroid hormones on the gingival tissues. Thesis, The University of Michigan, 1967.
24. Levin, M.L., et al.: Hepatitis B transmission by dentists, J.A.M.A. 228:1139, 1974.
25. Löe, H., and Silness, J.: Periodontal disease in pregnancy. I. Prevalence and severity, Acta Odont. Scand. 21:533, 1963.
26. Lyon, W.H., Coward, R.A., and Glassford, K.F.: Long-term intraoral findings in humans after exposure to total body irradiation, J.A.D.A. 68:30, 1964.
27. Mardner, M.Z.: AIDS: Control of dental office situations, N.Y. J. Dent. 56:170, 1986.
28. Milkovich, L., and Van den Berg, B.J.: Effects of prenatal meprobamate and chlordiazepoxide hydrochloride on human embryonic and fetal development, N. Engl. J. Med. 291:1268, 1974.
29. Nahmias, A.J., and Roizman, B.: Infection with herpes simplex viruses 1 and 2, N. Engl. J. Med. 289:667,719,781, 1973.
30. Nichols, C., et al.: Gingival bleeding: The only sign in a case of fibrinolysis, Oral Surg. 38:681, 1974.
31. O'Leary, T.J., et al.: The effect of ascorbic acid supplementation on tooth mobility, J. Periodontol. 40:284, 1969.
32. Pearlman, B.A.: An oral contraceptive drug and gingival enlargement; The relationship between local and systemic factors, J. Clin. Periodontol. 1:47, 1974.
33. Prichard, J.F.: Periodontal case management in hemorrhagic disease, J. Periodont. 26:247, 1955.
34. Rateitschak, K.H.: Tooth mobility changes in pregnancy, J. Periodont. Res. 2:199, 1967.
35. Ross, R., and Benditt, E.P.: Wound healing and collagen formation. IV. Distortion of ribosomal patterns of fibroblasts in scurvy, J. Clin Biol. 22:365, 1964.
36. Safra, M.J., and Oakley, G.P.: Association between cleft lip with or without cleft palate and prenatal exposure to diasepam, Lancet 2:478, 1975.
37. Saxen, I.: Associations between oral clefts and drugs taken during pregnancy, Int. J. Epidemiol. 4:37, 1975.
38. Smith, M.J.H., and Smith, P.K.: The Salicylates. New York: John Wiley and Sons, 1966.
39. Soderholm, G., Lysell, L., and Svensson, A.: Changes in the jaws in chronic renal insufficiency and hemodialysis. Report of a case, J. Clin. Periodontol. 1:36, 1974.
40. Stahl, S.S.: The effect of a protein-free diet on the healing of gingival wounds in rats, Arch. Oral Biol. 7:551, 1962.
41. Svanberg, G., et al.: Effect of nutritional hyperparathyroidism on experimental periodontitis in the dog, Scand. J. Dent. Res. 81:155, 1973.
42. Sznaider, N., et al.: Clinical periodontal findings in trisomy 21 (mongolism), J. Periodont. Res. 3:1, 1968.
43. Wade, A.B., and Stafford, J.L.: Cyclical neutropenia, Oral Surg. 16:1443, 1963.
44. Waldrep, A.C., Jr., and McKelvey, L.E.: Oral surgery for patients on anticoagulant therapy, Oral Surg. 26:374, 1968.
45. Weigler, J.M., Seldin, R., and Minkowitz, S.: Gaucher's disease involving the mandible: Report of a case, Oral Surg. 25:158, 1967.
46. Weiss, H.J.: Aspirin—a dangerous drug? J.A.M.A. 229:1221, 1974.
47. Wentz, F.M.: Oral manifestations of the blood diseases, J.A.D.A. 44:698, 1952.
48. Williams, R.C., Jr., and Mahan, C.J.: Periodontal disease and diabetes in young adults, J.A.M.A. 172:776, 1960.

17

SCALING AND ROOT PLANING

The word *scaling* refers to removal of accretions from the tooth surface, and *root planing* refers to procedures for removing contaminated surface cementum or dentin and for making the entire exposed tooth surface smooth and hard.

About 1000 years ago, Albucasis designed a set of instruments to remove calculus, stating that all calculus had to be removed to make the mouth healthy. Pierre Fauchard, "the father of modern dentistry," also recommended careful scaling of the teeth to remove calculus as an essential prerequisite for the cure of gum disease, and developed instruments for this purpose.[28]

Nearly 100 years ago, Riggs stressed the significance of tooth scaling for the treatment and prevention of periodontal disease.[73] He stated, "When you find a tooth with a characteristic concentration of tartar upon it, the first principle of surgery demands that you clean the tooth thoroughly . . . and in three days you will notice a marked improvement for the better."

Rationale for scaling

A beneficial effect of calculus removal upon gingival health has been noted in reports from numerous clinical and histopathological studies.[42,50,61,68,76,78,91,95]

Calculus on enamel, and supragingival calculus in general, can usually be dislodged from the tooth surface fairly easily. Access to such locations is good, and calculus on enamel is deposited on a hard, well-defined smooth surface without intermixing of calculus crystals with the enamel crystals.[82] The physical hardness of supragingival calculus is far less than that of the underlying tooth structures[69] and thus permits mechanical removal of the calculus without injury to the tooth. Electron microscopic studies[100] have revealed disarrangement of crystals and hyper- or hypomineralization of cementum exposed to the oral cavity.[81] During calcification of calculus on the root surface,

apatite crystals may be deposited onto the cemental surfaces as well as into the calculus matrix, thus interconnecting these 2 structures in a very intimate and firm relationship.[82]

A microscopic roughening of the root surface also occurs during the formation of periodontal pockets.[36,43,84] This roughening may be the result of exposed insertion sites of Sharpey's fibers and/or resorptive processes during the pocket formation. Crystallization of calculus into such surface roughnesses will establish a very firm mechanical union between the calculus and the tooth, and it becomes impossible to remove all of the calculus mechanically without some removal of surface cementum.[76] Calculus removal is further complicated by the fact that the subgingival calculus is more than twice as hard as cementum.[69] The fact predisposes to cemental injury during attempts to dislodge the calculus.

The subgingival calculus deposits have been described as forming patching and tongue-like projections, rather than occurring as an even surface glaze.[24] Consequently, selectively applied removal of subgingival calculus is necessary to dislodge these flakes, rather than an indiscriminate removal of surface substance, which may remove exposed cementum at a much faster rate than the harder subgingival calculus.

Rationale for root planing and polishing

It has been demonstrated that the root surface bordering a periodontal pocket is much more rough than the part of the root that has not been exposed in a pocket.[36] Focal resorption lacunae in such areas have been shown to contain plaque,[79] and thus would serve as foci for reinfection if not eliminated during scaling and root planing. It has become apparent that such defects containing plaque and calculus may often be observed by careful inspection following routine scaling and root planing,[22,39,64,88] even if flap surgery has been used to expose the root surface. Residual plaque in small resorption lacunae may be a common source of failure in pocket therapy, and the trend is toward use of fiber optic illumination and magnifying glasses for inspection of the root surface during instrumentation.[70] If the root surface in the pocket is not exposed by surgery, one has to rely on feel, by exploring for smoothness, for elimination of plaque containing lacunae.

Another reason for root planing is elimination of contaminated cementum.[37] Cementum-bound lipopolysaccharide endotoxins[1] may prevent normal cell adhesion to the root surface after treatment, unless the surface cementum has been removed or treated by phenol extraction of toxins.[2] The depth of toxic penetration into cementum has never been determined, but clinical observations indicate that only a very thin surface layer has to be removed to make the tooth biologically acceptable to the surrounding tissues.

Residual calculus after scaling is most apt to be present in root irregularities.[97] When the roots have been planed completely, no residual calculus has been observed,[76,78] indicating that the feel of a smooth, well-planed root surface is a hopeful signal for complete calculus removal.

A smooth tooth surface is also easier to keep clean than a rough surface,[32] and has a lesser potential to accumulate both supra- and subgingival plaque and calculus.[87,92,94] Experimental roughening of the subgingival tooth surface has revealed that subgingival plaque penetration[94] and calculus formation[92] are enhanced by surface roughness.

Polishing is the ideal way to finish root planing, if access can be gained. The polishing should remove scratch marks from scaling[97] and provide a hard, glossy surface. It will also remove minute specks of residual plaque and pellicle, which may contain irritating substances. A "smearing effect" with reorientation of surface crystals of enamel following polishing has been observed,[15,97] but the clinical significance of such a surface layer is unknown.

Instruments and devices for scaling and planing of teeth

A large number of different instruments and devices are available for scaling and planing of teeth. In this chapter, only instruments commonly used for the purposes of scaling and root planing, without causing undue harm to the tooth and/or the surrounding structures, will be considered. As there is no patent on or quality control over the great majority of the dental hand instruments, instruments with the same name may vary considerably in size, shape, and quality of steel from one manufacturer to another. Therefore, it is important that the clinician know the basic principles of instrument design in order to purchase instruments with desired specifications for special purposes and to see to it that optimal angulations of the working surfaces of the instruments are maintained when the instruments are sharpened.

In principle, calculus can be dislodged from the tooth surface (1) by scraping or pulling strokes, (2) by pushing or wedging strokes, or (3) by a mechanical

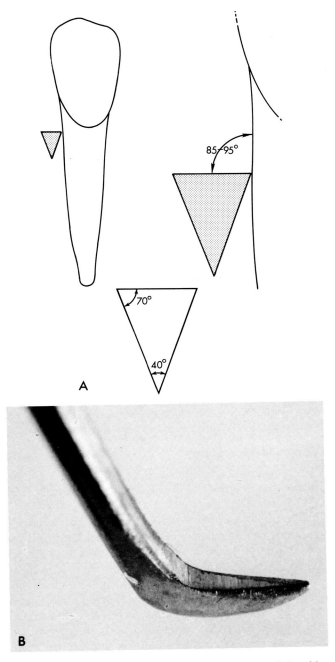

Fig. 17-1. *A,* Schematic drawing of the working relationships between a sickle and the surface of a tooth. *B,* Photograph of a sickle. Note that the tip and the nonworking edge have been rounded slightly to avoid soft tissue injury.

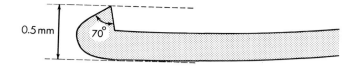

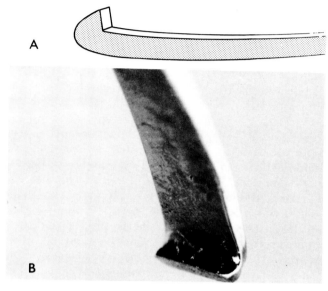

Fig. 17-2. *A,* Schematic drawing of a hoe. The working face of the hoe should make a 90° angle with the root surface. *B,* Photograph of a hoe. Note the rounded corners.

surface abrasion such as with ultrasonic or rotary instruments. Chemical means of calculus removal are unsafe, since they attack the surface of the tooth in-

discriminately along with chemically and structurally similar calculus.

Hand instruments

Among the oldest types of periodontal instruments are the scalers or sickles,[52] which in cross section are triangular in shape, with the angles between the face and the two other working surfaces approximately 70°. These instruments are designed to be used for pull strokes in such a way that the face of the instrument should make an angle of approximately 90° with the surface of the tooth (Fig. 17-1). The relatively obtuse angle of 70° between the face and the outer surfaces of the instrument permits application of considerable force against the tooth surface and the calculus without causing the instrument to dig into the tooth. An angle of approximately 70° between the surfaces that meet at the edge of the instrument should be used for all pull stroke instruments. Some sickles are designed with the blade and shank in a straight line with the handle. Other sickles, called *jackettes,* have angulated shanks to facilitate accessibility to all tooth surfaces. The sickle-shaped scalers are used mainly for supragingival and slightly subgingival calculus. They are especially suited for interproximal areas close to the contacts between the teeth.

Another type of scaler is the hoe, which is used to gain access to the root surface for removal of calculus in deep pockets.[93] The angle between the face and the outer cutting surface of a hoe should be about 70°, with a slight rounding at the corners of the edges. The shank is slightly bowed so that it can maintain contact on two points on the convex tooth surface (see Fig. 17-2 for illustration of a hoe). At least four different hoes are needed to provide access to all circumferential surfaces of the teeth.

The most commonly used instrument both for scaling and root planing is the curette. This spoon-shaped instrument has an inner surface or face that is flat, and curved outer surfaces that meet with the face in two cutting edges. Again, the angulation between the outer surfaces and the face should be about 70° for the pull stroke type of curette (Fig. 17-3). Pull-stroke

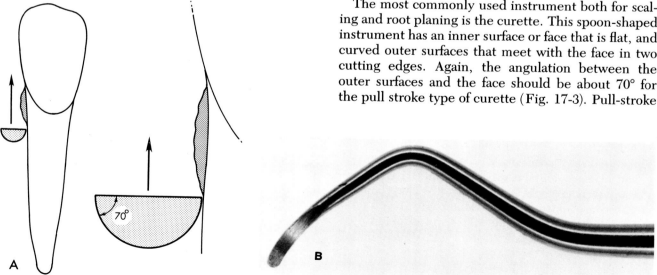

Fig. 17-3. *A,* The working position of a curette. *B,* A typical curette for pull strokes.

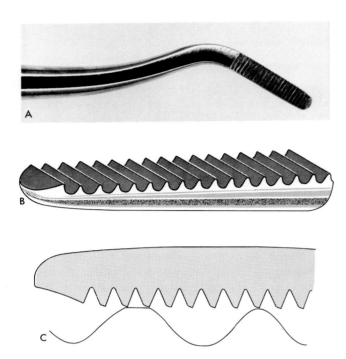

Fig. 17-4. *A, B,* Bunting periodontal file. *C,* A file will selectively remove the protruding roughness.

curettes work best for calculus removal when an 85-to-95° angle is used between the face and the tooth surface as the instrument is pulled along the tooth surface with a scraping action. If curettes are used for root planing, an angle of 60 to 80° to the tooth surface may be used to prevent undue removal of tooth substance.

Periodontal files have basically the design of a series of hoes separated by multiple and rather shallow serrations. Files are used to selectively remove the top of gross roughness (Fig. 17-4), such as at the cementoenamel junction, or to remove single small specks of calculus. They are excellent instruments for initial planing of very rough surfaces; however, there is a tendency for streaking to occur when files are used, and the tooth surface should be planed with a curette or sickle following the use of a file.[33] Because the blade of a file is thin, files may be used to gain access for removal of calculus and surface cementum at the bottom of deep periodontal pockets, where the space is so narrow that hoes or curettes cannot be brought into proper working position.

Various periodontal hand instruments have been designed for push stroke or wedging. The most common of these are chisel scalers. The blades are slightly curved, with a straight cutting bevel of about 40 to 45°. This instrument is activated with a push motion, and the flat side of the blade is held firmly against the root of the tooth while the cutting edge engages the calculus. This is a very effective instrument for removal of interproximal calculus, especially in the man-

dibular anterior region; however, chisels carry the inherent danger of causing gouging and streaking, and are therefore not recommended for general use.

A number of curettes have also been designed for push strokes. Most commonly used are the Gracey's curettes. These curettes are thinner than the pull stroke type of curettes and have a more acute angle, of about 30 to 40°, between the face and the outer surface. When properly used with a wedging action and applied at an angle of 15 to 20° between the face of the curette and the tooth surface, they are efficient instruments for removing small specks of calculus or for root planing (Fig. 17-5). However, with such an acute working angle, there is a danger of cutting too deeply into the tooth surface and of severing soft tissue attachment. For safety reasons, the pull instruments are usually preferred to the push type of scaling and root planing. The application of the instrument is often referred to in terms of a positive or negative *rake angle,* which is defined as the angle between the top cutting surface of an instrument and a plane perpendicular to the long axis of the tooth.[25] A positive rake angle, which is an acute one, occurs in the use of all cutting instruments, such as chisels and push curettes. Pull curettes, sickles, hoes, and files, on the other hand, have a zero or obtuse negative rake angle, and have been called scraping instruments. Efficient scaling and root planing are facilitated by sharp instruments, but a smooth root surface may also be obtained with a dull instrument.[34] Instruments with any roughness in the edge and outer surface, e.g., carbide par-

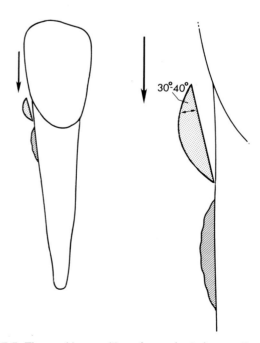

Fig. 17-5. The working position of a push stroke curette.

ticles fused on steel instruments,[49] should not be used if they have serrated edges.

Because scaling and root planing are performed in close proximity to the gingival tissues, possible harmful effects of instrumentation on soft tissues must be considered. The epithelial attachment is severed by routine subgingival scaling with curettes, and a good part of the junctional and sulcular epithelium will become dislodged.[56,65] Unless the scaling is done very carefully, some connective tissue fiber attachment to the tooth may also be severed at the bottom of a pocket.[65] It would appear likely, although it has not been proven experimentally, that the zone of degenerated connective tissue at the bottom of the epithelial attachment in active periodontitis[78] will be penetrated by routine scaling. The healing of gingival lesions following scaling is discussed in chapter 21 under curettage. However, it should be emphasized that unless scaling and root planing are done very carefully, especially in cases of severe gingival inflammation, these procedures may be potentially harmful to the attachment apparatus of the teeth.

Another hazard of subgingival instrumentation is bacteremia,[98] and proper precautions must be taken for patients with predispositions to bacterial endocarditis or other systemic infections.

Sharpening of instruments

The sharpness of an instrument is checked by examining the edge in reflected light. In a dull instrument, the edge presents a definite surface from which the light is reflected. As the instrument is sharpened, the light reflection from the edge is reduced until it appears as a fine, almost invisible line. The sharpness of the cutting edge should be restored without changing the original angles between the face and outer surfaces of the instrument.

Sharpening stones with a fine grit should be used to sharpen periodontal instruments. A relatively coarse stone may be used for initial sharpening of a very dull instrument or instruments with nicks in the edge that must be ground out; otherwise, all instrument sharpening should be done with a fine Arkansas stone, either mounted for use in a handpiece or in the form of flat stones or hand stones (Fig. 17-6). Lubricate the stone with oil or water before using it. Although the fine Arkansas stone is still preferable, a new type of aluminum oxide sharpening stone (Surgihone Stones, Miter, Inc.) is very effective for sharpening, but must be used carefully, since it may easily remove too much substance from the instrument. Surgihone stones should be scrubbed clean with soap and water and sterilized by autoclaving. Do not use oil to lubricate Surgihone stones.

Instruments should always be sharpened from the lateral or outer surfaces, rather than from the face, in

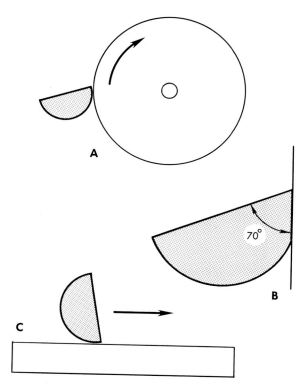

Fig. 17-6. Illustration of the positions of a curette and the round or flat sharpening stone.

order to avoid change in the working angulation of the instruments. Be sure to establish and maintain the proper angle between the stone and the surface of the instrument to be ground, so as not to create a new bevel at the cutting edge. After a sickle-shaped scaler has been sharpened, the ridge opposite the face should be dulled to prevent cuts from being made in the gingival tissue when the instrument is used subgingivally. Hoes and curettes should also be sharpened from the outer surface. A common mistake is to sharpen curettes from the face (Fig. 17-7). This approach will eventually weaken the instrument, making it more flexible. In addition, such sharpening will make the angle between the face and the outer surfaces more acute, with a greater potential for injury to hard and soft tissues. Such faulty sharpening also tends to produce a curved rather than a flat face, thus decreasing the "biting" capacity of the instrument against calculus. Sharpen instruments with a light touch, avoid heat, and inspect the edge frequently during the sharpening to avoid excessive removal of steel from the instrument. If a coarse stone is used and the instrument is oversharpened, there may be a tendency to produce what has been called a "wire edge" of sawtooth-like projections of metal. If a wire edge has been produced, it has to be eliminated with a fine Arkansas stone; otherwise, it will streak the tooth surface.

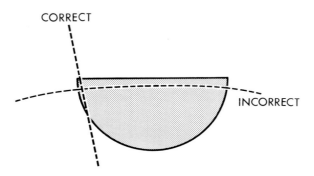

Fig. 17-7. The design of a curette may be changed and the instrument weakened if it is sharpened from the face.

The surfaces of sharpening stones have a tendency to become blackened and clogged with metal particles and should be cleaned frequently. Arkansas or other oil stones should be cleaned with solvents, such as chloroform, and sterilized by autoclaving. The Arkansas stone should not be permitted to become dry but should always be covered with a film of oil. The use of diamond hones for sharpening is discouraged, since it results in a serrated edge that will cause streaking of the tooth surface when the instrument is used.

Devices for scaling and root planing

Manual scaling and root planing are time-consuming and tedious procedures, and many attempts have been made to design mechanical equipment that could facilitate the scaling and planing procedures. The most commonly used device is the Cavitron Ultrasonic Dental Unit.[18,26] This instrument has a variety of scaling tips attached to a stack of ferromagnetic metal, which has the ability to change its length by shortening in a magnetic field. The stack will resume its original length if the magnetic field is shut off. The frequency of application and removal of such a field is around 25,000 cycles per second, and the total shortening of the tip is only about 0.004 mm, depending to a certain extent upon the power setting of the unit.

Because of the heat generated by the vibrating tip, the contact between the tip and the hard or soft tissue must be cooled by a stream of water. The tip should be blunt and applied very lightly, with constant movement.[18,78] Improper pressure or uneven speed of movement will produce a gouging and roughening of the root surface.

It was first believed that the calculus could be removed by formation of local cavities in the water with decreased local pressure caused by the motion of the tip, a phenomenon that was called "cavitation." However, it now appears that the deposits must be touched for removal, and the action is probably strictly mechanical.[13,44] It is also generally agreed that the working tip should be applied at a small angle, about 15°, to the tooth surface in order to be effective.[18]

Most of the studies done on the ultrasonic unit report that it is effective in the removal of calculus,[53,57] especially gross deposits.[18] However, the tactile sense from the tip of the instrument is almost completely lost when the unit is activated, and there is a tendency to remove more tooth substance than with hand instruments.[3,12] The Cavitron should not be used for removal of hard subgingival calculus, because this type of calculus is harder than the underlying or surrounding cementum[69] and a gouging effect of the cementum may easily result; in addition, the uncontrollable action, with inadequate tactile sensation and with the operator being unable to see the field, does not permit efficient and safe operation.

The Cavitron also produces a stippled tooth surface, rougher than is achieved by proper use of hand instruments,[44] and should therefore not be used for root planing. If it is used on cementum for scaling, the surface should be planed with curettes afterwards. The roughness scores of teeth planed with ultrasonic instruments have been reported to be twice those of teeth planed with hand curettes.[44] Opinions differ regarding the effectiveness of ultrasonic instruments[16,53] for removal of stains compared with conventional methods of dental prophylaxis. However, it is not practical to use the Cavitron first for stain removal and then have to plane with hand instruments and polish the root surface to gain smoothness afterwards.[85]

Soft tissue damage from ultrasonic scaling has been reported to be similar to that from hand instruments.[77,85] Edema, hydropic degeneration of the epithelium, and superficial coagulation necrosis indicating thermal injury have been reported.[59] A separation between the epithelium and the connective tissues following the use of the ultrasonics has been described.[77] However, the soft tissue healing following ultrasonics has been reported to be as prompt[77] or prompter than that following use of hand instruments.[31] Longer term results[31] for single-rooted teeth have been as good after the Cavitron as after hand-scaling.[8]

Bacteremia has been found to be as prevalent following ultrasonic instrumentation as following regular scaling.[9] Ultrasonic instruments are easy to operate, just as effective in removal of supragingival calculus as hand instruments, and well-accepted both by operators and patients. However, the action of an ultrasonic instrument subgingivally is poorly controllable, has a tendency to remove more tooth substance than do hand instruments, and leaves a pitted surface on cementum and dentin. Thus, the use of the Cavitron should be limited to removal of supragingival calculus on enamel, but such removal is not much of a problem using conventional hand instruments.

A number of other mechanical devices have been marketed for calculus removal and root planing, with-

involved furcations are often done most efficiently with fine diamond points or burs in the contraangle, if proper access can be provided. However, for safety reasons, such instruments should not be used on subgingival tooth surfaces unless these surfaces have been exposed by periodontal surgery, and polishing should follow the use of the diamond points, either by polishing burs or other devices.

Problems related to scaling and root planing

It has been claimed that proper root planing would result in complete removal of the cementum[71] and

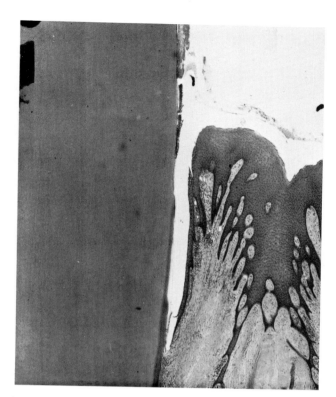

Fig. 17-8. Human specimen obtained 72 days after scaling and subgingival curettage. Note residual cementum on part of the instrumented subgingival root surface, whereas all of the cementum has been removed on the supragingival surface. Recurrent plaque and calculus are evident supragingivally. There is mild chronic gingivitis, but no inflammation at the bottom of the junctional epithelium.

out any demonstrated qualities superior to the Cavitron's: Dynacaire,[103] Rotosonic,[23] and Orbison.[99] The safety of these devices has not been established, and some of them are no longer available.

The most promising new vibrating apparatus for tooth planing is the EVA-system.[4] This device consists of a contraangle handpiece that can be attached to a regular handpiece. It works by mechanical vibrations in the long axis of the working tip when the tip is placed in the device. Triangular wedge-shaped diamond points with a smooth side opposite to a diamond-coated side are available for removal of overhangs on restorations, and fine plastic tips to hold abrasives or polishing material can be obtained in various sizes. This device is suitable for root planing, but will not improve on the results of good root planing with curettes, and does not result in quite as smooth a surface as that achieved by polishing with dental tape and fine polishing paste.[20] However, for removal of thick margins and small overhangs on fillings, the EVA-system with diamond points is recommended.

Planing of the cementoenamel junction, removal of overhangs, and reshaping and planing of periodontally

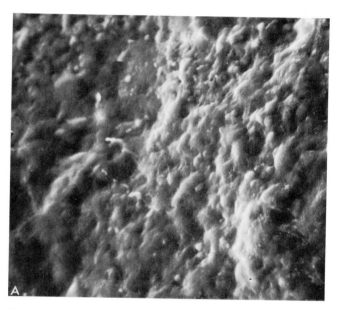

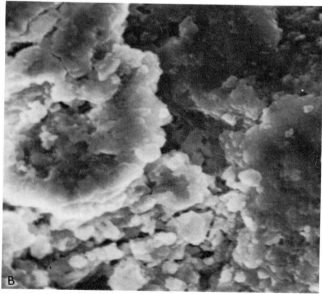

Fig. 17-9. *A,* Surface of subgingival calculus covered by bacteria (SEM, ×1000). *B,* Surface of subgingival calculus (SEM, ×3000).

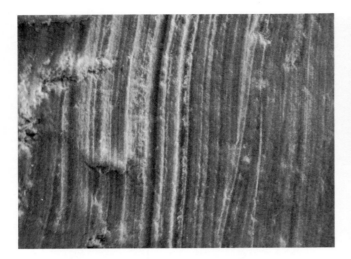

Fig. 17-10. Scratches following planing with sharp curette (SEM, ×300).

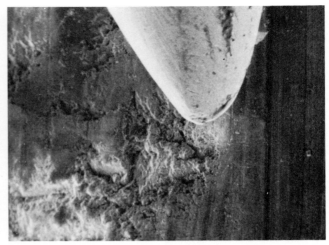

Fig. 17-11. Tip of #3 explorer testing a planed tooth surface that felt smooth clinically. Note residual roughnesses on the root (SEM, ×3000).

extend for various distances into the dentin.[72] However, a number of other investigators have found only partial or occasional complete removal of the cementum,[12,42,43,76,78] especially if the instrumentation has been close to the cementoenamel junction, where the cementum is thin (20 to 40 μm) (Fig. 17-8). It does not appear to be necessary to remove all cementum routinely to achieve a clinical feeling of a smooth tooth surface,[42] and because scaling often has to be repeated numerous times during the lifetime of an individual, it is important not to remove more tooth substance than is needed to obtain a clean, hard surface.

The surface of subgingival calculus is rough and covered by bacteria (Fig. 17-9A, B). Straight scratches following scaling may occur[11,45] (Fig. 17-10). Scanning electron microscopic studies[15,42,97] have reported small areas of calculus on scaled and planed root surfaces. These areas were so small that they could not be detected clinically (Fig. 17-11). In addition, there were small grooves 4-5 μm deep, which could not be felt clinically.[42] Thus, instruments may burnish the calculus without removing it completely (Fig. 17-12). Scaling may also produce a "smear" effect.

Because junctional epithelial cells may attach to minute specks of calculus[48] that cannot be located clinically, it may be assumed that such an occasional occurrence would not be of much clinical significance for epithelial reattachment or adaptation. Thus, after scaling and planing with sharp instruments, a root surface that feels completely smooth clinically is a fairly good indication that all significant calculus and contaminated surface cementum have been removed. Routine instrumentation should not be continued beyond that point unless pus secretion and bleeding to probing persist.

Certain anatomical features complicate successful scaling and tooth planing. By far the roughest surface area of a normal tooth is the cementoenamel junction.[36] Likewise, cementum exposed by periodontal disease is rougher than that attached to connective tissues[36,81] (Fig. 17-13). It has also been reported that the cementoenamel junction is the most common place for calculus retention both before and after scaling.[42,102] However, the root surface may already have been rough prior to pocket formation (Fig. 17-14). Calculus is often missed on the mesial root of the first mandibular molar because it may fill a natural concavity in the root.[29] Other areas with anatomical

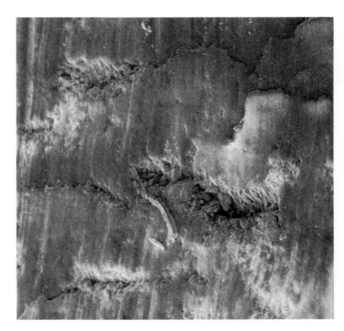

Fig. 17-12. Burnished calculus on root surface planed with dull curette (35 strokes) (SEM, ×300).

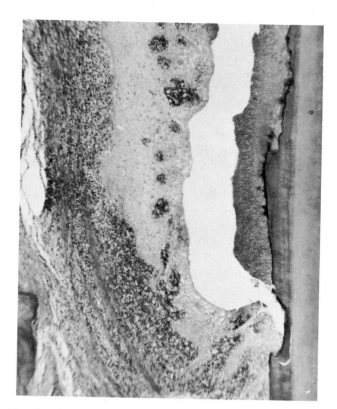

Fig. 17-13. Irregular cemental surface in periodontal pocket. There is pus in the pocket next to the root surface.

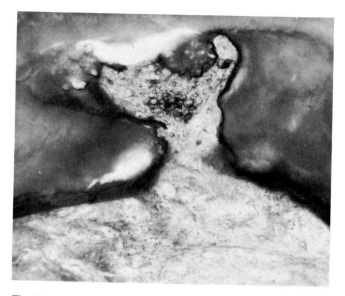

Fig. 17-15. Irregular cementum over enamel pearl in the furcation of a mandibular first molar.

problems preventing complete removal of calculus are[14,24,29,59] (1) a mesial concavity or depression in the maxillary bicuspids, (2) a distopalatal developmental groove in the root of maxillary lateral incisors, (3) mesial or distal developmental grooves of mandibular lateral and central incisors, cuspids, mandibular first bicuspids, and (4) numerous irregularities in the furcation areas[42,45] and adherent cementicles[39] (Fig. 17-15). In general, calculus at the cementoenamel junction[59] and interproximal areas[11] is often missed during scaling, and these areas should be given extra attention during tooth planing.

In summary, it appears that sharp hand instruments of suitable design are still superior to the available mechanical means for general scaling and root planing. Small instruments and a clear understanding of the root morphology are essential prerequisites for successful scaling and root planing. However, anatomical aberrations may require the use of mechanical devices, such as diamond points and the EVA-system, to achieve clean and smooth tooth surfaces.

Polishing devices and materials

Polishing is done to remove stains, plaque, cuticles, and pellicles from the tooth surfaces. Polishing will also reduce surface roughness to a point beyond that which can be achieved by root planing instruments,[20,97] and provide a surface gloss by an alteration of surface crystalline and possibly molecular patterns. It appears from experimental studies that polishing to a high gloss may inhibit plaque[87] and calculus formation.[10]

The most commonly used device for polishing is a rubber cup consisting of a moderately flexible rubber shell with web-shaped ridges in the hollow interior to carry polishing paste. This rubber cup is used in spe-

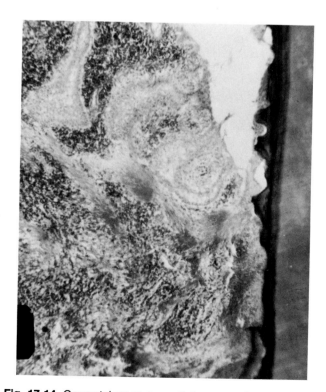

Fig. 17-14. Cemental spurs on partially exposed root surface.

cial prophylaxis contraangles or with a mandrel in regular contraangles. The thin flexible rims of the rubber cup permit polishing of the teeth partially into the gingival crevices buccally and lingually.

Rubber discs or wheels with abrasives incorporated into the rubber are also suited for stain removal, but these devices are usually highly abrasive and do not leave a well-polished surface. They should be used under water spray and with discretion, because they remove tooth substance rather fast. Polishing with a fine polishing paste should follow the use of these abrasive discs.

Various brushes for handpiece or contraangle, to be used with polishing pastes, have been advocated for polishing as part of prophylaxis procedures. However, the field of action of these brushes cannot be controlled as well as that of the rubber cups, meaning that they cannot be used as close to the free gingival margin and as far into gingival crevice as is possible with rubber cups. Because the contact area between the tooth and the gingiva is the critical zone for plaque and pellicle removal and for plaque retention, motor driven brushes are not recommended as prophylaxis instruments. The EVA-system[20] has plastic tips to carry polishing paste, which may be used interproximally where access is poor for rotating rubber cups.

Hand polishing may be done by wooden sticks and toothpicks of various shapes, usually in conjunction with abrasive or polishing pastes. Orangewood stick or porte-polishers with interchangeable wooden tip may be used interproximally or where access for mechanical polishing is poor. Dental tape with polishing paste,[20] or fine linen strips, also work well, but thei use is time consuming and they do not allow for acces to concave interproximal surfaces.

A very important consideration in polishing is wha agent to use as a polishing paste. Ideally, dental pro phylaxis paste should remove effectively all types c exogenous accumulations, including pellicle on th exposed tooth surface, without undue abrasion o scratching of enamel, cementum, or dentin.[63] In ad dition, the paste should have the potential to impar a smooth, highly polished appearance to the tooth

It has been shown that pumice of a larger particl size cleans more efficiently than that of a smaller par ticle size, but leaves a rougher surface. The most com monly used prophylactic pastes are effective cleanin; agents, but they are poor in polishing efficiency.' Therefore, if a rather coarse pumice paste has to b used for removal of tenacious stains, it should be use carefully, and the area should be polished afterward with a fine-particle polishing paste. In most instances use of anything coarser than flour of pumice for pol ishing associated with a dental prophylaxis is not ad vised, and it is best to follow up with a fine-particl polishing paste of chalk or tin oxide. Some of the fine

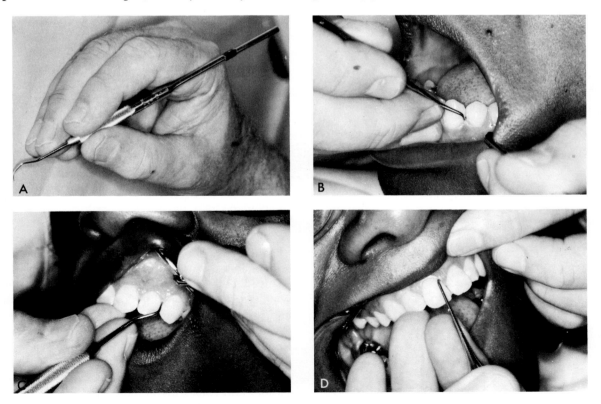

Fig. 17-16. *A,* The instrument is held with a slight pen grip, and the fourth finger used as rest and fulcrum. *B, C, D,* Use of finge rest and finger position in various areas of the mouth.

particle toothpastes may be used as polishing agents.

If root surfaces are exposed, use of acidulated fluorophosphate topically following the polishing is recommended.[19] This serves to harden the tooth surface and increase resistance to caries, and may reduce plaque accumulation and sensitivity.

Clinical procedures for scaling and root planing

Scaling and root planing are the most basic procedures in periodontal therapy and are indicated for every patient with accretions on the teeth and periodontal disease. The positions of the patient, the operator, and the operator's hands, as well as the use of a systematic approach, are all very important.

The patient should be reclining in the dental chair with the head kept at about elbow height of the operator when the patient is seated in an upright position. The patient should have been through an educational session regarding the significance of the scaling and planing, and, if indicated, should have been properly premedicated.

The instrument should be held with a light grasp between the fingertips of the first two fingers and touching the side of the fingertip of the middle finger. The tip of the fourth finger (ring finger) should be used as a rest and as a fulcrum when the instrument is activated (Fig. 17-16). If the area to be scaled appears highly inflamed and infected, applying iodine lotion over the field of operation, and dipping the instruments periodically into iodine lotion as they are introduced into periodontal pockets, are recommended. This is especially important for patients with diabetes or those with lowered resistance to infection from other causes.

The instrument should be moved along the surface of the tooth or the calculus and inserted into the gingival crevice with a light exploratory stroke until it is stopped at the bottom of the gingival crevice by definite soft tissue resistance. The insertion angle of the instrument should be adjusted in such a way that there is minimum soft-tissue interference with this exploratory stroke, thus permitting optimal sensitivity to roughness on the tooth surface. Then the instrument should be directed at the proper angulation, with the face at about an 85-to-90° angle with the surface of the tooth, and a short, forceful scaling stroke should be initiated (Fig. 17-17).

The pull motion of the instrument in the scaling stroke is derived from wrist and arm action rather than from finger movements. Planing strokes utilize the same basic movements, but with the face of the instrument at less than a 70-to-80° angle to the tooth surface, and with longer and more sweeping strokes than are used for calculus removal. The finger rest serving as the fulcrum should be as close to the working field as possible. Mouth mirrors should be used routinely for indirect vision and for retraction and direction of the light into areas of direct vision.

Surface characteristics of the tooth within the gingival crevice are assessed best with a thin explorer. A fine #17 explorer is the instrument of choice for areas where the access is convenient for this instrument. Place the bent tip part of the explorer almost flat to the tooth surface, with the sharp tip maintaining definite contact with the tooth. The instrument then can be moved safely into the gingival crevice without hurting the patient, because the dull back of the bent tip is contacting the soft tissues and can be used to displace the soft tissues gently until one is sure that the instrument has reached as close to the connective tissue attachment as is needed to locate calculus and significant tooth roughness in the crevicular area. When the bottom of the crevice is reached, turn the instrument slightly so that the tip is definitely directed toward the surface of the tooth as the exploratory stroke moves coronally. Interproximally, in the molar regions and for furcations, a #3 ("cowhorn") explorer may provide better access than the #17 instrument.

It is often difficult during subgingival exploration to differentiate between thick margins of dental restorations and calculus. If the tip of the explorer is kept in contact with the surface of the restoration as the explorer is moved in an apical direction, the operator will notice when the explorer makes an irregular movement from the margin of the restoration to the tooth surface, and it may be assumed that roughness on the root further apically is unrelated to the restoration and should be removed by periodontal hand

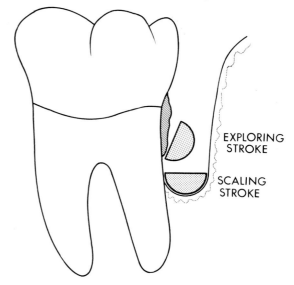

Fig. 17-17. The insertion of a curette into a pocket should be with a light exploring stroke, using the outer edge of the curette to explore calculus, fillings, and root surface. At the bottom of the pocket the instrument is turned so the face of the curette makes an 85 to 90° angle with the root surface before the powerful scaling stroke is executed.

instruments. The explorer should also be used to survey the tooth surface from the bottom of the gingival crevice in a coronal direction, since any roughness in this direction indicates potential interference with self-cleaning of the crevice and enhances plaque retention.

It is most important to hold the instrument with a very light pen grasp during exploration. A firm grip will dull the sensitivity of the operator's fingertips very quickly. The handle of the instrument should be thick enough to permit a suitable contact surface for the fingers, and should possess high surface friction. It should not be thin, smooth, or uniformly shaped.

During scaling and root planing, it is important to develop a rhythmic stroke routine, with complete finger and arm relaxation for exploration after each working power stroke. Forceful rubbing up and down on the tooth with hand instruments to be sure to "get it all off" may lead to unnecessary loss of tooth substance for the patient and fatigue for the operator, with numbness of the fingertips and backache.

Sequential order of scaling and root planing

Gross calculus and debris should be removed immediately after an educational orientation session with the patient has been completed and the patient has accepted the treatment plan. The presence of easily visible irritants and inflammation offers a great opportunity to educate the patient about the nature of his periodontal disease and to explain the need for patient involvement in plaque control.

The initial subgingival scaling should be done with great care, as the scaling stroke may easily be extended beyond the bottom of the junctional epithelium. Clinical and histologic observation of scaling being extended farther apically than intended[65,66] can easily be understood through the evidence of a zone of degenerated connective tissue attachment apically to the bottom of the junctional epithelium in active periodontitis.[75,80] Anesthesia should be avoided for this initial scaling of highly inflamed areas, since the risk of overextending the field of scaling is increased greatly in the absence of pain response from the patient. The scaling is performed best in "washed field," with the dental assistant providing a steady stream of water and evacuating the mouth. It is very important that the gingival crevices be flushed out well after completion of the scaling, since remaining debris may delay the healing.[65] Blowing air into the gingival crevice or pocket may be an unsafe procedure, especially at the lingual aspect of the mandibular molars and when there are deep buccal pockets on maxillary molars, since the air may enter into soft connective tissues and produce severe emphysema.[54]

Following the initial gross scaling and debridement, the teeth should be polished with a fairly coarse polishing paste (more for cleaning than for polishing), and the patient should assume plaque control by good oral hygiene.

If the patient has a highly active or acute periodontitis at the initiation of the treatment, it is advisable to wait for 3 to 4 weeks before performing the final scaling and root planing. The reason for the wait is that during this time a healing of the gingival tissues with initial maturation of the collagen fibers occurs, which means that definite landmarks for extension of the scaling and root planing are available even if anesthesia is used. Furthermore, the contraction of a collagenous gingival wall following scaling will help to close the gingival crevice to plaque formation and aid in establishing epithelial adaptation and reattachment to the tooth.

The second episode of scaling and root planing should be aimed at completing the scaling and root planing for the teeth that were included in each session. For deep pockets, local anesthetics are usually used and one or two quadrants are completed in one session. The polishing after this final planing should be done with a fine-particle polishing paste to achieve a high gloss, and topical application of acidulated fluorophosphate is recommended.

Healing following scaling and root planing

Immediately after scaling of teeth,[56,65,77] the epithelial attachment will be severed, and the junctional and crevicular epithelium partially removed. With severe inflammation, the scaling will often extend apically to the bottom of the epithelial attachment and create tears in the connective tissues. Strands of partially loosened epithelium and chronically inflamed connective tissue are commonly present in the crevice unless the soft tissue wall has been deliberately curetted (Fig. 17-18). The scaling also will split deep rete pegs in the wall of the pocket. If the scaling is done with hoes or files, much less injury occurs to the soft-tissue lining of the crevice.[61]

Two hours after scaling,[86] numerous polymorphonuclear cells can be observed between residual epithelial cells on the crevicular surface (Fig. 17-19). There is dilation of blood vessels, edema, and necrobiosis. The remaining epithelial cells show very minimal premitotic activity at this time. Similar findings can be seen at 5, 9, and 13 hours.

Twenty-four hours after scaling, a widespread and very intense labeling of epithelial cells has been found in all areas of the remaining epithelium, and in 2 days the entire crevice is covered by epithelium.

In 4 to 5 days, a new epithelial attachment may appear in the bottom part of the crevice. Depending on the severity of the inflammation and the depth of the crevice, complete epithelial healing may occur within 1 to 2 weeks (Fig. 17-20).

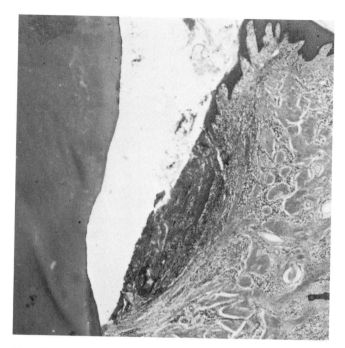

Fig. 17-18. Gingival crevice immediately following scaling with a curette. Note debris on soft tissue wall and complete severance of the junctional epithelium from the tooth surface.

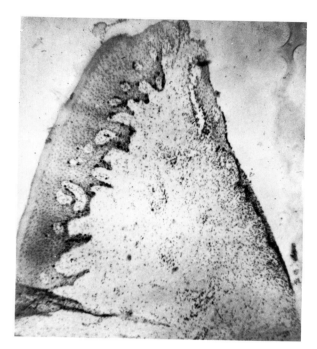

Fig. 17-19. Two hours after scaling in monkey, and ³ H thymidine labeling. Most of the junctional and crevicular epithelium has been removed during the scaling.

In a summary of tissue changes found in monkeys,[86] it was found that (1) the epithelial regeneration following scaling occurred mainly from remaining cells of the junctional and crevicular epithelium; (2) the regeneration of epithelium reached its peak 1 to 2 days following the scaling; (3) the connective tissue healing was most active 2 to 3 days after the scaling; and (4) a new epithelial attachment may be established as early as 4 to 5 days following the scaling. Although time intervals may differ, a few less detailed studies with humans indicate that the biological reactions after scaling are similar.[61,77]

It appears from limited investigations that the residual rete pegs in the crevice wall after scaling undergo involution,[95] and a normal epithelial attachment is formed.[91]

Complete healing may take as long as 9 months or more after scaling and root planing in deep periodontal pockets.[8] There is a profound change in the bacterial flora following scaling and root planing of periodontal pockets, with reduction in gram-negative organisms, motile rods, and spirochetes.[51,58] The recolonization of these organisms will occur in a month or 2 with poor oral hygiene,[51] but takes several months with good oral hygiene.[83,89] With repeated scaling and root planing every 3 months, such recolonization may be prevented.[90]

The visible clinical response to scaling and root planing depends much on the postoperative oral hygiene. Resolution of gingival inflammation always requires

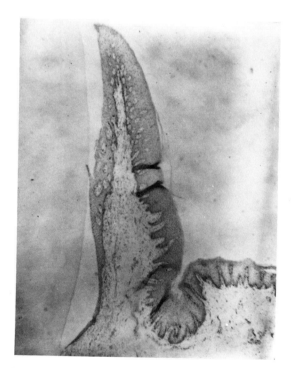

Fig. 17-20. Normal gingival crevice in monkey 2 weeks after scaling.

acceptable plaque control. However, there may be some healing and restitution of a new epithelial attachment following scaling, even in the absence of adequate oral hygiene. This newly formed epithelial attachment may for some time limit the toxic products of plaque from spreading in an apical direction and thereby prevent destruction of connective tissue fiber attachments apically to the new epithelial attachment. Thus, scaling and root planing may delay the progress of periodontitis even if the oral hygiene is inadequate.[17]

Incomplete scaling and root planing followed by good oral hygiene may result in apparent gingival health, but residual irritation and inflammation related to the inadequately instrumented root surface will reactivate the destructive periodontal disease and may even result in periodontal abscess formation.[96]

The ultrastructural changes of root surface structures following scaling have been studied by Selvig.[80] He found evidence of exchange of mineral and organic components across the tooth-saliva interface within a few weeks after thorough planing of cementum and root dentin. Increased mineral content was associated with increased perfection of the crystal structure, as well as organic changes suggestive of a subsurface cuticle. This hardening of the exposed root surface occurred within 3 to 4 weeks after the scaling. Active root caries with demineralization also could occur within 7 days. Thus, it is extremely important that the exposed root surfaces be kept clean following the scaling and polishing. Application of fluorides may facilitate the mineralization of exposed cementum.[30]

Clinical results of scaling, root planing, and oral hygiene

A striking reduction of gingival inflammation is commonly found following dental prophylaxis (Fig. 17-21). This improvement in gingival health is manifested as a change to more uniform color, reduction in bulk, increased density, reduced bleeding tendency upon probing, and decrease in crevicular depth.

Recent longitudinal studies indicate that for pockets 4 to 6 mm deep, an average reduction of pocket depth of 1 mm may be expected following such therapy, and for pockets 7 mm or deeper, the average reduction in depth is 2 mm.[55] Part of this decrease in pocket depth is due to recession of the free gingival margin, and part of it is due to gain of attachment as assessed with a thin probe and in relation to the cementoenamel junction.

The gain in attachment as probed clinically may change the bottom of the gingival crevice from a position apical to the mucogingival line to a position coronal to this line, and eliminate the need for mucogingival surgery.[40] The mucogingival line itself does not move in relation to the cementoenamel junction following scaling.

Role of scaling and root planing in periodontal therapy

Elimination of bacterial plaque and accretions is vital to the success of all periodontal therapy, and in fact constitutes the basic therapy for all patients with periodontal disease. Correction of defective restorations is usually included in the concept of root planing.

There is a consensus that scaling and root planing, plus control of bacterial plaque accumulation, possibly augmented by surgical recontouring of the gingival anatomy for esthetic reasons, is the treatment needed for gingivitis.

Traditionally, scaling and root planing plus oral hygiene instruction have been considered only as the initial or hygienic phase of treatment for periodontitis, to be followed by some modality of surgical therapy if the crevice depth exceeds 3 mm after completion of this initial phase.

Surgical treatment of periodontal pockets deeper than 3 mm after scaling and root planing has been recommended in order to (1) assure access for removal of accretions in inaccessible areas, (2) facilitate oral

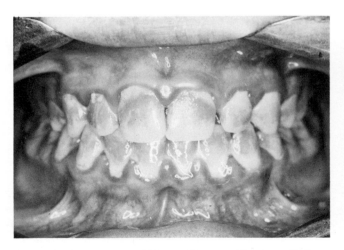 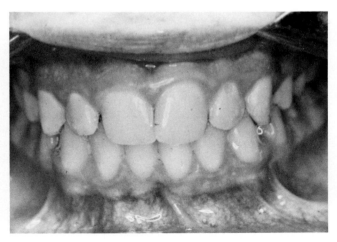

Fig. 17-21. Fifteen-year-old boy, with no oral hygiene. *B,* One week after prophylaxis and instruction in oral hygiene.

hygiene to the bottom level of the pockets, and (3) facilitate regeneration. However, a number of recent clinical trials conducted under well-controlled experimental conditions have found that scaling and root planing without subsequent surgical procedures may not only give excellent long-term results,[6] but, even in cases of deep pockets, lead to results as favorable as those obtained following surgical procedures.[38,47,62] It seems that post-scaling measurable pocket depth is not as critical as previously believed, and at least for shallow pockets less than 6 mm, scaling and root planing appear to be the treatment of choice.[38,47,62] However, access for elimination of calculus and plaque has to be gained, and, if following scaling and root planing there is pus or bleeding from a pocket, or inaccessible furcation involvement exists, surgery should be used to gain access to the involved root surface.

Thorough scaling and root planing should be the initial treatment for all cases of gingivitis and periodontitis. If this treatment is found not to be successful after 4 to 6 weeks (if pus and/or bleeding on probing is evident), then initial scaling and root planing should be augmented by surgical exposure of the root for further root planing.

It has been shown that for prevention of periodontal disease,[5,46] and for optimal results of maintenance care following all forms of periodontal therapy, it is essential to institute periodic professional cleaning of the teeth.[60] It appears that recall for professional prophylaxis and instruction in home care only once or twice a year following periodontal surgery is not adequate for most patients.[60,74] The thoroughness of the professional tooth cleaning seems to be a very significant factor in the success of such recall programs.[7]

REFERENCES

1. Aleo, J.J., et al.: The presence and biologic activity of cementum-bound endotoxin, J. Periodont. 45:672, 1974.
2. Aleo, J.J., DeRenzis, F.A., and Farber, P.A.: In attachment of human gingival fibroblasts to root surfaces, J. Periodont. 46:639, 1975.
3. Allen, E.F., and Rhoads, R.H.: Effect of high speed periodontal instruments on tooth surfaces, J. Periodont. 34:352, 1963.
4. Axelsson, P.: EVA-systemet. et nytt hjälpmedel for approximal rengöring, puts och polering, Sv. Tandlforb. Tidn. 61:1086, 1969.
5. Axelsson, P., and Lindhe, J.: The effect of a preventive programme on dental plaque gingivitis and caries in school children. Results after one and two years, J. Clin. Periodontol. 1:126, 1974.
6. Axelsson, P., and Lindhe, J.: Effect of controlled oral hygiene procedures on caries and periodontal disease in adults. Results after 6 years, J. Clin. Periodontol. 8:239, 1981.
7. Axelsson, P., and Lindhe, J.: The significance of maintenance care in the treatment of periodontal disease, J. Clin. Periodontol. 8:281, 1981.
8. Badersten, A., Nilveus, R., and Egelberg, J.: Effect of nonsurgical periodontal therapy. II. Severely advanced periodontitis, J. Clin. Periodontol. 11:63, 1984.
9. Bandt, C.L., Korn, N.A., and Schaffer, E.M.: Bacteremias from ultrasonic and hand instrumentation, J. Periodont. 35:214, 1964.
10. Barnes, G.P., Stookey, G.K., and Muhler, J.C.: In vitro studies of the calculus-inhibiting properties of tooth surface polishing agents and chelating agents, J. Dent. Res. 50:966, 1971.
11. Barnes, J.E., and Schaffer, E.M.: Subgingival root planing: A comparison using files, hoes and curettes, J. Periodont. 31:300, 1960.
12. Belting, C.M., and Spjut, P.J.: Effect of high-speed periodontal instruments on the root surface during subgingival calculus removal, J.A.D.A. 69:578, 1964.
13. Björn, H., and Lindhe, J.: The influence of periodontal instruments on the root surface. A methodological study, Odontol. Revy 13:355, 1962.
14. Bodecker, C.F.: The difficulty of completely removing subgingival calculus, J.A.D.A. 30:703, 1943.
15. Boyde, A.: The tooth surface. In Prevention of Periodontal Disease, ed. J.E. Estoe, D.C.A. Picton, and A.G. Alexander. London: Henry Kingston Publishers, 1971.
16. Burman, L.R., Alderman, N.E., and Ewen, S.J.: Clinical application of ultrasonic vibrations for supragingival calculus and stain removal, J. Dent. Med. 13:156, 1958.
17. Chawla, T.N., Nanda, R.S., and Kapoor, K.K.: Dental prophylaxis procedures in control of periodontal disease in Luchnow (rural India), J. Periodont. 46:498, 1975.
18. Clark, S.M.: The ultrasonic dental unit: A guide for the clinical application of ultrasonics in dentistry and dental hygiene, J. Periodont. 40:621, 1969.
19. Council on Dental Therapeutics: Accepted Dental Therapeutics. 35th ed. Chicago: American Dental Association, 1973.
20. Doyle, P.T.: The polishing effect of the EVA-system and dental tape. Thesis, The University of Michigan, 1971.
21. Dudding, N.J., Stookey, G.K., and Muhler, J.C.: Techniques for the preparation and use of zirconium silicate as a cleaning and polishing agent, J. Indiana Dent. Assoc. 44:54, 1965.
22. Eaton, E.A., Kieser, J.B., and Davies, R.M.: The removal of root surface deposits, J. Clin. Periodontol. 12:141, 1985.
23. Ellman, J.A.: Comparative safety of the rotosonic scaler and the curette, J. Periodont. 35:410, 1964.
24. Everett, F.G., and Potter, G.R.: Morphology of submarginal calculus, J. Periodont. 30:27, 1959.
25. Everett, F.G., Foss, C.L., and Orban, B: Study of instruments for scaling (planing). The rake angle, Parodontologie 16:61, 1962.
26. Ewen, S.J., and Tasher, P.J.: Clinical use of ultrasonic scalers, J. Periodont. 29:45, 1958.
27. Ewen, S.J.: A photomicrographic study of root scaling, Periodontics 4:273, 1966.
28. Fauchard, P.: The Surgeon Dentist. Translated from the 2nd ed. (1746) by Lillian Lindsay. London: Butterworth, 1946.
29. Frumker, S.C., and Gardner, W.M.: The relation of the topography of the root surface to the removal of calculus, J. Periodont. 27:292, 1956.
30. Furseth, R.: A study of experimentally exposed and fluoride treated dental cementum in pigs, Acta Odont. Scand. 28:833, 1970.
31. Goldman, H.M.: Histologic assay of healing following ultrasonic curettage, Oral Surg. 14:925, 1961.
32. Graham, C.J.: Home care effectiveness upon planned teeth and scaled teeth following surgery, J. Periodont. 37:43, 1966.
33. Greene, E., and Ramfjord, S.P.: Tooth roughness after subgingival root planing, J. Periodont. 37:396, 1966.
34. Greene, E.: Root planing with dull and sharp curettes, J Periodont. 39:348, 1968.
35. Guerini, V.: History of Dentistry. Philadelphia: Lea and Febiger, 1909.

36. Harvay, B.L.C., and Zander, H.A.: Root surface resorption of periodontally diseased teeth, Oral Surg. 12:1439, 1959.

37. Hatfield, C.G., and Baumhammers, A.: Cytotoxic effects of periodontically involved root surfaces, J. Dent. Res., abstr. no. 203, 1970.

38. Hill, R.W., Ramfjord, S.P., Morrison, E.C., Appleberry, E.A., Caffesse, R.G., Kerry, G.J., and Nissle, R.R.: Four types of periodontal treatment compared over two years, J. Periodont. 52:655, 1981.

39. Holton, W.L., Hancock, E.B., and Pellen, G.B.: Prevalence and distribution of attached cementicles on human root surfaces, J. Periodontol. 57:321, 1986.

40. Hughes, T.P.: Changes in the gingiva following scaling and root planing. A biometric evaluation. Thesis, The University of Michigan, 1975.

41. Hunter, R.K., O'Leary, T.J., and Kafrawy, A.H.: The effectiveness of hand versus ultrasonic instrumentation in open flap root planing, J. Periodont. 55:697, 1984.

42. Jones, S.J., Lozday, J., and Boyde, A.: Tooth surfaces treated in situ with periodontal instruments, Br. Dent. J. 132:57, 1972.

43. Kerr, D.A.: The cementum: Its role in periodontal health and disease, J. Periodont. 32:183, 1961.

44. Kerry, G.J.: Roughness of root surfaces after use of ultrasonic instruments and hand curettes, J. Periodont. 38:340, 1967.

45. Kopezyle, R.A., and Conroy, C.W.: The attachment of calculus to root planed surfaces, Periodontics 6:78, 1968.

46. Lindhe, J., Hamp, S.E., and Löe, H.: Plaque induced periodontal disease in beagle dogs. A 4-year clinical roentgenographical and histometric study, J. Periodont. Res. 10:243, 1975.

47. Lindhe, J., Westfelt, E., Nyman, S., Socransky, S.S., and Haffajee, A.D.: Long-term effect of surgical/nonsurgical treatment of periodontal disease, J. Clin. Periodontol. 11:448, 1984.

48. Listgarten, M.A., and Ellegaard, B.: Electron microscopic evidence of cellular attachment between junctional epithelium and dental calculus, J. Periodont. Res. 8:143, 1973.

49. Littlefield, T.W.: Root surface roughness after planing with various tungsten carbide curettes. Thesis, The University of Michigan, 1971.

50. Lövdal, A., et al.: Combined effect of subgingival scaling and controlled oral hygiene on the incidence of gingivitis, Acta Odont. Scand. 19:537, 1961.

51. Magnusson, I., Lindhe, J., Yoneyama, T., and Liljenberg, B.: Recolonization of a subgingival microbiota following scaling in deep pockets, J. Clin. Periodontol. 11:193, 1984.

52. McCall, J.O.: The evolution of the scaler and its influence on the development of periodontia, J. Periodont. 10:69, 1939.

53. McCall, C.M., and Szmyd, L.: Clinical evaluation of ultrasonic scaling, J.A.D.A. 61:559, 1960.

54. McClencon, J.L., and Hooper, W.C.: Cervico-facial emphysema after air blown into a periodontal pocket, J.A.D.A. 63:810, 1961.

55. Morrison, E.G., Ramfjord, S.P., and Hill, R.W.: Short-term effect of initial non-surgical periodontal treatment (hygienic phase), J. Clin. Periodontol. 7:199, 1980.

56. Moskow, B.S.: The response of the gingival sulcus to instrumentation: I. The scaling procedure, J. Periodont. 33:282, 1962.

57. Moskow, B.S., and Bressman, E.: Cemental response to ultrasonic and hand instruments, J.A.D.A. 68:698, 1964.

58. Mousques, T., Listgarten, M.A., and Phillips, R.W.: Effect of scaling and root planing on the composition of the human subgingival microbial flora, J. Periodont. Res. 15:144, 1980.

59. Nissle, R.R.: Ultrasonic scaling: Effects on gingiva and root surface. Thesis, The University of Michigan, 1962.

60. Nyman, S., Rosling, B., and Lindhe, J.: Effect of professional tooth cleaning on healing after periodontal surgery, J. Clin. Periodontol. 2:80, 1975.

61. O'Bannon, J.Y.: The gingival tissues before and after scaling the teeth, J. Periodont. 35:69, 1964.

62. Pihlström, B.L., McHugh, R.B., Oliphant, T.H., and Ortiz-Campos, C.: Comparison of surgical and nonsurgical treatment of periodontal disease. A review of current studies and additional results after 6½ years, J. Clin. Periodontol. 10:524, 1984.

63. Putt, S.M., et al.: Physical characteristics of a new cleaning and polishing agent for use in a prophylaxis paste, J. Dent. Res. 54:527, 1975.

64. Rabbani, G.M., Ash, M.M., and Caffesse, R.G.: The effectiveness of subgingival scaling and root planing in calculus removal, J. Periodont. 52:119, 1981.

65. Ramfjord, S.P., and Kiester, G.: The gingival sulcus and the periodontal pocket immediately following scaling of teeth, J. Periodont. 25:167, 1954.

66. Ramfjord, S.P., and Costitch, E.R.: Healing after simple gingivectomy, J. Periodont. 34:401, 1963.

67. Ramfjord, S.P., et al.: Results following three modalities of periodontal therapy, J. Periodont. 46:522, 1975.

68. Rateitshak, K.H.: Therapeutic effect of local treatment on periodontal disease assessed upon evaluation of different diagnostic criteria. I. Changes in gingival inflammation, J. Periodont. 35:155, 1964.

69. Rautiola, C.A., and Craig, R.G.: The microhardness of cementum and underlying dentin of normal teeth and teeth exposed to periodontal disease, J. Periodont. 32:113, 1961.

70. Reinhardt, R.A., Johnson, G.K., and Tussing, G.J.: Root planing with interdental papilla reflection and fiber optic illumination, J. Periodont. 56:721, 1985.

71. Riffle, A.G.: The cementum during curettage, J. Periodont. 23:170, 1952.

72. Riffle, A.G.: The dentin: Its physical characteristics during curettage, J. Periodont. 24:232, 1953.

73. Riggs, J.M.: Pyorrhea alveolaris, Dent. Cosmos. 24:524, 1882.

74. Rosling, B., Nyman, S., and Lindhe, J.: The effect of systematic plaque control on bone regeneration in infrabony pockets, J. Clin. Periodontol. 3:38, 1976.

75. Saglie, R., Johansen, J.R., and Flötra, L.: The zone of completely and partially destructed periodontal fibers in pathological pockets, J. Clin. Periodontol. 2:198, 1975.

76. Schaffer, E.M.: Histological results of root curettage of human teeth, J. Periodont. 27:296, 1956.

77. Schaffer, E.M., Stende, G., and King, D.: Healing of periodontal tissues following ultrasonic scaling and hand planing, J. Periodont. 35:140, 1964.

78. Schaffer, E.M.: Periodontal instrumentation, scaling and root planing, Int. Dent. J. 17:297, 1967.

79. Schroeder, H.E., and Rateitschak-Pluss, E.M.: Focal root resorption lacunae causing retention of subgingival plaque in periodontal pockets, Schweiz. Monats. Zahnheilk. 93:1033, 1983.

80. Selvig, K.: Ultrastructural changes in cementum and adjacent connective tissue in periodontal disease, Acta Odont. Scand. 24:459, 1966.

81. Selvig, K.A.: Biological changes at the tooth-saliva interface in periodontal disease, J. Dent. Res. 48:846, 1969.

82. Selvig, K.A.: Attachment of plaque and calculus to tooth surfaces, J. Periodont. Res. 5:8, 1970.

83. Slots, J., Mashimo, P., Levine, M.J., and Gener, R.J.: Periodontal therapy in humans. I. Microbiological and clinical effects of a single course of periodontal scaling and root planing as an adjunct to tetracycline, J. Periodont. 50:495, 1979.

84. Stahl, S.S.: The nature of healthy and diseased root surfaces, J. Periodont. 46:156, 1975.

85. Stende, G.W., and Schaffer, E.M.: A comparison of ultrasonic and hand scaling, J. Periodont. 32:312, 1961.
86. Stone, S., Ramfjord, S.P., and Waldron, J.: Scaling and gingival curettage. A radioautographic study, J. Periodont. 37:415, 1966.
87. Swartz, M.L., and Phillips, R.W.: Comparison of bacterial accumulation on rough and smooth enamel surfaces, J. Periodont. 27:304, 1957.
88. Sweeney, P.L., Caffesse, R.G., and Smith, B.A.: Scaling and root planing with or without periodontal flap surgery, J. Dent. Res. (Special Issue) 63:205, 1984.
89. Syed, S.A., Morrison, E.C., and Lang, N.P.: Effectiveness of repeated scaling and root planing and/or controlled oral hygiene on the periodontal attachment level and pocket depths in beagle dogs. II. Bacteriological findings, J. Periodont. Res. 17:219, 1982.
90. Syed, S.A., Morrison, E.C., Loesche, W.J., and Ramfjord, S.P.: The bacterial flora of treated periodontal pockets, J. Dent. Res. (Special Issue B) 59: abst. 76, 1980.
91. Thilander, H., and Hugoson, A.: The border zone tooth-enamel and epithelium after periodontal treatment. An experimental electron microscopic study in the cat, Acta Odont. Scand. 28:147, 1970.
92. Turesky, S., Renstrup, G., and Glickman, I.: Histologic and histochemical observations regarding early calculus formation in children and adults, J. Periodont. 32:7, 1961.
93. Waerhaug, J., Arnö, A., and Lövdal, A.: The dimension of instruments for removal of subgingival calculus, J. Periodont. 25:281, 1954.
94. Waerhaug, J.: Effects of rough surfaces upon gingival tissue, J. Dent. Res. 35:323, 1955.
95. Waerhaug, J.: Microscopic demonstration of tissue reaction incidence to removal of subgingival calculus, J. Periodont. 26:25, 1966.
96. Waerhaug, J.: A method for evaluation of periodontal problems on extracted teeth, J. Clin. Periodontol. 2:160, 1975.
97. Walker, S.L., and Ash, M.M., Jr.: A study of root planing by scanning electron microscopy, Dent. Hygiene 50:109, 1976.
98. Winslow, M.B., and Kobernick, S.D.: Bacteremia after prophylaxis, J.A.D.A. 61:69, 1960.
99. Woodruff, H.C., Levine, M.P., and Brady, J.M.: The effects of two ultrasonic instruments on root surfaces, J. Periodont. 46:119, 1975.
100. Yamada, N.: Fine structure of exposed cementum in periodontal disease, Bull. Tokyo Med. Dent. Univ. 15:409, 1968.
101. Zamet, J.S.: A comparative clinical study of three periodontal surgical techniques, J. Clin. Periodontol. 2:87, 1975.
102. Zander, H.S.: The attachment of calculus to root surfaces, J. Periodont. 24:16, 1953.
103. Zander, H.A., Kohl, J.T., and Keller, H.: New tool for dental prophylaxis, J.A.D.A. 63:636, 1961.

The oral mucosal membranes protect the underlying connective tissues through structural features and the natural surface self-cleansing of the teeth that occurs through use, but these means are inadequate to prevent plaque accumulation. Attempts have been made to enhance the natural cleansing action by prescribing so-called "detergent" diets, including fresh fruit, roots, raw vegetables, hard bread, sugar cane, and other fibrous foods, but none of these diets has had any effect on the aggregation of plaque at the gingival border of the teeth.[77,93,136] Although fibrous food may remove some plaque from the coronal parts of the teeth, relying on detergent diets for adequate plaque control in prevention of periodontal disease is not feasible. Therefore, various means for artificial cleansing of the teeth have been practiced over the ages by both primitive and civilized people.

Rationale for Plaque Control

Clinical observations and epidemiological investigations have demonstrated a strong and consistent association between the amount of dental plaque and the severity of periodontal disease.[8,74,88,105,115] Furthermore, studies on experimental gingivitis have established beyond doubt that failure to remove plaque by artificial means, after starting with clean teeth, will result in gingivitis, and that plaque removal after an experimental period of 3 weeks will lead to cure of the gingivitis.[8,81] Thus, there is not only an association but a cause-and-effect relationship between dental plaque and gingivitis.[81,82] In beagle dogs, periodontitis has been shown to develop following long-term exposure to plaque and calculus.[78] The mechanisms whereby plaque causes periodontal disease, however, are not known. It has been demonstrated that an interaction between dental plaque and dietary carbohydrates produces caries,[61] and that, in the absence of plaque, frequent additions of sucrose to the diet fail to result in caries.[85] Thus, it appears that elimination of dental plaque is of utmost importance for prevention of both periodontal disease and caries.[83]

Complete prevention of plaque formation is not possible by conventional mechanical means[75] and not practical by current chemical means. Instead, the goal of clinical plaque control at present is periodic mechanical or chemical plaque removal at intervals spaced closely enough together to prevent recurrent plaque formation and any resulting significant pathological effects.

Complete mechanical plaque removal at intervals not exceeding 48 hours seems to be adequate for prevention of gingivitis.[75] No such time interval has been established for prevention of caries, but it is considered advisable to remove all plaque immediately after ingestion of any sucrose-containing food or drink. Increasingly, thick plaque may also interfere with the saliva's buffer systems. Thus, when sucrose is available, the potential for a low pH at the plaque-tooth interface may increase. Efforts to prevent caries by mechanical plaque control carried out by the patients have been only moderately successful. This success has been limited to the buccal and lingual surfaces,[32] which may in part be due to the inaccessibility of narrow pits and fissures, as well as inadequate interproximal cleaning. Mechanical plaque control has been able to prevent gingivitis,[81] but its effectiveness in checking already present caries and periodontal disease is questionable.[45]

Mechanical Means of Plaque Control
Toothbrushing

The use of toothbrushes probably originated with the ancient custom of chewing or hammering the end of a freshly cut twig of soft wood to create a tool for cleaning the teeth. This custom goes back several thousand years in China,[56] and it has been claimed

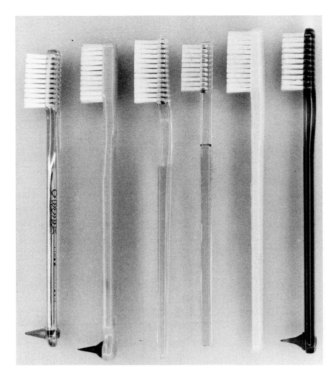

Fig. 18-1. A representative selection of a large variety of available multitufted toothbrushes. Number and diameter of filaments or bristles vary with the manufacturer.

that the first toothbrushes, made from pig's hair, also originated in China. Although toothbrushes were mentioned in early Roman literature (1st century A.D.), not much was said about toothbrushes until 200 to 300 years ago.[69]

Toothbrushes vary in size, shape, and texture, and may be manually used or motor driven (Fig. 18-1). There is no clear-cut evidence that one particular type of toothbrush is superior to other types for plaque removal and prevention of gingivitis.[48] The plaque-reducing effect of hard versus soft brushes is controversial; some investigators prefer the hard type,[118] while others have found no difference.[18] Several authors recommend the soft filament brushes, in view of the damage that hard filaments may cause.[67,69] Rounded bristle tips have been advised,[12] although the damage[54,56] from sharp tips probably is not significant, since nylon filaments become smooth with use.[67] The size of the brush head has generally been found to be an unimportant factor relating to cleaning ability.[71]

Some researchers have claimed that nylon filaments displace plaque particles, while natural bristles grip and pull them off.[91] Other researchers have found that nylon brushes are significantly better for plaque removal than natural bristles.[15] At the present time, practically all available toothbrushes have synthetic bristles of standard size. Because toothbrushes alone do not have any abrasive action on the tooth surface, there is no difference in abrasive potential between nylon and natural bristle brushes.[14] Abrasiveness depends on the properties of the dentifrice used with the toothbrush.[21,91] These properties will be discussed more fully later in this chapter. Multitufted, soft-filament nylon brushes with a filament diameter of 0.007 to 0.009 inch and well-finished filament tips are the most widely recommended toothbrushes at the present time. However, excellent oral hygiene without harmful side effects can be maintained with medium-hard and hard toothbrushes when suitable techniques are used.

A number of "interspace" toothbrushes (Fig. 18-2) are also available for cleansing of interproximal or furcation surfaces that provide poor access for regular toothbrushes.[52]

Methods for toothbrushing

A variety of methods for toothbrushing have been advocated, with no one method being universally superior. Any method of brushing that removes plaque effectively without harming hard and soft tissues is acceptable. Methods that are easy to learn and require minimum time and effort are favored.

The "roll," or "sweep," technique has been used extensively in the past with hard or medium-hard toothbrushes. The brush is placed on the attached gingiva close to the gingival margin of the teeth, with

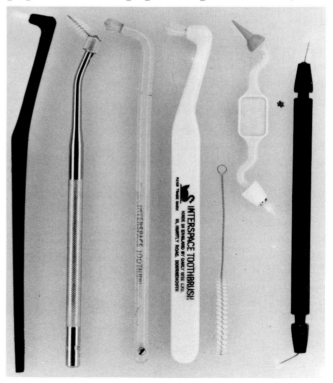

Fig. 18-2. "Interspace" brushes for cleansing of interproximal and furcation surfaces.

the bristles pointing apically in a 30-to-40° angle to the long axis of the teeth. Then, with a rolling or sweeping stroke, the brush is moved in a coronal direction until the bristles make a 90° angle with the tooth surface at the occlusal edge of the teeth. Only moderate pressure is applied, and the movements are repeated five to six times for each segment covered by the brush. On the lingual and palatal side, only a few teeth can be covered by each movement of the brush. The occlusal surfaces are scrubbed to complete the brushing.

This method works fairly well for patients with anatomically normal gingival tissues.[35] However, it is not a satisfactory method for patients who have lost interproximal tissues or have thick gingival margins. If a hard brush is used carelessly with these methods, mucogingival erosions and gingival clefts may be produced. This method is not used much anymore.

Charters' method. Another time-honored method of toothbrushing, one with special emphasis on interproximal cleaning, is Charters' method.[31] This method originally called for hard brushes, but medium-hard or soft brushes may be used. The bristles of the brush are pointed against the interproximal spaces and directed towards the outer tooth surfaces at a 45° apical angle with the long axis of the teeth. The sides of the bristles are pressed lightly against the gingival surface. If the interproximal spaces are open, the bristles may point perpendicularly to the long axis of the teeth to achieve maximum interproximal cleaning. The brushing is carried out with vibrating movements, pressing the brush in an interproximal direction and holding the sides of the bristles against the gingiva. This method of brushing is fairly effective, especially after periodontal surgery. However, it is time-consuming,[62] because on the lingual side each interproximal space has to be cleaned individually.

At present, the two most popular methods of toothbrushing are the Bass and the circular scrub techniques. Both methods utilize soft brushes.

Bass method. The Bass, or intrasulcular method, was initially proposed by Talbot in 1899. He wrote: "The bristles should be so passed in between the gum margin and the tooth as to remove the debris and exfoliated epithelial scales which have accumulated therein." However, the method was popularized and strongly promoted by Bass,[12,14] who also placed much emphasis on the uniform filament thickness of 0.007 inch and rounded filament ends (Fig. 18-3) to avoid gingival injury.

In the Bass method, the head of the brush is placed parallel to the occlusal plane, the bristles flat against the facial surface of the teeth and the ends of the bristles close to the free gingival margin. The brush is then turned to an almost 45° angle with the long axis of the teeth and the bristles pointed into the gin-

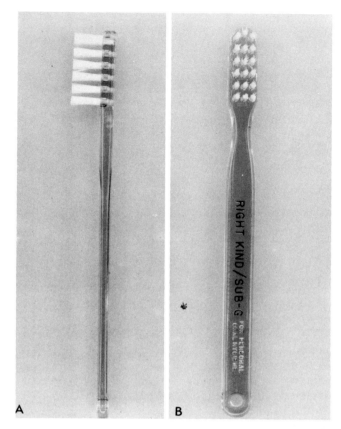

Fig. 18-3. Brush advocated by Bass for intrasulcular method of brushing.

gival sulcus and as far as possible into the interproximal spaces (Fig. 18-4 A, B). Gentle pressure is exerted on the long axis of the bristles, and the brush is activated with a short back-and-forth vibrating motion, ten times for each area. The motion is carried out without dislodging the tips of the bristles and without a back-and-forth movement of the bristle tips. During this action, the bristles should contact the teeth, the gingival sulcus, and the outer surface of the free gingiva.

The palatal and lingual surfaces of the molars and bicuspids can be brushed in a similar manner, but for the anterior teeth the brush should be inserted with the bristles held vertically and only part of the head of the brush inserted into the mouth (Fig. 18-4 C). Press the end of the bristles into the long axis of the teeth and activate the brush with short back-and-forth vibrating movements. A common error is to apply pressure that will bend the bristles against the surfaces of the teeth instead of directing the force in the long axis of the bristles into the gingival sulcus.

Brushing should begin with the buccal and distal surfaces of the last maxillary molar on the right side and cover all facial surfaces of the maxillary teeth, ending with the distal surface of the last maxillary molar on the left side. Be sure to allow for some overlap of brush coverage as the brush is moved from one position to another. The palatal side should then be brushed, starting with the palatal surfaces of the maxillary left molars and ending with the palatal surface of the last maxillary right molar.

Brushing in the mandible should begin with the distobuccal surface of the last mandibular molar on the right side. Then all facial surfaces should be brushed, ending with the last mandibular molar on the left side. Turn the brush to the distal and lingual surface of the same tooth and cover all lingual surfaces in a sequential order, ending with the distolingual surface of the last right mandibular molar. The occlusal surfaces of the posterior teeth should be cleaned with a vibrating and scrubbing action as the bristles are directed into the occlusal fissures.

The Bass technique is somewhat time-consuming to learn and to perform daily. The correct sulcular brushing on the lingual side is especially difficult to carry out.

The easiest method to learn is the horizontal scrub method, in which the buccal and lingual surfaces of the teeth are cleaned by a back-and-forth scrubbing action in the direction of the plane of occlusion. Unfortunately, this method has a high potential for both hard and soft tissue injury and cleans very poorly in the interproximal areas, so it cannot be recommended.

Circular scrub method. A practical combination of some principles from the Bass technique and others from the horizontal scrub technique has been adopted in the so-called circular scrub technique (Fig. 18-5). From recent studies, it appears that this technique has equal to or possibly better potential than the Bass technique for plaque removal and prevention of gingivitis.[10] The circular scrub method is easy to learn and requires a shorter time to perform than the Bass technique. Similar toothbrushes may be used for either technique.

For the circular scrub technique, place the brush parallel to the occlusal plane of the teeth, with the bristles pointing 70 to 90° in an apical axial direction and with the tips of most bristles contacting the outer surfaces of the teeth, but with some bristles extending several millimeters over the adjacent gingiva. Activate the brush with mild pressure in the direction of the bristles, and move the head of the brush in small (2 to 4 mm in diameter) circular movements, with the tips of the bristles moving on both the surfaces of the teeth and the gingiva. The combined piercing and scraping action of the tips of the bristles in the circular scrub method appears to be more effective in breaking up and removing plaque than the stationary vibration of the bristle tips in the Bass technique. This is especially true for the interproximal areas.

The positioning of the brush for the various parts of the dentition and the sequential procedures for clean-

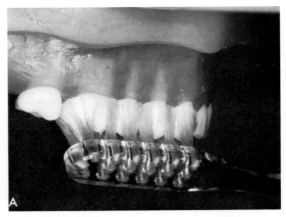

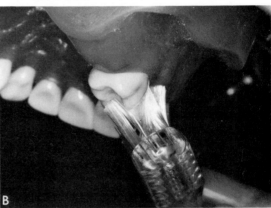

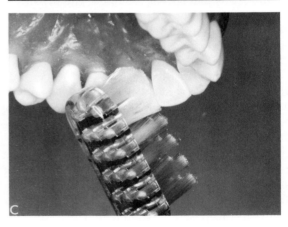

Fig. 18-4. Bass method of brushing as described in text. Brush filaments are pointed into gingival sulcus *(A)* and into the interproximal spaces *(B)*. *C,* Position of brush for palatal side, using only part of the brush.

ing the entire dentition are essentially the same for the circular scrub and the Bass technique. Five to eight circular scrub movements should be made for each brush position, and some overlap should be included as the brush proceeds in stepwise movements around the dental arch.

Without the addition of dental floss or other devices, the Bass or the circular scrub method of toothbrushing will provide adequate plaque removal for the main-

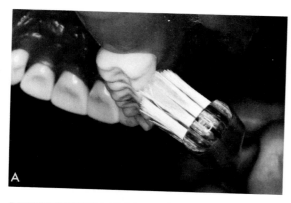

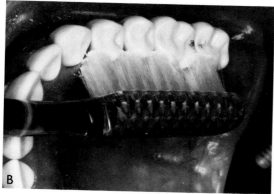

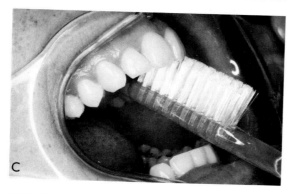

Fig. 18-5. Circular scrub method. The brush is positioned on the buccal *(A)* and palatal *(B)* surfaces of the teeth and several millimeters onto the adjacent gingiva. *C,* Position of brush for palatal surfaces of anterior teeth. Small circular movements of the tips of the bristles on the gingiva and teeth are made with mild pressure.

tenance of periodontal health in individuals with anatomically normal gingiva, as is often seen in children and young adults.[9,128] However, if there has been loss of periodontal tissues with resulting exposed interproximal tooth surfaces, or if the patient has irregular positions of the teeth or is fitted with various kinds of dental appliances, these basic methods of toothbrushing have to be augmented by other techniques to accomplish satisfactory plaque control. Even Charters' method,[31] which was originally developed for interproximal cleaning, is not adequate to this purpose, and proxibrushes[52] or other aids may have to be used. Proxibrushes are most effective for cleaning wide-

open interproximal spaces.[52]

A number of other techniques for toothbrushing have been used,[59] but none of them has any significant advantages over the Bass or the circular scrub technique,[46] and they usually have greater potential for harmful effects.

For a time, mechanical or motor-driven toothbrushes were promoted extensively. There is no conclusive evidence that these brushes and brushing methods have any advantage over manual brushes and brushing techniques,[7,96] and mechanical failures often limit their usefulness after some time. However, for handicapped people and persons with unusually low digital skill, mechanical toothbrushes may be indicated.[122]

Dental floss and tape

Dental floss or tape is usually the device of choice for removal of interproximal plaque,[51] which is inaccessible to toothbrushing (Fig. 18-6). The multifilamented dental floss that spreads out in a tapelike fashion when pressed against the tooth surface has replaced the previously popular dental tape for plaque control, although dental tape used with polishing paste still is best for interproximal polishing of teeth. Considerable sentiment has been expressed in favor of unwaxed dental floss over the waxed type,[13] with claims of more effective plaque removal for the unwaxed variety. However, in clinical trials, no difference in plaque removal was found between the two types of floss.[52,66,72] For teeth with tight interproximal contacts or rough restorations, it is usually easier to use waxed than unwaxed floss. Otherwise, no preference has been established.

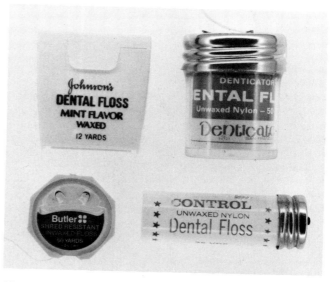

Fig. 18-6. Dental floss may be waxed, unwaxed, and flavored or unflavored. It may be prescribed in small pocket dispensers or large at-home dispensing units.

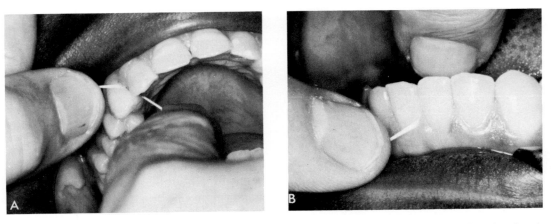

Fig. 18-7. Finger position and application of floss to interproximal areas. *A,* Floss is brought into crevice but closely adapted to tooth surface. *B,* Floss should spread out when moved back and forth slightly with light pressure.

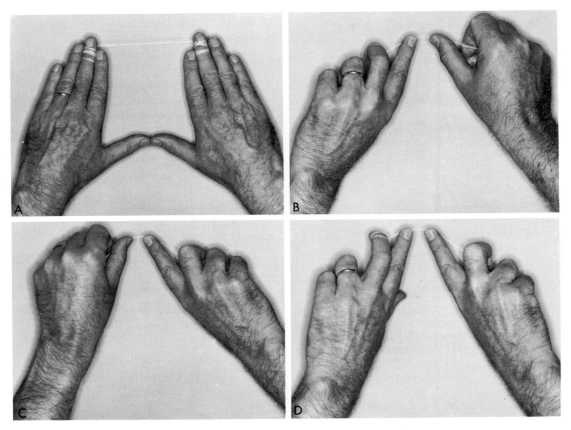

Fig. 18-8. *A,* Determining the length of floss and attachment to fingers. Position of fingers and thumb for flossing the right maxillary teeth *(B),* and left maxillary teeth *(C). D,* Position of fingers for flossing mandibular teeth.

Dental floss should be used as illustrated in Fig. 18-7. Cut off a 45-cm (18-inch) length of floss. Roll the cut ends around the terminal parts of each middle finger until the fingers point straight forward when the distended thumbs meet with the hands outstretched (Fig. 18-8 A). For the maxillary right teeth, hold the floss with the right thumb and the left fore-finger (Fig. 18-8 B). For the maxillary left side, hold the floss between the left thumb and the right forefinger (Fig. 18-8 C), and for all mandibular teeth hold the floss between the 2 forefingers (Fig. 18-8 D). The distance between the fingers guiding the floss should be 1.3 to 1.5 cm to provide secure control when the floss is passed between the teeth.

Pass the floss carefully through the contact area with an out-and-in motion, starting close to the fingers. Do not hold the fingers too far apart and do not snap the floss between the teeth, because this may cause injury to the gingiva. After the floss has passed the contact, move it up and down on 1 interproximal tooth surface at a time. Move it as far into the gingival crevice as it can go without causing gingival injury. A common mistake is to saw too much back and forth with the floss. This may cause tooth abrasions[39,69] or clefts in the gingival tissues. Move up and down on the tooth surfaces with only slight back-and-forth action of the floss. The tendency to cause abrasion is increased greatly if abrasive toothpaste is used with sawing movements of the floss.

Mechanical holders for dental floss (Fig. 18-9A) are recommended for persons who experience difficulty in manual use of floss (Fig. 18-9B), especially for the molar teeth. Special threaded devices are often used for areas with solder joints and for pontics of bridges (Fig. 8-10). Similar devices for interdental cleaning and for wide-open furcations are pipe cleaners[137] and knitting yarn.[123] No scientific data are available for evaluation of these devices, and they do not seem to offer any advantage over dental floss.

Toothpicks and interdental stimulators

Toothpicks of various materials and design have an old historical tradition, and it has been claimed that even monkeys have been observed to use sticks to remove food impacted between the teeth.[69] Except for removal of impacted food, which is actually not an oral hygiene but an occlusion problem, toothpicks are not as effective as dental floss for removal of interdental plaque,[51] and toothpicks do not remove more plaque from the lingual part of the interproximal surfaces than does an ordinary toothbrush.[52]

Concave interproximal surfaces that cannot be reached by dental floss are usually cleaned better with proxibrushes of various designs than with toothpicks. The end of a rounded toothpick[56] inserted in a special holder (Perio-Aid) has been recommended for augmentation of cleaning of the teeth at the dentogingival junction, especially where the access is poor for other devices, such as in furcations and narrow interproximal spaces (Fig. 18-11). This method appears to be cumbersome and has never gained wide acceptance.[48]

Toothpicks come in various shapes: round, flat, and triangular in cross section. They have been made from soft and hard wood, metal, and plastics. There is no evidence that any shape or material is generally superior to the others, although there is probably greater risk for harmful effects from metal, as well as less versatility for adaptation to interproximal spaces. Toothpicks should not be used where a normal interdental papilla fills the interdental space, because the

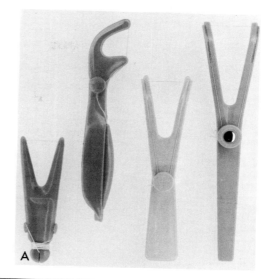

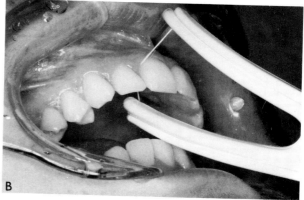

Fig. 18-9. *A,* Mechanical holders for dental floss. *B,* Use of floss holder on maxillary anterior teeth.

use of a toothpick in such an area may create gingival recession and an open interdental space. Such a space is neither anatomically normal nor desirable from a prevention standpoint.

The rationale for use of interdental stimulators was an alleged need for mechanical stimulation of the gingival tissues in order to maintain normal gingival structure and keep the metabolism protected by a well-keratinized epithelial surface.[128] Gingival keratinization may be increased by mechanical stimulation,[55,110] but this outer-surface keratinization has nothing to do with protection against gingivitis, which starts in the unkeratinized gingival sulcus.

It has been demonstrated very convincingly that gingival health may be maintained by periodic removal of plaque from the surfaces of the teeth without any specific gingival massage.[75,81] Alleged reduction of gingival inflammation associated with massage[54] is probably due to plaque removal from the tooth surfaces by the massaging devices and removal of bacteria and toxins from the gingival crevice by compression of the gingiva. There is no evidence that collagen for-

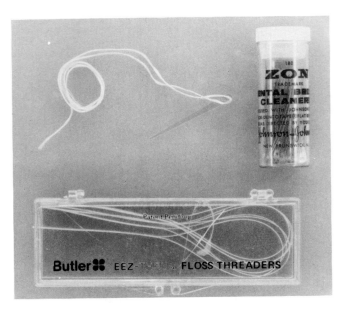

Fig. 18-10. Floss threaders used to pass floss beneath solder joints, splinted teeth, or teeth with heavy contacts.

mation is stimulated by massage, and massage of an inflammatory lesion in an infected environment does not seem to have a good therapeutic rationale, as was pointed out long ago.[89]

However, in spite of rational arguments against gingival massage, some benefit has been observed from use of interdental stimulators and toothpick combinations for patients with soft, swollen interdental gingiva who cooperate poorly in the regular use of dental floss. The use of dental floss is almost twice as time-consuming as the use of toothpicks or interdental stimulators,[52] and the patient's acceptance of dental flossing is often poor. Therefore, interdental stimulators or proxibrushes may be considered as a compromise solution for such individuals, although it appears that patients who clean well with one method also do the best with other methods, while poor performance with one method will lead to poor performance with another method.[138]

Rubber tips (Fig. 18-12) are the most popular devices for combined interdental cleaning and gingival stimulation, but triangular toothpicks of soft wood ("stimudents") have also been used extensively (Fig. 18-13). While the stimudents can be used only from the labial-facial approach, and do not work well for the molars, the rubber tips can be used both from the buccal and lingual approaches to the interproximal spaces of all of the teeth. However, the stimudents will clean the labial-facial part of the interproximal tooth surfaces better than the rubber tip, so a combination of the two modalities may be advisable, depending on the needs and abilities of the patient.

Semiflexible rubber tips with small surface ridges seem to clean better than hard and smooth cone-shaped tips, but it is most important that the tip be inserted into the interdental space along the contour of the gingiva, pointing about 45° coronally to the long axis of the teeth (Fig. 18-12B). The tip should then be vibrated with a mild pressure in the direction of the interdental space. As it is removed, it should be moved coronally along the interproximal surfaces of the teeth for cleaning action. Repeat the placement of the tip three or four times for each interproximal space from both the buccal and the lingual approach. Patients have a tendency to insert rubber tips and other interdental stimulators perpendicular to the long axis of the teeth. Although this may increase keratinization,[28] it has a tendency to result in an abnormal flat interdental papilla and should be avoided.

Dental irrigators

Dental or oral irrigation devices provide a steady or pulsating stream of water under pressure escaping through a nozzle. The pressure is from a pump or from a water faucet connection. For many years, water irrigators have been recommended on occasion for the treatment of periodontal disease,[92] but new, highly promoted commercial devices have now made this modality popular.[6]

It has been suggested that irrigation under pressure has a physical, mechanical, thermal, or chemicomedical effect,[108] depending on how it is used. However, the cleaning efficiency of irrigating devices is poor, in that only surface layers of soft plaque are removed[36,41,80] and only a slight reduction in severity of gingivitis may be expected. Therefore, these devices should not be used as a substitute for toothbrushing and can be expected to have only slight or not adjunctive value for persons with poor brushing habits. It has not been established that these devices are of any adjunctive value to patients who are brushing and flossing their teeth in prescribed manners.

Furthermore, the incidence of bacteremia among patients with periodontitis is greater after use of these devices than it is after regular toothbrushing.[40] Con-

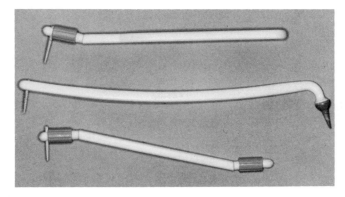

Fig. 18-11. Toothpick-holding devices.

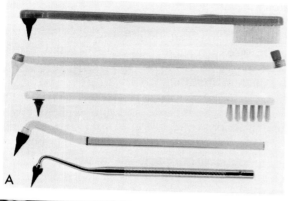

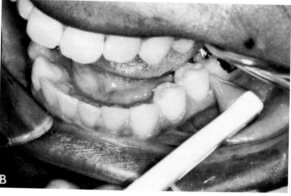

Fig. 18-12. *A*, Rubber tip holders. *B*, The position of a rubber tip during rotatory movement with light pressure for cleaning and gingival stimulation.

sequently, patients with rheumatic heart disease or a history of heart surgery, as well as those with diabetes in association with periodontitis, should be advised against using these devices.

Although the use of irrigation in patients with completely inadequate oral hygiene may have some benefit, greater and safer improvement of oral hygiene can be achieved by conventional methods. Patients using irrigation devices often tend to believe that these devices are more effective than has been proved, and consequently reduce their efforts in manual plaque control. The results are very disappointing. Even in patients with orthodontic or prosthetic appliances that complicate access for regular oral hygiene, the use of irrigation devices is of questionable or no value.

Oral irrigators have been recommended for application of chemical means of plaque control,[76] and have been found, in comparison to oral rinsing, to enhance the effectiveness of such means. The depth of penetration in periodontal pockets with oral irrigation by devices such as a Water Pik is only about ½ of the depth of the pocket.[38] Through use of a blunt needle and a hypodermic syringe, a greater part of the pocket may be reached,[63] but seldom the entire pocket. Antimicrobial irrigation of deep pockets to supplement

non-surgical periodontal therapy did not improve the results.[25]

Dentifrices

A dentifrice is a paste or powder used with toothbrushes or other mechanical cleansing devices for the purpose of cleaning the teeth. Dentifrices[56] contain abrasives such as calcium carbonate, calcium phosphate, aluminum, zirconium silicate, sodium bicarbonate, sodium chloride, and others.[101] They also contain soap or synthetic detergents for foaming action, humectants (glycerin, sorbitol, and water), and thickening agents such as carboxymethyl cellulose. Unsuccessful attempts have been made to make dentifrices truly therapeutic against gingivitis by adding antibiotics or other drugs. However, the only demonstrated therapeutic effect from adding preventive agents to dentifrices comes from addition of fluoride to protect against cavities.[70]

For plaque removal, the abrasiveness of the dentifrice does not appear to be important,[19,82,98] but abrasion may affect the dental pellicle, the tooth substance, and restorations. The surface pellicle, which is present on exposed tooth surfaces, has received much interest recently, since it was found that this pellicle is not removed by the patient's home care for plaque removal. The pellicle may harbor stains, calculus, and toxic products from bacterial plaque that has become attached to the pellicle, and may be partially responsible for the lack of cellular adaptation to exposed tooth surfaces demonstrated in tissue cultures.[2] One study reported a definite pellicle 24 hours after cleaning the teeth with pumice.[116] This layer increased in thickness with time. When nonabrasive dentifrices were used, compared with abrasive dentifrices, a thicker, smooth-surface pellicle developed. Cosmetic stain was found in the pellicle, and it often became mineralized and hard to remove. Some abrasives are needed in den-

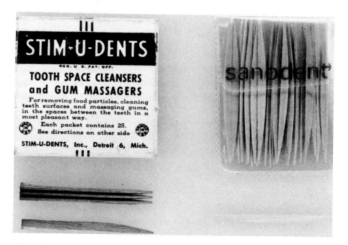

Fig. 18-13. Triangular toothpicks of soft wood used for interdental cleansing of facial tooth surfaces.

tifrices to keep the pellicle thin and thus avoid accumulation of surface stains.[19] However, dentifrice abrasives may cause harmful abrasions on teeth and restorations, and a standard level of desirable abrasiveness of a dentifrice has not been established. The Council on Dental Therapeutics of the American Dental Association has graded the abrasion of several popular dentifrices, based upon the removal of dentin in standardization brushing in an in vitro system.[107] However, this list should be used with some discretion, as its values may be different from those found in, for example, in vivo use with lubrication and dilution from the saliva. The potential abrasive effect of a dentifrice is not related solely to the abrasiveness of its particles.[64] Factors such as concentration, dilutants, brush brand, brush hardness, and temperature of testing have all been demonstrated to affect the abrasiveness of dentifrices. Hard brushes resulted in 3.5 times as much abrasion as soft brushes with the same dentifrice, and glycerin reduced abrasiveness as much as 88% compared to dilution with water.

Another longitudinal study over 54 months also reported lack of correlation between clinical results and laboratory values on the abrasiveness of the tested dentifrices.[131]

The ideal dentifrice, one that aids significantly in removal of plaque and surface pellicle without scratching or grooving teeth and restorations, has not been developed yet. There does not even seem to be a simple relation between the efficiency of cleansing and the kind and extent of abrasion.[95] Only a few nonconclusive studies have been reported on this polishing ability of dentifrices.[24] The subject needs further investigation.

At the present state of knowledge, it appears that abrasion from dentifrices can be minimized by the use of soft toothbrushes, use of small amounts of dentifrice with low abrasive potential (according to the results of the study by American Council of Dental Therapeutics), and avoidance of horizontal scrub movements of the toothbrush.

There is also a potential for chemical irritation to the mucosal membranes from ingredients present in most dentifrices;[3] however, due to the dilution with saliva in the mouth, there is usually no irritating effect. Nevertheless, the potential for chemical irritation or allergic reactions to a dentifrice should always be considered if manifestations of a stomatitis appear.

Chemical Plaque Control

Prevention of plaque formation, removal or dispersion of plaque, inhibition of calcification of bacterial accumulations, and even elimination of specific pathogenic organisms in the plaque are all goals of chemical plaque therapy.

General suppression of the oral bacterial flora by various broad-spectrum antibacterial compounds has been attempted. Substantial reduction of viable salivary bacteria has been demonstrated following use of a number of such agents, but, due to rapid reproduction of the bacteria in the mouth, this reduction has been of short duration.[125]

Various broad-spectrum antibiotics[82] have an inhibitory effect on both caries and periodontitis, but prolonged use of broad-spectrum antibiotics is not a practical solution to plaque control because of health hazards, in terms of resistance and allergic reactions, from such practice. Other antibiotics with a more narrow spectrum, such as vancomycin,[130] actinobolin,[4] kanamycin,[87] and others, have some plaque-inhibiting effects, but their effects are usually not as good as those derived from mechanical tooth cleansing, and are often of temporary efficacy.[82]

Efforts to inhibit plaque formation through use of dextranase[27] or fluoride mouthwashes[20] have not been successful in humans.

By far the most effective chemical agent for plaque control known today is chlorhexidine gluconate. Used twice a day as a mouthrinse in a 0.2% solution, it will prevent plaque formation,[84] dissolve newly formed plaque, and significantly reduce old plaque.[43]

A similar result may be obtained by topical application of 1% solution once daily.[84] Chlorhexidine salts are retained in the oral cavity for several days,[111] and by gradual release keep the teeth relatively free from bacteria over a prolonged time, in contrast to other short-acting oral disinfectants.[125] Chlorhexidine has been shown to prevent the development of gingivitis and cure experimentally induced gingival inflammation in humans.[84] However, when it was used as a supplement to habitual oral hygiene, only slight reduction in gingivitis occurred in patients with subgingival plaque and calculus.[43]

Although chlorhexidine has a very low toxicity effect,[84] it has some undesirable side effects. Complaints of bitter taste and of interference with taste sensation for some time after the application are common. Discoloration of teeth, of restorations, and of the tongue is often found. Desquamative lesions in the vestibular mucosa have been observed with prolonged exposure,[44] while in another study no side effects were observed after over 2 years of use of the drug.[85]

Chlorhexidine has recently been approved by the Food and Drug Administration for oral use in the United States. It is being used to some extent in Europe, mainly to facilitate healing after periodontal surgery and to prevent development of Dilantin gingivitis. A 0.12% solution is sold under the name of "Peridex" as a prescription drug.

Some antimicrobial effect has been found associated with the use of stannous fluoride.[94] The most noticeable benefit occurred following self-administered daily irrigation with stannous fluoride solution in a Water Pik device.[22] However, the stannous fluoride was not found to be as effective as Chlorhexidine.[65] Combined benefit from professional tooth cleaning and topical fluoride has been confirmed in larger scale clinical trials.[17]

A cationic disinfectant (Alexidine)[100] has a plaque-inhibitory effect, but not to the same degree as Chlorhexidine,[100] and with the same drawbacks as Chlorhexidine.

A new mouthrinse containing Sanguinarine will reduce plaque formation more than a placebo, but not as much as Chlorhexidine,[133,134] and may cause discoloration of tooth surfaces.

The use of sodium bicarbonate, salt, and hydrogen peroxide will not substantially improve oral health status beyond what can be expected from ordinary care,[29,60] although, when applied subgingivally in pockets after scaling and root planing, some benefit may occur.[114] A significant reduction in the rate of plaque formation has been demonstrated following the use of Listerine mouthwash,[42,57] but more long-term studies are needed.

The use of metronidazole, tetracycline, or non-steroidal anti-inflammatory drugs for preventive periodontics is still very controversial.[50,58,90,102,129,132] These drugs cannot be recommended for routine clinical use. It appears that the chemical means for plaque control may augment but not be substitutes for mechanical procedures.

Disclosing Agents

Staining of the bacterial plaque on the teeth to make it more visible both to the operator and to the patient has been recommended for a long time,[26] and a number of disclosing agents (Fig. 18-14) are available.[5,16,33,37,47,49]

For use in the dental office and for research involving plaque scoring, the Bismark brown solution is excellent.[37,104] In home use, tablets containing food color such as erythromin (FD7C Red No. 3)[5] have been used extensively, but this dye is now being replaced by other dyes.[33] It has been shown that the use of plaque-disclosing dyes can improve the effectiveness of oral hygiene instructions.[11] Although disclosing wafers may be a useful aid in oral hygiene instruction for a short time, they do not influence the long-term effect of an oral hygiene instruction program.[16] Showing the patient the existence of plaque in his or her own mouth, and reinforcing the presentation with repeated charting of stained plaque, may enhance the effectiveness of oral hygiene instruction. It is recommended that the patient use a disclosing wafer after his oral hygiene regimen every night for 8 to 10 nights following the initial instruction in oral hygiene. Then, he should use one wafer every 2 weeks in the future to check if the performance is satisfactory. Otherwise,

he should use it every night until an acceptable level is reached. Use of a suitable mirror system with the disclosing agents is recommended.[10]

Education and Motivation

Prior to learning oral hygiene techniques, the patient should be educated regarding the progressive nature of periodontal disease and the indisputable need for oral hygiene procedures in treatment and prevention of this disease. However, learning facts about the disease does not necessarily have much motivational impact on the patient's behavior. Therefore, the education of the patient should be slanted towards emphasis on what personal benefits the patient may derive from good oral hygiene.[30,139] Emphasizing only the prospect of a healthy mouth does not mean much to most patients, who very often have no symptoms of discomfort associated with their gingivitis or periodontitis. That they may lose their teeth in 20 to 30 years unless their oral hygiene is improved is in most instances not conceived by them as a serious threat. Preaching or scolding, and even demonstration of "creepy bugs" from their own mouth in phase contrast microscopes, have only a mild transient shock effect, which is rarely followed by long-term behavioral changes.[120]

Of all proposed approaches to patient motivation to long-term improvement in oral hygiene, two have proved more successful than the others. The first is to personalize the patient's education by making him personally involved and showing him tangible evidence of successes in achieving his goal of a healthy mouth. This is aided by the use of suitable mirrors,

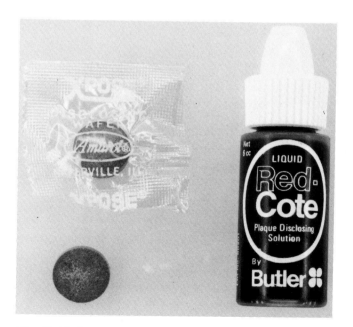

Fig. 18-14. Disclosing wafers and solution for the evaluation of plaque on the teeth in an oral hygiene instruction program.

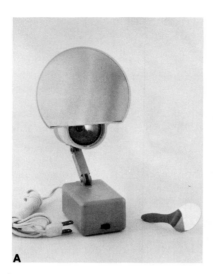
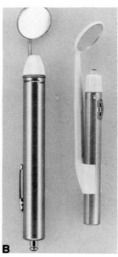

Fig. 18-15. *A,* Floxite light and mirror for patient self-examination of oral hygiene. *B,* Small pen-like lights and dental-type mirrors for self-examination before a mirror.

such as the Floxite (Fig. 18-15A), for self-examination, and of plaque-disclosing media, either for educational purposes before toothbrushing or for checking of performance after oral hygiene procedures.[9] The other effective motivational approach is to show the patient the monetary or social gain that can be derived from effective oral hygiene.[37] The monetary gain will be indirect, through less need for dental services. The social gain will come from having a good-looking and healthy dentition that can be displayed with pride and without fear of halitosis when "getting close."

With these motivational objectives in mind, an educational session for the patient should be scheduled prior to instruction in oral hygiene techniques. Booklets and self-teaching slides or film sequences can serve to present facts about plaque and periodontal disease and about their management. However, without the support of individualized explanations and the emotional appeal of a good teacher, very little, if any, behavioral benefit can be expected from such "canned" education.[119] A simple demonstration in the patient's own mouth, with the patient holding a hand mirror, is likely to have a much deeper impact on the patient than any pictures of other persons' mouths.

Start the educational session with demonstration of areas in the patient's mouth where there is minimal or no plaque or disease (Fig. 18-16A,B). If such areas are not present in the patient's mouth, the operator can demonstrate them in his or her own mouth or in the mouth of the dental assistant. Then show areas of periodontal disease with plaque and bleeding tendency. By far the most common symptom of periodontal disease is an increased bleeding tendency upon slight provocation, such as toothbrushing. Explain to the patient that the bleeding is from wounds

on the inner surfaces of the gums facing the teeth; the teeth are coated by bacterial plaque. Stress that these wounds, which they cannot see, are caused by large numbers of bacteria living on the uncleansed surfaces of the teeth and within the gingival sulcus. The gingival sulcus can be compared to the relationship between the fingernails and the skin. It is important to explain that the plaque on the teeth is an aggregation of bacteria, and that bacteria are sources of infection, rather than leftover food from the last meal. Explain how food particles adherent to the plaque will be digested away by oral enzymes, while the plaque, if left undisturbed, will grow by rapid bacterial proliferation. As some bacteria die, irritating and foul-smelling substances are released.

It is also helpful to point out with a periodontal probe where loss of attachment has occurred and to relate these areas to roentgenograms.

Then outline the goal of the proposed treatment: first, to establish tooth surfaces that are clean, promote healthy gingival tissues, and are accessible for effective oral hygiene; and second, to teach the patient how to maintain clean teeth by oral hygiene procedures. Explain that the only way to make the easily bleeding gingival wounds heal is to reduce as much as possible the bacterial infection associated with dental plaque, and that if in the future the gingiva starts to bleed during tooth-cleaning procedures, it indicates recurrence or active periodontal disease and the need for treatment. That periodontal disease is a bacterial infection resulting from lack of cleanliness of the teeth should be emphasized, as should the fact that effective cleaning procedures must be performed at least once every day in order to keep the mouth free of such infection.

It should be made clear to the patient that periodic prophylaxis in the dental office three to four times a year is helpful in the maintenance of oral health, but only by daily plaque removal at home can true periodontal health be attained and maintained. Teaching the patient why and how to cleanse his teeth is a more valuable health service than most other things done in dentistry. It has been demonstrated in a convincing scientific way that combining regular dental office visits with home oral hygiene will significantly reduce gingivitis and loss of supporting periodontal tissues.[126]

Beyond everything else, it should be understood clearly that teaching of oral hygiene should be based upon positive reinforcement and repeated during every visit to the dentist's office.

Instruction in Oral Hygiene

A number of studies have compared the effectiveness of self-instruction, individual instruction, and group instruction in teaching oral hygiene.[7,23,53,117,118,119] The results are highly controversial, which indicates that each of these approaches has some value and that they can be used singularly or in various combinations, according to the personality of the educator and the available facilities and circumstances.

Personal instruction tailored to the patient's need and ability is recommended. Such instruction may be supplemented by various visual aids, but with the clear understanding that the personal impact of the teacher is much more important than what can be achieved by various types of teaching machines.

Oral hygiene instruction should start with a demonstration of the favored toothbrushing technique on a cast or plastic model with the type of brush recommended to the patient (but not with the patient's brush, for sanitary reasons). Then plaque and plaque removal should be demonstrated in the patient's mouth. It is advisable to stain the plaque with a disclosing medium, with the explanation that the bacteria are colorless and hard to see even if present by the millions, but by a suitable stain they become visible when present in large aggregates. Give the patient a toothbrush of your choice and demonstrate how some of the plaque may be removed by the toothbrushing method just shown while the patient observes the procedure in a mirror. Explain also that interproximal plaque removal may necessitate the use of other means for complete removal. Then step by step teach the patient how to hold and how to use the toothbrush. This is a slow and painstaking procedure, and should

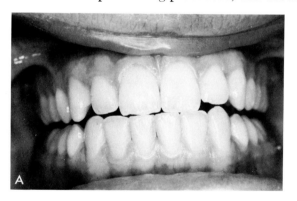

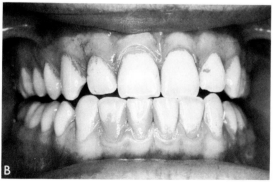

Fig. 18-16. Demonstration of plaque. *A,* Without disclosing solution, plaque is difficult to see. *B,* With use of disclosing solution, plaque is visible.

be made "achievement oriented" as much as possible by having the patient observe if he is removing the stained plaque or not, to show how he has to direct his efforts to become efficient in plaque removal. The cleansing of the teeth should be stressed, rather than any given method of toothbrushing. Even after extensive brushing, some interproximal stained plaque may remain, and the use of dental floss or other devices for removal of such plaque should be demonstrated.

At the end of this initial instruction session, encourage the patient to go through the recommended procedures in front of a mirror (the Floxite mirror is good)[10] at home at least once a day. Use disclosing tablets to check the result after completion of cleaning procedures. If stained areas appear, try to remove the stain.

When the patient returns for the second instruction, stain the teeth with disclosing solution and have the patient demonstrate with his own brush (which he should bring for every appointment, or one may be kept for him in the dental office) and with dental floss how he will remove the plaque and how he was instructed to perform plaque control procedures. This is often a very disheartening experience for the instructor, because what the patient demonstrates may be very different from what he was taught. It is important that the instructor be patient and understanding. Again, focus on the results rather than technical details. If the patient gets the plaque off and does not appear to do any harm to the gingiva or the teeth, technical finesse is of lesser importance. Repeated instructional sessions are always needed. Plaque scores may be used at the onset of every session as a measure of the patient's achievement, but such scores should be used with discretion and adjusted to the individual dental problems as well as to the technical ability of the patient. It should be understood that a zero plaque score is very seldom if ever obtainable and that there is an individual "permissible" plaque level that is compatible with clinical periodontal health. Thus, in evaluation of the patient, do not focus only on the plaque, but pay attention to the health status of the gingiva as well. If the gingiva appears to be healthy, the plaque control is adequate, although it may not be perfect. Some judgment must be exercised with regard to compromise between what is ideal and what is practically obtainable for the individual patient, with the understanding that frequency of recall for professional prophylaxis may be adjusted to the patient's level of oral hygiene performance to compensate for less-than-perfect plaque control.

Professional Tooth Cleaning

The concept of frequent professional cleaning of the teeth as a valuable approach in preventive dentistry was introduced by Axelsson and Lindhe.[9,79] They reported spectacular reduction in gingivitis and new caries lesions following polishing of children's teeth every 2 weeks, followed by topical fluoride application, compared with control groups with infrequent prophylaxis. The same investigators have also reported excellent results from frequent professional tooth cleaning during maintenance of patients after various modalities of periodontal therapy.[103,112,113,135]

Professional tooth cleaning removes plaque before it can mature and develop a more anaerobic bacterial flora that seems to be related to the development of gingivitis. It takes several weeks or a few months following scaling before the bacterial flora is reestablished in a pocket,[99] and it is important to remove the new plaque before it has reached the deep part of the pockets. With professional tooth cleaning about once every 3 months, it is possible to maintain periodontal support for treated teeth with periodontitis, even though the patient's oral hygiene may not be perfect.[106]

REFERENCES

1. Accepted Dental Therapeutics. 37th ed. Chicago: American Dental Association, 1977.
2. Aleo, J., DeRenzis, F., and Fabrer, P.: In vitro attachment of human gingival fibroblasts to root surfaces, J. Periodont. 46:639, 1975.
3. Allen, A.L., et al: An investigation of the clinical and histologic effects of selected dentifrices on human palatal mucosa, J. Periodont. 46:102, 1976.
4. Armstrong, P.J., and Hunt, D.E.: In vitro evaluation of actinobolin as an antibiotic for the treatment of periodontal disease, Appl. Microbiol. 23:88, 1972.
5. Arnim, S.S.: The use of disclosing agents for measuring tooth cleanliness, J. Periodont. 34:227, 1963.
6. Arnim, S.S.: Dental irrigators for oral hygiene, periodontal therapy and prevention of dental disease, J. Tenn. Dent. Assoc. 47:65, 1965.
7. Ash, M.M.: A review of the problems and results of studies on manual and power toothbrushes, J. Periodont. 35:202, 1964.
8. Ash, M.M., Gitlin, B.N., and Smith, W.A.: Correlation between plaque and gingivitis, J. Periodont. 35:424, 1964.
9. Axelsson, P., and Lindhe, J.: The effect of a preventive program on dental plaque, gingivitis and caries in school children. Results after one and two years, J. Clin. Periodontol. 1:126, 1974.
10. Baity, M.A.: Clinical evaluation of magnifying lighted mirror as an oral hygiene adjunct. Thesis, The University of Michigan, 1971.
11. Barrickman, R.W., and Penhall, O.J.: Graphing indexes reduces plaque, J.A.D.A. 87:1404, 1973.
12. Bass, C.C.: The optimum characteristics of toothbrushes for personal oral hygiene, Dent. Items 70:697, 1948.
13. Bass, C.C.: The optimum characteristics of dental floss for personal oral hygiene, Dent. Items 70:921, 1948.
14. Bass, C.C.: An effective method of personal hygiene (Part II), J. La. Med. Soc. 106:100, 1954.
15. Bay, I., Kardel, K.M., and Skougard, M.R.: Kvantitativ undersokelse of forskllige tandborstetypers plaque fjernende evne, Tandlaegebladet 71:103, 1967.
16. Bellini, H.R., Aanerud, A., and Moustafa, M.H.: Disclosing wafers in an oral hygiene instruction program, Odont. Rev. 25:247, 1974.
17. Bellini, H.T., Campi, R., and Denardi, J.L.: Four years of monthly professional tooth cleaning and topical fluoride application in Brazilian school children. I. Effect on gingivitis, J. Clin. Periodontol. 8:231, 1981.
18. Bergenholtz, A., et al: The plaque-removing ability of various toothbrushes used with the roll technique, Swen. Tandlak. Tidskr. 62:15, 1969.
19. Bergenholtz, A., Lignell, L., and Oberg, G.: Quantitative evaluation of the plaque-removing ability of four dentifrices. In Oral Hygiene, ed. A. Frandsen. Copenhagen: Munksgaard, 1972.
20. Birkeland, J.M., Jorkjend, L., and von der Fehr, F.R.: The influence of fluoride mouthrinsing on the incidence of gingivitis in Norwegian children, Community Dent. Oral Epidemiol. 1:17, 1973.
21. Bjorn, H., Lindhe, J., and Grondahl, H.G.: The abrasion of dentine by commercial dentifrices, Odont. Revy 17:109, 1966.
22. Boyd, R.L., Leggott, P., Quinn, R., Buchanan, S., Eakle, W., and Chambers, D.: Effect of self-administered daily irrigation with 0.02 SmF₂ on periodontal disease activity, J. Clin. Periodontol. 12:420, 1985.
23. Brandtzaeg, P., and Jamison, H.: The effect of controlled cleansing of the teeth on periodontal health in Norwegian Army recruits, J. Periodont. 35:28, 1964.
24. Brash, S.V., et al: The assessment of dentifrice abrasivity in vivo, Br. Dent. J. 127:119, 1969.
25. Broatz, L., Garrett, S., Claffey, N., and Egelberg, J.: Antimicrobial irrigation of deep pockets to supplement nonsurgical periodontal therapy. II. Daily irrigation, J. Clin. Periodontol. 12:630, 1985.
26. Bunting, R.W.: Oral Hygiene and the Treatment of Periodontal Diseases. Philadelphia: Lea and Febiger, 1936.
27. Caldwell, R.C., et al: The effect of a dextranase mouthwash on dental plaque in young adults and children, J.A.D.A. 82:124, 1971.
28. Canton, M.T., and Stahl, S.S.: The effects of various interdental stimulators upon the keratinization of the interdental col, Periodontics 3:243, 1965.
29. Cerra, M., and Killoy, W.: The effect of sodium bicarbonate and hydrogen peroxide on the microbial flora of periodontal pockets—a preliminary report, J. Periodont. 53:599, 1982.
30. Chambers, D., and Allen, D.: Computer analysis of oral hygiene habits, J. Periodont. 44:505, 1973.
31. Charters, W.J.: Immunizing both hard and soft mouth tissue to infection by correct stimulation with the toothbrush, J.A.D.A. 15:87, 1928.
32. Clark, C.A., Fintz, J.B., and Taylor, R.: Effects of control of plaque on the progression of dental caries: Results after 19 months, J. Dent. Res. 53:1458, 1974.
33. Cohen, W., et al: A comparison of bacterial plaque disclosants in periodontal disease, J. Periodont. 43:333, 1972.
34. Compton, F., and Beagrie, B.C.: Inhibitory effect of benzethamine and zinc chloride mouthrinse on human dental plaque and gingivitis, J. Clin. Periodont. 2:33, 1975.
35. Curtis, G.H., McCall, C.M., and Overa, H.I.: A clinical study of effectiveness of the roll and Charters' methods of brushing teeth, J. Periodont. 28:277, 1957.
36. Dabelsteen, I.: Undersogelse over den tandbelaegningfjernende og poche-rensende virkning av balneoterapeutisk apparatur, Tandlaegebladet 68:107, 1964.
37. Deo, B.A.: A modified Scanlon plan for oral hygiene motivation. Thesis, The University of Michigan, 1969.
38. Eakle, W.S., Ford, C., and Boyd, R.L.: Depth of penetration in periodontal pockets with oral irrigation, J. Clin. Periodontol. 13:39, 1986.

39. Everett, F.G., and Kunkel, P.W.: Abrasion through the abuse of dental floss, J. Periodont. 24:186, 1953.

40. Felix, J.E., Rosen, S., and App, G.R.: Detection of bacteria after use of an oral irrigation device in subjects with periodontitis, J. Periodont. 42:785, 1971.

41. Fine, D.H., and Baumhammers, A.: Effect of water pressure irrigation on stainable material on the teeth, J. Periodont. 41:468, 1970.

42. Fine, D.H., Letizia, J., and Mandel, I.D.: The effect of rinsing with Listerine antiseptic on the properties of developing dental plaque, J. Clin. Periodontol. 12:660, 1985.

43. Flötra, L.: The effect of chlorhexidine mouthwashes. Thesis, Oslo, Universitetsforlaget, 1970.

44. Flötra, L., et al: Side effects of chlorhexidine mouthwashes, Scand. J. Dent. Res. 79:119, 1971.

45. Flötra, L., et al: A four-month study on the effect of chlorhexidine mouthwashes on 50 soldiers, Scand. J. Dent. Res. 80:10, 1972.

46. Frandsen, A.: Oral Hygiene. Copenhagen: Munksgaard, 1972.

47. Friedman, L., et al: Bacterial plaque disclosure surgery, J. Periodont. 45:435, 1974.

48. Garfin, L.A.: Something old, something new. Toothpicks and toothbrushes, Dent. Surv. 40:102, 1964.

49. Garnick, J.: Use of indexes for plaque control, J.A.D.A. 86:1325, 1973.

50. Giedrys-Leeper, F., Selipsky, H., and Williams, B.L.: Effects of short-term administration of metronidazole on the subgingival microflora, J. Clin. Periodontol. 12:797, 1985.

51. Gjermo, P., and Flotra, L.: The plaque removing effect of dental floss and toothpicks: A group comparison study, J. Periodont. Res. 4:170, 1969.

52. Gjermo, P., and Flotra, L.: The effect of different methods of interdental cleaning, J. Periodont. Res. 5:230, 1970.

53. Glavind, L., Zeuner, E., and Attstrom, R.: Oral hygiene instruction of adults by means of a self-instructional manual, J. Clin. Periodontol. 8:165, 1981.

54. Glickman, I., Petralis, R., and Marks, R.: The effect of powered toothbrushing plus interdental stimulation upon the severity of gingivitis, J. Periodont. 35:519, 1964.

55. Glickman, I., Petralis, R., and Marks, R.: The effect of powered toothbrushing and interdental stimulation upon microscopic inflammation and surface keratinization of the interdental gingiva, J. Periodont. 36:108, 1965.

56. Glickman, I.: Clinical Periodontology. 4th ed. Philadelphia: W.B. Saunders Co., 1972.

57. Gordon, J.M., Lamster, J.B., and Seiger, M.C.: Efficacy of Listerine antiseptic in inhibiting the development of plaque and gingivitis, J. Clin. Periodontol. 12:697, 1985.

58. Gordon, J., Walker, C., Lamster, I., West, T., Socransky, S., Seiger, M., and Fasciano, R.: Efficacy of clindamycin hydrochloride in refractory periodontitis. 12-month results, J. Periodont., Suppl., p. 25, 1985.

59. Greene, J.C.: Oral health care for prevention and control of periodontal disease. In World Workshop in Periodontics, 1966, ed. S.P. Ramfjord, D.A. Kerr, and M.M. Ash. Ann Arbor, Michigan: The University of Michigan, 1966.

60. Greenwell, H., Bahr, A., Brossada, N., Debaune, S., and Rowland, D.: The effect of Keye's method of oral hygiene on the subgingival micro-flora compared to the effect of scaling and/or surgery, J. Clin. Periodontol. 12:327, 1985.

61. Gustafsson, B.E., et al: The Vipeholm dental caries study. The effect of different levels of carbohydrate on caries activity in 436 individuals observed for five years, Acta Odont. Scand. 11:195, 1954.

62. Hansen, F., and Gjermo, P.: The plaque removing effect of four toothbrushing methods, Scand. J. Dent. Res. 79:502, 1971.

63. Hardy, J.H., Newman, H.N., and Strahan, J.D.: Direct irrigation and subgingival plaque, J. Clin. Periodontol. 9:57, 1982.

64. Harte, D.B., and Manly, R.S.: Four variables affecting magnitude of dentifrice abrasiveness, J. Dent. Res. 55:322, 1976.

65. Ellden, L., Camosci, D., Hock, J., and Tianoff, N.: Clinical study to compare the effect of stannous fluoride and chlorhexidine mouthrinses on plaque formation, J. Clin. Periodontol. 8:12, 1981.

66. Hill, H.C., Levi, F.A., and Glickman, I.: The effects of waxed and unwaxed dental floss on interdental plaque accumulation and interdental gingival health, J. Periodont. 44:411, 1973.

67. Hine, M.K.: The use of the toothbrush in the treatment of periodontitis, J.A.D.A. 41:158, 1950.

68. Hine, M.K., Wachtl, C., and Fosdick, L.S.: Some observations on the cleansing effect of nylon and bristle toothbrushes, J. Periodont. 25:183, 1954.

69. Hirschfeld, I.: The Toothbrush. Its Use and Abuse. Brooklyn: Dental Items of Interest, 1939.

70. Horowitz, H.S.: A review of systemic and topical fluorides for the prevention of dental caries, Community Dent. Oral Epidemiol. 1:104, 1973.

71. Kardel, K.M., Olesen, K.P., and Bay, I.: Tandborstens evne til a fjerne plaque, Tandlaegebladet 75:189, 1971.

72. Keller, S.E., and Manson-Hing, L.R.: Clearance studies of proximal tooth surfaces. Parts III and IV. In vivo removal of interproximal plaque, Ala. J. Med. Sci. 6:399, 1969.

73. Koch, G., and Lindhe, J.: The state of the gingiva and the caries increment in school children during and after withdrawal of various prophylactic measures. In Dental Plaque, ed. W.D. McHugh. Edinburgh: E.S. Livingstone, 1970.

74. Kristoffersen, T.: Periodontal conditions in Norwegian soldiers—an epidemiological and experimental study, Scand. J. Dent. Res. 78:34, 1970.

75. Lang, N.P., Cumming, B.R., and Löe, H.: Toothbrush frequency as it is related to plaque development and gingival health, J. Periodont. 44:396, 1973.

76. Lang, N.P., and Raber, J.: Use of oral irrigators as vehicle for the application of antimicrobial agents in chemical plaque control, J. Clin. Periodontol. 8:177, 1981.

77. Lindhe, J., and Wicin, P.O.: The effects on the gingivae of chewing fibrous food, J. Periodont. Res. 4:193, 1969.

78. Lindhe, J., Hamp, S.E., and Löe, H.: Experimental periodontitis in the beagle dog, J. Periodont. Res. 8:1, 1973.

79. Lindhe, J., Axelsson, P., and Tollsbog, G.: Effect of proper oral hygiene on gingivitis and dental caries in Swedish schoolchildren, Community Dent. Oral Epidemiol. 3:150, 1975.

80. Lobene, R.R.: The effect of a pulsed water pressure cleansing device on oral health, J. Periodont. 40:667, 1969.

81. Löe, H., Theilade, R., and Jensen, S.B.: Experimental gingivitis in man, J. Periodont. 36:177, 1965.

82. Löe, H., et al: Experimental gingivitis in man. III. The influence of antibiotics on gingival plaque development, J. Periodont. Res. 2:282, 1967.

83. Löe, H.: A review of the prevention and control of plaque. In Dental Plaque, ed. W.D. McHugh. Edinburgh: E.S. Livingstone, 1970.

84. Löe, H., and Schiott, C.R.: The effect of mouthrinses and topical application of chlorhexidine in the development of gingivitis in man, J. Periodont. Res. 5:79, 1970.

85. Löe, H., von der Fehr, F.R., and Schiott, C.R.: Inhibiting experimental caries by plaque prevention. The effect of chlorhexidine mouthrinses, Scand. J. Dent. Res. 80:1, 1972.

86. Löe, H., et al: Two years oral use of chlorhexidine in man, J. Periodont. Res. 11:135, 1976.

87. Loesche, W., et al: The effect of topical kanamycin on plaque accumulation, I.A.D.R. Abstract No. 281, 1971.

88. Lovdal, A., Arno, A., and Waerhaug, J.: Incidence of clinical

manifestations of periodontal disease in light of oral hygiene and calculus formation, J.A.D.A. 56:21, 1958.

89. Lyons, H.: Fiction and facts in periodontology: An appraisal, J.A.D.A. 39:513, 1949.

90. MacAlpine, R., Magnuson, I., Kiger, R., Crigger, M., Garrett, S., and Egelberg, J.: Antimicrobial irrigation of deep pockets to supplement oral hygiene instruction and root debridement. I. Bi-weekly irrigation, J. Clin. Periodontol. 12:568, 1985.

91. Manly, R.S., and Brudevold, F.: Relative abrasiveness of natural and synthetic toothbrush bristles on cementum and dentin, J.A.D.A. 55:779, 1957.

92. Marshall, J.S.: Principles and Practice of Operative Dentistry. Philadelphia: J.B. Lippincott Co, 1901.

93. Marthaler, T.: Apfel, Gesundheit und Kauorgan, Schweiz. Mschr. Zahnheilkd. 78:832, 1968.

94. Mazza, J.E., Newman, M.G., and Sims, T.N.: Clinical and antimicrobial effect of stannous fluoride on periodontitis, J. Clin. Periodontol. 8:203, 1981.

95. McCornell, D., and Conroy, C.W.: Comparisons of abrasion produced by a simulated manual versus a mechanical toothbrush, J. Dent. Res. 3:224, 1968.

96. McKendrick, A.J.W., Barbenel, L.M.H., and McHugh, W.D.: A two-year comparison of hand and electric toothbrushes, J. Periodont. Res. 3:224, 1968.

97. McKendrick, A.J.W., McHugh, W.D., and Barbenel, L.M.H.: Toothbrush age and wear, Br. Dent. J. 130:66, 1971.

98. Moss, A.: Kliniske undersogelser over nogle tandpastaers og tanpulvers virkning over for plaqueforekomst, Tandlaegebladet 75:197, 1971.

99. Mousques, T., Listgarten, M.A., and Phillips, R.W.: Effect of scaling and root planing on the composition of the human subgingival microbial flora, J. Periodont. Res. 15:144, 1980.

100. Mühlemann, H.R., Hulss, D., and Steiner, C.: Antimicrobial rinses and proximal plaque on removeable gold crowns, Helv. Odont. Acta 17:89, 1973.

101. Muhler, J.C., and Stookey, G.K.: The development of an improved $ZrSiO^4$ prophylactic paste, J. Periodont. 41:290, 1970.

102. Newman, H.N., Young, F.I.S., Wan Ysof, W.Z.A.B., and Addy, M.: Slow release metronidazole and a simplified mechanical oral hygiene regimen in the control of chronic periodontitis, J. Clin. Periodontol. 11:576, 1984.

103. Nyman, S., Rosling, B., and Lindhe, J.: Effect of professional tooth cleaning on healing after periodontal surgery, J. Clin. Periodontol. 2:80, 1975.

104. Ramfjord, S.P.: Indices for prevalence and incidence of periodontal disease, J. Periodont. 30:51, 1959.

105. Ramfjord, S.: Survey of the periodontal status of boys 11 to 17 years old in Bombay, India, J. Periodont. 32:237, 1961.

106. Ramfjord, S.P., Morrison, E.C., Burgett, F.G., Nissle, R., Schick, R.A., Zann, G.J., and Knowles, J.W.: Oral hygiene and maintenance of periodontal support, J. Periodont. 53:26, 1982.

107. Report of the Council on Dental Therapeutics of the American Dental Association: Abrasivity of Current Dentifrices, J.A.D.A. 81:1177, 1970.

108. Reithe, P.: Prophylaxe parodontalen Erkerankungen im Rahmen der Konservativen Therapie, Dtsch. Zahnarztl. Zeitschr. 21:64, 1964.

109. Roberts, W.R., and Addy, M.: Comparison of the biskiguanide antiseptics alexidine and chlorhexidine. I. Effect on plaque accumulation and salivary bacteria, J. Clin. Periodontol. 8:213, 1981.

110. Robinson, H.B.G., and Kitchin, P.C.: The effect of massage with the toothbrush on keratinization of the gingiva, Oral Surg. 1:1042, 1948.

111. Rolla, G., Löe, H., and Schiott, C.R.: Retention of chlorhexidine in the human oral cavity, Arch. Oral Biol. 16:1109, 1971.

112. Rosling, B., Nyman, S., and Lindhe, J.: The effect of systematic plaque control on bone regeneration in infrabony pockets, J. Clin. Periodontol. 3:38, 1976.

113. Rosling, B., et al: The healing potential of the periodontal tissues following different techniques of periodontal surgery in plaque-free dentitions. A two-year clinical study, J. Clin. Periodontol. 3:233, 1976.

114. Rosling, B.G., Slots, J., Webber, R.L., Christersson, L.A., and Genco, R.J.: Microbiological and clinical effects of topical subgingival antimicrobial treatment on human periodontal disease, J. Clin. Periodontol. 10:487, 1983.

115. Russel, A.L., and Ayers, P.: Periodontal disease and socioeconomic status in Birmingham, Ala., Am. J. Public Health 50:206, 1960.

116. Saxton, C.A.: The effects of dentifrices on the appearance of the tooth surface observed with the scanning electron microscope, J. Periodont. Res. 11:74, 1967.

117. Schmid, M.O., and Curilovic, Z.: Die Wirkung von Instruktion und Motivation auf die Mundhygiene, Schweiz. Mschr. Zahnheilkd. 85:457, 1975.

118. Scully, C.M., and Wade, A.B.: The relative plaque-removing effect of brushes of different length and texture, Dent. Pract. Dent. Rec. 20:244, 1970.

119. Shiller, N., and Dittmer, J.: An evaluation of some current oral hygiene motivation methods, J. Periodont. 39:83, 1968.

120. Shulman, J.: Current concepts of patient motivation towards long-term oral hygiene: A literature review, J. Am. Soc. Prev. Dent. 4:7, 1974.

121. Skinner, E.W., and Tabata, G.K.: Abrasions of tooth surface by nylon and natural bristle toothbrushes, J. Dent. Res. 30:522, 1951.

122. Smith, J.F., and Blankenship, J.: Improving oral hygiene in handicapped children by the use of an electric toothbrush, J. Dent. Child. 31:198, 1964.

123. Smith, J.H., O'Conner, T.W., and Radentz, W.: Oral hygiene of the interdental area, Periodontics 1:204, 1963.

124. Sorrin, S., and Thaller, J.L.: The interproximal stimulator. An adjunct in periodontal therapy, J. Periodont. 30:44, 1959.

125. Stralfors, A.: Disinfection of dental plaque in man, Odont. Tidskr. 70:182, 1962.

126. Suomi, J.D., et al: The effect of controlled oral hygiene procedures on the progression of periodontal disease in adults: Results after third and final year, J. Periodont. 42:152, 1971.

127. Talbot, E.S.: Interstitial Gingivitis or So-called Pyorrhoea Alveolaris. Philadelphia: S.S. White Dental Mfg. Co., 1899.

128. Vogel, R.S., et al: Evaluation of cleansing devices in the maintenance of interproximal gingival health, J. Periodont. 46:745, 1976.

129. Vogel, R.J.: The experimental use of anti-inflammatory drugs in the treatment of periodontal disease. A review, J. Periodont. (Suppl.) p. 88, 1985.

130. Volpe, A.R., et al: Antimicrobial control of bacterial plaque and calculus and effects of these agents on oral flora, J. Dent. Res. 48:832, 1965.

131. Volpe, A.R., et al: A long-term clinical study evaluating the effect of two dentifrices on oral tissues, J. Periodont. 46:113, 1976.

132. Walsh, M.M., Buchanan, S.A., Hoover, C.I., Newbrun, E., Taggart, E.J., Armitage, G.C., and Robertson, P.B.: Clinical and microbiologic effects of single-dose metronidazole or scaling and root planing in treatment of adult periodontitis, J. Clin. Periodontol. 13:151, 1986.

133. Wennstrom, J., and Lindhe, J.: Some effects of a sanguinarine containing mouthrinse on developing plaque and gingivitis,

J. Clin. Periodontol. 12:867, 1985.

134. Wennstrom, J., and Lindhe, J.: The effect of mouthrinses on parameters characterizing human periodontal disease, J. Clin. Periodontol. 13:86, 1986.

135. Westfelt, E., Nyman, S., Socransky, S., and Lindhe, J.: Significance of frequency of professional tooth cleaning for healing following periodontal surgery, J. Clin. Periodontol. 10:148, 1983.

136. Wilcox, C.E., and Everett, F.G.: Friction on the teeth and the gingiva during mastication, J.A.D.A. 66:513, 1963.

137. Wilkins, E.M., and McCullough, P.A.: Clinical Practice of the Dental Hygienist. 2nd ed. Philadelphia: Lea and Febiger, 1964.

138. Wolffe, G.N.: An evaluation of surface cleansing agents, J. Clin. Periodontol 3:148, 1976.

139. Zaki, H.A., and Stallard, R.E.: An evaluation of the effectiveness of preventive periodontol education, J. Periodont. Res. Suppl. 3, 1969.

19

OCCLUSAL THERAPY IN PERIODONTICS

The elimination of periodontal injuries of a functional or dysfunctional origin requires occlusal therapy. Occlusal therapy thus constitutes an important part of the periodontal therapy for patients with traumatic periodontal injuries. Occlusion, as expressed in the morphological arrangement of the teeth, may in addition influence plaque retention, hygienic procedures, gingival morphology, and even the feasibility of successful pocket therapy. Occlusal therapy may also be indicated as part of the total periodontal treatment for esthetic reasons.

Occlusal therapy related to periodontics may be considered as comprising four categories: (1) orthodontic treatment, (2) temporary and provisional splinting, (3) occlusal adjustment, and (4) restorative dentistry and permanent splinting of teeth. The order in which these procedures are given is related to the sequence of therapy in the periodontal treatment plan.

ORTHODONTICS

Because there is no significant correlation between malocclusion according to Angle's classification and severity of periodontal disease,[16] orthodontic treatment of malocclusion should not be considered as a routine preventive or therapeutic procedure in periodontics. It has been shown that orthodontic treatment will not alter the periodontal prognosis for the better or the worse.[42] Even specific features of malocclusion, such as overbite, overjet, faulty intercuspidation, and anterior crowding, have been shown to be significant periodontal handicaps only for patients with poor oral hygiene.[2,3] Thus, malocclusion usually represents more of an esthetic and psychological problem than a periodontal one. However, there are a number of more specific aspects of combined malocclusion and periodontal disease in which orthodontic treatment may augment the periodontal treatment, or even be essential for optimal results.

Indications for othodontic treatment

1. *Impinging overbite* or shearing occlusion with trauma to the gingival tissues (Fig. 19-1). In order to eliminate the traumatic effect of the occlusion upon the gingival tissues, patients often need extensive orthodontic therapy or, in extreme situations, combined surgical and orthodontic therapy. The orthodontic treatment often must be augmented by occlusal adjustment and restorative procedures.[36]

2. *Extreme maxillary protrusion*, where the maxillary anterior teeth protrude between the lips (Fig. 19-2) and prevent normal lip seal.[12] Treatment of gingivitis associated with mouth-breathing in such patients is facilitated by elimination of the protrusion of the teeth.

3. *Functional anterior crossbite* or other unstable occlusal relationships, where the impact in closure moves the teeth in one direction while lip and tongue musculatures move the teeth in the opposite direction (Fig. 19-3). Such a jiggling of the teeth associated with occlusion seems to aggravate destructive periodontal disease,[28] and should be eliminated by occlusal adjustment or by orthodontic treatment, whichever is the more practical approach.

4. *Tipped teeth.* Trauma from occlusion is often seen in association with tipped teeth. Tipping causes formation of pseudopockets, and the deepened sulci often develop into true periodontal pockets. Uprighting tipped teeth orthodontically (Fig. 19-4) may increase the ability of the teeth to withstand occlusal forces and also reduce the depth of the pocket associated with the tipping.[7,27]

5. *Food impaction* associated with faulty contacts that may be eliminated by orthodontic treatment. Teeth that are rotated may not make contact with the neighboring teeth at the normal contact areas. Such faulty contacts may predispose to plaque retention, food impaction, and gingival irritation. Open contacts

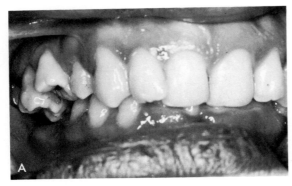

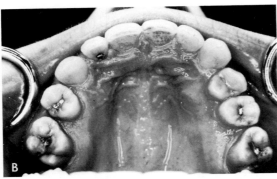

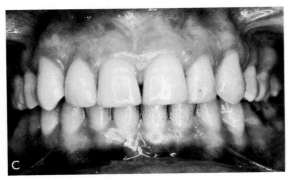

Fig. 19-1. *A,* Shearing malocclusion for right molars and impinging overbite in the anterior region. *B,* Palatal impingement. *C,* Good functional occlusion after orthodontic treatment.

are usually of concern in periodontal therapy only when food impaction occurs.

6. *Malposition of teeth* in relation to the alveolar process. Teeth in extreme labio- or linguoversion often develop a gingival dehiscence or cleft, which can be treated successfully and with favorable long-term prognosis only if the teeth are brought to a normal relationship with the alveolar process. If the recession associated with the malposition is not extreme, a normal gingival level may develop following the orthodontic repositioning of the teeth, and no specific periodontal therapy will be necessary.

7. *Fibrous gingival hyperplasia,* such as Dilantin gingivitis or hereditary gingival fibromatosis, often involves a very disfiguring malocclusion in the anterior region as a result of pressure from the hyperplastic tissues (Fig. 19-5). This malposition of the teeth should be treated orthodontically following removal of the hyperplastic gingival tissues, in order to achieve the optimal treatment results from both functional and esthetic standpoints and to facilitate good oral hygiene, which is essential for prevention or recurrence of the hyperplasia.

8. *Extensive open bites* associated with tongue habits and occlusal contact on only the last molars (Fig. 19-6) are often associated with severe periodontal disease around these molars.[36] Orthodontic treatment with or without surgery should always be considered for such patients.

9. *Extruded single-rooted teeth* with advanced periodontal disease may be moved back into the alveolar process orthodontically.[36] Such movement will create intrabony pockets, which may then be treated successfully with reattachment therapy. Forced orthodontic eruption of teeth with isolated intrabony pockets may also help in elimination of the pockets.[26]

Timing of orthodontics

A question often asked is, *When during a course of*

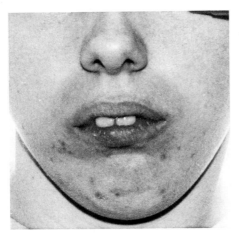

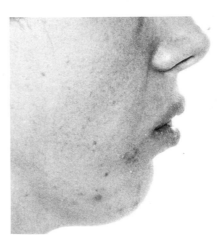

Fig. 19-2. Lack of lip seal associated with mouthbreathing and malocclusion. Note characteristic inactive, partially collapsed nostrils.

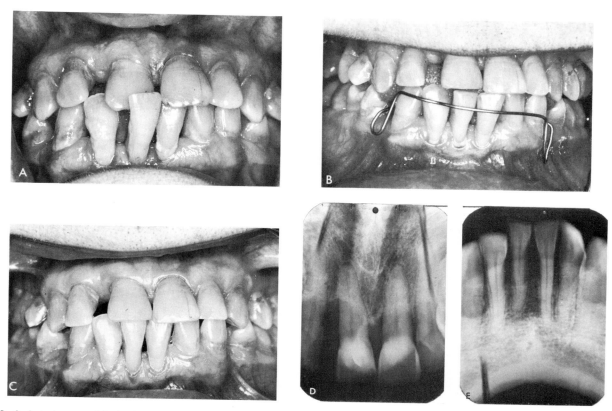

Fig. 19-3. *A,* Anterior crossbite in 60-year-old patient. *B,* Following scaling, the front teeth were reduced in length and the protruded mandibular right incisor brought lingually with a mandibular Hawley appliance. *C,* One year after orthodontic treatment, the occlusal function is good and the hypermobility has been eliminated. *D,E,* Roentgenograms one year after the orthodontic treatment show a well-defined lamina dura over the alveolar crest, indicating arrested bone loss. This patient has been observed for 17 years and no further bone loss has occurred. Further closure of the open contacts would have been impractical, because it would have required permanent splinting or orthodontic retention of the teeth.

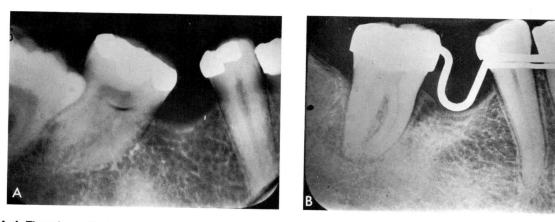

Fig. 19-4. *A,* Tipped mandibular second molar and partially erupted third molar, which later was extracted. *B,* Uprighting and intrusion of the tipped molar. Observe new bone formation at the mesial side of the molar.

periodontal therapy should orthodontic tooth movement be done? Orthodontic treatment should not be initiated until the teeth have been thoroughly scaled, the roots have been planed, and the patient has been instructed in oral hygiene.

Orthodontic treatment should be completed prior to a complete occlusal adjustment; however, in some instances, as with an anterior slide in centric and a forward impact on the maxillary incisor in centric occlusion, it is advisable to do a preliminary occlusal adjustment[36] to eliminate the slide in centric prior to the orthodontic tooth movement.

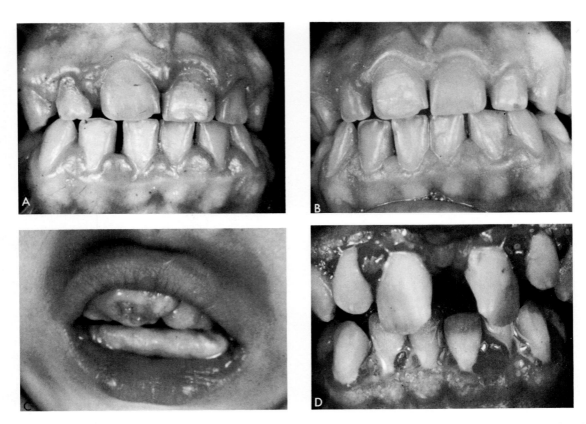

Fig. 19-5. *A,* Dilantin gingivitis with beginning separation of the anterior teeth. *B,* Following hygienic phase of the periodontal therapy, there is some reduction of the gingival hyperplasia and the distemas between the teeth. *C,* Severe Dilantin gingivitis. *D,* After removal of the hyperplastic gingiva, severe malposition of the teeth is evident.

The orthodontic treatment should be completed prior to the periodontal surgery, except in cases of fibrotic gingival hyperplasia, where the hyperplastic fibrotic tissues should be removed before beginning the orthodontic treatment. The main reason for postponing the periodontal surgery until completion of the orthodontic treatment is that the healing periodontal fibers will then be reoriented to the new tooth position, and thus, it is hoped, facilitate retention.[11] To allow for maturation of the new collagen fibers, the use of orthodontic appliances for splinting and retention for 3 to 4 months following the periodontal surgery is recommended. In addition, if the teeth were intruded into the alveolar process, the residual intrabony pockets following the orthodontic treatment will require reattachment therapy.

PERIODONTAL HAZARDS ASSOCIATED WITH ORTHODONTIC THERAPY
Periodontal abscesses

Orthodontic movement of teeth with periodontal pockets that have not had prior complete removal of subgingival calculus may result in periodontal abscesses, especially if a tooth is moved against the bony wall of an intrabony pocket. This hazard can be avoided by complete scaling and root planing, fol-

lowed by good oral hygiene. Orthodontic bands extended subgingivally are always a periodontal irritant.[57] The closer to the cementoenamel junction or to the attachment the bands are extended, the greater the hazard of loss of connective tissue attachment to the teeth from inflammation related to the margins of the bands. Conventional orthodontic treatment has actually been found to result in a slight but statistically significant loss of periodontal attachment in a group of children who were treated orthodontically, compared with a similar group that did not receive such treatment.[51,55,56] The new procedure of bonding orthodontic brackets to the teeth with adhesive materials makes it possible to carry out orthodontic treatment with less periodontal irritation.[58]

Faulty appliances

Faultily constructed removable orthodontic appliances can create gingival injury as a result of impingement (Fig. 19-7). Fortunately, periodontal lesions accidentally produced in this way have a fairly good prognosis for healing (Fig. 19-8).

Root resorption

Shortening of the root through root resorption is

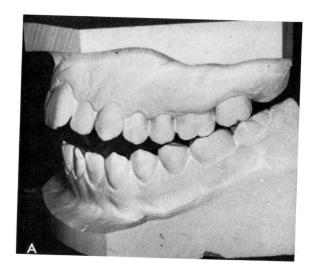

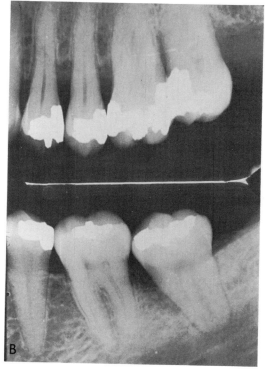

Fig. 19-6. *A,* Open bite with centric contacts only on the second molars. *B,* Severe bone loss on the mesial side of the mandibular second molar and around the maxillary second molar.

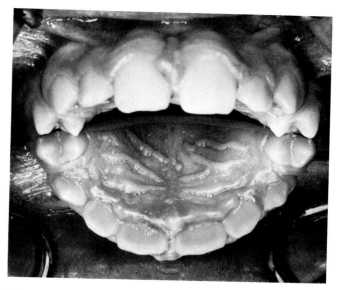

Fig. 19-7. *A,* Injury to the palatal and interproximal gingival tissues caused by a Hawley appliance that was forced against the gingiva by the occlusion.

another hazard of orthodontic treatment (Fig. 19-9) Root resorption is primarily apt to occur following use of heavy forces, which have a necrotizing effect on the periodontal membrane.[39] Since the force per unit of periodontal support may easily be high for teeth that have lost periodontal support, great restraint in application of force on such teeth is important.

Problems of age

Orthodontic treatment can be carried out successfully at any age, even advanced age. However, it is generally assumed that rebuilding of bone and reorientation of the trabecular system in bone takes place at a slower rate with increased age, thus requiring more time for orthodontic movement and retention in older than in younger individuals.

Newer appliances

The use of plastic-bonded brackets, lingually placed brackets, and coated-wire appliances has made the conventional unsightly orthodontic appliances unnecessary and thus made orthodontic treatment more acceptable to adults. However, it still appears true that whenever the objectives of the orthodontic treatment can be achieved by removable appliances, such appliances should be employed. They are safer, being less apt to cause gingival irritation and root resorption than are fixed appliances. Their main shortcoming is that they are essentially good only for tipping of teeth and maxillary expansion. For the technical aspects of orthodontic therapy, refer to textbooks in orthodontics[17,23] and occlusion.[36]

TEMPORARY AND PROVISIONAL SPLINTING

By definition, a *splint* is a rigid or flexible appliance used to stabilize and protect an injured part. In dentistry, splinting is used to gain occlusal stability. Splints may be classified as (1) temporary, (2) diagnostic or provisional, and (3) permanent. Each of these groups includes both fixed and removable appliances.[36] Splints engaging the crown of the teeth on the outside surfaces of the crown are called *external splints*, while those fitted or attached to the inside circumference of the teeth are called *internal splints*.

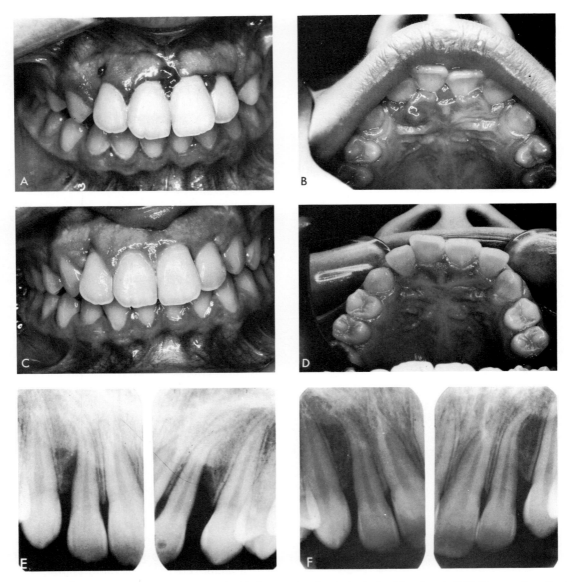

Fig. 19-8. *A,B,* Severe acute periodontitis associated with fragments of subgingival rubber band. *C,D,* Six months after removal of rubber band fragments during a mucoperiosteal flap procedure. Marked reduction of inflammation and pocket depth. *E,* Roentgenogram at the time of removal of the rubber band fragments. *F,* Six months after the flap operation. Considerable regeneration of bone on the distal aspects of both lateral incisors is apparent.

Indications for splinting

The purpose of a temporary splint is to reduce occlusal forces and stabilize teeth for a limited period of time. Temporary stabilization of teeth may be important (1) following accidental loosening of teeth by trauma, (2) as a supportive measure to facilitate periodontal therapeutic procedures for hypermobile teeth, (3) to avoid dislodging teeth prior to and during reconstruction procedures, and (4) for anchorage and temporary retention in orthodontic therapy.

The provisional or diagnostic splint has been recommended for borderline cases in which the final results of the periodontal treatment cannot be predicted

with certainty at the time of the initial treatment planning.[21] The alleged value of provisional splinting of teeth with regard to promotion of healing and regeneration of periodontal structures[14,21,30] has not been substantiated by research findings,[20,28,40,41] and reports indicate that such splinting may lead to ankylosis and resorption of traumatized teeth.[4,5] The results for reimplanted avulsed teeth were best if the teeth were not splinted. Splinting reduces the mobility of all of the teeth splinted together while the splint is in place, but when it is removed, even after 1 year, the mobility is the same as before the splinting.[41]

Mobility also is decreased following local treatment

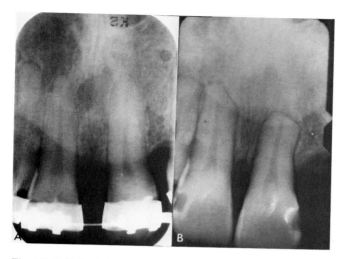

Fig. 19-9. At the initiation of orthodontic treatment in a 28-year-old male. *B,* After 6 months of orthodontic attempts to move the teeth together quickly. Root resorption evident on both central incisors.

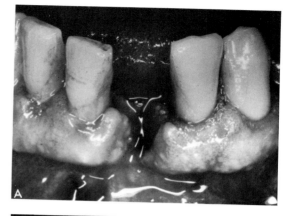

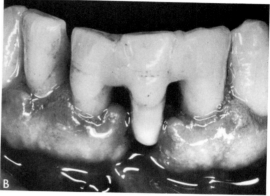

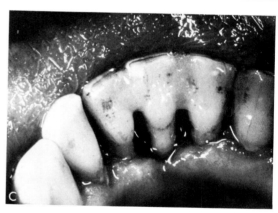

of periodontal disease even without splinting.[38,40,54] Thus, it is difficult to assess the need for splinting prior to periodontal treatment, and the value of the splinting as a component of the treatment.

Previous concepts concerning the significance of tooth mobility were based on the assumption that mobility beyond the normal level signified trauma from occlusion,[29] which tended to accelerate the progress of the pocket formation.[19] Since it has been shown in animal studies[48,53] that increased mobility may persist without actual trauma, and in longitudinal clinical trials that nonprogressive mobility does not seem to affect the periodontal prognosis,[37] elimination of the excessive mobility is not as important a goal of periodontal therapy as previously assumed.

Whether trauma from occlusion will interfere with healing following periodontal therapy is not known,[20,43] and it is possible that provisional splinting of teeth with progressive trauma from occlusion may be of benefit during the postoperative healing stage of periodontal therapy. However, using provisional splinting as a test of need for permanent splinting may produce meaningless results, because mobility of the individual teeth is not reduced by the provisional splinting.[40] There is some indication that abnormal mobility has an adverse effect on treatment results of periodontal pockets.[15]

Types of temporary splints

The *external wire ligature splint* has traditionally been the most popular splint for temporary stabilization of teeth. With the advent of self-curing acrylic, this type of splint became very effective in stabilization of teeth and esthetically less objectionable than when the wires were exposed.[36] Annealed stainless steel lig-

Fig. 19-10. *A,B,C,* Extracted loose mandibular incisor bonded temporarily to the adjacent remaining teeth. Even better is use of a plastic denture tooth for replacement of the missing tooth. With this, the gingival irritation from a conventional "flipper" is avoided.

ature wires (0.010 or 0.012 inch), single or double, may be adapted to the teeth facially and lingually, slightly gingivally to the contact areas (incisally to the cingulum of anterior teeth). The ends of the wire are tied together very loosely. Then wire loops (0.010 or 0.008 inch) are placed interproximally and tightened at the interproximal area, starting closest to the loop of the horizontal supporting wires. It is important to tuck the ends of the interproximal wire loops under the horizontal wire interproximally in order to avoid gingival irritation. The horizontal supporting wire is tightened after all the interproximal wires have been placed. Self-curing acrylic of the proper shade is then brushed over the wires and interproximally. This procedure should preferably be done under rubber dam in order to assure that the teeth are kept clean and dry and to avoid irritation of the gingival tissues from the acrylic monomer.

The recent advent of adhesive dental materials has made it possible to bond the interproximal contact areas of teeth together.[27] If the occlusion is reasonably well adjusted, the adhesive splint may function well for years, and can easily be repaired if the bond between the teeth is broken. It is important to allow adequate space for interproximal oral hygiene between the splint and the gingiva, regardless of the type of splint used.

External types of splints should always be used for temporary splinting, unless the teeth already have cavities or defective fillings in need of restorative procedures.[31] Making horizontal grooves in maxillary or mandibular anterior teeth[22] for wire-acrylic combination splints should be avoided unless one wants to commit the teeth to full crown splinting in the future. Full crowns extended subgingivally will contribute to gingival irritation and periodontal disease, even if they are made according to the best available principles.[46] For the same reason, it is not recommended that conjoint acrylic full crowns[50] be used for temporary splints, unless the teeth definitely need full crowns.

Temporary splinting of bicuspids and molars with various wire acrylic combinations, amalgam, or acrylic splints[36] is not recommended as part of periodontal therapy unless the splinting is related to hemisection of teeth or used to maintain teeth in a desired position until restorative dentistry can be done (Fig. 19-10).

Biteplanes as occlusal splints

The purposes for which biteplanes are used extensively in occlusal therapy are given in the following outline:

1. Eliminate trauma from occlusion.
2. Eliminate pain from temporomandibular joint and muscle dysfunction.
3. Facilitate registration of jaws in centric relation.
4. Control bruxism and prevent excessive wear of teeth.
5. Break occlusal habits (e.g., fingernail biting).
6. Stabilize mobile teeth.
7. Prevent hypereruption of teeth without antagonists.
8. Differential diagnosis of facial pain.
9. Maintain teeth in position after orthodontics.
10. Disocclude teeth during orthodontics.

A flat maxillary biteplane with cuspid rise[5,36] is the best universal appliance for prompt temporary elim-

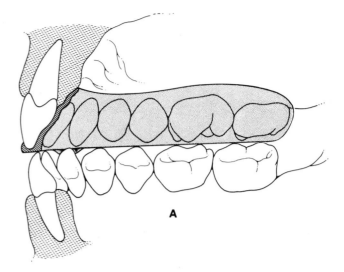

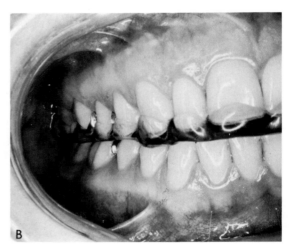

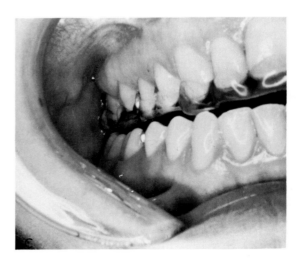

Fig. 19-11. *A,* Schematic drawing of the occlusal relationships of a maxillary biteplane. *B,* Clinical picture of the biteplane with the mandible in centric relation. *C,* "Cuspid raise" in right lateral excursion with disocclusion of all teeth except the mandibular working side cuspid against the acrylic.

ination of trauma from occlusion (Fig. 19-11). It is especially important to use biteplanes for patients with bruxism and advanced periodontal disease, since the biteplane will induce muscle relaxation and eliminate the bruxism—at least while the patient is wearing the biteplane—thus greatly reducing the potential for trauma from occlusion. A biteplane should always be used prior to occlusal adjustment for patients in whom pain or high muscle tonus makes it difficult to determine the normal centric relation.

Periodontically, a biteplane is a much more favorable device than a Hawley appliance[24] as a retainer for maxillary teeth with tendencies toward pathological migration or relapse following orthodontic therapy. A Hawley appliance often induces jiggling of such teeth between labially directed occlusal forces against maxillary anterior teeth and lingually directed forces from the appliance, while in a biteplane the occlusal forces are transmitted in an axial direction of the teeth, eliminating the jiggling forces.

Orthodontic tooth movements for patients with temporomandibular joint pain and/or muscle dysfunction syndrome both will often aggravate the pain and discomfort, unless the teeth are disoccluded by a biteplane during the orthodontic therapy. Freedom for the desired teeth to move then has to be established within the biteplane. The biteplane is usually made to cover the incisal and occlusal surfaces of all maxillary teeth, with occlusal stops for all the mandibular teeth on a flat surface area around centric relation and with sufficient cuspid rise to disocclude the posterior and anterior regions during lateral and protrusive excursions.[5,44]

OCCLUSAL ADJUSTMENT IN PERIODONTAL THERAPY
Objectives of occlusal adjustment

The objectives of occlusal adjustment that may be applicable to some aspects of the periodontal therapy are given in the following outline:
1. Eliminate trauma from occlusion.
2. Eliminate bruxism.
3. Reduce abnormal tooth mobility.
4. Enhance functional capacity and comfort.
5. Induce favorable wear patterns.
6. Stabilize occlusion after orthodontics.
7. Correct abnormal swallowing habits.
8. Establish optimal occlusion for restorations.
9. Eliminate food impaction and impingement.
10. Improve esthetic appearance.

Periodontal trauma from occlusion constitutes an aberration in periodontal health. Therefore, the treatment of traumatic lesions in the periodontium always should be included in the periodontal therapy.

Elimination of trauma from occlusion

A number of dental treatment procedures, such as orthodontic treatment, use of temporary splints and biteplanes, occlusal adjustment, restorative, procedures, and permanent splinting of teeth, are aimed at eliminating trauma from occlusion. Occlusal adjustment, however, is the modality of first choice if trauma from occlusion can be eliminated and a comfortable, stable occlusion can be established by moderate grinding on the teeth. Occlusal adjustment may also constitute an important part of other treatment modalities aimed at elimination of trauma from occlusion.

Primary trauma from occlusion is usually related to occlusal interferences and bruxism, whereas secondary trauma from occlusion is usually related to advanced loss of periodontal support. Secondary trauma may be manifested clinically as severe tooth mobility, which may interfere with normal occlusal function. This form of trauma may or may not be related to bruxism. Occlusal adjustment is indicated for patients with both primary and secondary trauma from occlusion. It should be understood that the majority of patients with incipient to moderate periodontitis may have occlusal interferences but no evidence of either primary or secondary trauma from occlusion or any other occlusal problems needing treatment. For such patients, occlusal adjustment is not a rational part of the periodontal treatment.

Control of bruxism

In order to eliminate primary or secondary trauma from occlusion, it is essential to curb bruxism. This sometimes can be accomplished by occlusal adjustment alone,[34] but may in other instances require the use of both biteplanes and occlusal adjustment.[36] In patients with bruxism, the normal neuromuscular protection against periodontal injury from occlusal forces is inactivated, and traumatic injury associated with faulty occlusion may occur to any part of the masticatory system. If such an injury is diagnosed, the patients should receive occlusal therapy for the bruxism, whether they have periodontal disease. However, bruxism assumes an additional significance in patients who have lost a considerable amount of periodontal support and have active periodontitis.

With advancing loss of periodontal support, there is an increasing chance that bruxism will have a traumatic effect on the periodontium (Fig. 19-12), and the combination of periodontal trauma and periodontitis may accelerate the rate of periodontal breakdown and pocket formation.[8] Comprehensive and meticulously accurate occlusal adjustment is indicated as part of the periodontal and dental therapy for all patients with signs and symptoms of trauma from occlusion association with bruxism.

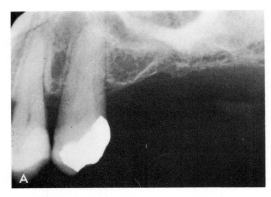

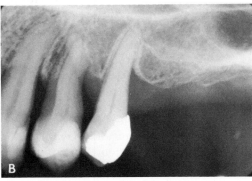

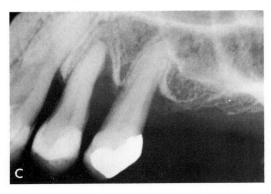

Fig. 19-12. *A,B,C,* There is a lapse of 1 year between each of these roentgenograms. Shortly after the first roentgenogram *(A)* was made, the patient came under severe psychic stress, started to grind his teeth, and the teeth became mobile. *B,* A year later, an unsuccessful attempt was made to adjust the occlusion. The mobility progressed until a biteplane was made one year later. *C,* The lamina dura is now well defined, but a marked widening of the periodontal space is evident at the distal aspect of both bicuspids.

Reduction of abnormal tooth mobility

Increased tooth mobility indicates that the optimal ratio between occlusal force and periodontal support has been exceeded. Although increase in tooth mobility does not always signify the presence of a traumatic injury, it indicates that a greater-than-normal functional demand has been placed on the remaining periodontal structures. This demand should be reduced whenever practical, in order to establish normal functional arrangement of the periodontal tissues.

With regard to a direct effect upon the periodontal therapy, reduction of hypermobility associated with secondary trauma from occlusion is of greater significance to the periodontal prognosis than is elimination of mobility related to primary trauma from occlusion. This is true because the secondary trauma occurs in teeth with a greater potential for accelerated periodontal destruction associated with the trauma[8] than teeth with normal periodontal support.

The essential approach to occlusal adjustment for patients with secondary trauma from occlusion is to assure that the biting forces in centric occlusion and centric relation are directed as much axially as possible and allow minimal or no eccentric contacts for teeth with abnormal mobility. All fremitus resulting from horizontal impact in complete centric occlusion closure should be eliminated. All functional guidance in lateral excursions beyond 1 mm from centric occlusion then is confined to the maxillary cuspids.

In many instances of secondary trauma from occlusion, the impact of the occlusal forces and the resultant tooth mobility can, by occlusal adjustment, be reduced to a level that is tolerated through a compensatory widening of the periodontal membrane without evidence of repeated or progressive traumatic injury. Although residual hypermobility does not represent the ideal outcome of the therapy, it may be preferable to permanent splinting of the teeth, which is the other alternative. Splinting must be used if repeated or progressive trauma from occlusion cannot be eliminated by occlusal adjustment.

On the basis of observations in a longitudinal study,[35,37] it appears that teeth with abnormal mobility after occlusal adjustment often maintain their residual periodontal support over an indefinite number of years, provided that good periodontal maintenance care is given and that there is sufficient support left for the teeth to permit mastication in a comfortable manner (Fig. 19-13). Many moderately severe mobility cases following occlusal adjustment may be maintained in a comfortable state without permanent splinting by the use of occlusal biteplanes.

Increasing functional capacity and comfort

In patients with advanced periodontitis and/or severe malocclusion, the masticatory system can be made to function more efficiently and comfortably following a well-planned and carefully executed occlusal adjustment. Reshaping of occlusal surfaces to enhance masticatory efficiency may also reduce both the forces required for mastication and the potential for trauma from occlusion, especially in patients with worn-out, flat occlusal restorations.

Induction of favorable wear patterns

It was shown in a longitudinal study by Beyron that

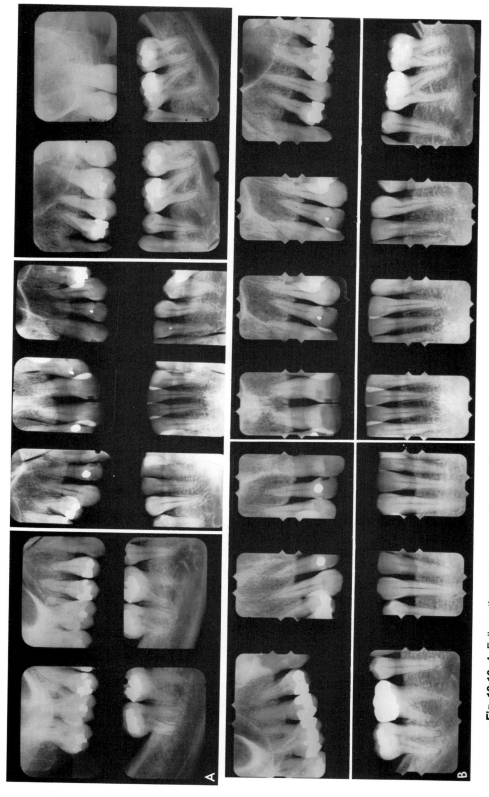

Fig. 19-13. *A,* Full mouth roentgenograms from a patient 37 years old. Moderately advanced bone loss with poorly defined alveolar crests and widened periodontal spaces. *B,* Fifteen years later. Occlusal adjustment, subgingival curettage, and recall for prophylaxis every 3 months had been done. Note the well-defined alveolar crest over the interproximal bone, and closure of contacts without orthodontic treatment.

multidirectional occlusal wear patterns tend to have a favorable long-term influence on the teeth and the periodontium, whereas restricted patterns gradually result in serious occlusal interferences and plunger cusp effects.[6] Multidirectional function is especially important for comfort and avoidance of trauma in patients who have lost a considerable part of their periodontal support. It is also assumed, based on animal experimentation[32] and observations in humans, that nonfunction has an unfavorable effect on periodontal health. Changing occlusal patterns so that multidirectional function is convenient to the patient will often extend functional activity to teeth that previously were not used because of occlusal interferences, thus reducing plaque and calculus retention on such teeth.

Stabilization of occlusion following orthodontic treatment

For the stability and function of the occlusion in patients who have received orthodontic treatment as part of their periodontal therapy, it is very important that comprehensive occlusal adjustment be done at the completion of the orthodontic treatment. The need for long-term or permanent retention of the teeth following orthodontic treatment can be greatly reduced by judicious occlusal adjustment.

Correction of abnormal swallowing habits

It has been reported that several patients with a "teeth-apart swallow" have developed a normal "teeth-together swallow" following occlusal adjustment.[36] This has been observed mainly in patients with considerable lateral discrepancy between centric relation and centric occlusion, as sometimes may occur following inadequate orthodontic therapy or faulty bite registrations in restorative dentistry. Such abnormal swallowing habits, often associated with a faulty tongue posture, may result in an unfavorable positioning of the teeth. The sequelae of abnormal swallowing and tongue habits tend to become progressively worse in patients with advanced periodontal bone loss, and occlusal therapy may be needed to stabilize the teeth.

Establishment of optimal occlusal relations prior to extensive restorative dentistry or splinting of teeth

By careful occlusal adjustment, optimal functional pathways for dental restorations may be established and the need for splinting of teeth minimized. Occlusal adjustment also allows teeth to move into optimal functional positions before preparation and placement of restorations.

Elimination of food impaction and impingement upon the gingival tissues

Gingival irritation from food impaction, impinging overbite, and faulty dental restorations or appliances may occasionally be eliminated by occlusal adjustment, although correction of such conditions often requires other modalities of dental treatment.[37] Occlusal adjustment may also eliminate plunger cusp effects, functional opening of contacts, and food impaction associated with occlusal interferences.

Improved esthetic appearance

Pathological migration of maxillary anterior teeth is often associated with advanced periodontal disease. Elimination of fremitus and shortening of the length of the teeth will often improve both esthetic and functional aspects of the occlusion for such patients.

Timing of occlusal adjustment

The question, *When during the course of periodontal therapy should occlusal adjustment be performed?* is an important one. A preliminary occlusal adjustment to eliminate painful or grossly disturbing occlusal interferences should be done on an emergency basis at the onset of the periodontal therapy. However, the teeth have a tendency to move back to a more normal position following scaling and instruction in oral hygiene, so for patients who need comprehensive occlusal adjustment, this adjustment should be postponed until the completion of the hygienic phase of the periodontal therapy. If the patient needs orthodontic treatment, this treatment should be completed prior to the occlusal adjustment, although minor corrections may be done during the orthodontic treatment. Occlusal adjustment should definitely be done prior to periodontal surgery and prior to extensive restorative dentistry involving occlusal surfaces of the teeth. A final check of occlusion with readjustment, if needed, should be done at the completion of the periodontal and dental therapy.

Methods of occlusal adjustment

Occlusal adjustment should be performed according to accepted principles and methods.[36] However, occlusal adjustment for patients with extensive loss of periodontal support and secondary trauma from occlusion may require specific measures, such as temporary stabilization of teeth during the adjustment and disocclusion of mobile teeth in excursions.

RESTORATIVE DENTISTRY AND PERMANENT SPLINTING OF TEETH IN THE TREATMENT OF PERIODONTAL DISEASE

Food impaction

Food impaction must be eliminated in order to maintain periodontal health. In some cases, this can be achieved through orthodontic therapy or occlusal adjustment, while in others restorative dental procedures will be needed.[37] Open contacts without food impaction and with stable occlusal relations do not constitute a periodontal handicap and thus do not require restorative treatment. Placement of restorations with accentuated contour to protect the gingiva against contact with food in areas of gingival recession is not recommended, because rolled gingival margins against a flat root surface are compatible with health when proper toothbrushing techniques are applied, and claims of bruising of the gingival margin by food have not been substantiated.

Impinging overbite

Deep overbite with traumatic impingement of the anterior teeth against the palatal and labial gingival tissues may require dental restorations to eliminate the trauma to the gingiva.[37] The traumatic impingement usually becomes critical following loss of posterior teeth and subsequent loss of vertical occlusal dimension.[36] Grinding off the incisal edges of the maxillary incisors may eliminate the trauma to the labial mandibular gingiva, provided that the position of these teeth can subsequently be stabilized; however, grinding off the incisal edge of the mandibular front teeth and/or raising the bite on the remaining posterior teeth or edentulous ridges will not stabilize the vertical dimension of occlusion, and usually aggravates the periodontal disease by causing overeruption of front teeth and intrusion of posterior teeth, accompanied by ridge resorption and recurrence of the anterior impinging overbite. In addition to minor orthodontic treatment, including intrusion and retrusion of the anterior teeth, followed by occlusal adjustment, the anterior impingement can be alleviated by pinledge inlays placed on the palatal aspect of the maxillary teeth. Such inlays should have flat palatal ledges to receive the closure impact of the mandibular incisors in an axial direction and thus stabilize the occlusion.[37]

Palatal ledges should be placed on maxillary anterior teeth whenever there is a mobility problem in the maxillary anterior region. Especially effective in aiding stabilization of occlusion are palatal ledges or lingual cusps on maxillary cuspids, because the axial load on the teeth associated with such restorations is well tolerated and helps maintain the vertical dimension for the patient. In order to obtain the full benefit from these restorations, the palatal aspect of the maxillary anterior teeth must be sufficiently hollow ground to avoid interfering contacts or restrictive guidance when combined lateral and protrusive excursions are performed.[36] The incisal edges should make contact in protrusive excursion, which should disocclude the posterior teeth. In cases where there is a tendency for forward tipping of the maxillary anterior teeth, it is recommended to have cuspid guidance only, without a functioning incisal guidance in lateral excursions.

Tipped molars

A number of periodontal hazards have been related to tipping of molars and loss of vertical dimension following loss of adjacent teeth.[25]

The ideal solution to such cases would be to bring all the remaining teeth back to their original position orthodontically and then replace the lost teeth by fixed bridgework. However, this may involve excessively complicated and time-consuming procedures, and it is in most instances more practical to make occlusal adjustment and establish as favorable a plane of occlusion as possible, then stabilize the tipped teeth with fixed bridges.[37] The restorations for the tipped teeth should be shaped to resemble the crowns of upright teeth, in order to avoid having the mesial surfaces overlie the gingival tissues and thus enhance plaque formation and induce periodontal pockets. If a second mandibular molar has tipped close to the second bicuspid, it is not advisable to close the contact and attempt to stabilize the occlusion by tacking an overcontoured mesial inlay on the second molar, since such a restoration would induce the formation of a deep gingival crevice with poor access for oral hygiene, and, further, the molar could still tip lingually.

Permanent splinting with reduced periodontal support

The purposes of permanent splinting of teeth are to eliminate or prevent trauma from occlusion and to enhance functional stability and esthetics. However, there are a number of disadvantages to splinting, such as technical difficulty, cost, added problems related to plaque control, and iatrogenic periodontal disease related to subgingival margins, faulty contours, and other aspects of faulty dentistry.[47,52] Unquestionably, splinting of teeth may eliminate trauma from occlusion[37] and render a dentition ravished by advanced periodontal disease and tooth loss healthy, functional, and esthetically acceptable. Because of the already mentioned drawbacks, however, splinting should not be applied unless absolutely necessary to establish and maintain periodontal health and comfortable function. When it is needed, only the minimal amount of splinting required for health and function should be utilized. Splinting should be accomplished with minimal interference with normal gingival physiology, which means that preferably restorations should not contact the gingival tissues[46] and should not interfere with optimal oral hygiene procedures. Splinting of teeth does not eliminate the potential for periodontal trauma from occlusion,[18] and good occlusal relations and good oral hygiene are most important whether or not teeth are splinted.

The big controversy over splinting of teeth is how to determine whether the teeth need to be splinted. It has been widely assumed that clinically detectable increase of mobility signifies the presence of trauma from occlusion (traumatic lesions) in the periodontium, indicating a need for treatment,[10] and implies that if the mobility were not eliminated the alleged trauma would lead to progressive breakdown of the periodontal support.

It has now been established that hypermobility of teeth may persist over a prolonged time without actual evidence of trauma from occlusion,[49,53] and that in such a situation the hypermobility does not signify an etiologic factor in the development of destructive periodontal disease and does not require splinting as part of periodontal treatment.

However, progressive trauma from occlusion following occlusal adjustment, expressed as soreness of the teeth to pressure or percussion during and after function, continuous migration or tipping of teeth, and radiographic evidence of ongoing resorption of the alveolar bone (lamina dura) several months after occlusal adjustment, are all indications of permanent splinting of the teeth, since these findings are diagnostic of periodontal lesions. Splinting may also be indicated for maintenance of the teeth in the desired position following orthodontic treatment, as well as for esthetic considerations.

In order to assess whether mobile teeth should be splinted, it is also important to determine if the mobility is limited, within defined boundaries, or if it is progressive. A limited mobility is often seen as a jiggling of mandibular anterior teeth where the interproximal contacts stop the lingual movements of the teeth during function and the constant tongue pressure brings the teeth anteriorly to a constant position when the jaws are apart.

Another example may be posterior with buccolingual mobility, where disoccluding the teeth in all eccentric excursions may restrict the influence of the components of the occlusal forces that produce the mobility, thus limiting the mobility to a small area close to centric relation and centric occlusion. Such limited mobility may persist at a constant level without producing traumatic injury and without the need for splinting.

Examples of progressive mobility and persistent trauma from occlusion are seen in the maxillary anterior region, especially with deep overbite and loss of periodontal support; or associated with mesial tipping of posterior teeth, where loss of neighboring teeth has eliminated the possibility of self-stabilization of the occlusion. Such cases of progressive trauma from occlusion require splinting of the teeth. In the presence of cuspid-guided occlusion and with firm cuspids, there is very seldom a need for splinting of mobile posterior teeth, unless the mobility is extreme or some teeth are missing, with subsequent drifting and/or instability of the occlusal relations. Splinting of mandibular anterior teeth because of a moderate or even considerable increase in mobility that is not accompanied by discomfort is rarely indicated, because such mobility is usually not due to continuous occlusal trauma but is related to a well-defined and self-limited widening of the periodontal spaces.

Maxillary anterior teeth with advanced loss of periodontal support need splinting more often than mandibular teeth with a similar loss of support. The reason is that, especially with deep overbite or inadequate cuspid guidance, these teeth do not have a definite labial limitation to the movement pattern, meaning that drifting may occur, indicating repeated episodes of traumatic injuries. Malposition of teeth may become unacceptable, from both a functional and an esthetic standpoint, unless they are retained by permanent splinting.[37]

Mobility of teeth in an axial direction is poorly controlled by occlusal adjustment, and is usually associated with severe mobility in lateral directions. Such cases often require splinting in order to establish a comfortable and stable occlusion.

Pin-ledge restorations with no contact with the gingival tissues are preferable for splinting of anterior teeth, provided that the labial surfaces of the teeth are fairly intact. With multiple mobile abutments, full crown restorations have been considered to provide the best retention,[33] but from a periodontal standpoint these restorations are poor unless they are placed completely coronally to the free gingivae.

Splinting of teeth with advanced loss of periodontal support has often been used as a type of "shotgun therapy" to compensate for inadequate understanding of occlusal dynamics, with a resulting lack of accuracy in occlusal adjustment and construction of single restorations. With refinement of techniques for occlusal adjustment and increasing emphasis on essential features of occlusal anatomy, periodontal irritation, and plaque control associated with extensive restorative dentistry, the current trend is toward less and less splinting of teeth and toward covering smaller and smaller areas of the teeth with restorations.

Current trends are to deemphasize the need for replacement of every lost tooth, and to stabilize occlusal function and maintain periodontal health, preferably with fixed restorations. Partial dentures and removable appliances have produced controversial results regarding gain or loss of occlusal stability.[8,13,45] A main reason for loss of periodontal attachment in partial denture abutments seems to be increased gingival irritation with such appliances.[6] Lost anterior teeth obviously should be replaced for both functional and esthetic reasons; however, there is considerable difference of opinion over indications for replacement of lost posterior teeth.

Clinical experience indicates that satisfactory function and occlusion, as well as neuromuscular stability, usually can be established if all bicuspids and anterior teeth are present, even if these teeth have lost a considerable amount of periodontal support. Even if some of the anterior teeth and/or biscuspids are lost, the occlusion can often be stabilized with the remaining teeth, and replacement of lost molars is more of an esthetic than a functional problem. Refinements in occlusal therapy, including occlusal adjustment, orthodontics, and restorative dentistry, have made it possible to treat advanced periodontal disease successfully, and occlusal therapy should be considered a very important aspect of periodontal treatment.

Summary

Elimination of trauma from occlusion is an essential part of complete periodontal therapy. This can be achieved by orthodontic treatment, temporary or provisional splinting, biteplanes, occlusal adjustment, and permanent splinting of teeth.

While splinting may eliminate trauma and enhance functional stability and esthetic appearance, disadvantages related to plaque retention, technical difficulty, and cost mean that splinting should be kept to the minimum needed to eliminate progressive trauma from occlusion.

Moderately increased mobility without signs and symptoms of trauma from occlusion or impediment to adequate function usually does not require treatment by splinting.

If continuous tipping or extrusion of the remaining teeth can be avoided, a satisfactory prognosis for the dentition often may be secured without replacement of lost molars.

REFERENCES

1. Adair, R.: Practical Oral Hygiene, Prophylaxis and Pyorrhea Alveolaris. 2nd ed. Atlanta: Oral Hygiene Publ. Co., 1915.
2. Ainamo, J.: Relationship between malalignment of teeth and periodontal disease, Scand. J. Dent. Res. 80:104, 1972.
3. Alexander, A.G., and Tipnis, A.K.: The effect of irregularity of teeth and the degree of overbite and overjet on the gingival health. A study of 400 subjects, Br. Dent. J. 128:539, 1970.
4. Andreasen, J.O.: The effect of splinting upon periodontal healing after replantation of permanent incisors in monkeys, Acta Odont. Scand. 33:313, 1975.
5. Ash, M.M. and Ramfjord, S.P.: Introduction to Functional Occlusion. Philadelphia: W.B. Saunders Co., 1983.
6. Beyron, H.L.: Characteristics of functionally optimal occlusion and principles of occlusal rehabilitation, J.A.D.A. 48:648, 1954.
7. Brown, D.S.: The effect of orthodontic therapy on certain types of periodontal pockets. I. Clinical findings, J. Periodont. 44:742, 1973.
8. Carlsson, G.E.: Studies in partial denture prosthesis. IV. Final results of a 4-year longitudinal investigation of dentogingivally supported partial dentures, Acta Odont. Scand. 23:443, 1965.
9. Chaiken, B.S.: Temporary splinting in periodontal therapy, Alpha Omega 47:97, 1953.
10. Cross, W.G.: The importance of immobilization in periodontology, Parodontologie 8:119, 1954.
11. Crum, R.E., and Anderson, G.F.: The effect of gingival fiber surgery on the retention of rotated teeth, Am. J. Orthod. 65:626, 1974.
12. Emslie, R.: The incisal relationship and periodontal disease, Parodontologie 12:15, 1958.
13. Fenner, W., Gerber, A., and Mühlemann, H.R.: Tooth mobility changes during treatment with partial denture prosthesis, J. Prosthet. Dent. 6:520, 1956.
14. Fiachetti, F.J.: Temporary splinting in periodontal therapy. Part 2, Dent. Dig. 64:265, 1958.
15. Fleszar, T.J., et al.: Tooth mobility and periodontal therapy, J. Clin. Periodontol. 7:495, 1980.
16. Geiger, A.M., et al.: Relationship of occlusion and periodontal disease. Part V. Relation of classification of occlusion to periodontal status and gingival inflammation, J. Periodont. 43:554, 1972.
17. Geiger, A., and Hirschfeld, L.: Minor Tooth Movement in General Practice. 3rd ed. St. Louis: C.V. Mosby Co., 1974.
18. Glickman, I., Stein, R.S., and Smulow, J.B.: The effect of increased functional forces upon the periodontium of splinted and non-splinted teeth, J. Periodont. 32:290, 1961.
19. Glickman, I.: Clinical significance of trauma from occlusion, J.A.D.A. 70:607, 1965.
20. Glickman, I., et al.: The effect of occlusal forces on healing following mucogingival surgery, J. Periodont. 37:319, 1966.
21. Glickman, I.: Clinical Periodontology. 4th ed. Philadelphia: W.B. Saunders Co., 1972.
22. Goldman, H.M., and Cohen, D.W.: Periodontal Therapy. 4th ed. St. Louis: C.V. Mosby Co., 1973.
23. Graber, T.M.: Orthodontics: Principles and Practice. 3rd ed. Philadelphia: W.B. Saunders Co., 1972.
24. Hawley, C.A.: A removable retainer, Int. J. Orthod. 5:291, 1919.
25. Hirschfeld, I.: The missing tooth: A factor in dental and periodontal disease, J.A.D.A. 24:67, 1937.
26. Ingber, J.S.: Forced eruption. Part I. A method of treating isolated one or two wall infrabony osseous defects. Rationale and case report, J. Periodont. 45:199, 1974.
27. Lang, N.P.: Das präprothetishe Aufrichten von gekippten untern Molaren im Hinblick auf den parodontalen Zustand, Schweiz Maschr Zahnheilk 87:560, 1977.
28. Lindhe, J., and Svanberg, G.: Influence of trauma from occlusion on progression of experimental periodontitis in the beagle dog, J. Clin. Periodontol. 1:3, 1974.
29. Mühlemann, H.R.: Tooth mobility. V. Tooth mobility changes through artificial trauma, J. Periodont. 25:202, 1954.
30. Neumann, R.: Die Alveolarpryorrhoe ihre Behandlung. 3rd ed. Berlin: H. Meusser, 1920.
31. Obin, J., and Arvins, A.: The use of self-curing resin splints for the temporary stabilization of mobile teeth due to periodontal involvement, J.A.D.A. 42:320, 1951.
32. Pihlström, B.L., and Ramfjord, S.P.: Periodontal effect of nonfunction in monkeys, J. Periodont. 42:748, 1971.
33. Prichard, J., and Feder, M.: A modern adaptation of the telescopic principle in periodontal prosthesis, J. Periodont. 33:360, 1962.
34. Ramfjord, S.P.: Bruxism, a clinical and electromyographic study, J.A.D.A. 62:21, 1961.
35. Ramfjord, S.P., et al: Subgingival curettage versus surgical elimination of periodontal pockets, J. Periodont. 39:167, 1968.
36. Ramfjord, S.P., and Ash, M.M., Jr.: Occlusion. 3rd ed. Philadelphia: W.B. Saunders Co., 1983.
37. Ramfjord, S.P.: Aesthetics, periodontology and restorative dentistry, Quintessence Int. 16:581, 1985.
38. Rateitschak, K.H.: The therapeutic effect of local treatment on periodontal disease assessed upon evaluation of different diagnostic criteria. I. Changes in tooth mobility, J. Periodont. 43:540, 1963.

39. Reitan, K.: Biomechanical principles and reactions, In Current Orthodontic Concepts and Techniques, ed. T. M. Graber and B.F. Swain. 2nd ed., Vol. I. Philadelphia: W.B. Saunders Co., 1975.

40. Renggli, H.H.: Splinting of teeth—an objective assessment, Helv. Odont. Acta 14:129, 1971.

41. Renggli, H.H., and Schweizer, H.: Splinting of teeth with removable bridges. Biological effects, J. Clin. Periodontol. 1:43, 1974.

42. Sadovsky, C., and BeGale, E.A.: Long-term effects of orthodontic treatment on periodontal health, Am. J. Orthod. 80:156, 1981.

43. Scharer, P., Butler, J.H., and Zander, H.A.: Die Heilung parodontaler Knockentaschen bei okklusaler Dysfunktion, Schweiz. Mschr. Zahnk. 79:244, 1969.

44. Shulman, J.: A technique for bite plane construction, J. Prosthet. Dent. 29:334, 1973.

45. Seeman, S.K.: A study of the relationship between periodontal disease and the wearing of partial dentures, Aust. Dent. J. 8:206, 1963.

46. Silness, J.: Periodontal conditions in patients treated with dental bridges. III. The relationship between the location of the crown margins and the periodontal conditions, J. Periodont. Res. 5:225, 1970.

47. Simring, M., and Posteraro, F.F.: Hazards and shortcomings of splinting, N.Y. Dent. J. 30:19, 1964.

48. Svanberg, G., and Lindhe, J.: Vascular reactions in the periodontal ligament incident to trauma from occlusion, J. Clin. Periodontol. 1:58, 1974.

49. Svanberg, G., and Lindhe, J.: Influence of trauma from occlusion on the periodontium of dogs with normal or inflamed gingiva, Odontol. Revy. 25:165, 1974.

50. Talkov, L.: Temporary acrylic fixed bridgework and splints, J. Prosthet. Dent. 2:693, 1952.

51. Vonesh, E.M.: Correlation between extensive orthodontic treatment and periodontal disease, Thesis, The University of Michigan, 1968.

52. Waerhaug, J.: Justification of splinting in periodontal therapy, J. Prosthet. Dent. 22:201, 1969.

53. Wentz, F.M., Jarabak, J., and Orban, B.: Experimental occlusal trauma imitating cuspal interferences, J. Periodont. 29:117, 1958.

54. Wüst, B.P., Rateitschak, K.H., and Mühlemann, H.R.: Der Einfluss der lokalen Paradontal Behandlung auf die Zahnlocherung und der Entzündungsgrad des Zahnfleisches, Helv. Odont. Acta 4:58, 1960.

55. Zachrisson, B.U., and Alnaes, L.: Periodontal conditions in orthodontically treated and untreated individuals. I. Loss of attachment, gingival pocket depth, and clinical crown height, Angle Orthod. 43:402, 1973.

56. Zachrisson, B.U., and Alnaes, L.: Periodontal conditions in orthodontically treated and untreated individuals. II. Alveolar bone loss: Radiographic findings, Angle Orthod. 44:48, 1974.

57. Zachrisson, B.U.: Cause and prevention of injuries to teeth and supporting structures during orthodontic treatment, Am. J. Orthod. 69:285, 1976.

58. Zachrisson, B.U. and Brobakken, B.O.: Clinical comparison of direct versus indirect bonding with different bracket types and adhesives, Am. J. Orthod. 74:66, 1978.

20

OBJECTIVES AND PRINCIPLES OF PERIODONTAL SURGERY

The word *surgery*, by definition, is "the act and art of treating injuries or diseases by manual operation."[42] If this broad definition were to be used, nearly all periodontal treatment practices would fall under the heading *periodontal surgery*. However, by common use, the term *periodontal surgery* is applied to surgical manipulation of periodontal soft tissues and bone and does not refer to the accompanying scaling and root planing of teeth, although these latter procedures play an important part in the success or failure of periodontal surgery.

OBJECTIVES OF PERIODONTAL SURGERY

The proceedings from a recent large workshop on Surgical Therapy for Periodontitis state, "Periodontal surgery is an appropriate therapeutic procedure to gain visibility and to provide access for root preparation and for removal of subgingival micro-organisms and other local irritants adjacent to deep or tortuous periodontal pockets or in furcation involvement."[21] They state further, "Periodontal surgery is also indicated to create optimal conditions for regeneration, replacement, or reconstruction of lost periodontal structures."

Periodontal surgery may also be indicated for esthetic reasons, such as tissue overgrowth or recession, to provide access for restorative dentistry, or to establish draining of an abscess.

In the past, the main objectives of periodontal surgery were (1) to eliminate pockets deeper than 3 mm, and (2) to provide optimal contour of the alveolar process and the gingiva. These two objectives have proven to be of no value for the future maintenance of the teeth in health and normal function.[21] They complicate periodontal treatment with unfavorable root exposure and discomfort, and should not be considered as viable objectives anymore. Periodontal surgery in itself is valueless unless it is followed by adequate plaque control.[35]

CONTRAINDICATIONS TO PERIODONTAL SURGERY

As a general principle, periodontal surgery is contraindicated for persons who have any systemic illness in which surgery may endanger their health.

Bleeding disorders

Periodontal surgery involves disruption of the tissues and necessarily some bleeding. Any hemorrhagic disorder of severe nature, such as hemophilia and thrombocytopenic purpura, usually constitutes a contraindication to periodontal surgery, unless the bleeding can be controlled. Bleeding disorders may also be manifestations of systemic diseases, drug therapy (such as with anticoagulants), or drug effects on the liver with fibrogenesis as seen in chronic alcoholism[33] and sometimes following the use of aspirin.[17] In addition, periodontal surgery should be avoided during the first 2 days of the menstrual period because of alterations of the clotting mechanism sometimes found in women at that time.

Lowered resistance to infection

Periodontal surgery is contraindicated for some patients with impaired defense mechanisms against bacterial infection. Such impairment is seen in neutropenia and acute monocytic and myelogenous leukemia or AIDS. Uncontrolled diabetes and prolonged heavy cortisone therapy may also interfere with the normal antibacterial response to surgery.

Specific contraindications

Patients with nutritional deficiency, which is usually due to chronic disease, should have periodontal surgery only if their deficiencies can be controlled.

Patients with short life expectancy owing to malignant diseases or severe cardiovascular impairment are candidates for palliative periodontal procedures rather than periodontal surgery.

Patients under severe mental stress or with mental or physical handicaps should not be subjected to periodontal surgery unless the mental stress can be relieved and their handicaps compensated for by extra care.

Periodontal surgery is usually avoided in pregnancy at the time of the missed 2nd and 3rd menstrual periods and during the last month of gestation. Without compelling reasons, periodontal surgery should be postponed until after delivery.

Poor oral hygiene

It has often been stated that periodontal surgery is contraindicated for persons who will not keep their teeth clean after the surgery. However, recent concepts of reparative periodontal surgery and professional maintenance care may justify certain modalities of periodontal surgery for patients with poor oral hygiene if they are willing to appear for frequent recall appointments.[34] Similarly, a very high caries rate may influence the selection of modality of periodontal surgery and the recall program, but is not a definite contraindication to the surgery, inasmuch as the main objective of the surgery is to eliminate subgingival irritants.

TIMING OF PERIODONTAL SURGERY

Except for emergency drainage of a periodontal abscess, all periodontal surgery should be postponed until at least one month after completion of the hygienic phase of the periodontal treatment. The reasons for this postponement will be discussed in this section.

Scaling and good home care will result in shrinkage and fibrosis of the gingival tissues, followed by reattachment of junctional epithelium. This reattachment may restore a physiologic gingival crevice in areas that had periodontal pockets at the time of the initial examination. Periodontal surgery always constitutes a traumatic insult, which should be avoided whenever possible. In many instances, the need for mucogingival surgery cannot be assessed properly at the time of the initial examination, because the relationship between the bottom of the pocket and the mucogingival line is often altered so favorably by scaling and improved oral hygiene that mucogingival surgery may not be necessary.[20]

Observing the patient during the hygienic phase will give an indication of what cooperation in oral hygiene can be expected from the patient in the future. Such information is essential in selecting the modality of periodontal surgery that will yield the best results for that particular patient, and in determining if specific arrangements will have to be made for professional postoperative care. Conventional types of periodontal surgery may do more harm than good if adequate cooperation and plaque control cannot be established.[34] In patients with high caries rates, the hygienic phase of treatment provides an opportunity to assess the patient's nutritional and hygienic commitment to caries control. Such information may influence greatly how much of the root surface should be left exposed following periodontal surgery.

The chances of harmful sequelae, such as loss of attachment associated with periodontal surgery, are reduced when the surgery is done on fibrous, firm gingival tissues, with the root surfaces devoid of calculus. When gingivectomy is performed on highly inflamed tissues, there is a tendency to extend root planing apically to the bottom of the epithelial attachment. At least initially, the new epithelial attachment will grow down to the apical level of the root planing, and the result may easily be a loss of fiber attachment to the tooth.[37] It has also been reported that fragments of calculus may be left under the periodontal flaps if the flap surgery is done without prior calculus removal.[24]

If the teeth need temporary splinting and/or occlusal adjustments, these procedures should be completed prior to the periodontal surgery, because occlusal therapy will help to stabilize the teeth and prevent dislodgment of periodontal dressings. Stability of the teeth may have a beneficial effect on periodontal healing.[12] Occlusal therapy may also allow multidirectional function and provide an opportunity for the patient to masticate using teeth not involved in the surgical procedure.

In patients with hyperplastic gingivitis needing orthodontic therapy, the surgical procedures should be performed prior to the orthodontic therapy, but in all other cases the orthodontic therapy should be completed prior to the periodontal surgery. The attachment of the regenerated periodontal fibers will then help to maintain the teeth in their postorthodontic position.[8]

It is very important that the periodontal surgery be done prior to restorative dental procedures whenever these procedures are to involve parts of the tooth close to the gingival margin.

PREPARING FOR PERIODONTAL SURGERY
Need for periodontal surgery

A thorough clinical examination, including probing of all crevices, should determine the need for periodontal surgery. The evaluation should be done 4 to 6 weeks after completion of scaling, root planing, and instruction in oral hygiene. If there is no clinical evidence of inflammation and no bleeding on light probing to the base of the crevices, there is no immediate need for further periodontal treatment.[32]

If plaque has induced marginal gingivitis, further plaque control should be implemented. If bleeding or an exudate is provoked from gentle probing to the base of the gingival crevice, the implication is that residual irritants are present on the subgingival root surfaces. Such situations are most often found with deep or tortuous pockets, and with furcation involvement.

The clinician may want to give scaling and root planing another chance, depending on the anatomic situation. However, in most instances, such pockets are scheduled for periodontal surgery, which allows for optimum access and visibility of the root surfaces.

Crevicular depth in itself should not dictate the need for surgical therapy, although it is a factor in access and visibility. Other reasons to schedule surgery may relate to regenerative procedures, esthetic and functional corrections of the gingiva for covering of exposed root surfaces, and facilitating restorative treatment.

Presurgical appointment

Presurgical charting should be done approximately 1 week before surgery. Psychological and pharmacological factors, nutrition, diet, and blood pressure should be considered.

Periodontal surgery may have an ominous implication to many patients, but, carried out with aseptic and atraumatic precautions, it is accompanied by very minimal pain or discomfort. The psychological preparation for periodontal surgery, therefore, should start with careful education and reassurance at the time the treatment plan is presented to the patient. It is a common observation that complaints of postsurgical pain and discomfort are greatly reduced when the patients are well informed regarding the purpose and extent of the surgery, as compared with patients who approach the periodontal surgery as a mysterious and crucial event.

An appointment prior to surgery provides an opportunity to discuss the surgery with the patient and to prescribe drugs needed to prevent harmful effects from bacteremias, which are unavoidable during the surgery. If at this time the patient exhibits anxiety regarding the surgical treatment, or has a history of syncope associated with past episodes of dental treatment, premedication with barbiturates or other drugs with tranquilizing effects is recommended.

No specific nutritional regime is indicated for periodontal surgery; however, the patient should avoid fibrous or tough foods for about a week following the periodontal surgery. The need for adequate fluid intake should always be emphasized.

It is advisable to record the patient's blood pressure at the time of the presurgical appointment and at the time of surgery. Just before surgery, the patient's blood pressure may be abnormally elevated, due to fear, or may have been lowered by premedication. Therefore, it is important to have a normal recording close to the time of surgery for reference in case serious complications involving alterations of the blood pressure should occur during the surgery.

INSTRUMENTS AND MATERIALS FOR PERIODONTAL SURGERY

Special instruments are available for the kind of surgery that is planned. All instruments and materials to be used during the periodontal surgery should prepacked and presterilized. Prior to sterilization, all instruments should be inspected carefully and sharpened when indicated. Usually a standard set of instruments is prepared for each surgical procedure, with a variety of additional instruments, sterilized in sealed paper bags, available if needed. Prepacked new disposable syringe needles, scalpel blades, and sutures should be used.

Following is a representative list of a standard kit of instruments, and another list of some instruments that are packed separately and may be requested during the surgery if needed.

STANDARD SURGICAL TRAY

Alabama Tray (Custom Equipment, Inc.)
Cotton pliers (HuFriedy)
Mouth mirror 5 (Kerr)
Explorers 3 and 17 (HuFriedy)
Pocket measuring probe M.1. (HuFriedy)
Columbia scalers 13 and 14 (Starlite)
Plastic instrument (Tarno, S.S. White)
#7 Wax instrument (Cleve-Dent)
Tissue scissors, Goldman Fox (HuFriedy)
Suture scissors, Lockin 11 (HuFriedy)
Needle holder, Crile-Wood 5-inch carbide (HuFriedy)
Mosquito Hemostat, curved (HuFriedy)
Tip for saline syringe
Aspirator tip
Rubber hose
Napkin chain
Orban knives 1 and 2 (HuFriedy)
Bard-Parker knife holders (2)

AVAILABLE IN STERILE WRAPPING

Bard-Parker blades 11, 12B, and 15
Atraumatic sutures, 3/0, 4/0, 5/0, 6/0 with curved ⅜ in.
regular or ½ in. reverse bevel needles
2 in. × 2 in. sponges
Bennett elevator, 12S (HuFriedy)
Rongeurs, Friedman 5 ½ in. (HuFriedy)
Ochsenbein bone chisels, 1 and 2 (HuFriedy)
Handpiece and round burs #8, small pointed diamonds + polishing bur
Bunting 5 and 6 scalers (Tarno, S.S. White)

Electrosurgical instruments

Electrosurgery has been recommended as an expedient and safe modality for gingival exision, and the healing pattern after electrosurgical soft tissue incisions has been reported to closely resemble the healing following conventional knife surgery.[2,27]

The electrosurgical unit should deliver a smooth, fully rectified, high-frequency current of unmodulated waves resulting from full-wave rectification and adequate filtering.[28] The electric current should be adjusted to the lowest setting that allows cutting without appreciable resistance to the electrode tip. A thin electrode tip cuts with the least amount of burning. The main advantages of electrosurgery over regular surgery are (1) that the cutting is followed by minimal hemorrhage, and (2) that the angle between the cutting needle and the handle can be adjusted by bending, so that the instrument is suitable for cutting gingival tissues at a desired angle anywhere in the mouth.

A recent study of electrosurgical gingival resection using apparently fully rectified current on monkeys indicated that the use of electrosurgery resulted in a statistically significant recession of the free gingival margin and loss of connective tissue attachment to the teeth, associated with apical migration of the junctional epithelium.[44] The surface of the cementum (Fig. 20-1) appeared to have been altered following contact with the activated electrosurgical needle, and only in exceptional cases did connective tissue reattachment occur in the surface of the cementum that had been touched by the electrosurgical needle.[44]

It has also been reported that bone may be altered following contact with an electrosurgical needle.[14] Thus, electrosurgery can be used safely in periodontics only for gingivoplasty[14] and with contact only with the enamel of the tooth. Contact with bone, cementum, and the cementoenamel junction must be avoided. Also, to avoid pulpal damage, contact between the electrode tip and metallic restorations should be avoided or the duration of the contact made less than ⁴⁄₁₀ of a second.[24]

Suture needles and suture material

Atraumatic suture needles of the ⅜ inch or ½ inch semicircular reverse cutting or conventional cutting

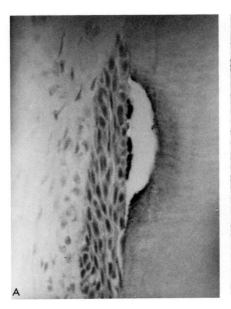
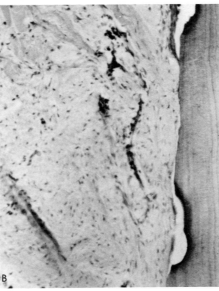
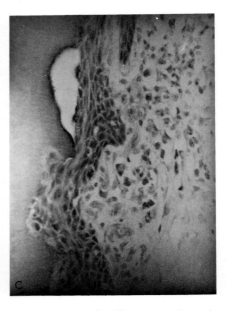

Fig. 20-1. *A,* Six months after electrosurgery. Altered cementum following contact of electrosurgical needle. The apparent empty space following decalcification indicates that the organic material in the cementum has been altered by the electrosurgery. *B,* Three months after electrosurgery. Two burn marks from contact with the electrosurgical needle. No new cementum formed over the burned cementum on the root surface. *C,* Six months after electrosurgery. Resorption of cementum with ingrowth of epithelium (monkey specimens).

types are commonly used for periodontal surgery. Sutures and needles come in sizes of 3/0, 4/0, 5/0, and 6/0, with silk or synthetic suture material. Commonly used is a silicone-treated silk suture number 4/0, a noncapillary-type suture that is swaged to a ⅜ inch or ½ inch half-circle reverse cutting needle. However, for very thin laterally repositioned flap or grafts, it may be advisable to use 5/0 or 6/0 sutures. For fibrous, thick gingival tissues, a 3/0 suture may be used.

Black silk suture is preferred to plastic materials because it is easy to tie and is easy to see. However, it has the disadvantage of acting like a wick, providing entry for bacteria and bacterial products into the tissues. Such contaminations can be counteracted by use of topical antibiotics.[26] If synthetic material is used, the braided type is recommended over the monofilament type, inasmuch as the monofilament is very difficult to tie and does not hold a knot well. However, the braided material (e.g., polyglycolic acid) will always be more irritating than the monofilament synthetic sutures. Resorbable synthetic materials are not recommended, because this type of suture often causes considerable irritation.

Surgical dressing

Periodontal dressings are used to protect the wound created by periodontal surgery and to maintain close flap adaptation to the bone and the teeth during the initial stage of healing. The traditional type of periodontal dressings or packs consists of zinc oxide-eugenol preparations with various additives for physical strength and bactericidal effects. Ward's Wondr-Pak[41] and a large number of other periodontal dressings fall into this group.[15] Powder preparations consist mainly of zinc oxide, powdered rosin, and tannic acid flakes. They may also contain asbestos fibers for added strength; however, dressings containing asbestos are no longer accepted by the Council on Dental Therapeutics.[16] Liquid preparations usually consist of eugenol and olive or peanut oil, and some antiseptic (such as thymol) is usually added to the liquid.

Another variety of dressings includes noneugenol-containing preparations with various types of bactericidal or bacteriostatic agents added.[36] Coe-Pack and Peripak are examples of this variety. Other dressings are fat-containing dressings with antibiotics such as bacitracin added to the zinc oxide and rosin powder.[4]

A number of cyanoacrylate dressings have been recommended;[13] however, these materials seem to cause considerable irritation to connective tissues.[46] A good multipurpose dressing, which causes minimal irritation and is easy to handle, is the Recorder 8226 Non-Asbestos Dressing. This type can be made up in large batches, divided into small portions, wrapped in foil, and kept refrigerated until needed. For patients sensitive to eugenol, Coe-Pack is recommended.

SETUP FOR PERIODONTAL SURGERY

Although complete asepsis cannot be maintained during periodontal surgery, every precaution should be observed in order to avoid contamination from sources other than the patient's own saliva. Fortunately, saliva does not seem to be a deterrent to wound healing. It is recommended that the dental assistant follow a routine checklist such as the following when preparing for the surgery.

Outline of presurgical procedures for dental assistants

Preparation of the Operatory
  Wash hands thoroughly.
  Refill towel and soap dispensers.
  Wash all standing equipment—counters, dental unit, chair, light, instrument panel, and all unit and chair attachments.
  Monitor all mobile equipment—oxygen, vacuum, electrosurgery, etc., for proper function.
  Post radiographs, records, and charts
Preparation of Assistant
  Cover hair with net and cap.
  Remove all rings or other jewelry.
  Scrub hands—use sterile handbrush and wash from elbows to fingertips for 3 minutes.
  Put on operatory gown.
Preparation of Surgical Area
  Wash hands with sponge (E-Z scrub sterile surgical brush).
  Attach all sterile instruments to panel—suction tip, aspirator, evacuators.
  Arrange medications.
  Arrange instrumentation packages and keep covered with sterile towel.
Preparation of Patient
  Have patient remove glasses (and earrings if appropriate).
  Have patient wash hands.
  Drape the patient.
  Wash patient's face with four PhisoHex sponges, dry with sterile towel.
  Place sterile towel and towel chain.
Final Preparation
  When ready for surgery, put on sterile gloves.
  Uncover surgical instruments.

The dental assistant should be trained in aseptic surgical procedures and know how to prepare the patient, arrange the instruments, pass instruments, and use suction in an efficient manner. Routine surgical scrubbing of the hands and use of surgical gloves are recommended. The instruments should be arranged and maintained in a definite order in the instrument tray during the surgical procedures.

PRINCIPLES OF ATRAUMATIC SURGERY

Psychological preparation of the patient should protect him against psychological trauma associated with the surgery. Careful presurgical preparation of the instruments, the settings of the operation, the patient, and the personnel involved in the surgical treatment should protect him against preventable physical injury associated with the surgery.

Preparation of surgical site

The site of the operation and the adjacent teeth and soft tissues should be washed liberally with an antiseptic solution, such as iodine lotion or mild tincture of iodine, to reduce the bacterial flora in the area of the surgery. An attempt should be made to introduce the antiseptic into the periodontal pockets and the gingival crevices. If the operation is to be performed in the maxilla, the surgical field can usually be isolated by sterile sponges placed in the mucobuccal fold, but in the mandible this is not always practical.

A profound, long-lasting (2 to 3 hours) anesthesia with vasoconstriction is desirable for most types of periodontal surgery. A relatively long-lasting anesthetic with 1:50,000 adrenalin is recommended. The site of the injection should be properly prepared with an antiseptic and a topical anesthetic.

Use of surgical instruments

A surgical operation always entails trauma; however, the traumatic impact on the surrounding tissues and vascular supply depends very much on the sharpness of the instruments and the operator's skill. Small oscillating movements with a scalpel cause much less trauma to the surrounding tissues than pressing the edge of the scalpel directly against the tissues in a forceful manner. Heavy pressure against soft tissues or bone, and tearing of the tissues, should be avoided because such procedures inflict a deeper zone of tissue destruction than does an incision with a sharp instrument.

The same principles requiring sharp instruments for soft tissues also apply to bone surgery. A chisel is much less traumatic to the underlying bone tissues during bone removal than is crushing with a rongeur or maceration with diamond stones or burs. In addition, postsurgical healing is more favorable following the use of chisels than of burs or ultrasonic instruments.[18]

TISSUE MANAGEMENT

Curetting soft-tissue attachment from the teeth involves a potential risk of permanently detaching some of the tissue.[25] Any flap procedure, split- or full-thickness,[45] will disturb the metabolism of the underlying bone as well as of the flap, and thus involves the risk of losing support for the teeth. Therefore, root planing should be confined only to the parts of the roots that have lost their fibrous attachment, and periodontal flaps should be extended only over the minimum area needed for access to exposed root surfaces. Remove only the minimum amount of tissue that has to be removed to attain the objective of the surgery. Whenever possible cover the wound with gingival epithelium.

Flaps and grafts should be handled gently, and mucoperiosteal elevators or tissue retractors should be used in such a way that they do not tear or unduly compress soft tissues. It is preferable to use suction during periodontal surgery rather than to compress the tissues with a dry sponge in order to gain better vision. The use of sponges also may result in cotton fibers being left in the wound, which may constitute a source of future irritation.[23]

Avoid undue drying of bone, which will cause necrosis of surface bone, and do not try to create a very smooth bone surface by extensive instrumentation. With such a smooth surface, healing will be delayed and complicated compared with a bony surface with residual soft tissue cells on the surface.[7] Use sterile saline solution rather than tap water for rinsing the wound area; tap water is neither sterile nor isotonic with body fluids.[30] Do not blow air into the field of surgery, as it may induce cervicofacial[29] or mediastinal emphysema, or even air emboli, which can be fatal.[38]

Suturing

Interrupted, direct, or figure-8 sutures allow the most precise positioning of flaps and grafts. Continuous sling sutures can be extended to close a flap for an entire quadrant of a dental arch by inserting separate sling sutures in the buccal and lingual mucoperiosteal flaps.[11] However, this type of suture will not allow as accurate placement of the flap as interrupted sutures, and the sutures very often get under the flap or between the flap and the teeth, preventing optimal healing of the flap to the teeth. If one of the suture loops tears loose, the entire suture may become slack and the precise adaptation of the flap may be lost. The only time a continuous sling suture may be used is in cases of buccal flap and palatal gingivectomy; however, even here the palatal loop of the suture irritates the gingival margin at the site of the gingivectomy and is therefore not recommended.

The fit of the flap should be tested prior to suturing. Do not try to pull the flap beyond its natural position with tight sutures, because the sutures then will work through the flap. In addition, the tension on the flap will interfere with the blood supply, which is essential to optimal healing. Take as small stitches as possible with the suture needle at the margin of the flaps. For thin, delicate flaps, it is advisable to use a suture needle with a reserve bevel and 4/0 to 6/0 sutures. It is technically more difficult to use a suture needle that has a reverse bevel than one that has a regular bevel, but with the reverse bevel needle the sutures do not have to be engaged deep in the tissues of the flap.

Occasionally, anchor sutures may be used for lateral sliding flaps, although the position of the flap is usually achieved more accurately with a direct suture. Mattress sutures may be used to hold large flaps in close interproximal contact, as, for example, after implant of bone interproximally.

COMPLICATIONS ASSOCIATED WITH PERIODONTAL SURGERY

Most, but not all, of the complications that may be associated with periodontal surgery are preventable by proper diagnosis and attentive preoperative and postoperative care by a concerned and skillful surgeon.

Therefore, it is important to have a comprehensive knowledge of the complications that may be encountered, how they may be prevented, and how they are best managed if they occur. The most significant complications are

1. Shock; syncope.
2. Hemorrhage.
3. Pain.
4. Swelling; hematoma.
5. Delayed healing.
6. Allergic reactions to dressings.
7. Sensitivity of the teeth.

Shock; syncope

The most serious of all complications is anaphylactic shock to an administered drug. This is a life-threatening state, one which requires immediate attention. It usually develops within about one half hour following administration of a drug. The patient first feels uneasy, has difficulty in breathing, has nausea, becomes pale, then cyanotic, perspires heavily, and goes into collapse. The blood pressure becomes very low and the pulse fast and weak, or it may not be felt at all, while the respiration becomes asthmatic. The assistant should be instructed to call emergency service whenever it is suspected that the patient is going into shock. The emergency telephone number to be called should appear in large numbers on a sign on the wall above the telephone. Place the patient in Trendelenburg's position, clear the air passages, and administer oxygen. If the blood pressure is very low, give 0.5 ml epinephrine (1:1000 injectable form) intramuscularly, preferably in the tongue muscles; however, it may be given in any large muscle. Do not inject epinephrine subcutaneously; that way, it is absorbed very slowly.

If the patient's heart has stopped completely, emergency external heart massage should be introduced, and if the breathing has also stopped, artificial respiration should be given until emergency help arrives.

All the personnel in the dental office should receive training periodically in cardiopulmonary resuscitation (CPR) procedures so that they can assume an active role in an emergency situation.

If the patient shows signs of agitation and chest pain, oxygen should be administered and the emergency service called, since these symptoms may indicate a heart attack. Administration of epinephrine would be contraindicated for such a patient.

Other causes of shock-like symptoms may be hypoglycemia of insulin shock in diabetes. Because the diagnosis may be difficult without an immediate past history, do not administer insulin to a comatose patient. Individuals with hypoglycemia may require a sugar-containing beverage prior to and during periodontal surgery.

Shock may also be the result of loss of blood, internal hemorrhage,[6] or cardiovascular accidents. The most important actions in any shock-like reaction are to call in emergency help immediately and to administer supportive emergency therapy.

Fortunately, by far the most common cause of loss of consciousness in the dental chair is simple syncope. The situation is unpleasant and embarassing to the patient and disruptive to the treatment procedures, but it does not involve danger to the patient's life.

If the patient starts to become abnormally pale, perspires heavily, and is restless, place the chair in a horizontal position with the head below the level of the body. Take the patient's pulse and observe his breathing. If the pulse becomes noticeably weaker than normal, record the blood pressure. As long as the patient's breathing is fairly normal, the pulse is regular, and the blood pressure does not go far below the normal level for the patient, one may be reasonably assured that the loss of consciousness is simple syncope. Be sure that the collar is not too tight around the neck. Aromatic ammonia may help prevent syncope. If the patient is in deep syncope and making slow recovery, oxygen should be administered. While the patient is regaining consciousness, he should be kept in a horizontal position and should not be allowed to sit up until his normal color has returned and he is fully recovered from a feeling of dizziness and nausea.

A number of precautionary measures will usually prevent syncope. It is important to allay the patient's fears through psychological and pharmacological preparation before the surgery. Instruments and blood should be kept outside the patient's field of vision.

A reassuring attitude on the part of the operator, slow and careful administration of anesthetics, and a controlled and quiet atmosphere in the operating room are all important precautions in the management of nervous patients. Avoid any sign of disappointment or disgust if things do not go as expected during the operation, as this might increase the patient's anxiety. In addition, avoid conversation with the personnel in the office about subjects not related to the surgery, because it may upset the patient that the operator's attention is not devoted entirely to the surgical procedures at hand. A general atmosphere of empathy and reassurance is very helpful in prevention of syncope.

Hemorrhage

Because periodontal surgery ordinarily severs only small blood vessels, significant hemorrhage is not a frequent complication of periodontal surgery when local anesthetics and vasoconstrictor drugs are used. The average amount of blood loss during one session of periodontal surgery has been reported to be 37 ml.[5] Periodontal surgery has usually been ruled out during the treatment planning for patients with bleeding disorders, and in borderline cases tests would have been made of the bleeding, clotting, and clot-retraction time. However, there is still the possibility that a patient may have acquired some bleeding disorder; for instance, from heavy intake of aspirin or other drugs after the systemic and hygienic phases of the treatment. Abnormal bleeding may be related to unexpected onset of a menstrual period. There may also be accidental severing of larger blood vessels during surgery, provoking extensive bleeding.

A distinction is usually made between primary, intermediate, and secondary types of bleeding. Primary postoperative hemorrhage starts at the time of the surgery. Intermediate hemorrhage starts soon after the surgery, after having stopped temporarily following surgery. It is usually due to the breakdown of an incomplete clot, such as is associated with loss of the vasoconstrictor effect of anesthesia. The secondary type of postsurgical hemorrhage may start from 24 hours to 10 days postoperatively. The patient should be instructed to contact the dentist who did the surgery immediately if intermediate or secondary hemorrhage occurs.

Whenever there is unusual bleeding, it is important first to reassure the patient and control the patient's emotional concern about the bleeding. A mild, oozing type of bleeding can usually be controlled by a pressure pack, using gauze moistened in steril saline solution and held firmly in position for 2 to 3 minutes. Injection of local anesthetics along with a 1:50,000 vasoconstrictor drug may also be helpful in controlling bleeding. If the bleeding is an arterial spouting of light red blood, as may be seen with encroachment on the palatal arteries, one may try to crush the cut artery with a hemostat. Hold the hemostat in position for several minutes and remove it very carefully. If there is not enough soft tissue to grasp with a hemostat, one may attempt to seal the vessel by crushing the bone

of the nutrient bone channel. If the cut surface is in soft tissue, cautery may be tried, either by a hot instrument or by a ball electrode from an electrosurgical machine. If the bleeding is severe, it may have to be stopped by tying a suture around the bleeding vessel.

A slow, oozing, venous bleeding (dark blood) may be stopped by the use of Gelfoam or Oxycel; however, these preparations are somewhat irritating and definately have to be removed before a periodontal dressing is placed over the wound.

The placement of a periodontal dressing helps to stop bleeding, and there is no need to have an absolutely dry surgical field, with complete stoppage of all bleeding, prior to the placement of a dressing. A thin layer of coagulated blood under the periodontal dressing actually affords a natural protection to the wound and eliminates direct contact between the materials of the dressing and the wounded tissues.

The patient should never be allowed to leave the dentist's office until all gross hemorrhaging has stopped. If the dentist cannot stop the hemorrhage, he should be responsible for transferring the patient to a hospital or some facility where further care can be provided.

If intermediate or secondary hemorrhage occurs, administration of local anesthetics with vasoconstrictors centrally to the wound is recommended. Then remove the periodontal dressing, clean and inspect the wound, and treat the bleeding similarly to a primary type of bleeding. It is psychologically reassuring to the patient, and in his best interests, that the person who did the surgery and who knows the patient's medical and dental history at least attempt to handle the complications of intermediate and secondary postoperative hemorrhage, rather than that the patient be referred directly to an emergency hospital service. Such emergency service is very rarely necessary.

Pain

Beyond some soreness during the first 24 hours following the periodontal surgery, there should be only minimal pain and discomfort if the basic principles of atraumatic surgery were observed carefully. Pain within the first few days following periodontal surgery usually results from mechanical trauma during the surgery, drying of the bone, traumatic bone surgery, or incorrectly placed periodontal dressing.

A very common source of postoperative pain is impingement from the postsurgical dressing, either upon the interproximal bone and soft tissue or at the mucosal and frenum levels. Alternatively, a dressing may interfere with masticatory function or cause bruxism. The patient should be instructed to contact the dentist if significant postoperative pain develops. The individual should be seen immediately. At the emergency appointment, the surgical area should be anesthetized, the dressing removed, and the cause of the pain identified. When the cause has been eliminated, a new, carefully fitted dressing should be placed in position. The dressing that is placed interproximally should be soft, so that it can cover the wound without pressure.

Do not prescribe pain-relieving medication without reexamining the wound, as the pain may be a warning that the dressing has had a traumatic effect upon the tissues in the area of the surgery. After the dressing has been changed, the patient may be given pain-relieving medication; however, medication usually is needed for only a few days.

Postsurgical pain related to infection usually does not start until 2 to 4 days following surgery. Such pain is usually accompanied by lymphadenopathy, and there may be a slight elevation in temperature. If not treated promptly, the lymphadenopathy and the elevation in temperature will increase. The patient should be examined, the temperature recorded, and the periodontal dressing removed. Perform a percussion test of the teeth in the area of the surgery. If the temperature is not significantly elevated and the teeth are not noticeably sore to percussion, place a topical antibiotic ointment (e.g., 3% Achromycin) over the wound and apply a new dressing. The patient should be instructed to take his temperature the next day and return if it has risen. If the temperature is significantly elevated or the teeth in the area of the surgery are noticeably sore to percussion, the patient should be placed on systemic antibiotic therapy. Fever and soreness of the teeth to percussion may indicate a developing osteomyelitis, and the patient should be treated with large doses of antibiotics, preferably penicillin. Doubling the normal dosage for at least 10 to 14 days is recommended for osteomyelitis. However, severe infections are extremely rare following the modalities of periodontal surgery commonly used at present.

Swelling; hematoma

Significant swelling or the formation of a hematoma is usually a sequela of traumatic periodontal surgery. Extensive soft-tissue surgery, such as for high mucoperiosteal flaps or distal wedge operations behind the last mandibular molar, may result in swelling. Infections associated with periodontal surgery also may induce swelling. Ice packs or ice cubes held in the mouth have traditionally been used to reduce swelling, but neither is very effective. Use of antihistamines has not been found to be effective except following extraction of impacted 3rd molars.[9] If there are symptoms of infection, such as elevation of temperature and lymphadenopathy, antibiotics should be prescribed; however, antibiotics do not have any immediate effect upon the swelling.

A hematoma will have to go through the various stages of resolution. If there is no evidence of infection, no specific therapy is indicated. Facial hematomas may result from direct trauma to the field of surgery; they may also be the result of bruising contact by the operator to the skin surfaces of the jaws. Facial hematoma is an annoying, but fortunately a rare, sequela to carefully performed periodontal surgery.

Delayed healing

In areas where part of the alveolar process has been left exposed following periodontal surgery, where severe trauma to the bone has occurred during the surgery, or where there has been heavy direct pressure on the bone from the periodontal dressing, so-called "bare bone" may develop (Fig. 20-2). Such areas of exposed bone may become infected on the surface, so that granulation tissue will not attach to it. This necrotic bone then will have to be resorbed by an inflammatory process in the underlying tissues, starting from the marrow spaces or the periodontal membrane. The dead bond is broken up by the resorptive process and finally expelled as sequestra. Such a delayed healing may take several weeks, and during this time the area should be kept covered by a periodontal dressing to minimize infection and discomfort. Fortunately, such an episode of delayed healing does not seem to have any detrimental long-term effect on the tissue attachment level of the teeth, although it may lead to permanent loss of bone.[8] The chance of "bare bone" developing is much greater following gingivectomy with electrosurgery.

If excessive granulation tissue develops as a result of poorly fitting periodontal dressing or loss of the dressing shortly after the surgery, the granulation tissue should be removed with a sharp instrument. This can usually be accomplished without pain, since newly formed granulation tissue is not as yet innervated. A well-fitting periodontal dressing then should be placed over the wound and left for one week.

Reactions to periodontal dressings

Allergic reactions to periodontal dressings sometimes occur, especially in patients who have been wearing dressings over a prolonged period of time due to multiple episodes of surgery or delayed healing. The sensitivity reaction is usually provoked by the eugenol in the zinc oxide-eugenol type of dressings. It also has been observed, although very rarely, with non-eugenol containing dressings.

The first symptom of a sensitivity reaction to periodontal dressing is a burning sensation in the buccal mucosa and on the surface of the tongue where contact with the dressing occurs. The patient should be told at the time of the surgery of the possibility of such symptoms occurring, and instructed to contact the

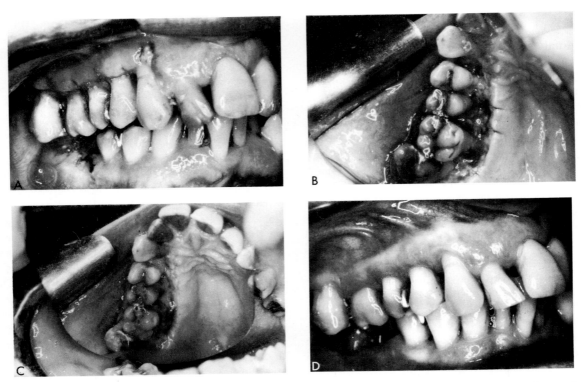

Fig. 20-2. *A,* One week after periodontal surgery. Releasing incision should not have been placed over buccal aspect of cuspid. Labial bone exposed over cuspid. *B,* Palatal view of same patient. Palatal flap too short. "Bare" necrotic bone. *C,* Same patient 2 weeks after surgery. Granulation tissue partially covering the exposed bone. *D,* Six months after surgery. Complete healing.

dentist immediately on experiencing them. If the dressing is not removed, the reaction progresses from erythema to vesicle formation and edema (which, especially in relation to the tongue, may be a serious complication, since epiglottal edema interferes with the air passage). If the patient is not treated, a generalized allergic reaction may develop, including a dermatitis, and the patient may become seriously ill. It is therefore very important that the surgical dressing be removed completely as soon as any of the initial symptoms of an allergic reaction appear (see Fig. 20-1). If a new dressing is needed, a non-eugenol-containing type of dressing, such as Coe-Pak or Peripak, may be used. The patient should also be given systemic antihistamines for at least 4 to 5 days in order to intercept the allergic reaction.

With severe allergic reactions, the patient may have to be hospitalized and given cortisone therapy. This type of treatment should be the responsibility of a qualified physician rather than of the dentist.

Sensitivity of the teeth

The root surfaces of the teeth that have been exposed to the oral environment as a result of periodontal surgery sometimes become extremely sensitive to heat and cold, as well as to mechanical and chemical stimuli. With optimal post-surgical plaque control, this sensitivity usually abates over a few weeks or months, but occasionally it may persist over a long period of time. A large number of procedures and medicaments have been recommended for treating such sensitivity; however, none is spectacularly effective. Toothpastes for reduction of sensitivity provide varying degrees of relief for long-term sensitivity.[40] Topical fluoride applications are often used,[19,31] but with only moderate success. Combining fluorides and electrical current[31,39] has been claimed to reduce sensitivity, but the reduction apparently is not dependent on the use of the electric current.[31] However, iontophoretic devices and dentifrices for root hypersensitivity should be prescribed as possible means of reducing discomfort, even though results may vary.[1,3]

It appears, from clinical observations, that vigorous plaque control is the most significant factor in long-term reduction of sensitivity, unless the sensitivity is related to occlusal dysfunction, which requires occlusal therapy.

PLACEMENT OF DRESSING

The periodontal dressing material should be mixed so that it is fairly hard and rolled into a long thin roll, like a thin pencil. The surgical field should be dried by suction; use sponges only if the hemorrhage cannot be controlled by suction. A dressing may be placed on a wound with a slight oozing type of bleeding. Place dressing material first interproximally using a plastic instrument. Do not use pressure against the wound. Then place the elongated roll of dressing buccally and lingually and press the buccal and lingual portions lightly together with the fingers. If the surgery included the distal aspect of the terminal tooth in the arch, shape the roll dressing into a U shape prior to insertion, and place the closed end of the U distally to the last tooth. Press the rolls of dressing lightly together interproximally with a plastic instrument. With a slight amount of Vaseline on the fingertips, smooth the surface of the dressing.

Dental floss tied to the teeth prior to placement of the dressing may help to hold the dressing in place, especially if there are open spaces between the teeth.

Check carefully for possible interference with occlusion and mucogingival structures.

Besides protecting the wound, another important function of the periodontal dressing is to hold flaps and grafts in close contact with the underlying bone or soft tissue. A correct consistency and careful manipulation of the surgical dressing is therefore important, both for avoidance of pain and discomfort and for promotion of optimal healing.

POSTOPERATIVE CARE

At the completion of the surgery, the patient should be informed about what to expect in terms of symptoms after surgery and what precautions to take. Following the oral explanation, the same instructions should be given to the patient in writing.

Instructions to Patients

The dressing covering the area of the surgery will harden in approximately ½ hour. Do not rinse your mouth, drink, or eat during this time.

The dressing protects and guides healing of the area operated on and reduces discomfort. It is important that the dressing remain in place until your next appointment. If a dressing, or a portion of the dressing, is lost during the first week following surgery, please telephone us. In order to avoid dislodging the dressing:

Do not chew in the area of the dressing.

Do not use your toothbrush on the dressing.

Do not chew hard foods, but do eat a well-balanced soft diet and be sure to drink an adequate amount of fluid (2 quarts a day).

Teeth not covered by the dressing should be brushed as previously instructed. The biting surfaces of teeth covered by the dressing may be brushed with a soft brush. Warm salt water (¼ teaspoon of salt per cup of water) or a diluted mouthwash may be used to rinse your mouth, including the area of the dressing.

Highly seasoned foods, tart fruit juice, or concentrated alcoholic beverages may temporarily cause some discomfort.

Avoid strenuous exercise for a few days.

You may expect a slight oozing bleeding, some swelling, and some soreness. If necessary, you may take 2 tablets for pain every 4 hours to relieve discomfort, but if there is considerable pain for more than 24 hours after the surgery, call for an appointment. If there is definite bleeding in an area, take a piece of gauze or clean cloth, moisten it with water, squeeze it out, and hold it directly against the bleeding area for ½ hour. If this does not stop the bleeding, call (telephone: Office; Home).

If you develop any fever or a burning sensation in the mouth, call for an appointment.

Change of dressing and removal of sutures

The initial dressing should be removed after 7 days. Break the dressing loose with periodontal curettes. Always direct the force away from the wound. Remove all sutures. To loosen soft debris, use cotton dipped in 1½% hydrogen peroxide (3% hydrogen peroxide plus an equal volume of warm water) to wipe over the teeth and the gingiva that had been covered by the dressing. Then rinse with warm water.

Curettes and dental floss should be used to remove any plaque or debris on the surface of the teeth.

Observe the area of the surgery very carefully for bits of calculus, periodontal dressing, soft debris, or outgrowths of granulation tissue. If any irritants are present, remove them with curettes.

If the wound is not completely epithelialized, replace the dressing and schedule another appointment in a week to remove the new dressing.

Postsurgical care

The success or failure of periodontal surgery depends to a great extent upon the immediate[37] and long-term postoperative care of the patient.[33] Only concern with the healing after the surgery is considered here.

At the time of the final dressing removal, the teeth should be polished and oral hygiene should be reviewed with the patient. Acidulated flurophosphate should be applied (or, if ceramic crowns are present, use non-acid fluorides). See the patient once a week for professional plaque removal for 3 to 4 weeks after the dressing removal. Then place the patient on recall for prophylaxis every 3 months. Another successful regime recommended by Westfelt et al. is recall every 2 weeks for 6 months, then a 3-month recall schedule[43] (see chapter 28 on maintenance care).

Summary

Establish specific objectives prior to the periodontal surgery.

Avoid surgery when it may constitute a health hazard to the patient.

Prepare the patient both mentally and physically for the surgery.

Take proper precautions against surgical infections.

Follow the principles of atraumatic surgery.

Be prepared to handle emergency situations.

Give proper postoperative and maintenance care, which is essential for the success of periodontal surgery.

REFERENCES

1. Addy, M., and Donell, P.: Dental hypersensitivity—a review. Clinical and *in vitro* evaluation of treatment agents, J. Clin. Periodontol. 10:351, 1983.
2. Aremband, D., and Wade, A.: A comparative wound healing study following gingivectomy by electrosurgery and knives, J. Periodont. Res. 8:42, 1973.
3. Ash, M.M.: Quantification of stimuli, Endod. Dent. Traumatol. 2:153, 1986.
4. Baer, P.N., Summer, C.F., III, and Scigliano, J.: Studies on hydrogenated fat-zinc bacitracin periodontal dressings, Oral Surg. 13:494, 1960.
5. Berdon, J.K.: Blood loss during gingival surgery, J. Periodont. 36:102, 1965.
6. Byrne, J.J.: Shock, New Engl. J. Med. 275:543, 1966.
7. Caffesse, R.G., Ramfjord, S.P., and Nasjleti, C.E.: Reverse bevel periodontal flaps in monkeys, J. Periodont. 39:219, 1968.
8. Costich, E.R., and Ramfjord, S.P.: Healing after partial denudation of the alveolar process, J. Periodont. 39:127, 1968.
9. Cranin, A.N., and Cranin, S.L.: Study of the effects of antihistamine on oral surgical sequelae, Oral Surg. 18:432, 1964.
10. Crum, R.E., and Anderson, G.F.: The effect of gingival fiber surgery on the retention of rotated teeth, Am. J. Orthod. 65:626, 1974.
11. Dahlberg, W.H.: Incisions and suturing: Some basic considerations about each in periodontal flap surgery, Dent. Clin. North Am. 13:149, 1969.
12. Fleszar, T.J., et al.: Tooth mobility and periodontal therapy, J. Clin. Periodontol. 7:495, 1980.
13. Forrest, J.O.: The use of cyanoacrylate in periodontal surgery, J. Periodont. 45:225, 1974.
14. Glickman, I., and Imber, T.: Comparison of gingival resection with electrosurgery and periodontal knives. A biometric and histologic study, J. Periodont. 41:142, 1970.
15. Glickman, I.: Clinical Periodontology. 4th ed., Philadelphia, 1972, W.B. Saunders Co.
16. Hazards of asbestos in dentistry. Reports of Councils and Bureaus, J.A.D.A. 92:777, 1976.
17. Hirsh, J., et al.: Relation between bleeding time and platelet connective tissue reaction after aspirin, Blood 41:369, 1973.
18. Horton, J.E.: The healing of surgical defects alveolar bone produced with ultrasonic instrumentation, chisel and rotary bur, Oral Surg. 39:536, 1975.
19. Hoyt, W.H., and Bibby, B.G.: Sodium fluoride for desensitizing dentin, J.A.D.A. 30:1372, 1943.
20. Hughes, T.P., and Caffesse, R.G.: Gingival changes following scaling, root planing and oral hygiene. A biometric evaluation, J. Periodontol. 49:245, 1978.
21. Kakehashi, S., and Parakkal, P.F.: Surgical therapy in periodontitis, J. Periodontol. 53:476, 1982.
22. Knowles, J.W., et al.: Results of periodontal treatment related to pocket depth and attachment level. Eight years, J. Periodontol. 50:225, 1979.

23. Kohler, C.A., and Ramfjord, S.P.: Healing of gingival mucoperiosteal flaps, Oral Surg. 13:89, 1960.
24. Krejai, R.F., et al.: Effect of electrosurgery on dog pulp under cervical metallic restorations, Oral Surg. 54:575, 1982.
25. Levine, H.L., and Stahl, S.S.: Repair following periodontal flap surgery with the retention of gingival fibers, J. Periodont. 43:99, 1972.
26. Lilly, G.E., et al.: Reaction of oral tissues to suture materials, Oral Surg. 33:152, 1972.
27. Malone, W.F.: Electrosurgery in Dentistry. Springfield, Il.: Charles C. Thomas, 1974.
28. Malone, W., Eisenmann, D., and Kusek, J.: Interceptive periodontics with electrosurgery, J. Prosthet. Dent. 22:555, 1969.
29. McClendon, J.L., and Hooper, W.C.: Cervico-facial emphysema after air blown into a periodontal pocket, J.A.D.A. 63:810, 1961.
30. McEntegart, M.G., and Clark, A.: Colonization of dental units by water bacteria, Br. Dent. J. 134:140, 1973.
31. Minkov, B., et al.: The effectiveness of sodium fluoride treatment with and without iontophoresis on reduction of hypersensitive dentin, J. Periodont. 46:246, 1975.
32. Morrison, E.C., et al.: Short-term effects of initial, nonsurgical periodontal treatment (hygienic phase), J. Clin. Periodontol. 7:199, 1980.
33. Nichols, C., et al.: Gingival bleeding: The only sign in a case of fibrinolysis, Oral Surg. 38:681, 1974.
34. Nyman, S., Rosling, B., and Lindhe, J.: Effect of professional tooth cleaning on healing after periodontal surgery, J. Clin. Periodontol. 2:80, 1975.
35. Nyman, S., et al.: Periodontal surgery in plaque-infected dentitions, J. Clin. Periodontol. 4:240, 1977.
36. Persson, G., and Thilander, H.: Experimental studies of surgical packs. I. In vivo experiments on antimicrobial effect, Odont. Tidskr. 76:147, 1968.
37. Ramfjord, S.P., and Costich, E.R.: Healing after simple gingivectomy, J. Periodont. 34:401, 1963.
38. Rickles, N.H., and Joshi, B.A.: Death from air embolism during root canal therapy. Possible care in a human and an investigation in dogs, J.A.D.A. 67:397, 1963.
39. Schaeffer, M.L., Bixler, D., and Yu, P.L.: The effectiveness of iontophoresis in reducing cervical hypersensitivity, J. Periodont. 42:695, 1971.
40. Smith, B.A., and Ash, M.M., Jr.: A study of desensitizing dentifrice and cervical hypersensitivity, J. Periodont. 35:222, 1964.
41. Ward, A.W.: Surgical eradication of pyorrhea, J.A.D.A. 15:2146, 1928.
42. Webster's New School and Office Dictionary. Ed. J. Devlin. New York: World Publishing Co., 1943.
43. Westfelt, E., et al.: Significance of frequency of professional tooth cleaning for healing following periodontal surgery, J. Clin. Periodontol. 10:148, 1983.
44. Wilhelmsen, N.R., Ramfjord, S.P., and Blankenship, J.R.: Effects of electrosurgery on the gingival attachment in rhesus monkeys, J. Periodont. 47:3, 160, 1976.
45. Wood, D.L., et al.: Alveolar crest reduction following full and partial thickness flaps, J. Periodont. 43:141, 1972.
46. Woodward, S.C., et al.: Histotoxicity of cyanoacrylate tissue adhesive in the rat, Ann. Surg. 162:113, 1965.

21

CURETTAGE

By definition, *curettage* is the scraping of a bodily cavity by means of a curette in order to clean its surface, to obtain material for diagnostic purposes, or to remove a lesion or foreign body. For nearly 100 years, numerous articles and textbooks have extolled the value of curettage in periodontal therapy, but it has always been a controversial procedure, with equally vociferous advocates and adversaries.[16,31,39] However, recent clinical research[15] has failed to demonstrate any benefit from gingival curettage beyond results that may be obtained by scaling and root planing only. However, since this old modality of periodontal treatment is still used widely, it will be described and discussed briefly.

In periodontics, the word *curettage* should be used strictly to mean the scraping or removal of soft tissues within the gingival crevice or periodontal pocket. Scaling and root planing (considered as a single process) may unintentionally include various degrees of curettage,[28] may be done at the same time as curettage (even with the same instruments), and is of decisive importance for the success of the curettage; however, the rationale is different for these two procedures. Therefore, they should be considered as two separate aspects of periodontal therapy.

Scaling and root planing during the hygienic phase of the therapy is aimed at the elimination of irritants on and within the surface of the tooth; curettage is aimed at surgical elimination of altered periodontal tissues in order to facilitate healing to a tooth surface that previous scaling and planing have made biologically acceptable to the soft tissues.

CURETTAGE IN THE TREATMENT OF GINGIVITIS

Gingival curettage has been recommended for patients with recalcitrant gingivitis when the gingival tissues are edematous, soft, and swollen.[12,13] The rationale for gingival curettage may be discussed under the following categories: (1) removal of crevicular debris; (2) elimination of obstacles to a normal epithelial attachment; (3) facilitation of connective tissue healing and maturation; and (4) promotion of a normal gingival vascular plexus.

During scaling and root planing, debris such as fragments of calculus may become adherent to the soft tissue surface or clefts in the wall of the gingival crevice[28] (Fig. 21-1). Curettage will remove this debris, but so will crevicular rinsing with a water spray.

Deep projections of crevicular epithelial ridges are commonly seen in severe gingivitis. Scaling will often produce clefts in these ridges;[23,28] these clefts could interfere with epithelial reattachment. It has also been assumed that residual projections of epithelium in the crevicular wall may prevent the formation of a long, thin epithelial attachment after scaling.[12] Such ridges are present shortly after scaling[26] (Fig. 21-2), but apparently they may undergo evolution, because a long, thin epithelial attachment after scaling has been reported after longer-term observation.[34]

Gingival curettage has been recommended as a means of eliminating the chronically inflamed connective tissues in the crevicular area, under the assumption that toxic and histolytic products associated with the inflammatory process would delay or interfere with healing.[12] This contention overlooks the fact that periodontal inflammation is basically a defensive response provoked by bacteria in the gingival crevice and on the surface of the tooth; when the bacteria are eliminated from the gingival crevice, the chronic inflammation will undergo resolution, with no need for the removal of inflamed tissues.

Another proposed need for gingival curettage has arisen over concern for the reconstitution of a normal gingival plexus of blood vessels in tissues that have been altered by chronic inflammation. The changes in the subcrevicular vascular patterns associated with

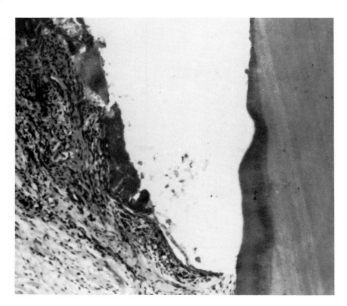

Fig. 21-1. Debris adherent to the crevicular wall immediately after scaling (human specimen).

gingivitis have been well documented.[10,25] It is not known whether the looped vasculature associated with gingivitis will revert completely to a normal gingival capillary network plexus following hygienic therapy; it has also been suggested that the enlarged vessels associated with chronic gingival inflammation may not allow for the normal metabolic interchange associated with small vessels in a healthy gingiva. Gingival curettage would solve these problems by providing optimal revascularization of the regenerated gingiva. However, these theoretical speculations have not been supported by clinical observations, which indicate that normal gingival physiology can be reinstituted simply by removing the irritants and maintaining good plaque control.[20]

Shrinkage of the gingival tissues, with recession of the free gingival margin and reduction of crevice depth, unquestionably can be induced by the gingival curettage of soft, swollen gingivae. However, if the cause of the gingival inflammation is removed from the surface of the teeth, the gingivae will also shrink as the inflammation subsides.[15] Gingival curettage will add insult to previously injured tissues.

Furthermore, if curettage is attempted while the periodontal tissues are weakened by active inflammation, the chances are great that permanent damage may ensue should the curettage be inadvertently extended beyond the apical border of the epithelial attachment.[35]

The common recommendation that gingival curettage should be performed in cases of edematous and highly inflamed gingivae[12,13] scientifically is not well founded. Although curettage under such conditions may result in an apparent clinical success, especially

in cases in which the cementoenamel junction is exposed about 1 mm into the gingival crevice, a much safer alternative would be to plane the cementoenamel junction and institute acceptable plaque control, without adding the risk of permanent loss of periodontal support that could result from the curettage. With extensive gingival curettage of an inflamed gingiva, postcurettage gingival recession will place the cementoenamel junction (and the associated bacterial retention site) supracrevicularly and thus reduce the gingivitis. A smoothing of the cementoenamel junction and the entire subgingival tooth surface may also result from the scaling, which is usually done in association with the curettage.

If for esthetic or functional reasons recontouring or reduction in crevice depth is desired, these processes can be carried out in a much easier and more predictable way by gingivoplasty than by curettage of fibrous gingival tissues present at the completion of the hygienic phase.

On the basis of current concepts of etiology, pathology, and healing following treatment, there does not appear to be any well-established rationale for gingival curettage as a separate, distinct procedure in the treatment of gingivitis.

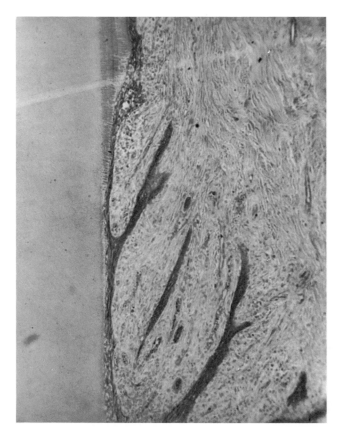

Fig. 21-2. Ten days after scaling and root planing. New epithelial attachment to cementum and dentin. Long epithelial projections. Mild chronic inflammation.

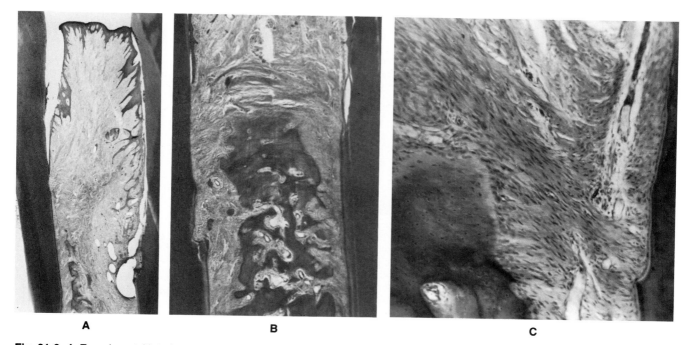

Fig. 21-3. *A,* Experimental intrabony periodontal pocket in rhesus monkey. *B,* After curettage and phenol treatment, connective tissue reattachment and regeneration of bone in pocket similar to *A.* Notch on root surface indicates the depth of the previous pocket. *C,* Higher magnification of reattachment coronally to notch in root surface. Note cementoblastic and osteoblastic activity.

Curettage in the treatment of periodontitis

Traditionally, the main purpose of using curettage in periodontal pockets was to eliminate the epithelial lining of the pocket in order to induce connective tissue attachment to the root surface, along with the formation of new cementum and bone. A large number of experimental studies in animals, and clinical, as well as histological and roentgenologic, studies in humans, have been concerned with periodontal responses to curettage when it is performed in conjunction with or in addition to scaling and root planing. Only recently have a few studies compared the clinical results of scaling and root planing with or without soft tissue curettage.[15]

It now appears that the reported excellent clinical results after gingival curettage have nothing to do with the soft tissue curettage,[15] and that the results would have been as good with scaling and root planing without the added curettage. However, a brief review will be offered here to explain how the current views were established.

Healing after curettage in pockets

Histologic evidence (Fig. 21-3) has been presented showing new attachment of periodontal fibers that are embedded in new cementum and new alveolar bone coronally to marks created on the surface of teeth during preceding subgingival curettage.[6] However, this evidence does not conclusively prove that reat-tachment to a root surface previously exposed in the pocket takes place due to curettage, because the new attachment may only represent the healing of a surgical detachment that took place during the curettage.[35] The subject of reattachment will also be discussed in chapter 23, which is on flap procedures.

Experimental studies on healing and reattachment in animals have indicated a high potential for spontaneous healing of nonepithelialized surgically created pockets; in contrast, epithelialized and clinically inflamed artificial pockets have a tendency to persist or become deeper if not treated.

Claims of connective tissue reattachment after curettage, based on evidence from roentgenograms, cannot be accepted (Fig. 21-4 A, B), because clinically the penetration of the probe does not relate in a decisive manner to the coronal border of the connective tissue attachment,[8,21] and alveolar bone may fill into intrabony lesions that are separated from the tooth by junctional epithelium.[9] The most spectacular claims of reattachment, supported by clinical and roentgenographic findings, are based on the healing of periodontal abscesses,[2] which will occur with or without curettage (Fig. 21-5). It appears that immediately after curettage, there is clinical loss of attachment, which will be followed by a slight gain of about 0.5 mm in 1 month. In addition, shrinkage reduces the height of the free gingiva margins by about 1 mm; with periodic prophylaxes, these results may be maintained.[15]

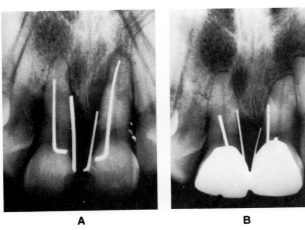

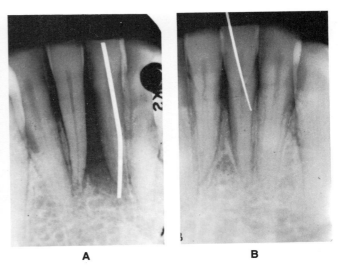

Fig. 21-4. *A,* Silverpoints placed in deep palatal pockets prior to subgingival curettage. *B,* Same patient as in *A* 1 year later. Orthodontic treatment and splinting of the central incisors was done after the curettage. Note that the silverpoints cannot be placed as far apically as in *A.*

Fig. 21-5. *A,* Abscess in deep periodontal pockets with silverpoint in the lingual pocket. *B,* One year after subgingival curettage. Note wide periodontal space on lateral incisor. No pocket could be probed at this time.

Roentgenographic evidence has been reported for the regeneration of alveolar crest height following curettage, but without controls that establish what would have happened if only scaling and root planing had taken place.

The soft tissue response to curettage has been studied extensively in both humans[6,38] and animals.[34] Immediately following curettage, only fragments of epithelium are seen, along with blood and polymorphonuclear cells. There is also some hemorrhage within the traumatized connective tissue. Within 1 day, epithelial proliferation starts at the borders, and the crevicular wound is covered by a band of polymorphonuclear cells. Seven to 9 days are needed to establish a new crevicular lining and junctional epithelium. In 2 to 3 weeks, the junctional and crevicular epithelium appears and behaves as it would in a normal, untouched control crevice, aside from the immature nature of the collagen fibers that are found directly below the newly formed epithelium. Epithelial reattachment has been reported to occur even to well-planed and sterilized calculus in small areas.

It has been suggested that the regeneration of crevicular epithelium would be slowed down by blood clots.[6,30,39] However, this concept has been refuted. Occasionally, connective tissue contact with the tooth will induce some areas of root resorption. A "creeping attachment," with coronal movement of the junctional epithelium without removal of the crevicular lining, appears very rarely, and the biologic basis for this phenomena is not understood.[19]

Instruments and techniques for curettage

The instruments and techniques for curettage should be suited to (1) removing the entire epithelial lining of the crevice or pocket; (2) removing the chron-ically inflamed connective tissues underlying and surrounding the epithelial projections; (3) affording control for selective tissue removal; (4) afflicting minimal trauma on the residual tissues; and (5) removing all debris from the pocket.

The following instruments or agents have been recommended for curettage: (1) varying types of curettes; (2) abrasive stones; (3) ultrasonics; and (4) caustics followed by curettage.

Gingival or subgingival curettage is definitely a surgical procedure,[6] requiring local anesthesia and sharp instruments used in a careful manner.

Use of curettes

The operator may choose a curette of the design he prefers so long as the instrument is small enough to afford access to narrow and deep periodontal pockets. Curettage should start from the bottom of the pocket, which should be located by careful exploration with the instrument. The old approach of extending the curettage apically to the bottom of the clinically determined pocket as discerned by probing was based on the false assumption that regular scaling extends only to the coronal aspect of the epithelial attachment.

It has been shown that routine scaling with a curette will separate the entire epithelial attachment from the tooth and will also remove most of the epithelial cells in that region (Fig. 21-6). If root planing is extended beyond the apical border of the epithelial attachment, permanent loss of connective tissue attachment may be the result. Thus, it is important that curettage be performed in a coronal direction, starting from the bottom of the pocket as located by the back edge of the curette. The curettage should gradually dissect the epithelial lining loose with strokes in a coronal or lateral direction.

The face of the curette should be directed at nearly a right angle to the pocket wall and moved with light pressure against the soft tissues. Holding a finger on the outside of the gingiva and pressing lightly against the pocket being curetted may help in scraping off the epithelial lining and the underlying chronically inflamed connective tissues. Using eight to twelve strokes for each area of the pocket, or scraping for a certain time interval for each tooth, has been recommended.[30,32] However, the angulation of the instrument, and the sharpness, force, and, above all, the character of the tissues, will determine how many strokes or how much time is needed.

If gingival tissues have been given time to heal following the removal of the calculus, the curette will glide on top of the mature collagen fibers without further tissue removal after the epithelial lining and the inflamed tissues are scraped. This is the best way to determine whether the curettage has been adequate.[6]

There is considerable controversy in reports concerning the possibility of complete removal of the epithelial lining of pockets by curettage without doing

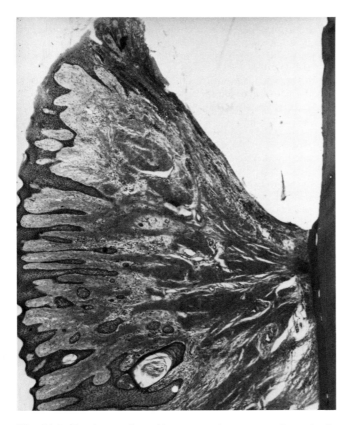

Fig. 21-6. Routine scaling with a curette has removed practically all of the junctional epithelium and part of the crevicular lining (human specimen immediately after scaling).

extensive harm. The reports vary, from claims that the epithelial lining could not be completely removed and that considerable damage was inflicted during curettage[35] to reports of consistent and complete elimination of the pocket epithelium by curettage.[5] Some reports indicate complete removal of the epithelium in most instances, but with some epithelium toward the gingival margin being retained in a few cases.

Special instruments such as the Pollock curette and the Berliner[3] scalpel have been recommended for subgingival curettage. However, the control of adequate tissue removal with minimal trauma is more difficult with these instruments than with conventional curettes, and the Berliner knife is not recommended when complete removal of the epithelial lining is desired.[38]

Abrasive stones

Rotating diamond stones have also been used for removal of the pocket lining. Although such instruments may remove the epithelium in most cases, their action is poorly controlled and they provide an obstructed field of vision; therefore, they cannot be recommended.

Ultrasonics

Ultrasonic curettage has been found effective in removing the epithelial lining of the pocket.[11,24,32] In some instances, the ultrasonic curettage had led to complete removal of the epithelial lining and left a smooth, non-traumatized connective tissue wall of the pocket, whereas in other instances some epithelium remained, especially toward the gingival margin.[24,32] It appears that the heat associated with the ultrasonic curettage does not have deep penetration if proper cooling is used,[11] and the healing after ultrasonic curettage progresses at approximately the same rate as the healing after the use of curettes.[32]

Caustics followed by curettage

A number of caustic agents have been recommended for necrosis of the epithelial lining of the pocket and to facilitate curettage. Lactic acid, mineral acids, and antiformin with sulfuric acid have been recommended for use following curettage since the turn of the 20th century.[14] Since that time, a number of non-demineralizing caustics, such as sodium sulfide[22] and camphor phenol,[1] have been used. However, none of these drugs is a specific "epithelial solvent,"[4,17,36] and all are strong irritants. The use of camphor phenol (3 : 1 strength) may facilitate the curettage.[36] A complete debridement of the pocket is required following the use of such drugs.

The main objection to the use of caustics is the poor control of their field and depth of action. Thus, direct curettage may be preferable to the combined use of caustics and curettes.

Current concepts of curettage

Until very recently, gingival or subgingival curettage was enjoying a renaissance when its results were compared with the results of other surgical approaches in periodontal therapy.[29] However, it now appears that the good results credited to curettage can be duplicated with less effort by scaling and root planing only.[15] Both longitudinal clinical studies[18,27] and histological investigations[8] have shown that there is actually no demonstrable benefit from removal of epithelium and inflamed connective tissue from the wall of the periodontal product. The advantages claimed in several clinical trials for subgingival curettage compared with other surgical techniques can apparently be attributed to scaling and root planing only.[15,29] The limitations of subgingival curettage are related to the limitations of access to the root surface exposed in the periodontal pockets and poor vision in the field of operation, which may be improved by using surgical flap procedures. Curettage does not provide any improvement in access for root planing. The only advantage curettage may have over scaling and root planing only would be in the treatment of juvenile periodontitis,[33] in which curettage may remove more bacteria lodged within the gingival tissues than would scaling and root planing alone. If antibiotics are used as support therapy, scaling and root planing alone would probably be as effective as curettage.

REFERENCES

1. Barkann, L.: A conservative technic for the eradication of a pyorrhea pocket, J.A.D.A. 26:61, 1939.
2. Bell, D.G.: A case of reattachment, J. Periodontol. 8:30, 1937.
3. Berliner, A.: Elimination of periodontal pockets, Dent. Dig. 56:397, 1950.
4. Beube, F.E.: An experimental study of the use of sodium sulphide solution in treatment of periodontal pockets, J. Periodont. 10:3, 1939.
5. Beube, F.E.: Treatment methods for marginal gingivitis and periodontitis, Texas Dent. J. 71:427, 1953.
6. Box, H.K.: Treatment of the Periodontal Pocket. Toronto: University of Toronto Press, 1928.
7. Bunting, R.W.: The control and treatment of pyorrhea by subgingival surgery, J.A.D.A. 15:119, 1928.
8. Caton, J., and Zander, H.A.: The attachment between teeth and gingival tissues after periodic root planing and soft tissue curettage, J. Periodontol. 50:462, 1979.
9. Caton, J., and Zander, H.A.: Osseous repair of an intrabony pocket without new attachment of connective tissue, J. Clin. Periodontol. 3:54, 1976.
10. Egelberg, J.: The blood vessels of the dentogingival junction, J. Periodont. Res. 1:163, 1966.
11. Ewen, S.J.: Ultrasonic sound—some microscopic observations, J. Periodont. 32:315, 1961.
12. Goldman, H.M., and Cohen, D.W.: Periodontal Therapy. 5th ed. St. Louis: C.V. Mosby Co., 1973.
13. Grant, D.A., Stern, I.B., and Everett, F.G.: Orban's Periodontics. 4th ed. St. Louis: C.V. Mosby Co., 1972.
14. Hecker, F.: Pyorrhea Alveolaris. St. Louis: C.V. Mosby Co., 1913.
15. Hill, R.W., et al.: Four types of periodontal treatment compared over two years, J. Periodontol. 52:655, 1981.
16. Hopewell-Smith, A.: Pyorrhea alveolaris—its interpretation. II. Concluding note, Dent. Cosmos 53:981, 1911.
17. Johnson, R.F., and Waerhaug, J.: Effect of antiformin on gingival tissues, J. Periodont. 27:24, 1956.
18. Lindhe, J., and Nyman, S.: Scaling and granulation tissue removed in periodontal therapy, J. Clin. Periodontol. 12:374, 1985.
19. Listgarten, M.A., et al.: Progressive replacement of epithelial attachment by a connective tissue junction after experimental periodontal surgery in rats, J. Periodontol. 53:659, 1982.
20. Löe, H., Theilade, E., and Jensen, S.B.: Experimental gingivitis in man, J. Periodont. 36:177, 1965.
21. Magnusson, I., and Listgarten, M.A.: Histologic evaluation of probing depth following periodontal treatment, J. Clin. Periodontol. 7:26, 1980.
22. McCall, J.D.: An improved method of inducing reattachment of the gingival tissues in periodontoclasia, Dental Items of Interest 48:342, 1926.
23. Moskow, B.S.: The response of the gingival sulcus to instrumentation: A histological investigation. I. The scaling procedure, J. Periodont. 33:282, 1962.
24. Nadler, H.: Removal of crevicular epithelium by ultrasonic curettes, J. Periodont. 33:220, 1962.
25. Nuki, K., and Hock, J.: The organization of the gingival vasculature, J. Periodont. Res. 9:305, 1974.
26. O'Bannon, J.Y.: The gingival tissues before and after scaling the teeth, J. Periodont. 35:69, 1964.
27. Pihlstrom, B.L., et al.: Comparison of surgical and nonsurgical treatment of periodontal disease. A review of current studies and additional results after 6½ years, J. Clin. Periodontol. 10:524, 1984.
28. Ramfjord, S.P., and Kiester, G.: The gingival sulcus and the periodontol pockets immediately following the scaling of teeth, J. Periodontol. 25:167, 1954.
29. Ramfjord, S.P., et al.: Results following three modalities of periodontal therapy, J. Periodont. 46:522, 1975.
30. Raust, G.T.: What is the value of gingival curettage in periodontal therapy? Periodont. Abstr. 17:142, 1969.
31. Riggs, J.M.: Pyorrhea alveolaris, Dent. Cosmos 24:524, 1882.
32. Schaffer, E.M., Stende, G., and King, D.: Healing of periodontal pocket tissues following ultrasonic scaling and hand planing, J. Periodont. 35:140, 1964.
33. Slots, J., and Rosling, B.G.: Supression of the periodontopathic microflora in localized juvenile periodontitis by systemic tetracycline, J. Clin. Periodontol. 10:465, 1983.
34. Waerhaug, J.: Microscopic demonstration of time reaction incident to removal of subgingival calculus, J. Periodont. 26:26, 1955.
35. Waerhaug, J.: The gingival pocket. Anatomy, pathology, deepening and elimination, Odont. Tidsk. 60:Suppl. 1, 1952.
36. Waerhaug, J., and Löe, H.: Effect of phenol camphor on gingival tissue, J. Periodont. 29:58, 1958.
37. Webster's Third New International Dictionary. Ed. P.B. Grove. Springfield, Mass.: G. and C. Merriam Co., 1961.
38. Wertheimer, F.: Effectiveness of "Berliner epithelial scalpel" in removing the epithelial lining in periodontal pockets, J. Periodont. 25:264, 1954.
39. Younger, W.J.: Some of the latest phases in implantation and other operations, Dent. Cosmos 35:102, 1893.

22

GINGIVECTOMY WOUND HEALING

Surgical removal of the soft tissue wall of a periodontal pocket has been recommended for a long time. It used to be assumed that the gingiva, soft tissues, and the bone were infected, and had to be removed to achieve healing. This operation was given the name of *gingivectomy* by Pickerill in 1912.[34] Later, providing access for the patient to practice plaque control was added to the rationale for gingivectomy. Then Kronfeld (1935) showed that the bone under the pocket was neither necrotic nor infected.[23] Orban, in about 1940, introduced the more modern uses of gingivectomy for surgical pocket elimination and gingival recontouring.[27,28,29] Recontouring of the alveolar process as part of the gingivectomy operation was suggested by Black in 1915.[3] All these variants of gingivectomy are only of historical interest. Except for the description of surgical recontouring of the gingiva for esthetic reasons[11,12] and for access for placement or correction of dental restorations, none of these variants will be discussed in this book.

Gingivectomy for surgical reduction of periodontal pockets is not an acceptable procedure anymore, and access for root planing can be gained more efficiently by flap procedures. One consideration in favor of gingivectomy for access to the tooth surface coronally to the bottom of the epithelial attachment is that gingivectomy carefully done does not lead to the bone resorption and loss of attachment commonly found with flap procedures.

Extent of tissue removal

The gingival tissues should be excised to the bottom of the gingival crevice as located by probing, and the surgical contour should be made to resemble the normal gingival contour, or approximately 45° to the tooth surface. It has been shown by several investigators that excision of the gingiva to the bottom of the probing will include complete removal of the epithelial attachment as well as of the entire wall of the periodontal pocket.[37,46]

Ideally, the tissue removal during gingivectomy should follow the contour line of the cementoenamel junction and expose a similar distance of the root surface buccally, lingually, and interproximally from the cementoenamel junction to the incision. This will mean a curved, convex buccolingual interproximal contour in the anterior part of the mouth, and an almost flat interproximal contour on the posterior segments. As pointed out by Black long ago, in order to achieve surgical pocket elimination, the tissue removal may have to include some removal of bone. Even osteoectomy of buccal and lingual supporting bone may be needed to eliminate interproximal craters and to avoid reverse architecture.[13,39] However, if bone surgery is contemplated, gingivectomy is not the technique of choice. Bone removal can be accomplished better through other procedures. It has been postulated that a zone of attached gingiva is essential for maintenance of gingival health, prevention of gingival recession, and an unaltered level of the connective tissue attachment.[8] However, a number of recent studies have documented that, with good plaque control and good health, the attachment levels can be maintained unaltered without attached gingiva.[47,48] Thus, the old assumption that gingivectomy would be contraindicated if pockets extended apically to the mucogingival line[10] is not necessarily true, although there is hardly any good reason for doing gingivectomy under such circumstances anyway.

A second approach to gingivectomy has been to remove all soft gingival tissues interproximally and surrounding the neck of the teeth buccally and lingually down to the alveolar process.[32] Although such an extensive surgical wound will heal, and even provide reorganization of body contour with filling of some intrabony defects, this procedure leads to unnecessary

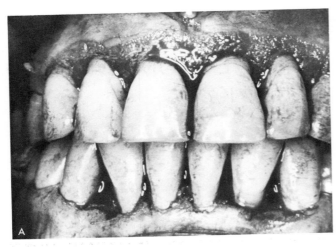

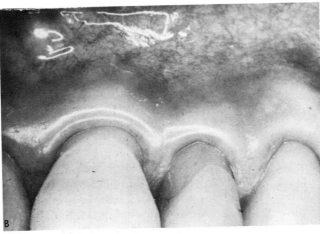

Fig. 22-1. *A,* Proper contouring of the gingiva during gingivectomy. *B,* Two years after the gingivectomy there are thick rolled gingival margins where the gingiva contacts flat root surfaces. However, the plaque control is good and the gingiva is healthy.

postoperative discomfort and loss of some connective tissue attachment around the neck of the teeth. Such supracrestal stripping of the gingival tissues is not recommended. Other recommended forms of gingivectomy have involved either following the bone contour with the incision[8] or doing partial pocket removal,[46] but these are not used anymore.

The long-term postoperative gingival contour is not entirely determined by the contour given the gingiva during a gingivectomy. The initial postsurgical contour changes considerably over some weeks or months, depending on the environment provided by tooth surfaces, bone, and the height of the palatal vault,[21,36] and such changes go on for years after the surgery.[21] Apparently, the free gingival margin becomes thick and rolled if the free gingiva after the surgery contacts a flat tooth surface (Fig. 22-1).

Partial gingivectomy followed by subgingival curettage[40] is an outmoded procedure, as are buccal flap and palatal gingivectomy.[7] These were esthetic

compromise procedures during an era that believed in a 3 mm crevice as prerequisite for health.

TECHNIQUES OF GINGIVECTOMY

In the selection of instruments and techniques for gingivectomy, certain requirements should be considered: (a) The techniques and instruments should permit precise removal of the minimal amount of gingival tissue required for pocket elimination and establishment of optimal gingival contour; (b) the instruments and techniques should inflict minimal surgical trauma to the soft and hard tissues; (c) there should be no hazard to the patient's periodontal, oral, or systemic health from commonly accepted usage of the instruments and techniques; and (d) instruments and techniques that do not interfere with optimal healing should be used.

Recommended procedures

According to accepted principles of periodontal surgery (chap. 20), the hygienic phase and occlusal adjustment, if indicated, should have been completed prior to the gingivectomy. The area of the surgery should be anesthetized, swabbed with an antiseptic solution, such as iodine lotion or tincture of iodine, to reduce the bacterial flora, and blocked off with cotton rolls.

Measure the depths of the pockets with a probe at the distobuccal and mesiobuccal line angle of each tooth and with the probe directed parallel to the long axis of the tooth. Then place the probe on the outside of the gingiva, pointing in the same direction as when the pockets were measured. Then, at a distance the same number of millimeters from the gingival margin, measure to the same point as when the pocket depth was recorded. Make a puncture mark with the tip of the probe at this level. Unless the buccal pockets are deeper than the interproximal pockets, the puncture marks should be made only for the interproximal pockets. Similar measurements and puncture marks should be made on the lingual or palatal aspects. These puncture marks correspond to the apical border of the epithelial attachment. The use of so-called "pocket markers"[13] is not recommended, because any tilt of the instrument will give false markings.

For the buccal incision, use a Bard-Parker #12B knife (Fig. 22-2). Begin the incision 1 to 2 mm apically to the puncture mark and with the blade directed at an angle of approximately 45° to the labial surface of the teeth. The tip of the knife should be aimed at the bottom of the pocket as recorded by the probe. Thus, if the gingiva is thin, the incision should be started about 1 mm apically to the puncture mark, but if the gingiva is thick, the incision must be started farther apically in order to contact the tooth at the bottom of the pocket. The incision should begin at the most

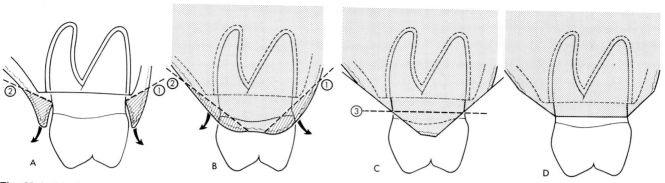

Fig. 22-2. Gingivectomy. *A,* Make buccal and palatal incision (*1* and *2*) to the bottom of the pockets. *B,* Buccal and palatal incisions *1* and *2* will not eliminate the interproximal pockets. *C,* Make interproximal incision *3* to the bottom of the pockets. *D,* Soft tissue walls of the pockets have been eliminated and interproximal contour is almost parallel to the cementoenamel junction.

distal aspect of the surgical field and be carried mesially, guided by the puncture marks, in a straight-line, continuous incision with light sawing movement. Do not try to make individual scalloping or discontinuous incisions for each tooth, since the fine contour is determined by the healing, not the incision.

The lingual or palatal incision should be made with an Orban #1 or #2 knife. However, if the palate has a low vault, it may not be practical to attempt a 45° angle with the teeth, and the incision can be guided by the contour present before the surgery, which may mean a different gingival contour for different teeth. The incision should be started from the distal aspect of the most distal tooth in the field of surgery and move mesially. Be sure to move the knife as far as possible into the interproximal areas, and retrace the incision, moving the knife from the mesial to the distal aspect. Do not hesitate to include the incisive papilla in the excision if required for optimal contour. The assistant should use suction continuously during the operation.

The excised tissues should be removed with curettes, starting from the most distal part of the incision. Then probe to assure that all pockets have been removed on the buccal and palatal aspect of each tooth, beginning at the distal line angle and working to the mesial line angle. If there are residual pockets present in these areas, they should be removed with an additional incision at the same bevel angle as the initial incision. The contour should be checked at this time; often it will be necessary to make an extra contouring incision in the palate to make the surgical contour blends properly with the palatal contour.

Probe for residual interproximal pockets, which should be eliminated by secondary interproximal incisions parallel with the cementoenamel junction of the teeth. In the molar and maxillary bicuspid regions, this means an almost straight incision at a right angle to the long axis of the teeth. The commonly recommended triangular shape of the interdental areas following gingivectomy[13] is not a realistic goal in pocket elimination, except to some extent for the anterior teeth. The interproximal secondary incisions from both the buccal and the lingual aspects should be made with a narrow interproximal spear-shaped knife, such as Goldman-Fox knives #8, #9, and #11,[13] or Orban knives that have been sharpened many times, leaving a narrow pointed blade.[13]

The excised tissues should be removed with sharp curettes, and the interproximal areas surveyed for further residual pockets. These incisions should have eliminated the pockets if proper screening was done, because crater-shaped interproximal lesions should not be treated by gingivectomy.

Elimination of interproximal craters will often necessitate some removal of bone. If a gingivectomy has been started in such a case, the pocket elimination and contouring should be completed. However, instead of removing periosteum and bone directly by stones, chisels, or burs, lay a small periosteal flap to expose the bone and proceed to remove the bone by chisels or files. Then place the periosteal flap back over the scraped bone.

Also remove any small tissue tags that may have resulted from overlapping incision or from tears associated with incomplete incisions. Small surgical scissors[13] (Goldman-Fox) or soft-tissue rongeurs (nippers) may be used. Holding the tissue tag up from the wound surface by the suction tip facilitates the removal. A sharp curette may also be used if the tissue tag is attached close to the tooth and can be pinched against the tooth. Tearing of tissues should be avoided.

Finally, the teeth should be meticulously planed. If the cementoenamel junction is rough, or there are prominent rough edges on the root surfaces, use periodontal files to remove all protruding rough areas, then plane the surfaces with curettes. Continue the planing until the surfaces feel absolutely smooth when tested with a #17 explorer. Use magnifying glasses to inspect root surfaces.

Placement of the surgical dressing and postoperative care should follow the general recommendations in chapter 20.

OTHER TECHNIQUES FOR GINGIVECTOMY
Electrosurgery

A general discussion of electrosurgery is presented in chapter 20. Before electrosurgery is used for gingivectomy, it should be evaluated on the basis of the 4 requirements for optimal techniques listed at the beginning of the previous section. It will then become apparent that electrosurgery fulfills only the 1st requirement regarding precise tissue removal as well as conventional surgical methods do.

There is definitely a greater danger of immediate and permanent damage to the periodontium from electrosurgery[9] than from the use of steel knives. Electrosurgery has been attractive as a technique for gingivectomy mainly because of its convenience: the tip of the needle can be bent to achieve ideal contour anywhere in the mouth. Achieving that may be a problem with knives, especially on the lingual aspect of lingually tipped mandibular anterior teeth. There is also less bleeding with electrosurgery than with knives.

Electrosurgery may be used for convenience when access for knives is poor, provided that the cutting needle is not brought into contact with cementum or bone,[9] and provided that other precautions for safety have been fulfilled (for example, that no explosive anesthetics are being used and no one involved in the process has a heart pacemaker). Electrosurgery is not recommended as a routine method for gingivectomy.

Diamond stones

Rotating abrasives for gingivoplasty and gingivectomy were first recommended in 1955[6] and have been used extensively for contouring of both soft tissues and bone.[13,35] Even with high speed, copious flow of water, and light touch, the stones have a tendency to shred the soft tissues, and the wound must subsequently be trimmed with surgical scissors. There also seems to be some delay in healing of bone following the use of diamond stones,[4] and permanent damage to the tooth surfaces may occur if the stones accidentally touch the tooth during the operation. Although diamond stones can be used to refine gingival contour, especially with firm gingival tissues, such refinement, including refinement of buccal spillways between the root eminences,[13] is of questionable significance to future gingival health. The gingival junction with the teeth cannot be precisely finished with a diamond stone.

Thus, based on the previously listed requirements, the diamond stone technique is not as effective and safe a tool as sharp knives for gingivectomy or gingivoplasty.

Chemical gingivectomy

Orban described a chemical method for gingivectomy using 5% paraformaldehyde.[30] Other caustics, such as potassium hydroxide,[15] have also been recommended.

However, it has been shown that these methods may lead to pain, deep necrosis, and loss of attachment, as well as poor gingival contour.[25] Thus, chemical gingivectomy cannot be recommended.

Wound healing

Since the classical paper on wound healing by Hartwell was published in 1929,[16] innumerable reports have added detailed information on wound healing. In addition, a large number of publications have been specifically devoted to the healing of the gingivectomy wound and to the reestablishment of the gingival crevice following the healing, both in humans[31,37] and in animals.[5,33,38] Traditionally, histological wound healing studies consider epithelial regeneration and connective tissue healing separately,[16] although they are interdependent.

Epithelium

Detailed information regarding the dynamics of healing of gingivectomy wounds have been gained from combined histological and autoradiographic studies in animals.[5,38] In one study, the epithelium at the wound margin did not show any increase or decrease in premitotic labeling 1 hour after incision.[5]

Five hours after the gingivectomy, many cells in the spinous layer were enlarged and pale-staining, and exhibited indistinct intercellular bridges, whereas the basal cells appeared normal and the radioactivity index had not changed. A "poly-band" was forming on the wound surface.

By 9 to 13 hours after the surgery, migration of cells over the wound surface had started[5,19] between the surface of the blood clot, including some necrotic debris, and the underlying vital connective tissue. The migrating epithelial cells did not show any premitotic labeling.[5] These cells have been described as moving by means of pseudopodia,[16] and they may have phagocytic ability.

Between 12 and 24 hours after surgery, the premitotic labeling in the epithelium extending from the wound margin[5] to about 2 mm, was increased markedly (more than 12 times that of the control area), while the number of labeled cells in the epithelium at a distance greater than 2 mm from the wound was normal.

Thirty-six hours postsurgically, the premitotic labeling had started to decrease compared with the 24-hour specimens.

Forty-eight hours following surgery, epithelial labeling rate still was high at the wound margin, but

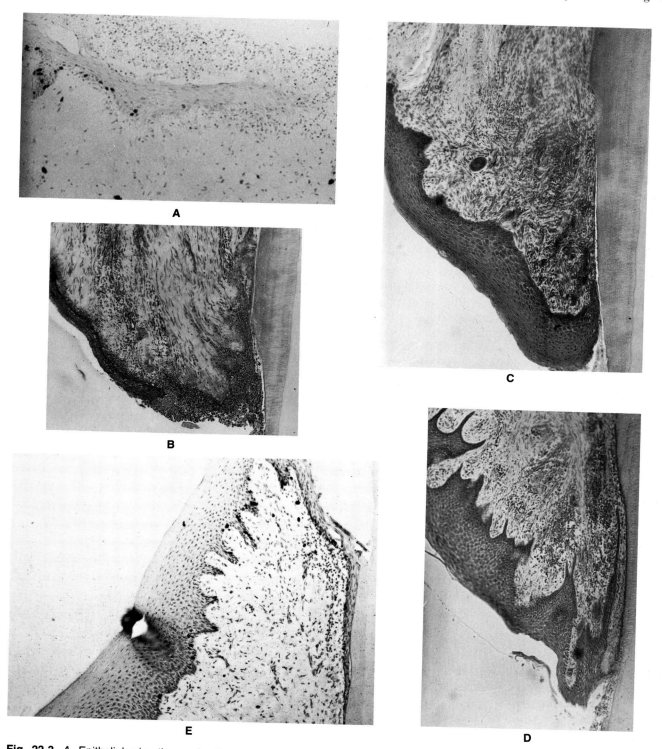

Fig. 22-3. *A,* Epithelial migration under the "poly-band" but over the wound surface 48 hours after surgery. *B,* Five days after gingivectomy (human specimens). The migrating epithelium has not quite reached the tooth surface. *C,* Seven days after gingivectomy, a new gingival sulcus is forming. *D,* Seven days after gingivectomy. Downgrowth of epithelium into the newly formed gingival sulcus. *E,* Thirty-five days after gingivectomy. New thin junctional epithelium. Mild chronic inflammation and minimal proliferative activity in the junctional epithelium (monkey specimen).

some labeled cells also appeared in the basal cell layer of the migrating epithelium (Fig. 22-3A).

From the 2nd to the 5th postoperative days, the epithelium migrated toward the tooth at a rate of about 0.5 mm per day (Fig. 22-3B). The new epithelium covering the wound was several cell layers thick and was not keratinized at this early stage. Labeled cells appeared in the basal cell layer along the length of the new epithelium. If any residual sulcus epithelium remained following the gingivectomy, these cells behaved in the same manner as the gingival surface cells.

An upgrowth of the connective tissue started to create a gingival sulcus 5 to 7 days postoperatively (Fig. 22-3C). This sulcus was first covered by a thin layer of epithelium showing considerable proliferative activity, and if the root planing had extended apically to the previous epithelial attachment, the new epithelial cells proliferated over the scraped root surface (Fig. 22-3D). Electron microscopic studies have revealed hemidesmosomes and a distinct basal lamina behind the first five to six cells of the migrating front of regenerating epithelium.[20] This migrating front contacted the blood clot without intervening desmosomes.

The establishment of the new epithelial attachment following gingivectomy has been described at the ultramicroscopic level by Listgarten.[24] Two months after the surgery, he observed a new epithelial attachment consisting of hemidesmosomes and a basal lamina. In some areas, the attachment apparatus connected the cells directly to the tooth surface. In other areas, a cuticular structure was interposed between the attachment and the tooth.

Although the outer surface epithelium appears to be normal[5,45] and keratinized in 2 to 3 weeks, the complete healing of the sulcular epithelium and the establishment of a new epithelial attachment take at least 4 to 5 weeks following the gingivectomy[5,44] (Fig. 22-3E).

Connective tissue

The connective tissue component of the healing tissues has been studied by histology and autoradiography.[38] In one study, the connective tissue part of the wound was covered by a blood clot two hours after the surgery. There was a marked migration of polymorphonuclear cells into the clot and to the wound surface. A thin layer of connective tissue (approximately 0.2 mm) immediately adjacent to the surgical incision showed widely spaced, pale-staining cells. In 5- and 9-hour specimens, it was observed that this thin layer of degenerating cells gradually became filled with polymorphonuclear cells, so that 13 hours after surgery there was a band of polymorphonuclear cells covering the entire wound. This "poly-band" included the superficial, degenerated, and necrotic connective tissue damaged by the surgery, and also part of the surface blood clot. The cementoblasts appeared to be disrupted and absent from the cemental surface for a depth of about 0.2 mm from the surgical wound. Osteoblasts on the alveolar crest were also missing in some areas after the surgery.

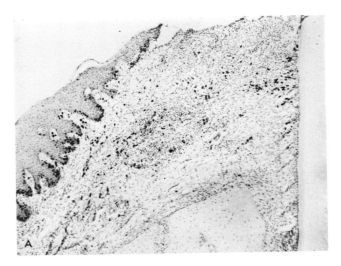

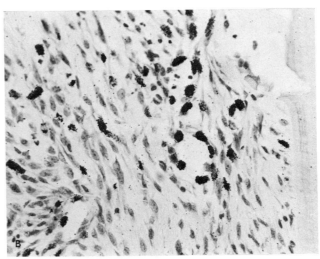

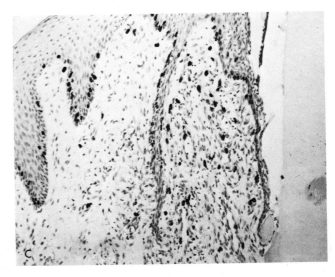

Fig. 22-4. *A, B,* Fibroblastic and angioblastic proliferative activity 3 days after gingivectomy. *B,* High magnification of same specimen as in *A* (monkey specimens). *C,* Seven days after gingivectomy. Intensive proliferation in the granulation tissues bordering the new gingival crevice.

The first significant increase in number of labeled cells were seen 0.3 to 0.5 mm below the "poly-band." Most of the early labeled cells appeared to be angioblasts, which were found either within the walls or in the immediate vicinity of the walls of small blood vessels.

Three days postoperatively, there was marked increase in angioblastic and fibroblastic activity (Fig. 22-4A,B). In addition to polymorphonuclear cells, a number of lymphocytes appeared. After 3 days, the labeled connective tissue cells had spread toward the basal cell layer of the regenerating epithelium. The connective tissue proliferation and reached a peak 3 to 4 days after the surgery, compared to the epithelial peak regeneration 24 to 36 hours after the surgery. Inflammatory infiltration of lymphocytes increased up to 5 to 7 days postoperatively.

The number of labeled connective tissue cells decreased noticeably between the 5th and 7th days. At 7 days, a definite free gingiva had formed on top of the wound (Fig. 22-4C).

Fourteen to 21 days after the surgery, the new sulcus was lined by epithelium, but a large number of lymphocytes and polymorphonuclear cells were present, indicating residual irritation. Only in the 35-day specimens did the sulcal lining and the junctional epithelium appear normal and with minimal subepithelial inflammation[5,43] (Fig. 22-3E).

Most of the regeneration of the free gingiva apparently takes place from the 3rd to the 9th days postsurgically, and consists initially of vascular granulation tissue. Functional orientation and collagenous maturation of the gingival connective tissue fibers require more than 5 weeks. It appears that a functionally sealing epithelial attachment to the tooth requires the support of firm fibrous gingival connective tissues. Collagen formation does not take place very actively until 14 to 21 days after surgery,[45] and continuous repair activity, evident as a significant increase in young connective tissue elements, has been demonstrated up to 28 days after the surgery.[42] Thus, the total healing time of a gingivectomy wound is at least 5 to 6 weeks,[38,44] although in the majority of cases, the surface epithelium is fully regenerated in 14 days. If the new free gingiva is formed in part by downgrowth of epithelial attachment on a planed root surface apically to the pocket and the gingivectomy incision, part of the new free gingiva will be old collagenous tissues, which may provide firm support for the regenerating new epithelial attachment.

Studies of the blood vessels in the healing gingivectomy wound[26] indicated that it took 5 weeks following the operation to regain a normal gingival fluid flow.[1] This finding tends to confirm the concept of a slow healing process.

Although some studies have found no effect on the healing response related to age, sex, location, and depth of pockets in humans,[42] other reports indicate a slower speed of healing in older rats[41] and humans[17] than in younger individuals. The rate of collagen mat-

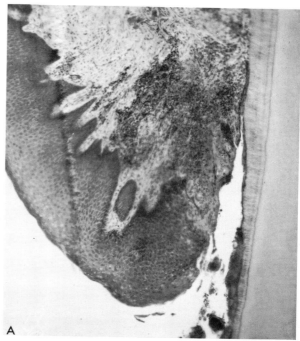

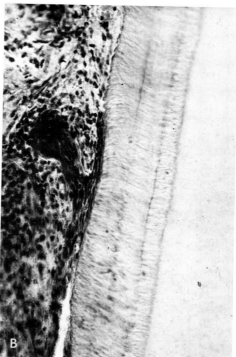

Fig. 22-5. *A,* Forty-four days after gingivectomy. Inadequate oral hygiene. Plaque extending into the gingival sulcus. Severe chronic inflammation. *B,* High magnification from the bottom of the junctional epithelium. Epithelial proliferation on uninstrumented root surface indicating epithelial extension beyond the zone of the surgery.

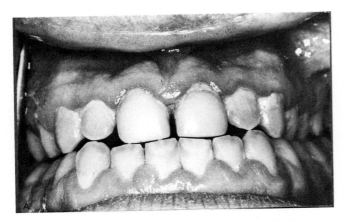

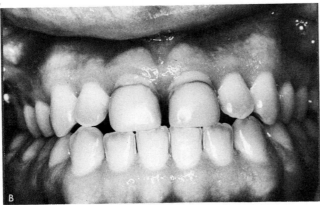

Fig. 22-6. *A,* Recurrent necrotizing ulcerative gingivitis treated repeatedly with penicillin. There is interproximal necrosis, but buccal and lingual hyperplastic pseudopapillae. Following debridement, gingivectomy was done. *B,* One year after the gingivectomy. Healthy gingiva with normal regenerated interproximal papillae.

These principles of wound healing described for gingivectomy also apply to other modalities of periodontal surgery.

Indications for Gingivectomy

The classical purposes of gingivectomy were surgical elimination of periodontal pockets and providing access for plaque control by the patient. Because it has been documented that pocket elimination is not essential for the maintenance of the dentition or for plaque control,[22] and because there are several drawbacks to the results of gingivectomy (esthetics, sensitivity, etc.), this surgical modality is not indicated for treatment for periodontal pockets anymore. However, it is still a useful procedure for gingival recontouring[11] (Fig. 22-6) to gain access for restorative procedures and correction of overhanging margins. It provides access to the root surfaces in suprabony pockets, with less subsequent bone resorption than following flap procedures. But such pockets are best treated by scaling and root planing without any surgery. Big masses of hyperplastic gingival and tuberosity tissues can be removed by gingivectomy, but the healing is slower and more painful than following flap procedures. Thus, in modern periodontics, there is very little use for gingivectomy.

uration appears to be increased in older individuals, as revealed by increasing denaturing temperature of the collagen.[18] However, the wounds of young individuals show greater tensile strength,[18] elastic stiffness, and energy absorption, which indicates that the faster rate of healing observed in younger individuals may be due to a better organization of the collagen fiber meshwork. The restitution of the microvascular system also appears to be slower in wounds of older individuals.[18]

While inflammation associated with wound healing normally will decrease markedly after 7 to 9 days,[43] it has been observed that inflammation in the area of a gingivectomy has a tendency to increase with time if the oral hygiene is not good.[42,43] Thus, the inflammation is often worse 4 to 5 weeks after the gingivectomy than it was before, and rapid downgrowth of the new epithelial attachment has been observed 5 to 6 weeks postsurgically in cases of poor oral hygiene[37] (Fig. 22-5).

The width of the attached gingiva has been reported to decrease slightly following gingivectomy.

REFERENCES

1. Arnold, R., et al.: Alterations in crevicular fluid flow during healing following gingival surgery, J. Periodont. Res. 1:303, 1966.
2. Bernier, J.L., and Kaplan, H.: The repair of gingival tissues after surgical intervention, J.A.D.A. 35:697, 1947.
3. Black, G.V.: Special Dental Pathology, Chicago, 1915, Medico-Dental Publishing Co.
4. Calderwood, R.G., et al.: A comparison of the healing rate of bone after the production of defects by various rotary instruments, J. Dent. Res. 43:207, 1964.
5. Engler, W.O., Ramfjord, S.P., and Hiniker, J.J.: A radioautographic study of healing following simple gingivectomy. I. Epithelialization, J. Periodont. 37:298, 1966.
6. Fox, L.: Rotating abrasives in the management of periodontal soft and hard tissues, Oral Surg. 8:1134, 1955.
7. Frisch, J., Jones, R.A., and Baskar, S.N.: Conservation of maxillary anterior esthetics: A modified surgical approach, J. Periodont. 38:11, 1967.
8. Gartsell, J.R., and Matthews, D.P.: Gingival recession. The condition, process and treatment, Dent. Clin. N. Am. 20:199, 1976.
9. Glickman, I., and Imber, L.R.: Comparison of gingival resection with electrosurgery and periodontal knives—a biometric and histologic study, J. Periodont. 41:142, 1970.
10. Goldman, H.M.: Gingivectomy: Indication, contraindications and method, Oral Surg. 22:323, 1946.
11. Goldman, H.M.: The development of physiologic gingival contours by gingivoplasty, Oral Surg. 3:879, 1950.
12. Goldman, H.M.: Gingivectomy, Oral Surg. 4:1136, 1951.
13. Goldman, H.M., and Cohen, D.W.: Periodontal Therapy, 5th ed., St. Louis, 1973, C.V. Mosby Co.
14. Grant, D.A., Stern, I.B., and Everett, F.G.: Orban's Periodontics, 4th ed., St. Louis, 1972, C.V. Mosby Co.

15. Gratzinger, M.: Elimination of periodontal pockets by chemical cautery, Dent. Dig. 51:120, 1945.

16. Hartwell, S.W.: Surgical wounds in human beings, Arch. Surg. 19:835, 1929.

17. Holm-Pedersen, P., and Löe, H.: Wound healing in the gingiva of young and old individuals, Scand. J. Dent. Res. 79:40, 1971.

18. Holm-Pedersen, P., and Viidik, A.: Maturation of collagen in healing wounds in young and old rats, Scand. J. Plast. Reconstr. Surg. 6:16, 1972.

19. Fejerskov, O.: Keratinized squamous epithelium of normal and wounded palatal mucosa in guinea pigs, J. Periodont. Res. (Suppl. 11)11:1, 1973.

20. Innes, P.B.: An electron microscopic study of the regeneration of gingival epithelium following gingivectomy in the dog, J. Periodont. Res. 5:169, 1970.

21. Jackson, D.B.: Gingival contour and coronal level changes following three periodontal treatment procedures. Thesis, The University of Michigan, 1973.

22. Knowles, J.W., et al.: Results of periodontal treatment related to pocket depth and attachment level. Eight years, J. Periodontol. 50:225, 1979.

23. Kronfeld, R.: The condition of the alveolar bone underlying periodontal pockets, J. Periodont. 6:22, 1935.

24. Listgarten, M.A.: Electron microscopic features of the newly formed epithelial attachment after gingival surgery, J. Periodont. Res. 2:46, 1967.

25. Löe, H.: Chemical gingivectomy. Effect of potassium hydroxide on periodontal tissues, Acta Odont. Scand. 19:517, 1961.

26. Novaes, A.B., et al.: Visualization of the microvascularization of the healing periodontal wound. III. Gingivectomy, J. Periodont. 40:359, 1969.

27. Orban, B.: Gingivectomy or flap operation, J.A.D.A. 26:1276, 1939.

28. Orban, B.: Indications, techniques, and postoperative management of gingivectomy in the treatment of periodontal pockets, J. Periodont. 12:89, 1941.

29. Orban, B.: To what extent should the tissues be excised in gingivectomy? J. Periodont. 12:83, 1941.

30. Orban, B.: The use of paraformaldehyde and oxygen in periodontal treatment, J. Periodont. 14:37, 1943.

31. Orban, B., and Archer, E.A.: Dynamics of wound healing following elimination of gingival pockets, Oral Surg. 31:40, 1945.

32. Patur, B., and Glickman, I.: Clinical and roentgenographic evaluation of the post-treatment healing of infrabony pockets, J. Periodont. 33:164, 1962.

33. Persson, P.A.: The healing process in the marginal periodontium after gingivectomy with special regard to the regeneration of epithelium (an experimental study on dogs), Odont. Tidskr. 67:593, 1959.

34. Pickerill, H.P.: Stomatology in General Practice, London, 1912, Henry Frowde, Hodder, and Stoughton.

35. Pollock, S.: Gingivoplasty technique using rotary diamond stones at ultra speed, Dent. Clin. North Am. p. 99, March, 1964.

36. Prince, J.P.: Gingival position and contour following gingivectomy, Paradontol. Acad. Rev. 2:153, 1968.

37. Ramfjord, S.P., and Costich, E.R.: Healing after simple gingivectomy, J. Periodont. 34:401, 1963.

38. Ramfjord, S.P., Engler, W.O., and Hiniker, J.J.: A radioautographic study of healing following simple gingivectomy. II. The connective tissue, J. Periodont. 37:179, 1966.

39. Schluger, S.: Osseous resection—a basic principle in periodontal therapy, Oral Surg. 2:316, 1949.

40. Shapiro, M.: Reattachment in periodontal disease, J. Periodont. 24:26, 1953.

41. Stahl, S.S.: The healing of gingival wounds in male rats of various stages, J. Dent. Med. 16:100, 1961.

42. Stahl, S.S., et al.: Gingival healing. II. Clinical and histologic repair sequences following gingivectomy, J. Periodont. 39:109, 1968.

43. Stahl, S.S., et al.: Gingival healing. IV. The effect of home care on gingivectomy repair, J. Periodont. 40:264, 1969.

44. Stahl, S.S.: Repair following a standardized gingivectomy in humans, Alpha Omega 63:175, 1970.

45. Stanton, G., Levy, M., and Stahl, S.S.: Collagen restoration in healing human gingiva, J. Dent. Res. 48:27, 1969.

46. Waerhaug, J.: Depth of incision in gingivectomy, Oral Surg. 8:707, 1955.

47. Wennström, J., et al.: The role of keratinized gingiva in plaque-associated gingivitis in dogs, J. Clin. Periodontol. 9:75, 1982.

48. Wennström, J., and Lindhe, J.: Role of attached gingiva for maintenance of periodontal health, J. Clin. Periodontol. 10:206, 1983.

23

PERIODONTAL FLAPS FOR SURGICAL POCKET ELIMINATION

According to one definition, a "flap is a piece of tissue partly severed from its place of origin for use in surgical grafting and repair of body defects."[59] In periodontics, flap procedures traditionally have been developed for three purposes: (1) for surgical elimination of periodontal pockets; (2) to induce adaptation, reattachment and bone regeneration in periodontal pockets; and (3) to correct gingival and mucogingival defects and deficiencies.

Obviously, a flap procedure developed originally for one of these purposes may also serve other objectives. For example, the Nabers apically repositioned flap[32] is used both for surgical pocket elimination and mucobuccal fold extension. In addition, a procedure may have been modified from its original purpose to serve mainly a different purpose—for example, the Widman flap procedure[60] was changed from surgical pocket elimination to the modified Widman flap procedure for root access and reattachment.[47,50]

All of the older reasons for doing flap surgery have been replaced by the single rationale of gaining access for efficient scaling and root planing.[24]

Periodontal flaps are designed as full-thickness or mucoperiosteal flaps when the periosteum is elevated from the bone with the flap, or as partial thickness or "split-thickness"[57] flaps when the flap is dissected free over the periosteum, leaving the periosteum and some contiguous connective tissues attached to the bone.[18]

History of Periodontal Flaps for Surgical Pocket Elimination

It has always been difficult to establish which dental procedures were the earliest to be developed, because oral communications have often preceded written descriptions (which were not necessarily by the same persons), and language barriers may have contributed to the numerous misinterpretations and disregard of historic data in the periodontal literature.

The following brief historical review does not pretend to be authoritative or complete, but is authentic to the extent that the sources cited have been reviewed carefully.

Neumann, in 1912 and 1915, described a semilunar incision in the gingiva for access to the root surfaces and the alveolar crest.[34] His description is vague and certainly does not delineate a flap operation for surgical pocket elimination. In the 3rd edition of Neumann's textbook in 1920, and later,[35] a mucoperiosteal periodontal flap procedure is well described. Following elevation of a crevicular mucoperiosteal flap, the inflamed tissues on the inside of the flap are removed with sharp spoons, as are tissues adherent to the teeth and the alveolar process. It is stressed that the surgery should result in a horizontal alveolar and gingival atrophy. Bony spurs and ledges are removed with a chisel until the alveolar process has the appearance of horizontal bone atrophy.

However, Neumann recognized the importance of scaling and planing, stating that if one wants the area that was operated on to heal well, it is beyond anything else important that all concretions be removed from the roots, and that the roots should appear as smooth as a mirror following planing and polishing. Widman, in 1916, appears to have been the first to describe flap surgery for pocket elimination,[11] although Cieszynski in a discussion in 1914 referred to periodontal flap surgery for access for scaling, removal of granulation tissue, and reduction of pocket depth.[6] However, he gave no description of methodology.

The English translation of Widman's article in 1918[60] gives a detailed description of a mucoperiosteal flap design, which leaves a collar of epithelium and inflamed connective tissues around the necks of the teeth from the gingival margin to the bone. Subsequently, this soft tissue collar is removed, and the bone is trimmed with round burs to reconstruct "the same anatomical form as in ordinary alveolar atrophy." Also emphasized was root planing and holding the flap close to the alveolar process and to the teeth with interproximal sutures. In the procedure described, the buccal and lingual flaps are not made to fit together interproximally and bare bone is left to granulate over in a way similar to common practice in current pocket elimination flap surgery.[43] Widman, in a modification of his original technique,[61] was the first person to describe the reverse incision, although it had been alluded to previously by Cieszynski.[6]

In 1918, Zentler described the use of a crevicular mucoperiosteal flap for access to remove infected bone and "infected granulomatous" tissues.[67] The method is very similar to what Neumann described in 1920.[34] However, Zentler's rationale for the flap surgery was removal of infected bone, whereas Neumann and Widman removed bone only for the purpose of eliminating sharp edges and introducing good contour comparable to horizontal atrophy of the bone. Other authors, such as Zemsky[66] and Berger,[2] used essentially the Zentler method of flap surgery[67] for pocket elimination.

During the 1930s and 1940s, gingivectomy became the most popular method of surgical pocket elimination, but, as pointed out by Schluger in 1949,[53] this operation did not offer an acceptable solution for the elimination of intrabony pockets and craters, and for pockets extending apically beyond the attached gingiva. Schluger recommended doing a gingivectomy first and then a mucoperiosteal flap to expose the alveolar crest and part of the alveolar process. This would be followed by a bone resection to produce "a graceful, gradual rise and fall in the proposed bony profile with the greatest curvature of the arc at the deepest point of the pocket." The narrow mucoperiosteal flap was placed back over the operated-bone and a surgical dressing applied. His goal for bone surgery corresponded with that of Neumann and Widman.

With deep periodontal pockets and pockets in areas of narrow attached gingiva, trimming the gingival margin enough to eliminate periodontal pockets will lead to a loss of all attached gingiva, and, in order to achieve pocket elimination combined with a favorable gingival response, the mucogingival line has to be moved in an apical direction. This consideration led to modifications of Schluger's initial approach.[14] Techniques he proposed were the "push back" and the "pouch" operations,[19] with an extensive exposure of the alveolar process and a mucobuccal fold extension following surgical remodeling of the bone for pocket elimination. These procedures caused a loss of bone[63] and were often very painful, and are therefore no longer used.

A new approach to surgical elimination of periodontal pockets extending beyond the mucogingival line was proposed by Nabers in 1954.[32] He used essentially the Neumann flap approach,[34] with a crevicular mucoperiosteal flap and trimming of the inside of the gingival margin of the flap. The main difference is that Nabers placed the flap in a more apical position following the bone contouring and held it in the new position by sutures and a dressing. As the attached gingiva was included in the flap, loss of the entire attached gingiva during the pocket elimination was avoided. This method was modified by Ariaudo and Tyrell[1] to include two instead of one vertical releasing incision suggested by Nabers. Later, Nabers modified the procedure by recommending Widman's reverse bevel incision as the initial approach to the flap design,[33] and Friedman suggested calling this procedure "the apically repositioned flap."[14]

The apically repositioned flap following a reverse bevel incision and some osseous removal, with or without flap coverage of the alveolar crest and the interproximal bone, has been the most common approach to surgical elimination of moderately deep periodontal pockets. However, in areas where pocket elimination may be achieved without extensive loss of attached gingiva, reverse bevel flap surgery may be used for pocket elimination without apically repositioning the gingiva—for example, the palatal pockets or distal wedge operations.

METHODOLOGY OF REVERSE BEVEL AND APICALLY REPOSITIONED FLAP SURGERY FOR POCKET ELIMINATION

Before making the inital reverse bevel incision, the surgeon must decide if the goal of the treatment is surgical pocket elimination. Only the pocket elimination approach will be discussed in this chapter.

The techniques for the surgery should (1) permit precise tissue removal; (2) result in minimal trauma to hard and soft tissues; (3) present no hazard for permanent loss of periodontal support; and (4) result in optimal healing.

Simple reverse bevel flap surgery

If no bone surgery or mucogingival correction is required for pocket elimination, the reverse bevel surgery can be done in the following safe and simple fashion.[25] Following routine preparation for surgery as outlined in chapter 20, make scalloped reverse bevel gingival incisions about 1 mm from the free gingival margin. The incision should deviate away from the long axis of the tooth sufficiently to create a thin flap, and should be extended to the alveolar technique buccally and lingually (Fig. 23-1A). Use Bard-Parker knives #11 or #12B, or Orban knives #1 and #2, selected on the basis of access. Raise mucoperiosteal flaps with elevators to about 2 mm apically to the alveolar crest (Fig. 23-1B). Deflect these flaps and do a regular gingivectomy from the alveolar crest to the

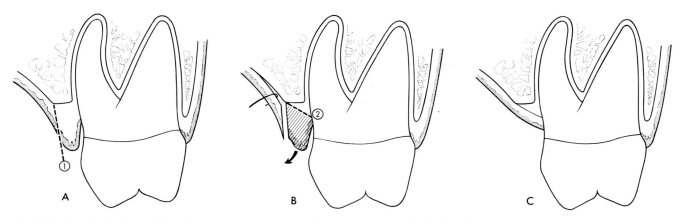

Fig. 23-1. *A,* Initial incision *(1)* on the palatal aspect of a molar with hyperplastic gingiva. *B,* A palatal mucoperiosteal flap has been raised from the initial incision. A gingivectomy incision *(2)* is made from where the initial incision met the alveolar process to the bottom of the palatal pocket, and the excised tissues are removed. *C,* The palatal flap has been replaced to the tooth.

bottom of the gingival crevice or pocket under the flap from both the buccal and lingual sides (Fig. 23-1B). Plane the exposed tooth surfaces, place the flap to contact the tooth (Fig. 23-1C), and suture the flaps together by interrupted interproximal sutures. Place dressing and treat postoperatively in the way described in chapter 20.

The operation just described will give essentially the same result as a gingivectomy, but without the open wound and delayed healing of a gingivectomy. The proper distance between the initial incision and the tooth depends on how deep the pockets are and how much tissue will have to be removed to eliminate the pockets. The angulation of the knife also has to diverge more from the surface of the tooth in an apical direction if the gingival wall of the pocket is thicker than if the pocket is thin-walled. The procedure may be called *gingivectomy under flap*.

The common procedures for surgical elimination of deep or moderately deep periodontal pockets are as follows: A reverse bevel incision is made at a distance from the teeth and at an angle depending on how deep the pockets are and the thickness of the pocket wall. If the pocket wall is thin, the inital incision is made at the free gingival margin or within the crevice. With a thick and bulky free gingiva, the inital incision is laid far enough from the tooth to create the desired dimension of the gingiva postsurgically (Fig. 23-2A,D).

If the pockets are deep or extend beyond the mucogingival line, the attached gingiva may have to be repositioned apically in order to eliminate the pockets. The initial reverse bevel incision then is made about 0.5 to 1 mm away from the free gingival margin, directed parallel to the tooth surface and extended to the alveolar process (Fig. 23-2D). In the palate, where the gingiva cannot be repositioned apically, the initial incision should be placed far enough from the tooth, with sufficient undermining bevel that the mucosal margin of the flap can be adapted to the tooth without any pockets appearing postsurgically. Although a scalloping incision is used, the middle interdental soft tissues become separated from the flap during this incision. Sufficient interdental projections may be included in the flaps to cover the interproximal alveolar process at the termination of the surgery, as recommended by Neumann.[35]

Another popular surgical flap procedure does not include the interdental tissues in the flap during the initial incision, so the interproximal bone will not be covered by the flaps after the surgery.[43,60]

Surgical procedures

For the *initial incision,* use Bard-Parker blade #11 or #12B if these blades can be directed at the desired angles to the teeth; otherwise, use Orban knives #1 and #2. Make releasing vertical incisions at the ends of the flap if apical repositioning is intended, or if the flap is to end in an area where pockets occur. Flap placement and suturing may be facilitated by having the releasing incision go through an interdental papilla. However, if there are interproximal pockets at the termination of the flap, it is better to lay the releasing incision at the distobuccal, mesiobuccal, or lingual line angles of the tooth where the flap is to terminate, thus including the entire involved interdental area in the flap. Do not make the releasing incisions on the midbuccal or midlingual surfaces of a tooth, as this may result in a gingival or bony dehiscense after the surgery.

Use mucoperiosteal elevators (Bennett or a #7 wax instrument) to raise a full-thickness flap from the alveolar process. If the flap is to be repositioned apically, it must be raised past the mucogingival junction, even

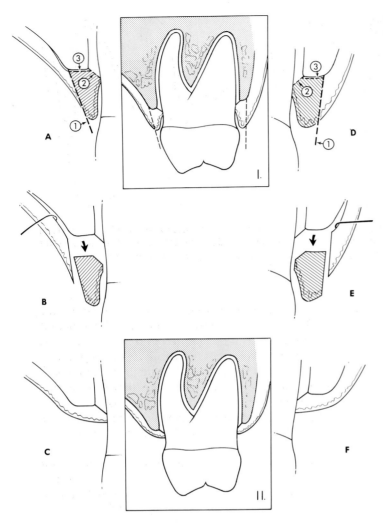

Fig. 23-2. *A-D,* The initial palatal reverse bevel incision *(1)* is made far enough away from the tooth so the thin flap will fit itself to the tooth without a residual pocket at completion of the surgery. Incision *(2)* is excised from the alveolar crest and the interproximal bone *(3)*. *B,* A mucoperiosteal flap is raised and the collar of gingival tissues is removed. *C,* The flap is sutured to the alveolar process and the tooth. *D,* The incisions are made in the same order buccally as described for the palatal side. *E,* A buccal mucoperiosteal flap is raised beyond the mucogingival line into the mucobuccal fold. The collar of gingival tissues is removed. *F,* The attached gingiva is positioned apically towards the mucobuccal fold, and the buccal flap is sutured in a position where it contacts the buccal surface of the tooth. This interproximal bone usually is not covered by the flap.

beyond the bottom of the mucobuccal fold if the vestibule is to be deepened (Fig. 23-2E). For pocket elimination without repositioning, raise the flap only sufficiently to obtain access to bone, which has to be removed for pocket elimination and necessary contouring. After the periosteum has been separated from the alveolar crest mechanically, the flap should be allowed to rest against the bone to protect the bone from drying.

Make the *second main incision* through the bottom

of the pocket along the tooth surface to the alveolar crest (Fig. 23-2A,D). Use the same knives as for the first incision. The root surface thus separated from the soft tissues should not be scratched or nicked.

Make the *third incision* on top of the alveolar process after deflecting the buccal and lingual flaps raised after the first incision (Fig. 23-2A,D). Use an interproximal spear-shaped knife, such as an old Orban knife that has been narrowed from previous sharpenings,[47] and cut carefully to the surfaces of the teeth. This last incision should follow the contour of the alveolar crest and the interdental septum as much as possible.

Following the third incision, remove the loosened collar of gingival tissues with a sharp curette (Fig. 23-2B,E). Use suction and irrigate the field of surgery with sterile saline solution when needed for vision. The part of the root surface that has been exposed in the periodontal pockets should be curetted and planed thoroughly. However, where there is residual periodontal membrane attachment to the roots of the teeth (close to the alveolar crest), no curettage should be done. Remove the soft tissues from the bony surface of intrabony lesions. Curettage should be done under the flaps without holding the flaps away from the bone for any length of time. The bone then may be trimmed to eliminate intrabony defects, interproximal craters, and deviations from normal contour of the alveolar process.[13,15,53,54]

Bone surgery

According to Friedman,[13] the contouring of bone without elimination of bone directly attached to the teeth is called *osteoplasty*, while removal of bone directly involved in the support of the teeth is called *osteoectomy* or *ostectomy*.

Osteoectomy of bone support extending to the bottom of intrabony lesions or craters may pose the problems of furcation exposures, unesthetic root exposure, and elimination of valuable support for the teeth. It also places anatomical restrictions on how deep pockets may be treated if the goal of surgical pocket elimination is to be achieved. Therefore, a number of modifications have been suggested to the basic requirements of surgical reinstitution of a bone contour similar to horizontal alveolar atrophy.[34,60] The two most commonly used modifications are (1) Prichard's suggestion to leave three wall bony lesions to granulate rather than perform complete surgical elimination;[42] and (2) Ochsenbein and Bohannan's recommendations to use the palatal approach for elimination of interproximal craters and intrabony lesions in order to avoid exposure of buccal furcations and esthetically unacceptable results.[37,38]

Bone may be removed by files,[34] burs,[60] chisels,[67] rongeurs, or diamond stones.[12] The method that accomplishes the desired bone removal with the least trauma to the remaining tissues should be used. Although the results of healing studies after bone surgery are controversial,[29,31] it would seem that a sharp chisel is the instrument that can accomplish the surgical separation of bony tissues with the least depth of injury to the underlying structures. Recent studies have confirmed this.[23]

In areas of osteoectomy, diamond stones should not be used to finish removal of bone adjoining the roots of the teeth, because this could easily scar the teeth. The final bone removal in osteoectomy is best accomplished by using chisels or by careful use of small fissure burs with ample cooling by sterile saline solution.

Following recontouring of the bone, the flaps are placed in contact with the bone and the buccal and lingual surfaces of the teeth (Fig. 23-2E,F). The buccal flap with the attached gingiva is moved apically until its border just touches the tooth after suturing. The flaps usually do not cover the interproximal bone.[43]

Flap management

Whether or not bone is removed, tissue flaps should be adapted over the alveolar process and toward the teeth before completion of the surgery, to assess whether further reshaping or repositioning will be required in order to achieve the goal of the surgery. To obtain optimal gingival contour after the healing, thinning of the flap may be indicated. A Bard-Parker #12B blade or fine surgical scissors may be used for this purpose. Thinning of the flap has to be done in a careful, nontraumatic manner, because, if the flap is made too thin or traumatized badly, it will necrotize and leave exposed bone, which takes a long time to heal. In order to assure pocket elimination, some authors recommend that the edge of the alveolar crest be left exposed,[1,19,33] while others adapt the flaps to touch the teeth on top of the bone.[14,20,34,60,67]

A common approach is to adapt a thin flap margin to touch the buccal and lingual surfaces of the teeth, and to leave the interproximal bone uncovered by the flap.[14,43,60] However, making the initial incision with exaggerated scalloping and including sufficient interproximal tissues with the flap to cover the interproximal bone following the surgery is recommended. Before such flaps are sutured in place, the interproximal papillary part of the flaps has to be thinned. This can usually be accomplished by fine, curved surgical scissors. An attempt should be made to have thin buccal and lingual interproximal flap extension meet when sutured together.[20,47] Such flap design will facilitate optimal postsurgical healing. However, if the attached gingiva was initially very narrow, the entire flap may have to be repositioned so far apically to gain sufficient attached gingiva that the alveolar crest and the interproximal bone cannot be covered by epithelialized soft tissues following the surgery.

The distal wedge operation

Applications of the reverse bevel flap surgery to eliminate pockets at the distal surface of the last molars or to correct pockets bordering edentulous spaces have been described by Robinson as "distal wedge"[51] operations and by Kramer and Schwarz as "proximal wedge" techniques.[27] These procedures eliminate pockets by removing the internal bulk of connective tissues often found in the maxillary tuberosity and the mandibular retromolar regions.

For distal surface pockets, a reverse bevel incision is started at the buccal or lingual aspects of the molars. The incision is started 1 to 3 mm away from the free gingival margin, depending on the depth of the pockets, and is directed to the alveolar crest around the neck of the tooth. From the distobuccal or distolingual aspect of the last molar, the incision is extended distally (Fig. 23-3A) toward the hamulus in the maxilla or the ascending ramus in the mandible and carried down to the alveolar process. Then another incision is started at the distal aspect of the molar 2 to 3 mm away from the first incision. It too is carried down to the alveolar process at an angle to join the first incision on the surface of the bone. The two incisions make a V-shaped wedge (Fig. 23-3B), which is extended distally to the end of the first distal incision. These two incisions may be in a straight line, or curved slightly to converge distally, or may be almost parallel. In the last case, they should be joined at the distal ends by a connecting incision. The initial reverse bevel incision should be completed for the lingual aspects of the molars if it was started buccally, or for the buccal aspects if it was started lingually. (All of these initial incisions, both for the reverse bevel and the distal wedge, are designated as incision #1 in the illustrations).

Incision #2 is made along the root surfaces of the teeth from the bottom of the pockets to the alveolar crest (Fig. 23-3C). This will separate the distal wedge adhering to the distal surface of the last molar, and the wedge of tissues (Fig. 23-3B) can be removed by a rongeur. The buccal and lingual wedges of pocket lining tissues should be removed at this time (Fig. 23-3C).

Incision #3 is a reverse bevel undermining incision to create thin buccal and lingual gingival mucosal flaps from the borders of incision #1 (Fig. 23-3D). This incision may be made with a Bard-Parker #12B or an Orban knife. The flaps should not be made thinner than 1 to 1.5 mm, and from where the incisions contact the alveolar process, a mucoperiosteal flap should be raised 2 to 3 mm to provide access (Fig. 23-3E).

Finally, the residual supracrestal and interproximal connective tissues should be dissected loose from the alveolar process with an Orban knife as incision #4 (Fig. 23-3D,F), and removed with curettes or ron-

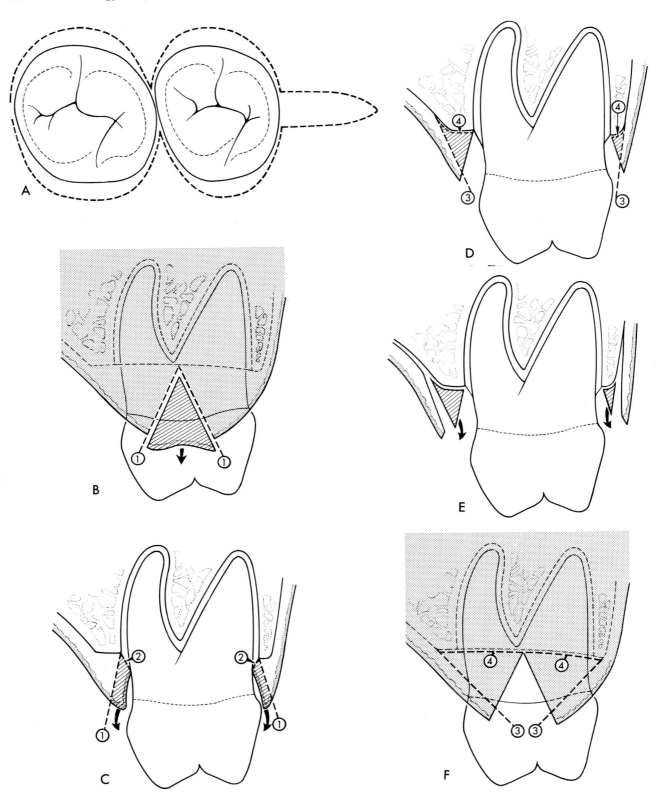

Fig. 23-3. *A,* The initial incisions are indicated by broken lines. The incisions should extend to the alveolar crest. *B,* The distal wedge created by the initial incision *(1)* is shown. *C,* A crevicular incision *(2)* separates the gingival tissues from the teeth. This will permit removal of the distal wedge and the buccal and lingual strips of gingival tissues. *D,* Palatal and buccal flaps are created by reverse bevel incisions *(3),* and the supracrestal tissues are dissected loose from the bone *(4). E,* Mucoperiosteal flaps have been raised and the supracrestal tissues are removed. *F,* The undermining incisions *(3)* in the distal wedge area are indicated, and *(4)* designates the dissection between the soft tissue wedges and the alveolar process.   *Continued*

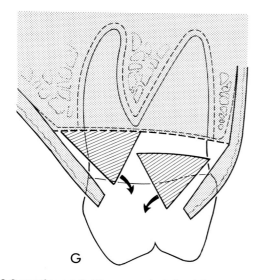

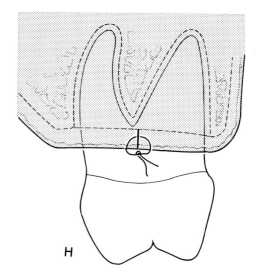

Fig. 23-3 continued *G*, The separated distal tissue fragments are removed. *H*, The wound has been sutured. The reduction in bulk of the retromolar tissues is evident.

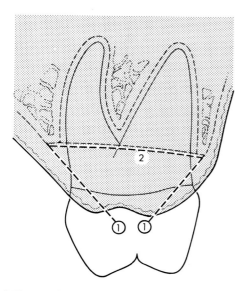

Fig. 23-4. Reverse bevel incisions *(1)*, creating buccal and lingual flaps in retromolar tuberosity. After reflection of these flaps, the suprabony retromolar soft tissues are dissected free from the alveolar process *(2)* and removed. This will allow suturing of the buccal and palatal flaps in a more apical position than previously.

geurs. This will permit the desired reduction in bulk of the retromolar tissues (Fig. 23-3G). The exposed root surfaces should be planed coronally to the fiber attachments and the flaps sutured in place (Fig. 23-3H). The flaps should fit closely together and contact both the bone and the surfaces of the teeth, including the distal surface of the last molar, when sutured.

Another method of surgical reduction of hyperplastic tissues at the distal aspect of the last molars[51] is to make distal reverse bevel incisions, creating thin flaps 2 to 3 mm apart (Fig. 23-4). Then the flaps should be deflected, and all the soft tissues between the 2 flaps removed from the alveolar process, and the flaps sutured together.

Both of the methods just discussed work well in the tuberosity region of the maxilla and for teeth bordering edentulous spaces that have sufficient attached gingiva to cover the wound. However, in the mandibular retromolar areas with distal pockets of mandibular third molars, the tissues are usually soft and are often glandular and friable. Under such circumstances, it has been suggested that whatever keratinized gingiva exists should be displaced laterally, a distal wedge incision made perpendicular to the retromolar bone, and the wedge held in a hemostat and dissected loose from the bone. Denude the bone for 2 to 3 mm distally and distobuccally from the tooth, and close the distal part of the wound with a suture so it does not gape open. Place a surgical dressing so it will contact the denuded bone in the surgical defect. Healing with scar tissue over the bone takes 3 to 4 weeks, with the dressing being changed weekly. This procedure involves postoperative pain or discomfort, and there is a tendency for relapse over years of postoperative observations.

A better, but technically more difficult, solution to the problem is to use a split-flap procedure and a free gingival graft (see movies recommended at the end of this chapter). Remove a distal wedge of soft tissues on top of the periosteum and excise the free gingiva from the buccal side (Fig. 23-5A). Dissect the alveolar mucosa free from the periosteum at the distobuccal and buccal aspects of the tooth toward the external oblique ridge to create a graft bed. Then place a free gingival graft from the palate to cover the distal and distobuccal graft bed on the periosteal surface of the bone (Fig. 23-5B). Let the graft contact the buccal and distal

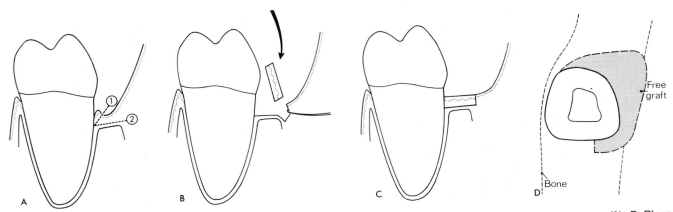

Fig. 23-5. *A,* Excise the free gingiva *(1)* on the buccal side, and dissect the alveolar mucosa free from the periosteum *(2). B,* Place a free graft from the palate on the prepared graft bed. *C,* The graft extends slightly over the external border of the mandible, since the graft will shrink. *D,* The free graft should be extended distally and mesially to create a border of attached gingiva in these areas.

marginal surfaces of the tooth (Fig. 23-5D). Insert a well-fitting periodontal dressing. This procedure will usually result in a narrow but adequate zone of attached gingiva, as well as in pocket elimination.

The retromolar and buccal and lingual aspects of mandibular third molars are the most difficult areas in the mouth for periodontal surgery. There are hazards connected with the close proximity to the lingual nerve, artery, and vein, and often there is considerable bleeding during the surgery. The cheek and the external oblique and the mylohyoid ridges also often interfere with pocket elimination for mandibular third molars.

Healing of gingival mucoperiosteal flaps

A crevicular gingival incision extended to the alveolar process, followed by elevation of a mucoperiosteal flap, is used routinely in conjunction with the extraction of teeth, periodontal flap operations, and other surgical interventions on the alveolar process. Following repositioning of such flaps to their original site, complete healing without any significant permanent loss of soft tissue attachment or bony support of the teeth in humans has been reported by several investigators.[3,8,26]

Histologic evidence of complete healing has also been obtained from animal studies.[17,21,44] Some loss of attachment and bone has been observed if the root surface corresponding to the fiber attachment has been instrumented.[30] However, partial or complete connective tissue healing has been observed against both uncuretted and curetted cementum and dentine. Cellular cementum and cementoid has been found to be deposited on all types of root surfaces, but was thickest over old cementum or in deep nicks on the tooth surface.[30] The degree of presurgical inflammation did not seem to affect the healing.[26] If the flap procedure has not injured the cemental surface in the area of surgical separation between the flap and the tooth, and the flap is closely readapted following the surgery, full restitution of both connective tissue and epithelial attachment will take place within 3 weeks[26] (Fig. 23-6). However, surgical flap separation from the bone will always induce some bone resorption (Fig. 23-7), which is usually regained after a few months.[5] Details of the healing process will be discussed here with reference to reverse bevel flaps, because the most extensive healing studies have been concerned with that type of flap. At the present time, it is the flap used most extensively in periodontics.

Healing following flap surgery leaving bone denuded

As explained earlier in this chapter, a commonly used method for surgical elimination of periodontal pockets during the 1950s involved surgical exposure of the alveolar process for bone removal and recontouring. Sometimes exposed bone was partially covered by a narrow mucoperiosteal flap,[53] while in other cases a wide area of alveolar process was left denuded of soft tissues in order to assure pocket elimination and a wide zone of attached gingiva after the surgery.[19]

Healing studies in both animals[63] and humans[7,40] have revealed severe periodontal reactions to denudation of a part of the alveolar process. Leaving alveolar process bone exposed (even though covered by surgical dressings) caused severe inflammation and necrosis of bone[7].

Although the denudation surgery usually does not lead to significant loss of connective tissue attachment, and the immediate postoperative bone loss may be completely regained interproximally[63] and partially regained buccally and lingually, this modality of surgery has been replaced by less painful and faster-healing procedures that are equally effective in pocket elimination.

Healing following exposure of the periosteum on the alveolar process

After it became apparent that exposure of the alveolar process caused extensive bone resorption, the *periosteal retention procedure*[62] was tried. Although this procedure seemed to cause less bone resorption than did denudation when the remaining periosteal layer was thick,[41] it definitely provoked some bone resorption. If the retained periosteum was thin or became nicked during the surgery, the resorption was severe. In a human study, it was found that the exposed periosteum offered only a limited protection to the underlying bone.[45] Inflammation and resorption of the alveolar process was similar and almost as severe as when the bone was denuded.

Thus, even with periosteal retention[62] and placement of a surgical dressing, serious inflammation and bone resorption, with subsequent slow or incomplete healing, is apt to occur. The procedure is therefore no longer used.

Healing of reverse bevel flaps

The histology of healing of full-thickness reverse bevel flaps in monkeys has been described in detail with regard to time intervals and flap adaptation.[5] The initial reaction within 2 hours is superficial necrosis at

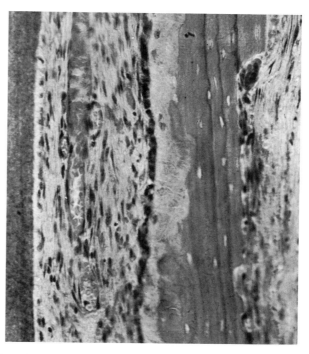

Fig. 23-7. Resorption and repair of necrotic alveolar process 3 weeks after mucoperiosteal flap surgery in human.

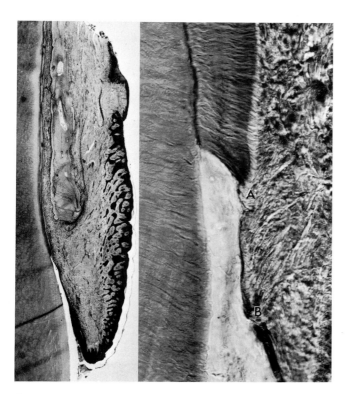

Fig. 23-6. Low and high magnification of block section, human specimen 3 weeks after mucoperiosteal flap surgery. There is new epithelial and connective tissue attachment to thin layer of cementoid material over the enamel from *A* to *B* close to the cementoenamel junction (high magnification).

the wound margins, clot formation if space is available, and accumulation of polymorphonuclear cells. Small patches of periosteal tissues may remain on the bone in spite of the attempt to perform complete periosteal separation from the bone.

After 24 hours, there is a fairly thick band of polymorphonuclear cells and superficial necrosis on the surgical surfaces of the flap and over uncovered interproximal bone. The inflammatory reaction is minimal where the flap is closely adapted to the bone.

After 2 days, slight epithelial and connective tissue proliferation is evident, and there is fibrosis and extension or inflammation into the marrow spaces close to the wound. The cementoblasts are disarranged or absent for about 1 mm from the wound surface.

The rest of the healing sequences vary with differences in flap adaptation to the tooth and bone. Fibroblastic and angioblastic activity is very intensive from the 3rd to the 7th or 8th day after the surgery, and originates from the periodontal membrane surface, from marrow spaces, and from the margin of the flap.

If there is close flap adaptation to the tooth, the epithelium grows down on the connective tissue surface of the flap, under the superficial area of necrosis including the "poly-band," and close to the tooth surface. A new epithelial attachment may appear within 7 days. If the flap adaptation was fairly close to the tooth, but did not make contact, connective tissue will grow up from the periodontal membrane and the inner surface of the flap. The epithelium will migrate from the flap margin, over the granulation tissue until it makes contact with the tooth, and then proliferate down along the tooth surface in essentially the same manner as healing of a gingivectomy wound. This type of healing is followed by much more severe inflammation than the healing after close flap adaptation.

By far the most undesirable sequela of healing occurs when the flap is 1 mm or more short of contacting the tooth, and thus leaves bone exposed. Connective tissues will grow out of the periodontal membrane, the marrow spaces, and the inner surface of the flap. However, this filling in of the defect by granulation tissue is accompanied by severe inflammation and bone resorption, both from the surface granulation tissues and from the periodontal membrane side. The epithelium may grow down on the side of the flap towards the bone, then extend over the granulation tissue protruding from the periodontal membrane, and finally reach the tooth and establish a gingival sulcus. This results in a ridge of epithelium between the flap and the new free gingival margin, and this ridge may interfere with normal gingival physiology.

The tissue reactions associated with poorly adapted flaps are essentially identical to the sequelae of denudation of the alveolar process. Spaces filled with blood between the flap and the bone, associated with poor adaptation, lead to delayed healing, more inflammation, and more bone resorption than with close flap adaptation.

The reaction of the bone to the surgery depended to a great extent on the presence or absence of a covering flap and to lesser extent on whether or not some bone had been removed surgically.[16,26,41,55,56]

Untraumatized bone covered by well adapted flaps[5] showed only slightly delayed and very superficial bone resorption as part of a late (2 to 3 weeks) stage of healing. Bone that had been traumatized by chisels or files developed more empty lacunae immediately following the surgery, indicating necrosis for a short distance under the surface even when covered with a well-adapted flap. This superficial necrosis was followed by slight resorption that started about 5 days after the surgery. Under a well-fitting flap, the resorption lasted only a few days, was superficial, and underwent prompt repair. After 9 days, there was a definite band of young connective tissue joining the flap to the bone and to the underlying connective tissue. New bone formation and periosteal reattachment sometimes took place on the surface of dead bone, but such areas underwent subsequent remodeling resorption. This resorption was still going on 72 days after the surgery.

The most severe bone reaction occurred at the alveolar crest when the flaps were repositioned apically from the neck of the teeth, exposing bone. In such areas, inflammation and bone resorption extended 1 to 2 mm into the periodontal membrane, and the healing was seriously delayed. It appeared that an overlying epithelial or thick connective tissue barrier was needed to prevent extension of inflammation into the periodontal membrane following flap surgery. However, both histologic observations and histometric measurements indicated that the resorbed bone had a tendency to regenerate to almost the preoperative level within 10 weeks.[5]

With ideal flap adaptation, healing appeared to be complete within 21 days, whereas with poor flap adaptation the wound was not completely healed within 72 days. Cementoblastic activity close to the wound does not reappear until healing is fairly complete.[5]

The long-term loss of bone at the alveolar crest following full-thickness reverse bevel flap surgery in humans certainly will vary with flap adaptation and surgical trauma as well as with thickness of the bone and the flap, but the loss will average 0.5 to less than 1.0 mm.[8,16,26,34,58,64] The most severe loss, of 2 to 3 mm, occurs in instances of thin labial bone (Fig. 23-8), and no loss takes place in patients with thick bone, or in the interproximal areas.

Partial thickness flaps

Initial reports indicated that partial-thickness or "split-thickness"[56] flaps healed very quickly and resulted in practically no adverse reactions from the bone on the alveolar process and at the alveolar

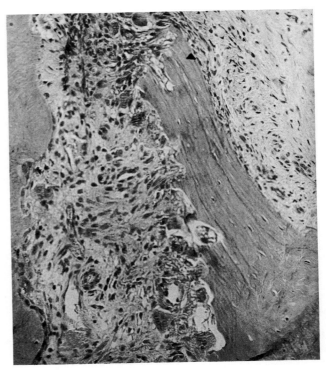

Fig. 23-8. Severe resorption of alveolar bone and cementum under poorly fitting flap 9 days after reverse bevel flap surgery (monkey specimen).

crest.[41,56] A study in dogs showed minimal tissue destruction, rapid repair, slight alteration of the dentogingival junction, and maximum preservation of periodontal supporting structures.[57] It also appeared from a study in monkeys that residual periosteum on the bone facilitated flap healing.[5] However, well controlled studies in humans have reported greater bone loss from partial-thickness than from full-thickness flaps,[64] and exposure of the periosteum[45] has been found to provoke almost as severe bone resorption as does complete denudation.[7] Clinical observations also indicate a tendency for more gingival recession following partial- than for full-thickness flaps, probably due to interference with the gingival blood supply during partial-thickness flap procedures. The most critical feature of partial flaps appears to be the thickness of the periosteum left on the bone. If this is less than 0.5 mm, the residual periosteum is apt to undergo necrosis and delay the healing. Thus, for success of a partial-thickness flap it is important that the gingiva be thick enough to allow adequate thickness of both the gingival mucosal part and the periosteal part of the flap. Under such favorable circumstances, the partial-thickness flap will probably heal faster and with fewer adverse reactions than a full-thickness flap. If the gingiva and mucosal covering on the alveolar process is thin, a partial-thickness flap is contraindicated.[64]

Whenever osseous defects are to be corrected, the full-thickness flap is recommended, in the interest of both access and preservation of good blood supply for healing. However, the exposure of the alveolar process should be limited to the minimum extent needed to gain access for the bone surgery, because at least a transient bone resorption will follow any surgical separation between the periosteum and the bone.

CURRENT STATUS OF POCKET ELIMINATION SURGERY

Both short-,[4,65] and long-term[46] results indicate that reverse bevel flap surgery, with or without bone surgery, and with or without apically repositioned flaps (depending on mucogingival considerations), is an effective method for elimination or reduction of periodontal pockets. However, with regard to preservation of attachment for the teeth, the results are not as favorable on a short-term basis as following some other method of treatment,[4,46,65] while on a long-term basis the results are similar whether the pockets are eliminated surgically or not.[46]

Of particular concern are the reports of loss of alveolar crest height following both full- and partial-thickness flap procedures.[64] It thus appears that in order to achieve pocket reduction with minimal loss of attachment and alveolar bone, the flap surgery should involve as small an area as possible of the alveolar process, the residual fiber attachment to the

roots should be left intact,[28] and complete flap coverage of the wound should be secured.[5]

A number of clinical trials have established that surgical pocket elimination does not contribute to the maintenance of the attachment level of teeth beyond what can be expected of non-surgical modalities of periodontal treatment.[22,49] A sulcus depth of 1 to 3 mm following therapy is as likely, if not more so, to lose attachment over time as is a sulcus of 4 mm,[49] and surgical pocket elimination has been shown to induce more recession than other techniques not aiming for pocket elimination.[50] Because there are obvious disadvantages to recession, such as esthetics, root sensitivity and caries, patients will usually prefer nonresective techniques if given a choice. Even with poor oral hygiene, the prognosis is not enhanced by pocket elimination surgery.[36] The fact that pocket depth does not have to be eliminated surgically in order to secure a good prognosis means that much more advanced periodontal disease than before may now be treated with assurance of a favorable prognosis.

Sometimes resective surgical techniques are indicated for elimination of gingival hyperplasia and to gain access for restorative dental procedures. These aspects are discussed in chapter 27.

REFERENCES

1. Ariaudo, A.A., and Tyrell, H.A.: Repositioning and increasing the zone of attached gingiva, J. Periodont. 28:106, 1957.
2. Berger, A.: The flap operation, J.A.O.A. 18:1459, 1931.
3. Borden, S.M.: Histological study of healing following detachment of tissues as is currently carried out in the vertical incision for the surgical removal of teeth, J. Can Dent. Assoc. 14:510, 1948.
4. Burgett, F.G., et al.: Short-term results of three modalities of periodontal therapy, J. Periodont., 48:131-135, 1977.
5. Caffesse, R.G., Ramfjord, S.P., and Nasjleti, C.E.: Reverse bevel periodontal flaps in monkeys, J. Periodont. 39:219, 1968.
6. Cieszynski, A.: Bemerkungen zur Radikal-Chirurgischen Behandlung der sogennante Pyorrhea Alveolaris, Deutsche Monatsschr. Zahnheilk. 32:575, 1914.
7. Costich, E.R., and Ramfjord, S.P.: Healing after partial denudation of the alveolar process, J. Periodont. 39:127, 1968.
8. Dedolph, T.H., and Clark, H.B.: A histological study of mucoperiosteal flap healing, J. Oral Surg. 16:367, 1958.
9. Donnenfeld, O.W., Marks, R.M., and Glickman, I.: The apically repositioned flap—a clinical study, J. Periodont. 35:381, 1964.
10. Ellegaard, B., and Löe, H.: New attachment of periodontal tissues after treatment of infrabony lesions, J. Periodont. 42:648, 1971.
11. Everett, F.G., Waerhaug, J., and Widman, A.: Leonard Widman: Surgical treatment of pyorrhea alveolaris, J. Periodont. 42:571, 1971.
12. Fox, L.: Rotating abrasives in the management of periodontal soft and hard tissues, Oral Surg. 8:1134, 1955.
13. Friedman, N.: Periodontal osseous surgery: Osteoplasty and osteoectomy, J. Periodont. 26:257, 1955.
14. Friedman, N.: Mucogingival surgery: The apically repositioned flap, J. Periodont. 33:328, 1962.
15. Friedman, N., and Levine, H.: Mucogingival surgery, current status, J. Periodont. 35:5, 1964.

16. Friedman, N., and Levine, H.: Experimental periodontal surgery on human beings. A clinical histologic (preliminary) study, J. Dent. Res. 43:791, 1964.

17. Glickman, I., and Lazansky, J.P.: Reattachment of the marginal gingiva and periodontal membrane in experimented animals, J. Dent. Res. 29:659, 1950.

18. Goldman, H.M., and Cohen, D.W.: Periodontal Therapy, 5th ed., St. Louis, 1973, C.V. Mosby Co.

19. Goldman, H., Schluger, S., and Fox, L.: Periodontal Therapy, St. Louis, 1956, C.V. Mosby Co.

20. Hiatt, W.: Regeneration via flap operation and the pulpal periodontal lesion, Periodontics 4:205, 1966.

21. Hiatt, W.H., et al.: Repair following mucoperiosteal flap surgery with full gingival retention, J. Periodont. 39:11, 1968.

22. Hill, R.W., et al.: Four types of periodontal treatment compared over two years, J. Periodont. 52:655, 1981.

23. Horton, J.E.: The healing of surgical defects in alveolar bone produced with ultrasonic instrumentation, chisel and rotary bur, Oral Surg. 39:536, 1975.

24. Kakehashi, S., and Parakkal, P.F.: Proceedings from the state-of-the-art workshop on surgical therapy for periodontitis, J. Periodont. 53:478, 1982.

25. Kardel, K.M.: Parodontal Kirurgi, Copenhagen, 1967, Dansk Tandlaegeforening.

26. Kohler, C.A., and Ramfjord, S.P.: Healing of gingival mucoperiosteal flaps, Oral Surg. 13:89, 1960.

27. Kramer, G.M., and Schwarz, M.S.: A technique to obtain primary intention healing in pocket elimination adjacent to an endentulous area, Periodontics 2:252, 1964.

28. Levine, G., and Stahl, S.: Repair following periodontal flap surgery with retention of gingival fibers, J. Periodont. 43:99, 1972.

29. Mazorow, H.B.: Bone repair after experimentally produced defects, J. Oral Surg. 18:107, 1960.

30. Morris, M.L.: The reattachment of human periodontal tissues following surgical detachment: A clinical and histological study, J. Periodont. 24:220, 1953.

31. Moss, R.W.: Histopathologic reaction of bone to surgical cutting, Oral Surg. 17:405, 1964.

32. Nabers, C.L.: Repositioning of the attached gingiva, J. Periodont. 25:38, 1954.

33. Nabers, C.L.: When is gingival repositioning an indicated procedure? J. West. Soc. Periodont. 5:93, 1957.

34. Neumann, R.: Die Alveolar-Pyorrhea and ihre Behandlung, 2nd ed., 1915; 3rd ed., 1920, Berlin, 1912, Hermann Meusser, 1912.

35. Neumann, R.: Die chirurgische Behandlung der Paradentose. In Die chirurgische Erkrankungen den Mundlhöhle, der Zähne und Kiefer, Partsch, C., ed., Munich, 1932, J.F. Bergmann.

36. Nyman, S., et al.: Periodontal surgery in plaque-infected dentitions, J. Clin. Periodont. 4:240, 1977.

37. Ochsenbein, C., and Bohannan, H.M.: The palatal approach to osseous surgery. I. Rationale, J. Periodont. 34:60, 1963.

38. Ochsenbein, C., and Bohannan, H.M.: The palatal approach to osseous surgery. II. Clinical application, J. Periodont. 35:54, 1964.

39. Pennel, B.M, et al.: Repair of the alveolar process following osseous surgery, J. Periodont. 38:426, 1967.

40. Pfeifer, J.: The growth of gingival tissues over denuded bone, J. Periodont. 34:10, 1963.

41. Pfeifer, J.S.: The reaction of alveolar bone to flap procedures in man, Periodontics 3:135, 1965.

42. Prichard, J.: The infrabony technique as a predictable procedure, J. Periodont. 28:202, 1957.

43. Prichard, J.F.: Advanced Periodontal Disease, 2nd ed., Philadelphia, 1972, W.B. Saunders Co.

44. Ramfjord, S.P.: Experimental periodontal reattachment in rhesus monkeys, J. Periodont. 22:67, 1951.

45. Ramfjord, S.P., and Costich, E.R.: Healing after exposure of the periosteum on the alveolar process, J. Periodont. 39:199, 1968.

46. Ramfjord, S.P., et al.: Longitudinal study of periodontal therapy, J. Periodont. 44:66, 1973.

47. Ramfjord, S.P., and Nissle, R.R.: The modified Widman flap, J. Periodont. 45:601, 1974.

48. Ramfjord, S.P., et al.: Results following three modalities of periodontal therapy, J. Periodont. 46:9, 522, 1975.

49. Ramfjord, S.P.: Surgical pocket elimination: Still a justifiable objective, J.A.D.A. 114:37, 1987.

50. Ramfjord, S.P.: Present status of the modified Widman flap procedures, J. Periodont. 48:558, 1977.

51. Robinson, R.: The distal wedge operation, Periodontics 4:256, 1966.

52. Rosling, B., Nyman, S., and Lindhe, J.: The effect of systematic plaque control on bone regeneration in infrabony pockets, J. Clin. Periodontol. 3:38, 1976.

53. Schluger, S.: Osseous resection. A basic principle in periodontal surgery, Oral Surg. 2:316, 1949.

54. Schluger, S.: Surgical techniques in pocket elimination, Texas Dent. J. 70:246, 1952.

55. Simpson, H.: The reattachment of mucoperiosteal flaps in surgical extraction wounds in Macacus rhesus monkeys, Aust. Dent. J. 4:86, 1959.

56. Staffileno, H., Wentz, F., and Orban, B.: Histologic study of healing of split thickness flap surgery in dogs, J. Periodont. 33:56, 1962.

57. Staffileno, H., Levy, S., and Gargiulo, A.: Histologic study of cellular mobilization and repair following a periosteal retention operation via split-thickness mucogingival flap surgery, J. Periodont. 37:117, 1966.

58. Tavtigian, R.: The height of the facial radicular alveolar crest following apically repositioned flap operation, J. Periodont. 41:412, 1970.

59. Webster's Third New International Dictionary, Groove, P.B., and staff, Ed., Springfield, Mass., 1961, S.C. Merriam Co.

60. Widman, L.: The operative treatment of pyorrhea alveolaris. A new surgical method, Sven. Tandl. Tidsk. (Special Issue) Dec. 1918.

61. Widman, L.: Einige Erinnerungen hinsichtlich der Arbeit von R. Neumann: Die radikal-chirurgische Behandlung der Alveolar-Pyorrhea, Vierteljahrschrift f. Zahnheilk. 39:18, 1923.

62. Wilderman, M.N.: Repair after a periosteal retention procedure, J. Periodont. 34:483, 1963.

63. Wilderman, M.N., Wentz, F.M., and Orban, B.J.: Histogenesis of repair after mucogingival surgery, J. Periodont. 31:283, 1960.

64. Wood, D.L., et al.: Alveolar crest reduction following full and partial thickness flaps, J. Periodont. 43:141, 1972.

65. Zamet, J.S.: A comparative clinical study of three periodontal surgical techniques, J. Clin. Periodontol. 2:87, 1975.

66. Zemsky, J.L.: Surgical treatment of periodontal diseases with the authors' open-view operation for advanced cases of dental periclasia, Dent. Cosmos 68:465, 1926.

67. Zentler, A.: Suppurative gingivitis with alveolar involvement, J.A.M.A. 71:1530, 1918.

24

FLAP SURGERY FOR REATTACHMENT AND ADAPTATION IN PERIODONTAL POCKETS

Concepts and histologic evidence of reattachment and readaptation of periodontal soft tissues following therapy were discussed in Chapter 21 under subgingival curettage. This chapter will concern the use of periodontal flap procedures for closing periodontal pockets to bacterial plaque, by epithelial and connective tissue reattachment or by close readaptation of the pocket wall to the surfaces of the teeth.

Initially, periodontal flap procedures were designed for surgical pocket elimination[27,51,54] rather than for reattachment, although healing and reattachment are terms used interchangeably in the articles cited here, as well as in later publications.

A definite differentiation should be made between healing after surgical separation of periodontal tissues, including artificially produced pockets, and results following treatment of pockets associated with chronic destructive periodontal disease (chronic periodontitis). As pointed out in chapter 23, surgical flaps will, when readapted to the tooth, heal back to the preoperative level of attachment,[19] provided that no harm has been inflicted on the root surface during surgery or the production of artificial pockets. However, if there has been instrumentation of the Sharpey's fiber attachment during the surgical separation, only partial connective tissue healing is apt to occur.[22,50] Also, the attachment that has been lost with periodontal or periapical abscesses and periodontal drainage often heals to the immediate predestruction level following elimination of the acute infection, even without specific periodontal therapy.

Rationale for Flap Procedures

The main reasons for choosing flap procedures rather than subgingival curettage to gain reattachment are (1) they facilitate access for root planing, elimination of pocket lining, and soft tissue lining of an intrabony defect; (2) there is less trauma to the pocket wall during elimination of the epithelial lining; and (3) the adaptation of the flap to the surface of the tooth is better with the flap procedure, and there is thus a better potential for healing of the tissues between the flap and tooth.

Flap Surgery for Reattachment

Flap surgery for reattachment has been called "surgical curettage by flap"[14] because the objectives in terms of both removal of tissues and healing sequences are essentially the same for the curettage and the flap procedures. However, such a phrase is somewhat cumbersome to use and has not been widely accepted.

Zemsky referred to a vertical "slit operation" followed by deflected flaps for access to root surfaces and granulation tissues.[53] He also made mesiodistal and vertical interproximal incisions, and raised flaps partially to allow efficient root planing and curettage of the inner surfaces of the pockets. After these procedures, the flaps were sutured together. Zemsky used another "open view operation" for pocket elimination, at which the interproximal alveolar crest was left bare. It is not clear whether his operations were aimed at reattachment.

Kirkland in 1931 described in detail the use of a rather conservative crevicular, gingival flap procedure.[17] This procedure may be considered an "open curettage" aimed at reattachment. He first scaled the teeth, and then at a subsequent appointment made an incision from the bottom of the pockets to the alveolar process with connecting interproximal incisions. Then he raised a flap only enough to gain access for removal of the epithelium and all inflamed connective tissues on the surface of the bone. After the procedure, he planed the roots and sutured the flaps together.

The current widespread interest in flap surgery for reattachment developed after Prichard's article on

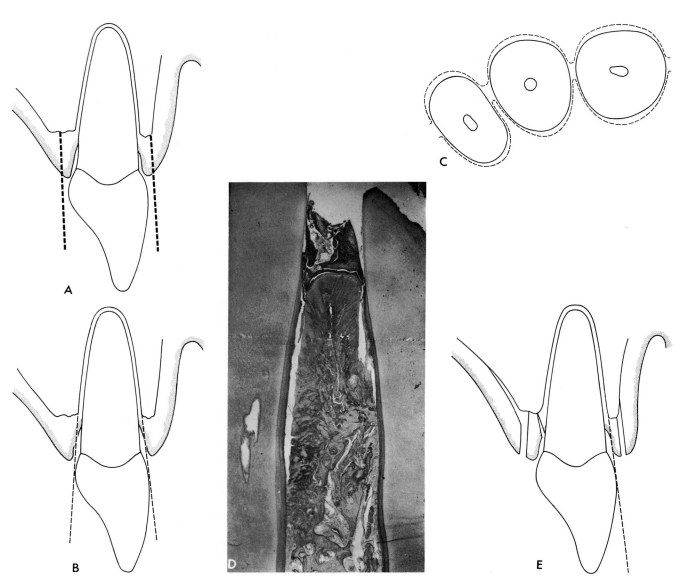

Fig. 24-1. *A,* The initial incision is made about 0.5 mm from the free gingival margin and directed parallel to the long axis of the tooth. It is extended to the alveolar crest. *B,* If the gingival sulcus is 2 mm or less in depth or the gingiva is extremely thin, the initial incision may be made from the bottom of the sulcus to the bone (an intracrevicular incision). *C,* Scalloping of the flaps and removal of some interproximal tissues is indicated if the teeth are situated close together and there are deep interproximal pockets. The separated buccal and lingual papillae will then act as pedicle grafts or flaps after suturing. *D,* Photomicrograph showing that the epithelial projections in the interproximal pockets cannot be removed without removing the interdental tissues entirely. *E,* After raising the buccal and lingual flaps for 2 to 3 mm, a second intracrevicular incision is made to the alveolar crest. *Continued*

predictable healing of intrabony pockets[32] and Carranza and Glickman's suggestion about complete removal of the soft tissue lining of intrabony pockets in order to gain reattachment.[4] Both these articles appeared in 1957, and since that time there have been numerous reports on partial or complete healing of intrabony periodontal lesions following flap surgery.

METHODS OF FLAP SURGERY

Two basically different methods of flap surgery for reattachment have been recommended. One is essentially to remove the free gingiva and expose the intrabony defect by flaps, plane to root surfaces, remove all soft tissues over the bone, and suture the flaps together, but not necessarily in such a way that the defect is covered by the flaps. After the surgery, tinfoil or Telfa is placed over the defects and covered with a periodontal dressing.[31,32,33] Roentgenologic documentation and reentry findings[31,32] have established that this approach may give good results, mainly for

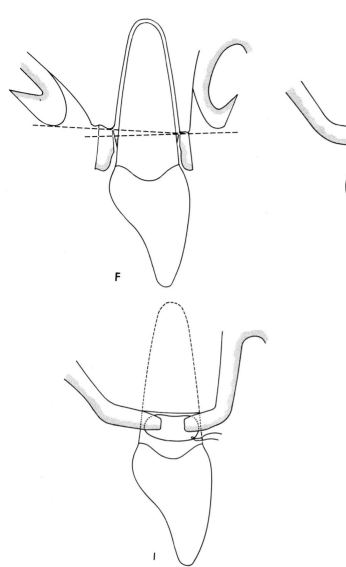

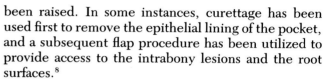

Fig. 24-1 continued. *F*, Deflect the buccal and lingual flaps and dissect the remaining collar of gingival tissues from the alveolar crest and the interdental bone with a third incision. *G*, The buccal and lingual flaps should be held together by an interrupted direct or figure-eight suture. *H*, Avoid folding the edges of the flap when suturing, because this would interfere with optimal healing. *I*, If the flaps are too short or they cannot be approximated properly, recontour the alveolar process slightly or place foil over the wound before the surgical dressing is applied.

the three-wall variety of intrabony lesions.[12] It appears that bone regeneration may occur in such intrabony pockets even if a postsurgical dressing is made to fill the intrabony lesions in such a way that there is no blood clot to act as a scaffold for regeneration.[20]

A second and more common approach to flap surgery for reattachment has developed from Kirkland's use of flap procedures for an "open subgingival curettage," or from application of the reverse bevel technique[26,34] instead of curettage after the flap has

been raised. In some instances, curettage has been used first to remove the epithelial lining of the pocket, and a subsequent flap procedure has been utilized to provide access to the intrabony lesions and the root surfaces.[8]

Several studies[44,50] have reported the basic gingival mucoperiosteal flap design of Neumann[27] for the initial flap. However, instead of trimming the flap for surgical pocket elimination as he did, researchers have attempted to gain some reattachment after elimination of the crevicular epithelial lining and the inflamed connective tissues by curettage of the flap, as recommended by Kirkland.[17] Judging from clinical probing, this method has provided a significant reduction in pocket depth, resulting from both gingival recession and reattachment (an average of 3 mm in one study).[49]

More often used for reattachment or readaptation therapy is a reverse bevel gingival mucoperiosteal flap[8,15,26,34,36,38,52] of the Widman[51] design, but without Widman's original attempt at a surgical pocket elimination, and without his recommended postsurgical exposure of the intradental bone.

Modified Widman Flap

The recommended unrepositioned mucoperiosteal flap[26] procedure, or "the modified Widman flap,"[38,40] is outlined in the following step-by-step description (Fig. 24-1A to I). The flap surgery should not be initiated until 1 to 2 months after completion of the hygienic phase of the periodontal therapy. The initial incision should be made following the preparation of the field of surgery with local anesthesia and application of disinfectant.

An initial gingival incision (Fig. 24-1A) is made with a Bard-Parker #11 blade or any other suitable knife that can be directed parallel to the long axis of the tooth. If the buccal or lingual pockets are deeper than

2 mm, this initial incision should be placed at least 0.5 mm away from the free gingival margin in order to assure complete removal of all crevicular epithelium, which otherwise would prevent connective tissue reattachment to the tooth following the surgery. The gingival epithelium is about 0.5 mm thick,[38] but rete pegs in the pocket wall may extend deeper. When the buccal crevice is 2 mm or less, or when esthetic considerations are of great importance, an intracrevicular incision or an incision at the free gingival margin may be used to minimize postsurgical gingival shrinkage (Fig. 24-1B).

The placement of the initial incision is influenced by the thickness of the gingiva and the alveolar process. If the gingiva and the alveolar process are thin, the incision should be made as close to the tooth as is practical, whereas with a thick gingiva and a heavy alveolar process, the postoperative gingival contour may be improved by placing the initial incision 1 to 2 mm away from the tooth in order to create a thin gingival margin of the flap. Do not end up with a very thin flap (less than 1.5 mm), because, without adequate connective tissue support and good circulation, the flap may undergo necrosis.

The initial incision is continued towards the interproximal areas with a scalloping outline of the flap (Fig. 24-1C). As the interproximal spaces are approached, the incision should be brought closer to the tooth, almost to the gingival margin, because the contour of the tooth will reach the alveolar process 2 to 3 mm away from the tooth surface, and thus also away from the pocket epithelium.

It is important, for postoperative flap adaptation, to remove the very minimum of interproximal tissues sufficient for elimination of the epithelial lining of the pockets. This is especially important from the palatal side, because there the flap cannot be stretched at all. However, in the middle of the interproximal areas, the epithelial projections in the pocket walls between the mesial and the distal aspects of the papillae often come close to touching (Fig. 24-1D). It is therefore advisable, when the roots of the teeth are situated closely together, to make the initial incision in such a manner that part of the very interproximal papillae will be separated from the flap and later removed.

In order to keep a sufficient amount of tissues with the flap to cover the interproximal bone following the surgery, it is often advisable to exaggerate the scalloping effect of the initial incision by staying 1 to 2 mm away from the midpalatal surface of the teeth when the incision approaches the surfaces of the teeth and is extended toward the interproximal areas.

Vertical gingival releasing incisions are seldom needed to gain access if the pockets are deep. Such incisions should be made at the mesial or distal line angles of the tooth where the flap ends, and extended for the minimal distance needed for access when the flap is elevated. Avoid vertical incisions in the palate in the region of the second bicuspid and of the first and second molars.

Use mucoperiosteal elevators to raise a full-thickness flap only for 1 to 2 mm, or the minimum needed to deflect the flap sufficiently to gain access to the root surfaces and the interproximal bone. After the periosteum has thus been separated from the alveolar crest mechanically, the flap is allowed to rest against the bone to protect the bone from drying.

A second incision is made around the neck of each tooth, from the bottom of the pocket to the alveolar crest (Fig. 24-1E). The knives used for the initial incision may also be used for the second incision, but these should stay clear of actually touching the root apically to the bottom of the pocket.

The third and final incision is done with a spear-shaped, narrow interproximal knife (for example, Orban knives that have been sharpened many times). The buccal or lingual flaps (or both) are pushed aside by the flat surface of the knife or deflected by the assistant so that the knife can be placed on top of the alveolar crest and used to cut loose the collar of gingival tissues. This collar has now been separated from the buccal and lingual gingival flaps and the teeth. This last incision should follow as much as possible the surface of the alveolar crest and the interproximal bony septum (Fig. 24-1F). Care should be taken not to nick the tooth surface with the knife.[35]

The separated collar of gingival tissues is then removed with curettes. The part of the root surfaces not covered by attached periodontal fiber endings should be carefully planed with curettes. Indiscriminate curettage of residual fiber attachment should be avoided, as this may interfere with connective tissue healing.[21,22] All soft tissues should be removed from the bony surface of intrabony lesions as recommended in 1931 by Kirkland.[17] This removal of suprabony soft tissues should be accomplished with sharp dissection, rather than as curettage of the bony surface, and as much as possible without prolonged deflection of the flaps. The presence of vestiges of residual periosteum over the alveolar process will facilitate rather than retard healing. Use sterile saline solution and suction when needed for a clear view of the field.

The flaps are adapted to the bone and to each other interproximally and held firmly in position with finger pressure on sterile gauze moistened in saline. If the adaptation of the flaps to the teeth or between the flaps interproximally is incomplete, the flaps may be thinned or some bone removed from the outer aspects of the alveolar process in order to enhance the flap adaptation. If the flaps have been cut too far away from the teeth, so that close contacts cannot be established, reattachment usually will not occur, except perhaps in two- and three-wall intrabony pockets. Under such circumstances, the main goal of the surgery may be changed to pocket elimination and osteoplasty, with establishment of thin flap margins.

The flaps are sutured together with individual interproximal sutures (Fig. 24-1G to I). The postoperative care, including placement of dressings, should follow the procedures outlined in chapter 20.

Advantages and disadvantages of the modified Widman flap

The main advantage of the modified Widman flap procedure is the possibility of establishing an intimate postoperative adaptation of healthy collagenous connective tissues and normal epithelium to all tooth surfaces. It has been shown in both animals[3] and humans[48] that with a close adaptation of gingival tissues to the tooth surface, a marginal new epithelial attachment forms. This attachment tends to seal off the deeper areas of separation between the tooth and the surrounding tissues. Thus the healing connective tissues may adapt as closely to the clean tooth surface as to an implant.[1] Reattachment with formation of the cementum may then develop gradually from the apical aspect of the lesion.[10] In such cases, minimal or no inflammation is present in the area of connective tissue adaptation, indicating that the pathologic periodontal pocket has been eliminated as a source of irritation. The new marginal epithelial attachment acts as a protective umbrella against bacterial penetration along the surface of the tooth. Apparently, such areas may gradually develop a long epithelial attachment,[22] which with persistent irritation may open up again as a pathologic pocket, but which can also be maintained in a state of health over many years.

It is well established that reattachment can occur following formation of lateral sliding flaps.[47] Because the interproximal tissues are biologically identical to the labial tissues, it appears that when flap adaptation is as good interproximally as it can be buccally, reattachment and readaptation should be attained as well interproximally as buccally.

An electron microscopic study by Listgarten[23] has elucidated the ultrastructural features of healing that occur between a surgical flap and the denuded tooth surface in monkeys. Similar findings in humans have been reported by Frank and associates.[10] Regeneration of the junctional epithelium occurred against both dentine and cementum. The ultrastructure of the re-formed epithelial attachment was in every way similar to undisturbed junctional epithelium, with hemidesmosomes, a basement lamina, and several layers of elongated epithelial cells parallel to the tooth surface. Connective tissue attachment and cemental regeneration over both exposed cementum and dentine were found.[11] The junction between the exposed tooth

surface and the newly formed cementum consisted of a densely stained granular layer free of collagen fibrils. This junction had a tendency to split during the preparation of sections. During early stages of healing, the collagen fibrils within the new cementum had no specific orientation, but at later stages, bundles of fibrils appeared to be connected to gingival fibers. Several groups of two or three collagen fibrils were covered by apatite crystals, indicating calcification. Other areas showed collagen fibrils extending into calcified, newly formed cementum. This indicated that calcification, occurring at the surface of the cementum along collagen fibrils, is responsible for connective tissue reattachment to the tooth following treatment.[10]

According to Frank and associates,[11] it appears that the first steps of connective tissue reattachment occur through a demineralization of the apatite crystals of the superficial dentine or cementum, followed by a fibroblastic matrix deposition establishing tissue continuity between the calcified tooth and the connective tissue. The cementum reattachment then follows through mineralization of the collagen fibrils.

Electron microscopic observations have been made of the dentogingival junction following a lateral sliding flap operation covering a previously denuded labial surface of a tooth. These operations have confirmed that healing similar to that obtained with the experimental flaps may occur on a pathologically exposed root surface.[24]

With the conventional types of reverse bevel flaps,[33] with or without apical repositioning, the interproximal bone and sometimes the root surfaces are left denuded at the termination of the surgery. Eventually, such an area will granulate over, and healing will occur at a more apical level than following a modified Widman flap procedure.[39] Therefore, in order to achieve pocket elimination and minimal return of pocket depth, the conventional type of reverse bevel flap surgery involves much more bone removal than does the modified Widman procedure. Although some reduction of pocket depth by shrinkage also follows the modified Widman flap surgery, the chief aim of this operation is maximum healing and reattachment of periodontal pockets, with minimum loss of periodontal tissues during and after the surgery.

Bone may heal into a intrabony lesion following a variety of periodontal procedures.[8] Such a result is most desirable. However, it has been found that in many instances when lost bone has not been regained to any appreciable extent (judged by repeated roentgenograms over several years), there may appear to be a consolidation of the bone crest and no indication of further bone loss. A thin probe may be inserted several mm. along the tooth surface without bleeding, exudation, or pain in the location of the previous pocket,[37] whereas, in other areas with obvious inflamed recurrent periodontal pockets, there is a continuous loss of bone with time. It thus appears that the modified Widman flap surgery may be successful in maintaining periodontal support and health by mechanisms of a long epithelial attachment, and in maintaining close connective tissue adaptation with or without reattachment of connective tissue and regeneration of bone.

A regeneration of bone in an intrabony lesion may also occur without connective tissue attachment and with a long thin epithelial attachment separating the tooth from the bone and connective tissues.[6]

The concept of epithelial reattachment and close connective tissue adaptation as a substitute for surgical pocket elimination in the maintenance of periodontal health and support has created some confusion in the mind of many clinicians. These clinicians were trained to equate success of periodontal therapy with pocket elimination as judged by clinical probing, and to consider areas where the probe could be inserted more than 3 mm during follow-up examinations to be failures. Rather than complete surgical pocket elimination, the key to success now seems to be optimal healing and prevention of subgingival plaque extension. These may be secured by good oral hygiene and frequent recalls for professional cleaning of the teeth.[28,43]

The obvious advantage of the modified Widman flap procedure, compared with conventional reverse bevel flap surgery including bone surgery,[33] is conservation of bone and optimal coverage of the root surfaces by soft tissues following the modified Widman surgery.[39] This procedure provides a more pleasing esthetic result, a favorable environment for oral hygiene, and potentially less root sensitivity and less root caries. It also tends to result in more pocket closure clinically[16] than occurs following the pocket elimination procedure when long-term follow-up is done (Fig. 24-2).

One apparent disadvantage of the modified Widman flap surgery is the flat or concave interproximal architecture immediately following removal of the surgical dressing, especially in areas of interproximal bony craters. Professional tooth cleaning in these crater areas is recommended once a week or once every 2 weeks for 4 to 5 weeks after the surgery to avoid the possibility that regenerating tissues may cover a plaque-infected root surface.

If meticulous oral hygiene is maintained, the interdental tissues will regenerate over a few months with gain rather than loss of attachment, as measured clinically from the cementoenamel junction with a calibrated probe.[39,40] The total gingival contour may appear less desirable following modified Widman flap surgery than following surgical pocket elimination; however, appearance does not have any significance with regard to plaque control, gingivitis, and maintenance of attachment levels.[52]

The modified Widman flap procedure represents a modification of subgingival curettage, and its merits can be compared with these of subgingival curettage. The flap procedure, however, provides better access to the root surface than does curettage, and permits removal of the epithelial lining of the pocket with less trauma and better postoperative adaptation than does curettage. However, curettage has the advantage of not directly affecting the bone and the subpocket connective tissue attachment to the root. The short-term results regarding maintenance of attachment are better following curettage than following the modified Widman procedure.[2,39] The long-term results are similar for both procedures.[18,36]

The selection of a procedure for individual cases should be based on convenience with regard to requirements of time and technical skill, as well as on esthetic and functional considerations.

Surgical elimination of interproximal bony craters is not justified for maintenance of attachment levels.[18,39] It may offer greater long-term reduction in pocket depth than do subgingival curettage or modified Widman flap surgery (Fig. 24-2), but leads to less gain in attachment, besides the loss of buccal and lingual bone that occurs in ostectomy.[30]

One large advantage of the modified Widman flap procedure over curettage is its feasibility when implantation of bone and other substances is contemplated. This aspect is discussed in chapter 26.

Indications for the modified Widman flap procedure

Whenever reattachment and/or minimal gingival recession is desired, the choice for the treatment of pockets is between the modified Widman flap procedure and subgingival curettage. There is no well-established basis for a definite choice between the two methods,[18] but modified Widman flap surgery is preferred for patients with (1) deep pockets (more than 5 mm) in the anterior and buccal maxillary posterior regions; (2) intrabony pockets and craters; (3) pockets with furcation involvement; (4) bone grafts; (5) high caries rate; and (6) severe root sensitivity.

In the mandibular posterior regions and the palatal aspect of the posterior maxillary teeth, more extensive soft tissue removal for pocket reduction is often included in the modified Widman flap approach than in areas where esthetics may be a problem (see chapter 23). Reattachment following mucogingival surgery is discussed in chapter 25.

PROPOSED PROCEDURES TO AUGMENT REATTACHMENT FOLLOWING FLAP SURGERY

Application of various acids has been proposed for 100 years to "condition" the exposed root surface to connective tissue reattachment. The most recently

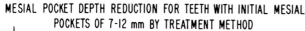

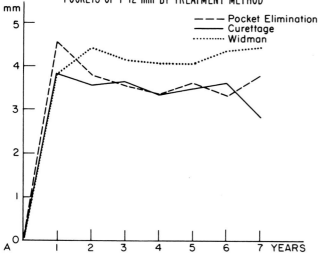

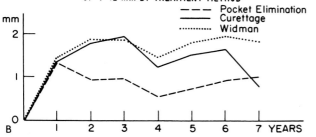

Fig. 24-2. Reduction of pocket depth for deep periodontal pockets is as good or better following modified Widman surgery as following pocket elimination surgery or subgingival curettage. There is more gain of attachment over several years following modified Widman surgery or curettage than following pocket elimination surgery.[18]

tried has been citric acid with a pH of 1. When experimental cases have been compared with controls without the acid both in animals and humans, a number of favorable reports have indicated significant gain in connective tissue reattachment and bone regeneration in the furcations.[7,41,42] However, recent well-controlled studies in humans have failed to show any benefit from citric acid compared to non-citric acid controls.[25,45]

Another adjunct to be added to the treated root surface, supposedly to encourage connective tissue attachment, is fibronectin; but there is no evidence of beneficial effect of this enzyme in the treatment of human periodontitis.

A new concept of guided tissue regeneration from the periodontal membrane, proposed by Nyman et al,[29] is more promising than any of the other pro-

cedures at the present time. Following a modified Widman flap procedure, a millipore or Gore-Tech filter is placed along the root surface. The filter is placed over the alveolar crest in such a way that it prevents downgrowth of the epithelium along the root surface, while it allows connective tissue from the periodontal membrane to regenerate in a coronal direction. Case reports have documented spectacular periodontal regeneration both in intrabony pockets and in exposed furcations, with clinical, roentgenographic, and histologic evidence[13] of new connective tissue attachment and new bone in regions of previous periodontal pockets. A search for suitable resorbable filter material is underway. The limitations of this form of therapy are not known as yet.

REFERENCES

1. Bodine, R.L., and Mohammed, C.J.: Histologic studies of a human mandible supporting an implant denture. Part II, J. Prosthet. Dent. 26:415, 1971.
2. Burgett, F.G., et al.: Short term results of three modalities of periodontal therapy, J. Dent. Res., Abstr. no. 553, p. 186, 1972.
3. Caffesse, R.G., Ramfjord, S.P., and Nasjleti, C.E.: Reverse bevel periodontal flaps in monkeys, J. Periodont. 39:219, 1968.
4. Carranza, F.A., and Glickman, J.: Some observations on the microscopic features of intrabony pockets, J. Periodontol. 28:33, 1957.
5. Caton, J., and Nyman, S.: Histometric evaluation of periodontal surgery. I. The modified Widman flap procedure, J. Clin. Periodontol. 7:212, 1980.
6. Caton, J., and Zander, H.A.: Osseous repair of an inflammatory pocket without new attachment of connective tissues, J. Clin. Periodontol. 3:54, 1976.
7. Cole, R., et al.: Clinical studies on the effect of topical citric acid application on healing after replaced periodontal flap surgery, J. Periodont. Res. 16:117, 1981.
8. Ellegaard, B., and Löe, H.: New attachment of periodontal tissues after treatment of intrabony lesions, J. Periodont. 42:648, 1971.
9. Ferynhough, W., and Page, R.C.: Attachment, growth and synthesis by human gingival fibroblasts on demineralized or fibronectin-treated normal and diseased tooth roots, J. Periodont. 54:133, 1983.
10. Frank, R., et al.: Gingival reattachment after surgery in man: An electron microscopic study, J. Periodont. 43:597, 1972.
11. Frank, R., et al.: Ultrastructural study of epithelial and connective gingival reattachment in man, J. Periodont. 45:626, 1974.
12. Goldman, H.M., and Cohen, D.W.: The intrabony pocket: Classification and treatment, J. Periodont. 29:272, 1958.
13. Gottlow, J., et al.: New attachment formation in the human periodontium by guided tissue regeneration. Case Reports, J. Clin. Periodontol. 13:604, 1986.
14. Grant, D.A., Stern, J.B., and Everett, F.G.: Orban's Periodontics, 4th ed., St. Louis, 1972, C.V. Mosby Co.
15. Harvey, P.M.: Management of advanced periodontitis. Part I. Preliminary report of a method of surgical reconstruction, N.Z. Dent. J. 61:180, 1965.
16. Kelly, G.P., et al.: Radiographs in clinical periodontal trials, J. Periodont. 46:7, 381, 1975.
17. Kirkland, O.: The suppurative periodontal pus pockets: Its treatment by the modified flap operation, J.A.D.A. 18:1462, 1931.

18. Knowles, J.W., et al.: Results of periodontal treatment related to pocket depth and attachment level: Eight years, J. Periodont. 50:225, 1979.

19. Kon, S., et al.: Visualization of the microvascularization of the healing periodontal wound. IV. Mucogingival surgery: Full thickness flap, J. Periodont. 40:5, 1969.

20. Kramer, G.M., and Kohn, J.D.: Postoperative care of the infrabony pocket, J. Periodont. 32:95, 1961.

21. Levine, H.L.: Periodontal flap surgery with gingival fiber retention, J. Periodont. 43:91, 1972.

22. Levine, H.L., and Stahl, S.S.: Repair following periodontal flap surgery with the retention of gingival fibers, J. Periodont. 43:99, 1972.

23. Listgarten, M.A.: Electron microscopic study of the junction between surgically denuded root surfaces and regenerated periodontal tissues, J. Periodont. Res. 7:68, 1972.

24. Listgarten, M.A.: Ultrastructural features of repair following periodontal surgery. In Periodontal Surgery, Biologic Bases and Technique, Stahl, S.S., ed., Springfield, Il., 1976, Charles C. Thomas.

25. Marks, S.C., and Mehta, M.R.: Lack of effect of citric acid treatment of root surfaces on the formation of new connective tissue attachment, J. Clin. Periodontol. 13:109, 1986.

26. Morris, M.L.: The unrepositioned mucoperiosteal flap, Periodontics 3:147, 1965.

27. Neumann, R.: Die Alveolar-pyorrhoe and ihre Behandlung, 3rd ed., Berlin, 1920, Hermann Meusser.

28. Nyman, S., Rosling, B., and Lindhe, J.: Effect of professional tooth cleaning on healing after periodontal surgery, J. Clin. Periodontol. 2:80, 1975.

29. Nyman, S., et al.: New attachment following surgical treatment of human periodontal disease, J. Clin. Periodontol. 9:290, 1982.

30. Olsen, C.T., et al.: A longitudinal study comparing apically repositioned flap with and without osseous surgery, Int. J. Periodont. and Rest. Dent. 4:10, 1985.

31. Patur, B., and Glickman, J.: Clinical and roentgenographic evaluation of posttreatment healing of infrabony pockets, J. Periodont. 33:164, 1962.

32. Prichard, J.: The infrabony technique as a predictable procedure, J. Periodont. 28:202, 1957.

33. Prichard, J.F.: Advanced Periodontal Disease, 2nd ed., Philadelphia, 1972, W.B. Saunders Co.

34. Ramfjord, S.P.: Reinsercion, Rev. Assoc. Odont. Argentina 47:275, 1959.

35. Ramfjord, S.P., and Costich, E.R.: Healing after simple gingivectomy, J. Periodont. 34:401, 1963.

36. Ramfjord, S.P.: Clinical trial of therapeutic measures in periodontics, Int. Dent. J. 21:16, 1971.

37. Ramfjord, S.P., et al.: Longitudinal study of periodontal therapy, J. Periodont. 44:66, 1973.

38. Ramfjord, S.P., and Nissle, R.R.: The modified Widman flap, J. Periodont. 45:601, 1974.

39. Ramfjord, S.P., et al.: Results following three modalities of periodontal therapy, J. Periodont. 46:9, 522, 1975.

40. Ramfjord, S.P.: Present status of the modified Widman flap procedure, J. Periodont. 48:558, 1977.

41. Register, A.A.: Bone and cementum induction by dentin, demineralized in situ, J. Periodontol. 44:49, 1973.

42. Rivie, C.M., et al.: Healing of periodontal connective tissues following surgical wounding and application of citric acid in dogs, J. Periodont. Res. 15:314, 1980.

43. Rosling, B., Nyman, S., and Lindhe, J.: The effect of systemic plaque control on bone regeneration in intrabony pockets, J. Clin. Periodontol. 3:38, 1976.

44. Shaw, J.F.: Treatment of multiple periodontal pockets by extended flap operation, Parodontologie 16:121, 1962.

45. Smith, B.A., et al.: The effectiveness of citric acid as an adjunct to surgical attachment procedures, J. Clin. Periodontol. 13:701, 1986.

46. Soehren, S.E., et al.: Clinical and histologic studies of donor tissues utilized for free grafts of masticatory mucosa, J. Periodont. 44:727, 1973.

47. Sugarman, E.F.: A clinical and histological study of the attachment of grafted tissues to bone and teeth, J. Periodont. 40:381, 1969.

48. Sullivan, H., Carman, D., and Dinner, D.: Histologic evaluation of the laterally positioned flap, I.A.D.R. Abstract No. 467, 1971.

49. Wade, A.B.: An assessment of the flap operation, Dent. Pract. 13:11, 1962.

50. Waerhaug, J.: The gingival pocket, Odont. Tidskr. Vol. 60, Suppl I, 1952.

51. Widman, L.: The operative treatment of pyorrhea alveolaris. A new surgical method, Sven. Tandlak. Tidskr. (Special Issue) Dec. 1918.

52. Zamet, J.S.: A comparative clinical study of three periodontal surgical techniques, J. Clin. Periodontol. 2:87, 1975.

53. Zemsky, J.L.: Surgical treatment of periodontal diseases. Open-view operation for advanced cases of dental periclasia, Dent. Cosmos 68:465, 1926.

54. Zentler, A.: Suppurative gingivitis with alveolar involvement, J.A.M.A. 71:1530, 1918.

25

MUCOGINGIVAL SURGERY

The goal of mucogingival surgery is to correct aberrations in the relationship between the attached gingiva and the alveolar mucosa. Such corrections will, by necessity, also affect gingival relationships to the underlying and contiguous tissues, including bone, muscle attachments, and the vestibular fold.[13]

RATIONALE FOR MUCOGINGIVAL SURGERY

A distinct boundary demarcates the attached gingiva from the alveolar mucosa. This border, called the *mucogingival line* or the *mucogingival junction*,[97] can easily be determined clinically as well as histologically and histochemically.[6,36] The junction can be made easier to distinguish clinically by painting with an iodine solution, but tissue movability tests tend to locate the junction slightly more apically than it is located by direct inspection of the surface mucosa.[6]

Histologically, the surface of the attached gingiva is highly keratinized, while the alveolar mucosa has minimal to no keratinization.[99] The attached gingiva has heavy collagenous fiber bundles, which tie the surface epithelium firmly to the bone and the teeth. The alveolar mucosa, on the other hand, is characterized by loose fibrous connective tissue containing numerous elastic fibers, which do not occur in the attached gingiva.[97] It has been postulated that the alveolar mucosa is not as well fitted anatomically to withstand injury from passage of food as is the attached gingiva,[80] and that the latter is more suited to dissipate pull from the adjacent muscles transmitted through the alveolar mucosa and frena, thus preventing the gingival margin from being retracted by lip and cheek action.[38] If this protective function of the attached gingiva has been lost either by recession, gingivectomies, abnormal frenum insertions, or a very shallow vestibule, proper oral hygiene procedures may be restricted,[96] and accumulation of debris during mastication may be enhanced.[23] Mechanical pull on the free gingiva has also

been suggested as a reason for inflammation related to lack of attached gingiva.[55,80,96]

It is generally assumed that an "adequate width" of attached gingiva is essential for the maintenance of periodontal health. However, why this is so, and what an "adequate width" would be, are still unsettled. Minimal widths have been stated to range from 3 mm[23] to less than 1 mm,[116] while some authors have suggested that, instead of a numerical value, the only true criterion for adequacy should be the ability to maintain gingival health with good oral hygiene.[39]

It has been observed that regions with less than 1 mm of attached gingiva (distance between the mucogingival line and the bottom of the gingival crevice as located by probing) could not be kept free of gingival inflammation, despite good oral hygiene, while areas with a width of 1 mm or more could be kept practically free of clinically visible inflammation.[65] Another investigation has complicated further the problem of how to assess the adequacy of the attached gingiva based on measurements.[57] Following scaling and root planing of teeth with gingival inflammation, the attachment level as assessed by probing frequently appeared to be at a more coronal level after the scaling, especially in areas with no bone underlying the mucogingival junction, while the position of the mucogingival line did not change when related to the cementoenamel junction. Thus, subjects that did not appear to have any functional attached gingiva at the time of the initial examination might have 1 mm of attached gingiva one month after the scaling and healing. The width of the attached gingiva also increases with age.[1]

It is usually stated in the literature that the objectives of mucogingival surgery are (1) to retain or create a gingival margin with an "adequate" width of attached gingiva; (2) to eliminate tension and pull on the free gingival margin; and (3) to provide sufficient vestibular

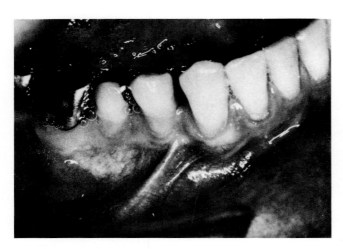

Fig. 25-1. Blanching of free gingiva on cuspid and first bicuspid from pull on lip. This situation has been observed to be stable (unaltered) for over 30 years.

depth and freedom from frena to permit efficient tooth-brushing and reflexion of food in mastication.[20,23,53,64,96] It appears that the crucial factor in determining the rationale and need for mucogingival surgery is whether, following removal of local irritants on the teeth and maintenance of good oral hygiene (using a soft toothbrush), the gingiva can be kept free from clinically visible inflammation.

Maintenance of the position of the free gingival margin without further recession or inflammation may be achieved by good oral hygiene without any augmentation of the gingiva.[29] Such observations have led to much controversy in the field of mucogingival surgery.[49] Manual pulling on the patient's lip or cheek to test the need for mucogingival surgery is meaningless and may be misleading, because it may produce blanching of the free gingival margin even if freedom of inflammation in these patients indicates a functionally adequate zone of attached gingiva (Fig. 25-1).

It has never been shown that a certain vestibular depth is needed for effective toothbrushing or for self-cleaning after mastication. Therefore, there is no valid reason for vestibular extension for that purpose.

DEVELOPMENT OF MUCOGINGIVAL AND VESTIBULAR EXTENSION SURGERY

Mucogingival surgery may be dated back to the work of Kazanjian[63,64] and Pichler and Trauner[86] between 1920 and 1930. Their procedures were aimed strictly at mucobuccal fold extension in preparation for prosthetic appliances. Hilming (1942) first suggested mucogingival surgery for periodontal treatment in an attempt to correct high frenum insertions and gingivectomy failures in patients with minimal residual attached gingiva.[54] His mucobuccal fold extension surgery was more or less an excision of frenula combined with deepening of the mucobuccal fold.[55]

Kazanjian's technique for vestibular extension was introduced into periodontic therapy in 1954 by Stewart.[105] This technique made it necessary for a band of novmovable attached gingiva to be between the gingival margin and the vestibular mucosa, and did not increase the width of the attached gingiva. A number of other techniques were also aimed primarily at frenectomy and deepening of the vestibule, although it was claimed that they also resulted in a wider zone of attached gingiva.[45,53] In these procedures, a horizontal incision was made to the periosteum at the mucogingival junction. A sharp dissection separated a mucosal flap from the periosteal surface, severing muscle and connective tissue attachments from the periosteum to the desired depth of the mucobuccal fold. Despite all attempts at maintaining a deepened vestibule following these procedures, there was a return of the tissues toward presurgical levels during the healing. A number of modifications of these methods, including denudation of a strip of labial bone, have been suggested.[23,96,102]

The early vestibular extension procedures usually started with an incision at the bottom of the vestibule, often leaving alveolar mucosa between this incision and the demarcation line from a gingivectomy done immediately before the extension incision. Later techniques removed all alveolar mucosa and attached gingiva over the alveolar process, leaving periosteum over the bone. Extensive investigations by Bohannan showed that neither of these procedures resulted in significant long-term deepening of the vestibule.[14,15] Alveolar denudation procedures were also tried. Fox's "pushback"[42] and Schluger's "pouch" operation[42] included denudation of the alveolar process with extensive bone exposure, which had to be kept covered by periodontal dressings for several weeks. This operation was followed by much pain, necrosis, and sloughing of bone. Although it appeared that this process led to gain of attached gingiva and deepened vestibule[13] histologic studies[17,46] showed that the regenerated tissues were often not true attached gingiva and that labial bone might be lost permanently.[119] It was shown later that denudation of the alveolar process, in addition to causing bone loss, could also lead to resorption on the underlying root surfaces[25] (Fig. 25-2).

Following a study in dogs, it was claimed that if, instead of denudation, a split flap was used, leaving the bone covered by periosteum, no loss of bone occurred.[103] However, studies in humans indicate that unless the soft tissue cover left over the bone in a split thickness flap is very thick, the bone loss is almost as extensive as following denudation.[89,121] Other studies did not report any difference in the postsurgical amount of attached gingiva between patients treated

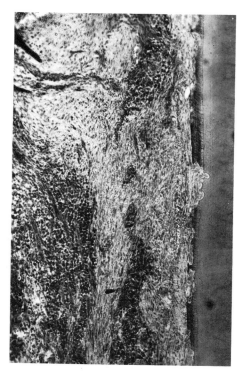

Fig. 25-2. Four weeks after denudation of the alveolar process, showing resorption of cementum and dentine. There was severe chronic inflammation (human specimen).

with denudation and those with periosteal retention.[21,40]

It appears that granulation tissues derived from remaining free or attached gingival connective tissue, or from the periodontal membrane, will become covered by keratinized gingival epithelium.[62] In contrast, granulation tissue originating from the connective tissues underlying the alveolar mucosa will induce a nonkeratinized epithelial coverage. Following denudation of the alveolar process, bone resorption is usually extensive on the labial surface, and much of the new granulation tissue will come from the periodontal membrane, especially if the labial bone plate is thin. This will result in a wide zone of attached gingiva, whereas with periosteal retention or thick labial bone, with only superficial resorption, less granulation tissue will originate from the periodontal membrane and there will be minimal or no gain of attached gingiva. It has been suggested that the results following mucogingival surgery would be more predictable if a strip of periosteum was removed leaving denuded bone at the mucobuccal fold.[75,93,94] However, this is not a recommended procedure.[27,33]

Because of the unpredictable results, risk of losing bony support for the teeth, painful and slow healing, and introduction of safer gingival repositioning and grafting procedures, none of the described techniques is used in current periodontal practice.

A number of investigations have been concerned primarily with extension of the depth of the mucobuccal fold rather than with the width of the attached gingiva.[4,13,14] However, these two parameters are not necessarily related, since there is no evidence to indicate a specific cause-and-effect relationship between a shallow vestibule and periodontal disease. A vestibular deepening procedure proposed by Edlan and Mejchar,[31] for example, is very effective in deepening the vestibule,[115] but does not increase the width of the attached gingiva. In this technically difficult procedure, a mucosal flap from the inside of the lip and the vestibule is placed over the alveolar process following separation of the periosteum from the alveolar process and suturing of this periosteal flap to the lip. Postoperative complications of obstructed glandular ducts and shortening of the lip makes this an impractical operation.[5]

APICALLY REPOSITIONED FLAPS

The first attempt to solve mucogingival problems associated with periodontitis was a proposal by Norberg to place a coronally repositioned flap over a periosteal scaffold on the alveolar crest when pockets extended beyond the mucogingival line.[76,77] However, this procedure never became well known, and the credit goes to Nabers for developing a method to move the patient's attached gingiva apically to solve mucogingival problems.[72] He raised a mucoperiosteal flap beyond the mucogingival line and trimmed off about 2 mm at the gingival margin. Then he repositioned the flap apically to gain width of attached gingiva (Fig. 25-3). Later he proposed an initial reverse bevel incision in order to thin the gingival margin and eliminate the pocket epithelium before moving the flap apically.[73] If the patient has a definite band of keratinized gingiva prior to the surgery, apically repositioned flap procedures are predictable for increasing

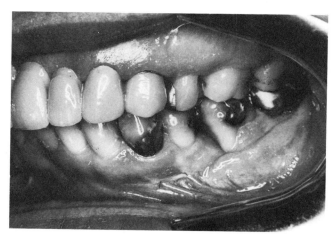

Fig. 25-3. Apically positioned flap, increasing the width of attached gingiva for the first molar. Six weeks after surgery.

the width of the attached gingiva and for pocket elimination.

Less vascular congestion and tissue necrosis occur with full-thickness than with partial-thickness flaps,[113] and as much or more crestal bone resorption occurs following the split-thickness compared with the full-thickness flap.[101] The split-thickness flap is also a more technically demanding procedure. Thus, there does not seem to be any reason to use the split-thickness flap for apical repositioning.

FRENUM OPERATIONS

A *frenum* is a mucous membrane fold containing muscle and connective tissue fibers. It attaches the lip and cheek to the alveolar mucosa, the gingiva, and the underlying periosteum.

It has been postulated that frena may jeopardize gingival health when they are attached too closely to the gingival margin either because of interference with proper placement of a toothbrush or through opening of the gingival crevice by muscle pull.[45,54,118] A frenum may be excised in a frenotomy (partial removal of the frenum), which involves localized vestibular extension surgery with an incision to the periosteum across the frenum as close to the attached gingiva as possible.[38] Dissection is extended laterally for at least one tooth on either side of the frenum, and the mucosal border of the incised frenum is sutured to the periosteum at the apical base of the incision. The wound is covered by a periodontal dressing. Others have recommended total frenectomies[20] instead of apical displacement of the frenum with a flap. The frenum may be held by a hemostat, and a V-shaped wedge of tissue is excised on both sides of the hemostat; the frenum attachment is then dissected loose from the bone with sharp dissection through the periosteum, and removed. This wound may or may not be sutured, and a protective dressing is placed interproximally over the wound and the denuded bone (Fig. 25-4). This wound may require two to three weekly changes of dressings and may be somewhat painful the first week after the surgery. Avoid pressure on the dressing or placing too much dressing. Frenum operations are often part of other mucogingival corrections and may involve grafting procedures to prevent recurrence of high frenum attachments, as will be discussed later in this chapter.

That a high frenum attachment will destroy gingival tissue through constant muscle tension and action[118] is unlikely. As with all mucogingival surgery, the indications for frenectomy should be based on whether gingival health can be maintained following scaling and proper oral hygiene, rather than on tests using pull on the lip or measurements of the attached gingiva. Labial frenectomies in children before complete eruption of the permanent cuspids are usually not indicated, because what appears to be a very heavy

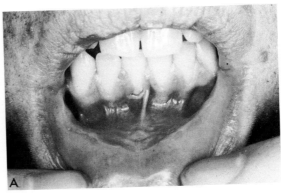

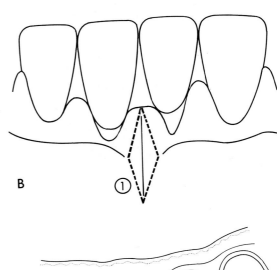

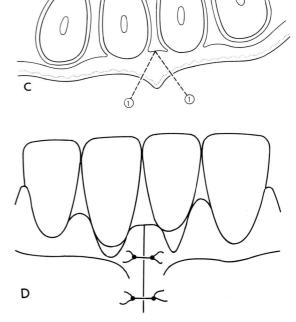

Fig. 25-4. *A,* High labial frenum. *B,C,* Incision to the bone on both sides of the frenum (1). Extend the incision well into the alveolar mucosa. *D,* Remove the frenum and suture the two wounds together.

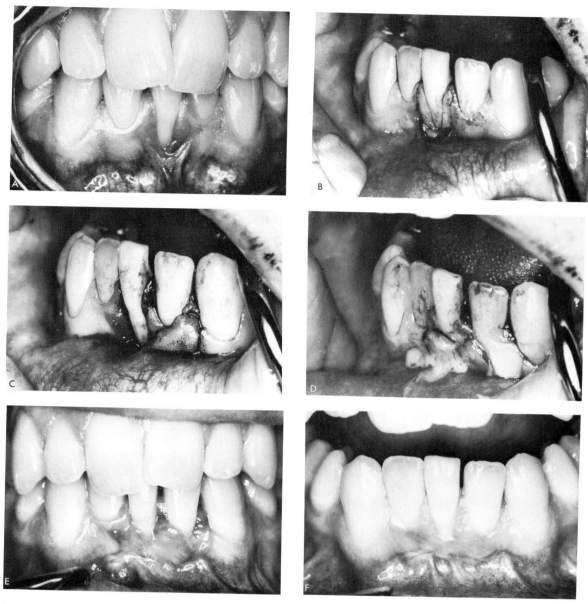

Fig. 25-5. *A,* Lack of attached gingiva and 4 mm pocket on the labial aspect of the mandibular central incisor. *B,* The free gingiva bordering the cleft is excised. *C,* The exposed root surface is planed and some of the protrusion reduced by removal of tooth substance. A full-thickness pedicle flap is separated from the incisor. Achronmycin ointment is placed over the wounds and the sutures. *E,* Three weeks after surgery. Healing is not complete. *F,* Three years after the surgery. There is adequate attached gingiva. No inflammation is present, and gingival crevices are less than 1 mm deep. However, some gingival recession is apparent both at the donor and recipient tooth.

frenum at the time of the eruption of the incisors usually regresses after the erupting cuspids close the diastema between the central incisors.

PEDICLE GINGIVAL GRAFTS

The first pedicle flap or "bridge flap" designed to cover areas of gingival recession was proposed by Kalmi and co-workers in 1949.[59] The bridge flap failed because of the stretch on both ends of the flap. In another investigation, a horizontal pedunculated strip of gingival tissues, detached at the mesial and left with undisturbed attachment at the distal end, was placed coronally to cover denuded root surfaces and sutured in place.[83] Unfortunately, the blood supply to this type of flap proved to be inadequate and severe necrosis with loss of the flap resulted. One modification of this technique to a single tooth has been reported,[111] but this procedure has not gained much acceptance.

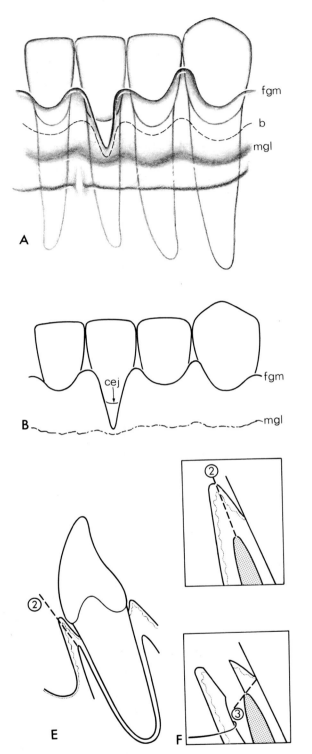

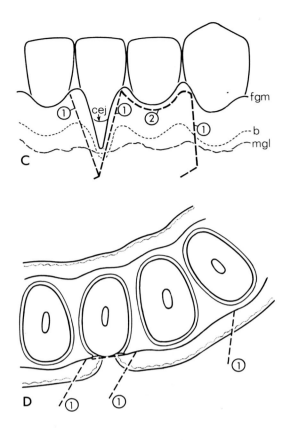

Fig. 25-6. *A,* Orientation drawing showing the structural relations of the gingival cleft on the central incisor. *B,* The cleft extending to the mucogingival line. *C,D,* Initial incisions (1) slanted for optimal flap adaptation. Boundaries of the flap are indicated by broken line *(2).* Bone crest is indicated by fine dashed line *(b).* *E,* Incision 2 is made from the free gingival margin of the alveolar crest of the donor tooth. *F,* Mucoperiosteal full-thickness flap is raised, and the remaining crevicular gingiva is excised *(3).*
Continued

Lateral Sliding Flap

Grupe and Warren introduced the lateral sliding flap in 1956 as a procedure to correct single defects of gingival dehiscence or cleft formation.[47] The original operation, as described by Grupe and Warren, consisted of one vertical gingival incision on each side of gingival cleft, excising the inflamed free gingiva, and a horizontal incision at the base of the cleft for the same purpose. Another vertical incision was made, including one papilla distally or mesially to the defect and extending well into the alveolar mucosa. A full-thickness flap was raised for part of the attached gingiva, but the apical part of the flap was dissected free from the periosteum in a split-thickness flap. The flap was positioned laterally over the area of the gingival cleft and sutured in this new position. A periodontal dressing was placed and changed at weekly intervals until healing had occurred (Fig. 25-5).

A number of modifications of this procedure have been proposed. Staffileno preferred to use a split-thickness, laterally repositioned flap to avoid the denudation of bone which followed the Grupe-Warren operation.[104] Grupe proposed a modification using a stair-step form of a lateral sliding flap, leaving the coronal half of the attached gingiva at the donor site undisturbed.[48] The flap was then laterally and coronally repositioned and sutured. This procedure required a very wide zone of attached gingiva at the

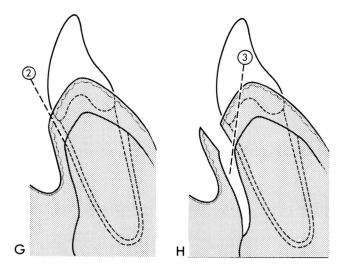

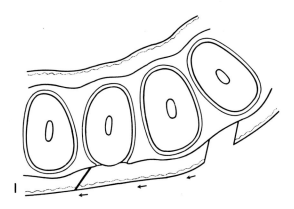

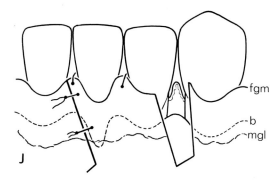

Fig. 25-6 continued. *G,H,* Drawings illustrating how incisions 2 and 3 affect the interproximal tissues, and indicate that the mucoperiosteal flap should be separated from the bone for a few millimeters apically to the mucogingival border. *I,* The pedicle flap has been moved in place over the recipient tooth. *J,* The flap is held in place by labial sutures and by a suspensory suture tied on the lingual aspect of the recipient tooth. Some denuded bone is present between the lateral incisor and the cuspid. As much as possible, avoid leaving labial bone over the donor tooth unprotected by the flap. Place dressing over the field of surgery (*fgm,* free gingival margin; *b,* bone crest; *mgf,* mucogingival line; *cej,* cementoenamel junction).

donor site, and Björn suggested another modification using a vertical curved incision instead of the step incision, and a widening of the zone of attached gingiva with a free gingival graft prior to the lateral sliding flap procedure.[12] The following procedures are recommended for the lateral sliding flap operation (Fig. 25-6).

Lateral sliding flap surgery

Preparatory treatment. Scaling and root planing followed by instruction in oral hygiene.

Orthodontic movement of teeth, if needed, to bring the tooth with the gingival cleft into favorable alignment with the other teeth and the alveolar process.

Surgical treatment. Administer local anesthesia.

Block off with gauze and swab the surgical area with iodine lotion or tincture of iodine.

Excise the free gingival borders of the cleft with two straight incisions that meet in a V in the alveolar mucosa apically to the bottom of the cleft.

Remove the excised free gingiva with curettes and plane the exposed root surface. Prominence of the tooth may be reduced by planing with sharp curettes.

Prepare the wall of the cleft which is to receive the graft. Make the surface beveled so that overlapping connective tissue contact can be made with the graft, and excise any frenum or mucobuccal fold attachment that will interfere with proper graft placement.

Make an undermining beveled incision at the donor border of the cleft in such a way that when the graft is later placed over the recipient site, the two meeting surfaces have similar bevels. Extend this incision through the periosteum.

Make the releasing vertical incision for the graft approximately at the proximal line angle of the tooth situated at least one tooth away from the defect. It is important that this incision be made in such a way that the entire interdental papilla and a slight amount of labial or lingual gingiva will be included with the graft. Tilt the scalpel so that this incision will produce a beveled thin connective tissue border on the graft. Extend the incision into the alveolar mucosa for 1 to 2 mm and make a small horizontal or slanted cut back toward the defect so that the flap can later be stretched to cover the recipient site.

Make an intracrevicular releasing incision at the tooth adjacent to the defect; extend the incision through the papilla and into the neighboring tooth crevice until it meets the vertical releasing incision.

Separate the graft from the bone as a mucoperiosteal flap extended apically to the mucogingival line. How far apically the flap has to be separated depends on how far apically the preparatory incisions in the cleft area had to be extended.

Remove with sharp dissection any residual soft tissue bulk that would interfere with close graft adap-

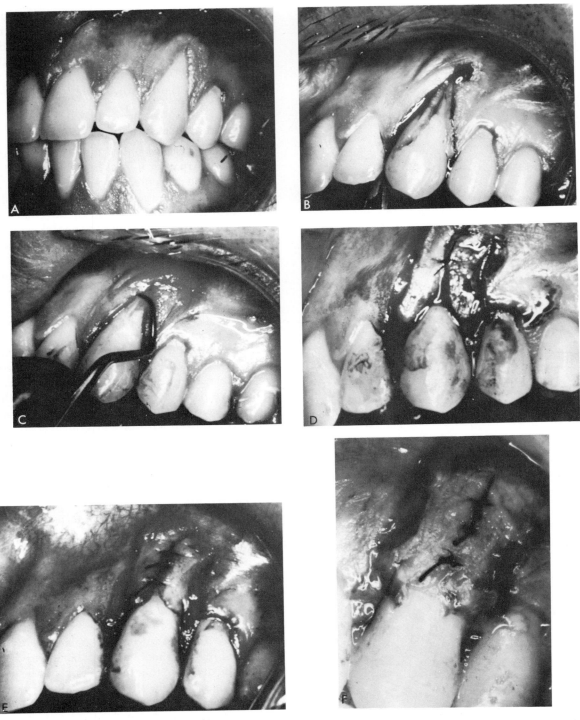

Fig. 25-7. *A,* Gingival recession over maxillary cuspid, posing an esthetic problem. *B,* The free gingiva is excised from the borders of the cleft. *C,* Thorough root planing is performed. *D,* Full-thickness papillary flaps from the mesial and distal borders of the cleft are extended into the alveolar mucosa and placed over the cleft. *E,* Flaps are sutured together. Achromycin ointment and a dressing are placed over the wound. *F,* One week after surgery. The sutures are removed and a new dressing applied.   *Continued*

tation at the border of the defect. Also remove epithelial remains from the donor tooth.

Slide the graft over to the recipient position. If there is any tissue pull on the graft, it may be necessary to increase the releasing cut-back. This should be done

with the flap reflected and with a very shallow sharp incision into the periosteum from the inner surface of the flap, avoiding interference with the blood supply.

Suture to secure the desired position of the graft with small needles and thin sutures (5/0 or 6/0). Apply

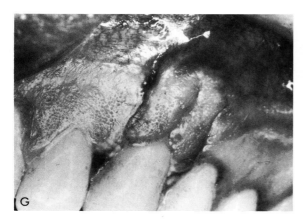 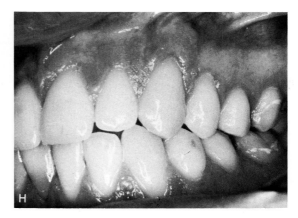

Fig. 25-7 continued. *G*, Three weeks after the surgery. The healing is not complete. *H*, One year after the surgery. The esthetic result is good and the gingival crevice is less than 1 mm in depth.

an initial suspensory suture to hold the flap in place, and a couple of sutures between the flap and the recipient wall of the former cleft.

Hold the sutured flap firmly against the graft bed with finger pressure on a piece of gauze moistened in sterile saline. This is done to assure close contact between the graft and the recipient bed tissues.

Place Achromycin ointment and a periodontal dressing over the graft. Make sure that the dressing covers the sutures and the interproximal spaces, on both the buccal and lingual sides.

Remove the dressing and the sutures after one week. Clean the wound with 1.5% hydrogen peroxide and warm water.

Place a new periodontal dressing.

Remove the dressing after another week. Polish the involved teeth with rubber cup and pumice. Place a new dressing if the area of denuded bone has not healed completely; otherwise, instruct the patient in good oral hygiene with a soft toothbrush and the circular scrub method.

Inclusion of more teeth to make a wider lateral sliding flap has been recommended,[2,38] but without any convincing advantage over the original design. Mucosal cut-back of the releasing incision and utilization of adjacent edentulous areas for donor tissues are other modifications.[24,95] Such pedicle grafts from edentulous ridges adjacent to gingival defects may provide a good source for new attached gingiva. It is important not to pull or twist the flap too vigorously, as this may jeopardize its blood supply. Mild pressure on the flap for a few minutes before and after it has been sutured in place will expel excess blood and prevent formation of hematoma under the flap.

Double Papillae Flap

Another modification of pedicle grafts is the double papillae flap,[22] which has been recommended for covering relatively wide labial or lingual gingival reces-

sion with normal papillae adjacent to the defect (Fig. 25-7). All crevicular gingival epithelium at the margins of the defect is removed with two incisions that meet in a V at the apical base of the defect. Vertical incisions are then made at the proximal line angles of the adjacent teeth and carried into the alveolar mucosa. Full-thickness mucoperiosteal flaps, including the papillae, are raised at both sides of the defect. Following thorough root planing, the two flaps are sutured together with a fine needle and thin suture material (5/0 or 6/0), held in position over the defect for a few minutes and covered by Achromycin ointment and a periodontal dressing (Fig. 25-7).

If this procedure is to be used, the proximal papillae have to be wide enough to cover the defect. Clinical experience indicates that the prognosis for this operation may be improved by raising full-thickness flaps in conjunction with the papillae instead of the originally recommended split-thickness flaps. The bone left exposed by the surgery is exposed interproximally, and no lasting defect is apt to occur. If sufficient donor tissues are available, healing between the two flaps over the tooth surface is more likely if the joining cut surfaces are slanted to overlap slightly, rather than meeting in cuts perpendicular to the tooth surface. Slanting the releasing incision for the two flaps will also provide better esthetic results than incisions perpendicular to the bone surface.

The idea of using interdental papillary gingiva to gain buccal or lingual attached gingiva was actually proposed by Hattler in 1967,[50] but his procedure never became popular. The double papillae flap procedure is technically demanding and often followed by relapse, with recurrent gingival recession, whereas the lateral sliding flap operation is easy to do and has a high success rate. The double papillae procedure therefore should be used only when, for anatomical reasons, the lateral sliding flap or other graft procedures are contraindicated.

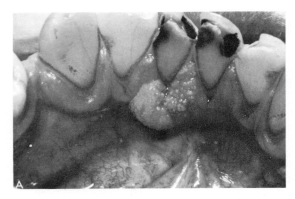

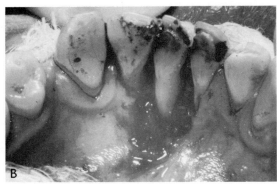

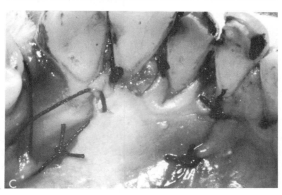

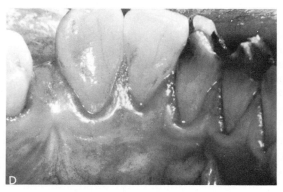

Fig. 25-8. *A,* Papilloma on the lingual aspect of mandibular lateral and central incisors. *B,* Large gingival defect after removal of the papilloma. *C,* Broad based full-thickness pedicle flap sutured in place to cover the gingival defect. Denuded bone now appears in the wide space between the cuspid and the bicuspid. *D,* One year after the surgery. The gingival crevices are not more than 1 mm deep.

Healing of Pedicle Grafts

A pedicle graft behaves like a regular mucogingival flap, and the histological features of healing of mucogingival flaps described in chapters 23 and 24 also apply to pedicle grafts.

Animal studies with experimentally produced gingival recession[120] and specimens from studies in humans[106,110] all indicate that connective tissue and epithelial reattachment to pedicle grafts may occur to root surfaces previously exposed to the environment of the oral cavity.

The healing sequence of pedicle grafts in dogs was described in detail by Wilderman and Wentz.[120] They found that during the first 4 days, the attachment of the flap to the tooth and bone is mediated by a thin fibrinous blood clot. At this time, connective tissue begins to proliferate from the flap into the clot and gradually fills the interface between the flap and the hard structure. Epithelial downgrowth along the tooth surface is most pronounced 8 to 10 days after the surgery. By 18 to 21 days, the flap appears to be firmly attached to the tooth, but functional orientation of the new connective tissue fibers attached to the root is not evident until 180 days. Sullivan and co-workers,[110] and Sugarman[106] have documented histologically as much as 2 to 3 mm of connective tissue reattachment following lateral sliding flaps in humans. They also often found a long and narrow new epithelial attachment, and in some instances connective tissue adaptation without evidence of reattachment and without inflammation. Listgarten described collagen fibrils within newly formed cementum on these previously exposed root surfaces.[67] During the early stage of the healing, the fibrils run a haphazard course, but as the new cementum grows in thickness, the single fibrils coalesce and appear as collagenous bundles with functional orientation.

Several authors have reported an average gain of clinical attachment of 2 to 3 mm following lateral sliding flap operations,[106,109,110] and a very high rate of success.[52,69] It has been claimed that application of citric acid to the denuded root surface would enhance the area of new connective tissue attachment,[70] but this assumption has not been confirmed by other studies.[58] The merits of full- versus split-thickness flaps for the lateral sliding flap procedure are still a controversial issue. It appears that split-thickness flaps have more vascular disruptions and are more prone to partial or complete necrosis than are full flaps.[113] Reattachment is more apt to occur with full-thickness flaps than with split flaps, and the entire healing is faster, with less recession at the recipient site, when a full-thickness flap is used.[10,85] The only disadvantage of the full-thickness flap is the denuded bone left at the border of the donor site at the completion of the surgery; with split flaps, this bone will be left covered by periosteum.

Although it is often stated that there is less bone resorption with a split thickness than with a full flap, this concept is not unequivocally supported by research findings.[121] If the procedure is carried out according to our recommended technique, the only exposed bone will be located interproximally. The chances for permanent bone loss are thus minimal with either method. An attempt to get the "best of both worlds" is a newly proposed technique,[91] in which the part of the flap that is to cover the denuded root is a full-thickness flap, and the more distant half of the flap is split-thickness, so that the periosteum will be left over the bone at the exposed donor area. Another variation is to apply a free gingival graft over the donor site for a lateral sliding flap.[32] All these methods give good clinical results with a minimal recession at the donor site. The simplest procedure is the full-thickness lateral sliding flap (Fig. 25-8), which may also be used lingually in the mandible.

The pedicle graft requires good alveolar bone and periodontal membrane support on both sides of the exposed root as a basis for reattachment of the graft. When there is loss of periodontal support for the adjacent teeth, a lateral sliding flap is not a practical procedure, since one may gain a new gingival cleft for the one treated. There is a potential danger of dehiscence over the donor tooth if the labial bone is very thin or there is none at all prior to the operation. In such instances, a double papillae flap may be safer than a lateral sliding flap. Prominence of the root associated with the cleft is another drawback. It should be reduced as much as possible; otherwise, the flap may heal, but the recession will recur for the same reason that it happened in the first place.

FREE GINGIVAL GRAFTS

Skin grafts have been used for nearly 200 years to enhance healing of burns or other superficial skin injuries. They gained general acceptance after Thiersch (1874)[112] showed that split-thickness thin grafts worked better than the thick, full-thickness grafts used previously. Split-thickness grafts include only part of the lamina propria, while those of full-thickness imply inclusion of the entire lamina propria. Intraorally, free skin grafts[88] have been suggested for alveolar ridge extension in denture patients.[44] Free mucosal grafts also have been recommended both for this purpose and for vestibular extension.[26]

Björn (1963)[11] first described the use of free gingival grafts in periodontal therapy. According to Prichard,[87] such grafts were first reported in the United States by King and Pennell in 1964. They transplanted palatal mucosa to the labial vestibular area over a maxillary cuspid, where it became marginal attached gingiva.

The present interest in free gingival grafts as a periodontal procedure, however, started with Nabers' de-

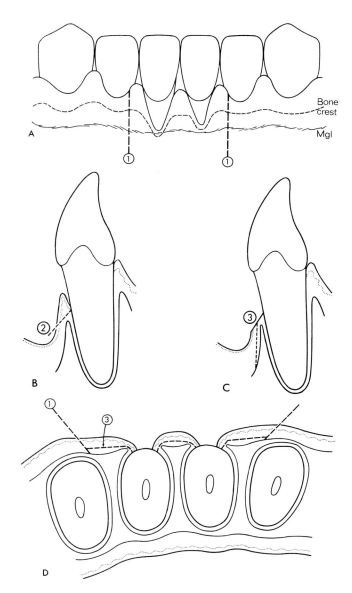

Fig. 25-9. *A,* Schematic drawing of gingival recession extending beyond the mucogingival junction. The initial vertical incisions are indicated (1). *B,* The free gingiva is excised (2). *C,* A split-thickness mucogingival flap is raised beyond the mucobuccal fold. *D,* Drawing illustrating the slanted vertical incisions (1) and the split-thickness flap dissections (3).   *Continued*

tailed description of this procedure for mucobuccal fold extension in 1966.[74,75] Tissues excised during gingivectomy were used for the graft, but later practice has been to obtain the free grafts from the palate confined to areas with no rugae. Free gingival grafts have been recommended for treatment of (1) an inadequate zone of attached gingiva,[108] (2) abnormal muscle attachment,[114] (3) shallow vestibular depth,[74] (4) gingival recession,[8,71,100,106] and (5) deep pockets to prevent rapid initial downgrowth of epithelium (Fig. 25-9, 25-10).

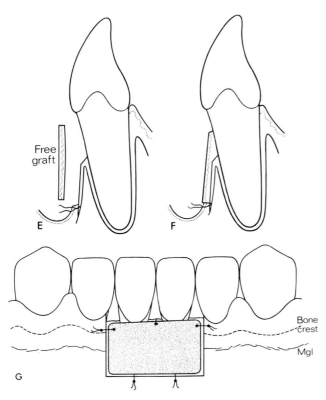

Fig. 25-9 continued. *E,* The split-thickness mucogingival flap has been sutured to the periosteum at the apical border of the flap. A free gingival graft is ready to be applied over the graft bed. *F,* The graft in place, covering 1 to 2 mm of the exposed tooth surfaces. *G,* The graft has been sutured into the desired position. Achromycin and a periodontal dressing are applied.

Procedures for Free Gingival Grafting

The first step is to prepare the recipient site for the graft. The ideal recipient site is a smooth periosteal surface whose residual periosteum has not been traumatized and is at least 0.5 mm thick. If the surgery is intended to involve the marginal gingiva, a gingivectomy may be done first. After this, make two vertical incisions to the bone, one at each end of the area to be covered by the graft. Make the incision beveled, with the tip of the blade directed toward the recipient site, and extend the incision as far apically as the graft is to go. Dissect the mucosal surface away from the periosteum in a split-flap procedure. Carry the dissection a couple of millimeters deeper than the desired boundary of the new attached gingiva. Removal of a strip of periosteum at the apical base of the flap has been recommended.[9] The mucosal border of the flap should be sutured to the periosteum at the apical border of the flap to avoid a gaping, painful wound when the lip is moved after the surgery.

If the free gingival margin is not to be involved in grafting, and there is some attached gingiva present,

make the same type of vertical incisions, but start the split-flap procedure from the mucogingival line instead of from the gingivectomy incision. Remove any surface roughness from the graft bed with sharp scissors. Also, be sure that no residual muscle attachment or pull from the lip will move the recipient bed tissues. Control bleeding with gauze sponges moistened in sterile saline solution. Make a template of the recipient site out of tinfoil, to be used as a pattern for the graft.

The graft is usually obtained from the palate, but other wide zones of attached gingiva or edentulous ridges may be used.[84,107] Place the tinfoil pattern over an area without palatal rugae. Make a shallow beveled incision, pointed to the graft from about 1 mm outside the borders of the template to make allowance for shrinkage. Let this incision extend only 1 to 1.5 mm under the mucosal surface. Dissect free a thin (1 to 1.5 mm) graft[101] without causing pinching or other trauma to the graft. Placing a suture in one border of the graft before it is dissected free from the donor site has been recommended.[3]

Place the graft on gauze moistened in sterile saline, with the cut surface up. Cut off with surgical scissors any roughness or area of the tissue that appears to be or contain glands or fat. The purpose of this cutting is to attempt to create a smooth surface and a graft of even thickness. Do not let the graft dry out under hot lights during this procedure. Place the graft over the prepared bed and press it gently into position for 2 to 3 minutes with a sponge moistened in sterile saline solution.

Suture the graft in place with 5/0 Teflon-coated Dacron[107] or 5/0 silk sutures. Use only the minimum number of sutures needed to assure the desired position of the graft. Do not suture the graft to the mucosal border. Hold the graft in place with mild pressure on moist gauze for 2 to 3 minutes.

Carefully apply a periodontal dressing. The use of rubber dam[108] or tinfoil[84] under the dressing has been recommended, but these measures do not seem to make any difference in the success or failure of the procedure. The donor site should also be covered by a surgical dressing. An acrylic palatal stent may be desirable to hold the dressing in place. Avoid too much pressure on the dressing, as this may precipitate pain and delay healing.

Remove the dressing after 1 week. Debride the wound and the teeth with saline solution. Clean the tooth surfaces bordering the graft with curettes, and allow a new dressing to remain for another week. Then remove the dressing and polish the teeth well with rubber cup and pumice. Instruct the patient in careful but thorough oral hygiene with a soft toothbrush (0.007 bristles).

With thick free gingival grafts and close suturing,

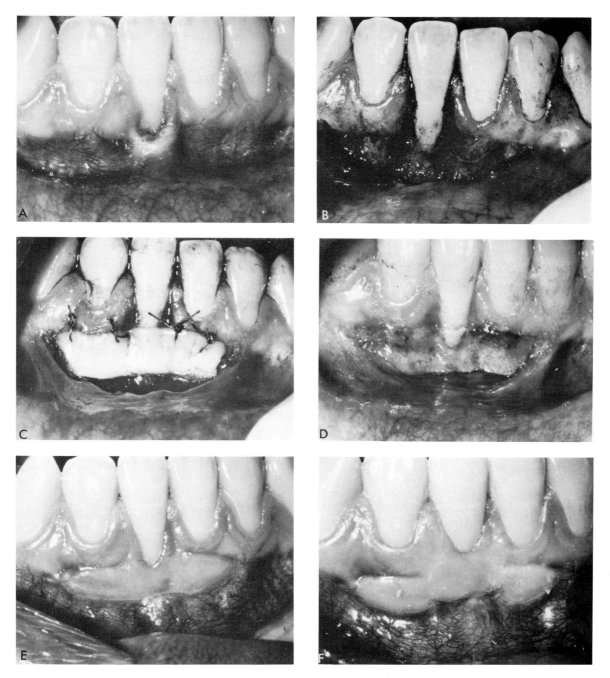

Fig. 25-10. *A,* Gingival inflammation on right mandibular incisor associated with lack of attached gingiva. *B,* Graft bed prepared for free gingival graft. *C,* Free gingival graft from palate sutured in place. In this case the mucogingival flap was not sutured to the periosteum, which is an optional procedure. Achromycin ointment and a periodontal dressing were placed over the graft area. *D,* One week after the surgery. The part of the graft that covered the exposed root surface is partially sloughing off. *E,* Two months after the surgery, the gingival tissues are healthy and there is ample attached gingiva. For esthetic reasons, a coronally repositioned flap procedure was done for the right mandibular incisor (see Fig. 25-11 for details). *F,* One year after the coronally repositioned flap surgery. Good esthetic results and shallow normal gingival crevices.

it is possible to get some root coverage over wide gingival clefts,[56] while thin grafts tend to slough off if the cleft is wider than 1 - 1½ mm.

It has been established that both free gingival grafts and split-thickness, apically repositioned flaps may reduce pocket depth and result in functionally adequate zones of attached gingiva if a preoperative margin of gingiva is present,[34] but with a preoperative margin of alveolar mucosa, free gingival grafts should be used to establish adequate attached gingiva.[35] It appears that a free graft provides a protective function for the underlying connective tissues and bone, and is more likely to prevent recession at the dentogingival margin than is the split-thickness, apically repositioned flap.[34]

Coronally Repositioned Flaps

The first report on coronal repositioning of a gingival flap to cover exposed root surfaces and gain attachment was by Norberg in 1926.[76] He recommended forming a mucoperiosteal flap, removing all granulation tissue from the inside of the flap and the bone, performing no corrective bone surgery, and making a shallow incision through the periosteum on the inside of the flap at its apical extension. The flap is then pulled coronally

to cover the exposed root surfaces and secured by sutures in that position for the healing period. Norberg's description of careful flap management to avoid necrosis and promote healing is classic. Modifications of this procedure were published later.[77,78,79,90] However, the technique never became popular until recently, when it was revived in a new form by Bernimoulin[7] on the basis of a report by Björn about combining free grafts and lateral sliding flaps.[12] The attached gingiva adjacent to gingival recession is often narrow in width, and, especially with multiple gingival recessions, there is often a lack of donor material. Free

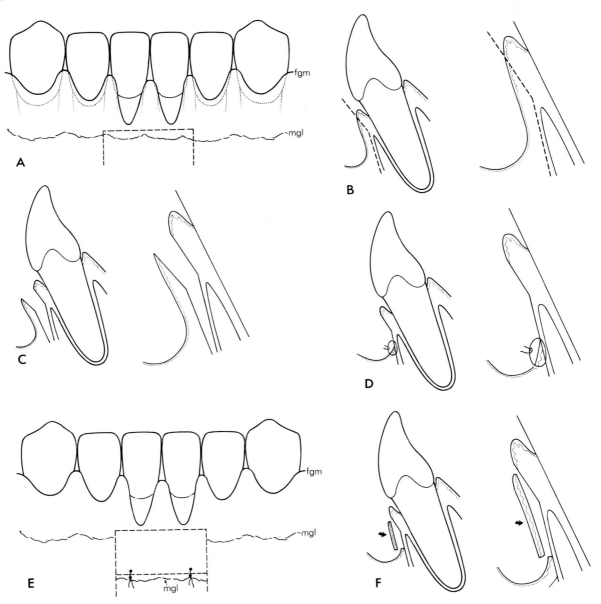

Fig. 25-11. *A-H,* First-stage surgery. *A,* Initial incisions (broken lines) for a two-stage operation to cover denuded root surfaces. *B,* Initial incision (broken lines) from the outer aspect of the free gingival margin to the alveolar crest, and a split-flap dissection on top of the periosteum over the labial aspect of the process. *C,* Raise a split-thickness mucogingival flap, and suture the gingival margin of the flap to the periosteum in an apical position *(D),* leaving a periosteal graft bed as indicated in *E. F,* A free gingival graft from the palate is fitted to the graft bed. *Continued*

gingival grafts can be used as a first-stage operation to establish a wider band of attached gingiva, which can later be moved coronally by a full-thickness flap procedure and an internal periosteal release incision (Fig. 25-11). Excellent results have been reported following this two-stage operation (Fig. 25-12).[8,19]

Healing of Free Gingival Grafts

Numerous studies have been reported on the healing and revascularization of free skin grafts. It is generally agreed that such free grafts are nourished by an avascular "plasmatic" circulation during the first 2

to 3 days following the surgery,[122] and that circulation is later slowly reestablished through formation of blood vessels. Extensive microscopic studies of the healing and revascularization of free gingival grafts have revealed a healing pattern similar to that of skin grafts.[81] The graft is initially separated from the recipient bed by a thin layer of fibrinous exudate with numerous polymorphonuclear cells. Cellular nutrition of the graft is maintained to some extent for the first few days by plasmatic seepage; however, this method of metabolic interchange is not sufficient to nourish the surface epithelium, whose outer layers undergo

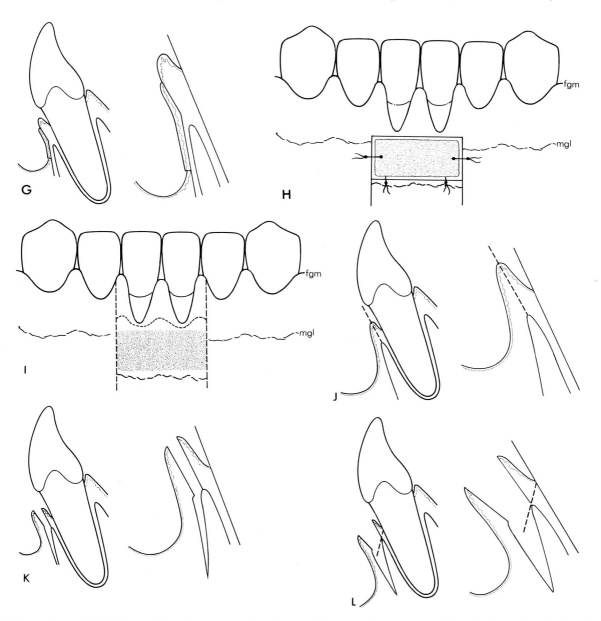

Fig. 26-11 continued. *G,H,* The graft has been sutured in place. *I-O,* Second-stage surgery. *I,* One to 2 months after the first-stage operation, the second stage surgery is initiated with 2 vertical incisions (broken lines). *J,* A second incision is made from the free gingival margin to the alveolar crest. *K,* A full-thickness mucoperiosteal flap is raised. *L,* The remaining free gingiva is excised.

Continued

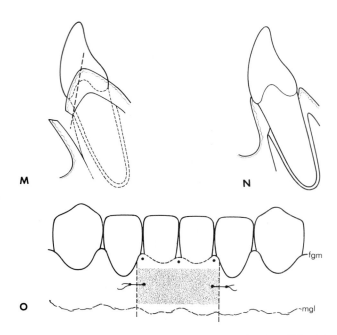

Fig. 25-11. continued *M*, A buccal interproximal graft bed is prepared by excision of the buccal aspect of the interdental papilla. *N*, The entire flap is positioned coronally. *O*, The flap is sutured in a coronal position to cover the previously denuded root surface (*fgm*, free gingival margin; *mgl*, mucogingival line).

degeneration, necrosis, and desquamation during the first 2 to 3 days. A few basal cells, especially in the epithelial ridges, may retain their vitality and later contribute, together with epithelium from the adjacent tissues, to the reepithelization of the graft. A surface layer of new epithelium is present after 4 to 5 days, with rete pegs formed after 7 to 14 days and keratinization after 28 days.[81]

The initial plasmatic circulation is rapidly replaced by a vascular system starting the 3rd or 4th day after the grafting.[81] Anastomoses form between vessels of the graft bed and the preexisting vessels in the graft. Capillary budding from the graft bed into the graft is also a prominent feature of early revascularization. Other studies have described capillary invasion into the graft as early as 2 days following the grafting.[16] By the 14th day, the vasculature has assumed a normal pattern, with a subepithelial plexus and loops extending into the connective tissue papillae between the epithelial ridges.[39,81] The thinner the graft, the faster the healing. Thick grafts have the highest degree of primary shrinkage, with the least secondary contracture during the healing and the best resistance to function. However, thin split-thickness grafts are more assured of "take," because of facilitated plasmatic circulation, and are preferred in spite of their considerable secondary contracture during healing.[107]

Very little osteoclastic activity appears under free grafts, indicating that the grafts protect the bone from extensive resorption. These grafts are therefore indicated for areas with thin labial bony plates.[16] Cementoid has been observed under free grafts after 14 days, with later maturation of cementum and collagen fiber attachment where the grafts cover root surfaces.[82]

In a study of healing, it appeared that the level of attachment to the tooth could be maintained more coronally if free grafts were placed at the bone margin, rather than farther apically.[41] If a free gingival graft is used to cover a denuded root surface, the lateral and apical margins of the graft should extend several millimeters away from the root onto vascular connective tissues. It has been claimed that in order to achieve lasting coverage of a root surface with a free graft, the denuded area has to be less than 3 mm deep and less than 3 mm wide; otherwise, there will not be enough plasmatic and collateral circulation for a "take" of the graft by bridging from the borders.[71] This is not always true.[56]

Although it is always desirable to have the entire recipient bed covered by periosteum, the "take" of grafts usually occurs even if small areas of periosteum are missing, making the graft partially contact denuded bone.[18] Again, revascularization will take place from the connective tissue margins of the periosteal defects or from contact with periodontal membrane.

Clinically, the graft assumes a gray-white appearance the first 2 to 3 days after the transplantation. Then, with the plasmatic circulation and the budding capillaries, the graft becomes edematous and swollen, with a pinkish-gray appearance that gradually changes to a shiny red after 7 to 12 days. Maturation brings a more normal-appearing surface after 3 to 4 weeks, but it may be months before the graft blends well with the adjacent gingiva. Favorable morphological transition between the graft and the surrounding tissues is enhanced by thin borders of the graft and beveled surfaces of the recipient bed.

Free gingival grafts have a very low failure rate if applied over a suitable graft bed. Loss of the graft may occur following failure to stabilize the graft in proper portion, inadequate hemostasis under the graft, or infection. If the graft was placed over mobile tissues, it will not provide attached gingiva, although the surface will be keratinized.

TISSUE SPECIFICITY AND INTERACTION IN MUCOGINGIVAL SURGERY

It has been assumed that the functional stimuli of the oral environment determine the characteristics of the attached gingiva during wound healing, with friction associated with mastication and toothbrushing being the most important stimuli to both keratinization and type of gingival connective tissues. The movement pattern imposed on the healing tissues by the

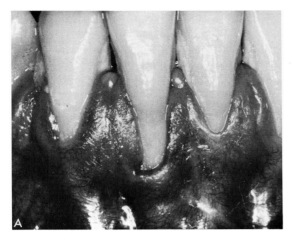

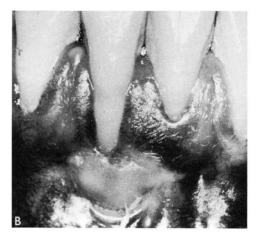

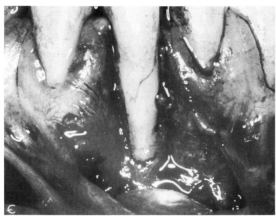

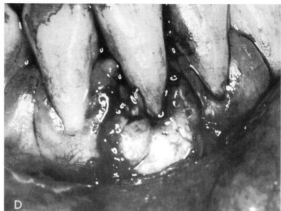

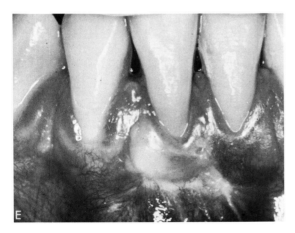

Fig. 25-12. *A,* Lack of attached gingiva. *B,* One month after a free gingival graft had been placed apically to the gingival recession. *C,* A pedicle flap is raised, including the healed free gingival graft. *D,* The pedicle flap is positioned coronally and sutured in place. *E,* Six months after the coronally repositioned flap procedure. Good esthetic and functional result, with healthy gingiva and shallow gingival crevices.

musculature has also been considered an important factor in determining the mucogingival demarcation.

In opposition to this functional hypothesis is the more recent concept that the type of gingival epithe-

lium that develops over a gingival wound is genetically determined by the type of underlying connective tissue. A number of studies have been done to determine whether functional adaptation of surface characteristics will occur in tissues that have been heterotopically transplanted. Smith, experimenting in dogs, moved gingival pedicle flaps into the mobile tissues of the alveolar mucosa or rotated mucosal flaps into an area with attached gingival base.[98,99] He found that after 12 months the transplanted flaps maintained their original morphological characteristics, except that a collar of attached gingiva formed around the neck of the teeth contacted by the alveolar mucosal graft.

His results were confirmed in a similar study in monkeys whose alveolar mucosa was transplanted heterotopically onto connective tissue of the attached gingiva.[60] A split-thickness gingival flap was transplanted onto a bed of connective tissue of the alveolar mucosa. The transplanted tissues maintained their original characteristics, even after observations for up to 1 year. The gingival graft placed on the movable base of the previous alveolar mucosa still displayed a high degree of keratinization and contained neither PAS-positive tissue nor elastic fibers, while the alveolar mucosal flap grafted over attached gingival base had numerous elastic fibers, PAS-positive epithelium, and no surface keratinization. Adjacent to the teeth contacted by the transplanted alveolar mucosa, a collar of new attached gingiva had developed, probably originating from the periodontal membrane. The concept that connective tissue determines the type of surface epithelium was developed further by transplants of free gingival connective tissue grafts into subepithelial pouches in the alveolar mucosa.[61] When these implanted grafts were unroofed after healing, the free gingival connective tissue grafts became covered by keratinized epithelium and assumed the characteristics of attached gingiva. Another report shows that free connective tissue grafts from the palate may be used routinely to increase the width of keratinized attached gingiva in humans.[30] Subepithelial strips of connective tissue have also been used for free gingival grafts to cover areas of gingival recession, with good results.[66]

The importance of the origin of the reparative granulation tissue in determining the type of regenerating gingival epithelium has also been shown experimentally,[62] and serves to emphasize further the genetic determinant in formation of attached gingiva. A change in the location of the mucogingival junction requires a change of the connective tissue underlying the epithelium.[51] Thus, it appears that if an increase in attached gingiva is sought, gingival connective tissue has to be transplanted to the area or to be provided through proliferation from the periodontal membrane. The latter is an impractical approach, because either it will provide a narrow band of gingiva at the neck of the teeth, or denuded thin bone will have to be lost through severe necrosis and new connective tissue will have to be formed from the underlying periodontal membrane[37] to gain a wide zone of attached gingiva. With pedicle flaps and free gingival grafts, connective tissue that is genetically associated with keratinized gingiva is transplanted directly to the site at which attached gingiva is desired, thus providing the most predictable and lasting solution to mucogingival problems.

DETERMINATION OF NEED AND SELECTION OF TECHNIQUES FOR MUCOGINGIVAL SURGERY

Mucogingival defects may be related developmentally to an abnormal frenum attachment, malposition of teeth, or a shallow vestibule. They may also be the result of periodontal disease, gingival atrophy, or periodontal treatment. Regardless of origin, the need for surgical treatment should be based on whether gingival health can be maintained following the hygienic phase of the periodontal therapy, or whether the desired pocket therapy and restorative dentistry can be implemented without complete loss of attached gingiva. The need for mucogingival surgery should not be based on measurements of the width of the attached gingiva or on tests of gingival response to pull on the

patient's lip or cheek. If a patient is able to keep a gingival area free from inflammation, the need for mucogingival surgery is highly questionable from a future health standpoint, regardless of any anatomical aberration that may be present. However, esthetic requirements may justify the surgery beyond strict considerations of health.

Because denudation or split thickness vestibular extension surgery, as well as periosteal fenestration, result in eventual loss of what originally appeared to be gain in attached gingiva, and because of the postsurgical sequelae of pain, bone resorption, and scarring, those procedures should be avoided. Because heterotopically transplanted tissues maintain their genetically determined specificity even if transplanted to a different environment, it seems that tissues to be transplanted should have the characteristics that are desired postsurgically.

When gain of attachment is sought, the most predictable methods are coronally or laterally repositioned flaps of various forms and free gingival grafts. The lateral sliding or coronally positioned flap is the best solution to isolated areas of gingival recession or defects, while free gingival grafts offer the best solution to a narrow zone or an area completely lacking attached gingiva or a shallow vestibule. Free gingival grafts work well for establishment of attached gingiva in areas with little or no attached gingiva prior to the surgery; as, for example, distobuccally to the second or third mandibular molar or buccally to mandibular cuspids and bicuspids with general gingival recession.

If coverage and attachment to denuded root surfaces is desired, the success is to a great extent dependent on a good blood supply to the grafted tissues. The first choice is a coronally positioned flap following a free gingival graft,[8] since this will not affect the neighboring teeth. In some instances, the free gingival graft may also provide coverage of the denuded root surface.[56]

It has been recommended to use free gingival grafts for children prior to orthodontics in the mandibular anterior region.[68] This should not be done, because the band of attached gingiva will increase in width when the teeth are moved on the alveolar ridge.[28]

REFERENCES

1. Ainamo, J., and Talari, A.: The increase with age of the width of the attached gingiva, J. Periodont. Res. 11:182, 1976.
2. Ariaudo, A.: Problems in treating a denuded labial root surface of lower incisor, J. Periodont. 37:274, 1966.
3. Becker, N.: A free gingival graft utilizing a presuturing technique, Periodontics 5:194, 1967.
4. Bergenholtz, A., and Hugoson, A.: Vestibular extension surgery in cases with periodontal disease, J. Periodont. Res. 2:221, 1967.
5. Bergenholtz, A., and Hugoson, A.: Vestibular sulcus extension surgery in the mandibular front region. The Edlan-Mejchar method. A five year follow-up study, J. Periodont. 44:309, 1973.

6. Bernimoulin, J.P., Son, S., Regolati, B.: Biometric comparison of three methods for determining the mucogingival junction, Helv. Odont. Acta 15:118, 1971.

7. Bernimoulin, J.P.: Deckung gingivaler Rezessionen mit koronaler Verschiebungs-plastik, Dtsch. Zahnarztl. Ztschr. 28:1222, 1973.

8. Bernimoulin, J.P., Luscher, B., and Mühlemann, H.R.: Coronally repositioned periodontal flap, J. Clin. Periodontol. 2:1, 1975.

9. Bessman, E., and Chasens, A.: Free gingival graft with periosteal fenestration, J. Periodont. 39:298, 1968.

10. Bhaskar, S.N., et al.: Full and partial thickness pedicle grafts in miniature swine and man, J. Periodont. 42:66, 1971.

11. Björn, H.: Fri transplantation av gingiva propria, Sven. Tandlak. Forb. Tidskr. 55:684, 1963.

12. Björn, H.: Coverage of denuded root surfaces with a lateral sliding flap. Use of free gingival grafts, Odont. Revy. 22:37, 1971.

13. Bohannan, H.M.: Studies in the alteration of vestibular depth. I. Complete denudation, J. Periodont. 33:120, 1962.

14. Bohannan, H.M.: Studies in the alteration of vestibular depth. II. Periosteum retention, J. Periodont. 33:354, 1962.

15. Bohannan, H.M.: Studies in the alteration of vestibular depth. III. Vestibular incision, J. Periodont. 34:209, 1963.

16. Brackett, R.C., and Gargiulo, A.W.: Free gingival grafts in humans, J. Periodont. 41:581, 1970.

17. Bradley, R.E., Grant, J.C., and Ivancie, G.P.: Histologic evaluation of mucogingival surgery, Oral Surg. 12:1184, 1959.

18. Caffesse, R.G., et al.: Healing of free gingival grafts with and without periosteum. Part I: Histologic evaluation, J. Periodontol. 50:586, 1979.

19. Caffesse, R.G., and Guinard, E.A.: Treatment of localized gingival recession. Part IV: Results after 3 years, J. Periodont. 51:167, 1980.

20. Carranza, F.A., and Carraro, J.J.: Mucogingival techniques in periodontal surgery, J. Periodont. 41:294, 1970.

21. Carraro, J.J., et al.: Effect of bone denudation in mucogingival surgery, J. Periodont. 35:463, 1964.

22. Cohen, W.D., and Ross, S.E.: The double papillae flap in periodontal therapy, J. Periodont. 39:65, 1968.

23. Corn, H.: Periosteal separation. Its clinical significance, J. Periodont. 33:140, 1962.

24. Corn, H.: Edentulous area pedicle grafts in mucogingival surgery, Periodontics 2:229, 1964.

25. Costich, E.R., and Ramfjord, S.P.: Healing after partial denudation of the alveolar process, J. Periodont. 39:127, 1968.

26. Cowan, A.: Sulcus deepening incorporating mucosal graft, J. Periodont. 36:188, 1965.

27. Diedrich, P., Jacoby, L., and Aba, F.: Untersuchungen ueber die Breite der Gingiva propria nach Vestibulumplastik mit und ohne Periostfenstrung, Dtsch. Zahnarztl. Ztschr. 27:346, 1972.

28. Dorfman, H.: Mucogingival changes resulting from mandibular incisor tooth movements, Am. J. Orthod. 74:286, 1978.

29. Dorfman, H.S., et al.: Longitudinal evaluation of free autogenous gingival grafts, J. Periodontol. 7:316, 1980.

30. Edel, A.: Clinical evaluation of free connective tissue grafts used to increase the width of keratinized gingiva, J. Clin. Periodontol. 1:185, 1974.

31. Edlan, A., and Mejchar, B.: Paradontologische indizierte Vertiefung des unteren Mundvorhofes, Parodontologie 18:87, 1964.

32. Espinal, M.C., and Caffesse, R.G.: Comparisons of the results obtained with the laterally positioned pellicle sliding flap. Revised technique and the laterally sliding flap with a free gingival graft technique in the treatment of localized gingival recession, Int. J. Periodont. and Rest. Dent. 1:31, 1981.

33. Elliott, J.R., and Bowers, G.M.: Alveolar dehiscence and fenestration, Periodontics 1:245, 1963.

34. Fagan, F., and Freeman, E.: Clinical comparison of the free gingival graft and partial thickness apically positioned flap, J. Periodont. 45:3, 1974.

35. Fagan, F.: Clinical comparison of the free soft tissue autograft and partial thickness apically positioned flap—preoperative gingival and mucosal margins, J. Periodont. 46:586, 1975.

36. Fasske, E., and Morgentroth, H.: Comparative stomatoscopic and histochemical studies of the marginal gingiva in man, Parodontologie 12:151, 1958.

37. Friedman, N.: Mucogingival surgery, Texas Dent. J. 75:358, 1957.

38. Friedman, N., and Levine, L.: Mucogingival surgery, Dent. Clin. N. Am. March 1964.

39. Gargiulo, A.W., and Arrocha, R.: Histoclinical evaluation of free gingival grafts, Periodontics 5:285, 1967.

40. Glickman, I., et al.: Healing of the periodontum following mucogingival surgery, Oral Surg. 16:580, 1963.

41. Glickman, I., et al.: Healing of apically positioned mucosal flaps and free gingival grafts, I.A.D.R. Abstract No. 468, 1971.

42. Goldman, H., Schluger, S., and Fox, L.: Periodontal Therapy, St. Louis, C.V. Mosby Co., 1956.

43. Gordon, H.P., Sullivan, H.C., and Atkins, J.C.: Free autogenous gingival grafts. II. Supplemental findings—histology of the graft site, Periodontics 6:130, 1968.

44. Gorney, H., Gorney, A., and Forman, S.: Creation of a mandibular ridge by deepening the labial sulcus and lining it with a skin graft, J.A.D.A. 29:751, 1942.

45. Gottsegen, R.: Frenum position and vestibule depth in relation to gingival health, Oral Surg. 7:1069, 1954.

46. Grant, J.: A histological study of repositioning the attached gingiva in periodontal therapy, Iowa Dent. J. 44:62, 1958.

47. Grupe, J.E., and Warren, R.F.: Repair of gingival defects by a sliding flap operation, J. Periodont. 27:92, 1956.

48. Grupe, J.E.: Modified technique for the sliding flap operation, J. Periodont. 37:491, 1966.

49. Hall, W.B.: Pure Mucogingival Problems, Chicago: Quintessence Publ. Co., 1984.

50. Hattler, A.: Mucogingival surgery: Utilization of interdental gingiva as attached gingiva by surgical displacement, Periodontics 5:126, 1967.

51. Heaney, T.G.: A reappraisal of environment, function, and gingival specificity, J. Periodont. 45:695, 1974.

52. Hiatt, W.: Regeneration via flap operation and the pulpal periodontal lesion, Periodontics 4:205, 1966.

53. Hileman, A.: Surgical repositioning of vestibule and frenums in periodontal disease, J.A.D.A. 55:676, 1957.

54. Hilming, F.: Om Betydningen av höjt insererende ligamenter i de marginaler paradentale lidelsers klinik, Odont. Tidskr. 50:602, 1942.

55. Hilming, F., and Jervoe, P.: Surgical extension of vestibular depth. On the results in various regions of the mouth in periodontal patients, Tandlaegebladet 74:329, 1970.

56. Holbrook, T., and Ochsenbein, C.: Complete coverage of the denuded root surface with a one-stage gingival graft, Int. J. Periodont. and Rest. Dent. 3:8, 1983.

57. Hughes, T.P.: Changes in the gingiva following scaling and root planing: A biometric evaluation. Thesis, University of Michigan, 1975.

58. Ibatt, C., et al.: Effects of citric acid treatment on autogenous free graft coverage of localized recession, J. Periodontol. 56:662, 1985.

59. Kalmi, J., Moscor, M., and Goranov, Z.: The solution of the aesthetic problem in the treatment of periodontal disease of anterior teeth: Gingivoplastic operation, Parodontologie 3:53, 1949.

60. Karring, T., Östergaard, E., and Löe, H.: Conservation of tissue specificity after heterotopic transplantation of gingiva and alveolar mucosa, J. Periodont. Res. 6:282, 1971.

61. Karring, T., Lang, N.P., and Löe, H.: The role of gingival connective tissue in determining epithelial differentiation, J. Periodont. Res. 10:1, 1974.

62. Karring, T., et al.: The origin of granulation tissue and its impact on postoperative results of mucogingival surgery, J. Periodont. 46:577, 1975.

63. Kazanjian, V.H.: Surgical operations as related to satisfactory dentures, Dent. Cosmos 66:387, 1924.

64. Kazanjian, V.: Surgery as an aid to more efficient service with prosthetic dentures, J.A.D.A. 22:566, 1935.

65. Lang, N.P., and Löe, H.: The relationship between the width of keratinized gingiva and gingival health, J. Periodont. 43:623, 1972.

66. Langer, B., and Langer, L.: Subepithelial connective tissue grafts technique for root coverage, J. Periodontol. 56:715, 1985.

67. Listgarten, M.A.: In Periodontal Surgery. Biologic Basis and Technique, ed. S.S. Stahl. Springfield, Il., Charles C. Thomas, 1976.

68. Maynard, J.C., and Ochsenbein, C.: Mucogingival problems, prevalence and therapy, J. Periodont. 46:543, 1975.

69. McFall, W.T.: Laterally repositioned flap. Criteria for success in periodontics, Periodontics 5:89, 1968.

70. Miller, P.D.: Root coverage using a free soft tissue autograft following citric acid application. Part I: Technique, Int. J. Periodont. and Rest. Dent. 2:65, 1982.

71. Milnek, A., Smukler, H., and Buchner, A.: The use of free gingival grafts for the coverage of denuded roots, J. Periodont. 44:249, 1973.

72. Nabers, C.L.: Repositioning of the attached gingiva, J. Periodont. 24:38, 1954.

73. Nabers, C.: When is gingival repositioning an indicated procedure? J. West. Soc. Periodont. 5:92, 1957.

74. Nabers, J.M.: Extension of the gingival fornix utilizing a gingival graft. Case history, Periodontics 4:77, 1966.

75. Nabers, J.M.: Free gingival grafts, Periodontics 4:243, 1966.

76. Norberg, O.: Är en utlakning utav vevnadsforlust otankbar vid kirurgisk behandling av. s. k. alveolar-pyorrhoe, Sven. Tandlak. Tidskr. 19:171, 1926.

77. Norberg, O.: Biologi och terapi i det marginala paradentiets sjukdomskomplex, Sven. Tandlak. Tidskr. 34:32, 1941.

78. Nordenram, A.: Parodontalkirurgisk rekonstruksjon av gingivalränder efter partiell gingivektomi i samma seans, Sven. Tandlak. Tidskr. 52:373, 1959.

79. Nordenram, A., and Landt, H.: Evaluation of a surgical technique in the periodontal treatment of maxillary anterior teeth, Acta Odont. Scand. 27:283, 1969.

80. Ochsenbein, C.: Newer concepts of mucogingival surgery, J. Periodont. 31:175, 1960.

81. Oliver, R.C., Löe, H., and Karring, T.: Microscopic evaluation of the healing and revascularization of free gingival grafts, J. Periodont. Res. 3:84, 1968.

82. Oliver, R.C., and Woofter, C.: Healing and revascularization of free mucosal grafts over roots, I.A.D.R. Abstract No. 469, 1971.

83. Patur, B., and Glickman, I.: Gingival pedicle flaps for covering root surfaces denuded by chronic destructive periodontal disease: A clinical experiment, J. Periodont. 29:50, 1958.

84. Pennel, B.M., et al.: Free masticatory mucosa graft, J. Periodont. 40:162, 1969.

85. Pfeifer, J.S., and Heller, R.: Histologic evaluation of full and partial thickness lateral repositioned flaps: A pilot study, J. Periodont. 42:331, 1971.

86. Pichler, H., and Trauner, R.: Die Alveolarkammplastik, Oesterr, Z. f. Stomat. 28:675, 1930.

87. Prichard, J.: Advanced Periodontal Disease, 2nd ed., Philadelphia, W.B. Saunders Co., 1972.

88. Propper, R.: Simplified ridge extension using free mucosal grafts, J. Oral Surg. 22:469, 1964.

89. Ramfjord, S.P., and Costich, E.R.: Healing after exposure of periosteum on the alveolar process, J. Periodont. 39:199, 1968.

90. Restrepo, O.J.: Coronally repositioned flap: Report of five cases, J. Periodont. 44:564, 1973.

91. Reuben, M.P., Goldman, H.M., and Janson, W.: Biological considerations fundamental to successful employment of laterally repositioned flaps and free autogenous gingival grafts in periodontal therapy. In Periodontal Surgery. Biological Basis and Technique, ed. S.S. Stahl. Springfield, Il., Charles C. Thomas, 1976.

92. Robinson, R.E.: Mucogingival junction surgery, J. Calif. State Dent. Ass. 33:379, 1957.

93. Robinson, R.E.: Periosteal fenestration in mucogingival surgery, J. West. Soc. Periodont. 9:107, 1961.

94. Robinson, R.E., and Agnew, R.G.: Periosteal fenestration at the mucogingival line, J. Periodont. 34:503, 1963.

95. Robinson, R.E.: Utilizing an edentulous area as a donor site in laterally repositioned flap, Periodontics 2:79, 1964.

96. Rosenberg, M.M.: Vestibular alterations in periodontics, J. Periodont. 31:231, 1960.

97. Sicher, H., and Bhaskar, S.M., eds.: Orban's Oral Histology and Embryology, 7th ed., St. Louis, C.V. Mosby Co., 1972.

98. Smith, R.M.: A study of the intertransplantation of gingiva, Oral Surg. 29:169, 1970.

99. Smith, R.M.: A study of intertransplantation of alveolar mucosa, Oral Surg. 29:328, 1970.

100. Snyder, A.J.: A technique for free autogenous gingival grafts, J. Periodont. 40:702, 1969.

101. Soehren, S.E., et al.: Clinical and histologic studies of donor tissues utilized for free grafts of masticatory mucosa, J. Periodont. 44:727, 1973.

102. Spirgi, M., Corti, M., and Held, A.J.: Les Vestibuloplasties dans la proplylaxie et la therapeutique des paradontolyses, Schweiz Mschr. Zahnk. 73:678, 1963.

103. Staffileno, H., Wentz, F., and Orban, B.: Histologic study of healing of split thickness flap surgery in dogs, J. Periodont. 33:56, 1962.

104. Staffileno, H.: Management of gingival recession and root exposure problems associated with periodontal disease, Dent. Clin. N. Am. p. 113, March 1964.

105. Stewart, J.: Reattachment of vestibular mucosa as an aid in periodontal treatment, J.A.D.A. 49:283, 1954.

106. Sugarman, E.F.: Clinical and histological study of the attachment of grafted tissue to bone and teeth, J. Periodont. 40:381, 1969.

107. Sullivan, H.C., and Atkins, J.H.: Free autogenous gingival grafts. I. Principles of successful grafting, Periodontics 6:5, 121, 1968.

108. Sullivan, H.C., and Atkins, J.H.: The role of free gingival grafts in periodontal therapy, Dent. Clin. N. Am. 13:133, 1969.

109. Sullivan, H., Dinner, D., and Carman, D.: Clinical evaluation of the laterally positioned flap, I.A.D.R. Abstract No. 466, 1971.

110. Sullivan, H., Dinner, D., and Carman, D.: Histological evaluation of the laterally positioned flap, I.A.D.R. Abstract No. 467, 1971.

111. Summer, C.F.: Surgical repair of recession on the maxillary cuspid: Incisally repositioning the gingival tissues, J. Periodont. 40:119, 1969.

112. Thiersch, K.: Ueber die feineren anatomischen Verankerungen bei Aufheilung von Haut auf Ganulationen, Arch. f. Klin. Chir. 17:318, 1874.

113. Tisot, R.J., and Sullivan, H.C.: Evaluation of survival of partial thickness and full-thickness flaps, I.A.D.R. Abstract No. 470, 1971.

114. Vander Voorde, H.E.: Gingival grafting and gingival repositioning, J. Am. Dent. Assoc. 79:1415, 1969.

115. Wade, B.A.: Vestibular deepening by the technique of Edlan and Mejchar, J. Periodont. Res. 4:307, 1969.

116. Waerhaug, J.: Review of Cohen. "Role of Periodontal Surgery", J. Dent. Res. 50:219, 1971.

117. Wennström, J., et al.: Role of keratinized gingiva for gingival health. Clinical and histologic study of normal and regenerated gingival tissues in dogs, J. Clin. Periodontol. 8:311, 1981.

118. Whinston, G.J.: The frenotomy and mucobuccal fold resection utilized in periodontal therapy, N.Y. Dent. J. 22:495, 1956.

119. Wilderman, M.N., Wentz, F.M., and Orban, B.J.: Histogenesis of repair after mucogingival surgery, J. Periodont. 31:283, 1961.

120. Wilderman, M., and Wentz, F.: Repair of a dento-gingival defect with a pedicle graft, J. Periodont. 26:218, 1965.

121. Wood, D., et al.: Alveolar crest reduction following full and partial thickness flaps, J. Periodont. 43:141, 1972.

122. Woodruff, M.: The Transplantation of Tissues and Organs, Springfield, Il., Charles C. Thomas, 1966.

26

TREATMENT OF INTRABONY POCKETS AND FURCATION INVOLVEMENT: BONE IMPLANTS

Although intrabony pockets and pockets extending into furcations have similar pathologic and histomorphologic features, approaches to management of these lesions may differ considerably. The approaches will be discussed individually here.

INTRABONY POCKETS

If a periodontal pocket extends apically to the adjacent alveolar crest, the pocket is referred to as an *intra-* or *infrabony pocket*[65] or *lesion,* while pockets whose bottoms are situated coronally to the adjacent alveolar crest are called *suprabony pockets* or simply *pockets.* In this book, no distinction is made between intra- and infrabony pockets. Following the suggestion of Goldman and Cohen,[30] intrabony pockets are often classified according to the number of bony walls associated with the pocket. For instance, a pocket that has bone in its mesial wall, but no bone in its buccal or lingual aspect, is called a *one bony wall pocket.* A pocket with a mesial bony wall and a lingual bony wall but no buccal bony wall is called a *two bony wall pocket,* and a pocket with mesial, buccal, and lingual bony walls is called a *three bony wall pocket.* Although this classification does not have any biologic or pathologic significance, it may have bearing on treatment modality and prognosis. The etiology and chronicity of the pockets may also affect the management. Pockets that developed as the result of an acute periodontal abscess or a pulpal infection draining through the periodontal membrane should be treated differently from, and have a much better prognosis than, pockets that developed slowly over a long period of time.

It also appears that the more closely the bony walls of the pockets are situated to the tooth, the better is the prognosis for reattachment and regeneration of the lost bone.

Principal Approaches to Therapy

As with other periodontal pockets, intrabony pockets may be treated by surgical eradication or by reattachment therapy followed by various degrees of bone regeneration. A third approach may be eliminating the pocket as a pathologic lesion, with subsequent epithelial reattachment and close epithelial adaptation to the clean, scraped tooth surface, but leaving a residual anatomical defect that may be partially penetrated by a thin periodontal probe.

Surgical elimination of intrabony pockets

Surgical elimination of intrabony pockets will always require bone surgery. The surgery will usually be of the osteoectomy type, involving removal of functional periodontal support both for the tooth with the intrabony pocket and for some adjacent teeth. In a few instances in which the intrabony pocket has one bony wall related to an edentulous ridge, the intrabony pocket can be eradicated by osteoplasty only.

Various types of intrabony pockets may be eliminated by routine periodontal flap procedures and bone surgery, as outlined in chapter 23. However, surgical elimination usually requires a considerable amount of both ostectomy and osteoplasty to establish an acceptable contour level in relation to the bottom of the intrabony lesion. In some instances, this leveling of contour would lead to exposure of previously unexposed furcations and cause considerable reduction of valuable periodontal support both for the involved tooth and for the adjacent teeth. Such sacrifice of periodontal support in hopes of a good prognosis cannot be recommended, since longitudinal studies show excellent results without surgical bone reduction.[67,68] In some instances, as with intrabony palatal pockets of maxillary bicuspids in patients with low palatal vaults, such pockets cannot be eradicated with bone surgery for anatomical reasons, and there is a marked tendency for return of previous gingival height and pocket depth if flattening of the palatal contour is attempted.[40]

Even authors who recommend surgical elimination of intrabony pockets[32,65] usually apply the elimination procedures only to one and two bony wall pockets and do not attempt to eliminate three bony wall pockets surgically. In cases of pockets having one or two bony walls at the coronal opening and three bony walls at the bottom, leveling the bone involved in the one and two bony wall part of the pockets and leaving the three bony wall defect to granulate following removal of the soft tissues in this area has been recommended,[29,65] but does not seem to be advisable.[73]

Reattachment or readaptation therapy

As pointed out in chapters 21 and 24, intrabony pockets, especially of the three bony wall type, provide the best opportunity for regaining lost periodontal attachment and bone. The technical procedures and biological principles of reattachment therapy have been described in these two chapters, and also in chapter 25 ("Mucogingival Surgery"). Of special importance to the success of reattachment or readaptation therapy of intrabony lesions is very close adaptation of the incised soft tissues to a clean tooth surface.

Following curettage or flap surgery, small pedicle-type gingival flaps may be used as a supplement to the regular reverse bevel flap procedure. To ensure close marginal adaptation with an edentulous ridge bordering an intrabony pocket (Fig. 26-1), it is often

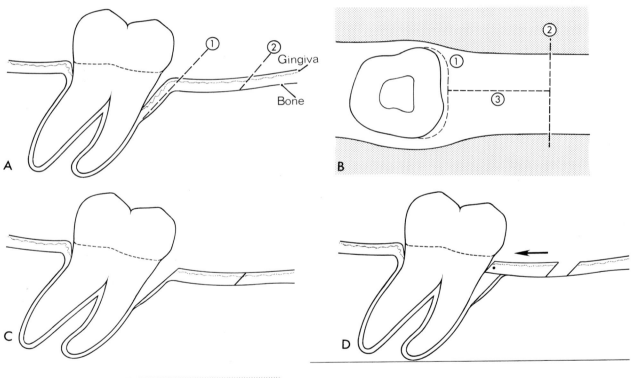

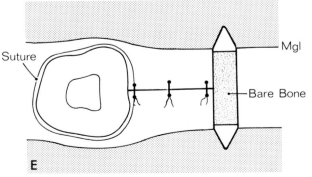

Fig. 26-1. *A,* Excise the soft tissue lining of the infrabony pocket *(1).* Remove the excised tissues with a curette, and plane the exposed tooth surface. Make a slanted incision *(2)* across the alveolar ridge and into the alveolar mucosa about 3 mm mesially to the first incision. *B,* Make a vertical incision on the top of the ridge *(3),* and raise the buccal and lingual mucoperiosteal flaps extending into the alveolar mucosa. *C,* The flaps are sutured together. *D,* The flaps are pulled distally and tied to the tooth with a suture going around the tooth. *E,* The flaps are sutured in place and some bare bone is left over the alveolar crest. The entire area of the surgery is covered by a dressing (*mgl,* mucogingival line). This is a modification of a procedure first described by Hiatt (*Periodontics* **5:**132, 1967).

advisable to release pedicle flaps by a buccolingual incision 2 to 3 mm away from the pocket. These pedicle flaps can be sutured close to the tooth. This procedure may leave a small portion of bone exposed on the edentulous ridge, which will heal with no loss of support for the teeth.

Emphasis has been placed on complete removal of soft tissue coverage of the bone in the intrabony lesions,[32] but the value of such procedures has not been established. However, by common usage, the soft tissue covering the bone in an intrabony lesion usually is removed. However, there does not seem to be much justification for curettage of the bony surfaces or for "stirring up" the bone by the use of burs to penetrate the surface layer of the bone.

Subgingival curettage or the Widman type of reverse bevel flap surgery is recommended as the treatment of choice for most chronic intrabony pockets. Treatment of intrabony pockets associated with periodontal abscesses has been discussed in chapter 15 as part of emergency treatment. Abscesses, however, may be an extension of old chronic pockets, and after allowing 4 to 6 weeks of healing time for the abscess, the remaining part of the pocket may require further surgical therapy.

Much emphasis has been placed on roentgenographic or reentry evidence of bone regeneration as a requisite to proving success in treating intrabony lesions.[65] Unquestionably, regaining lost bone support is the most desirable end result of all periodontal therapy. However, in recent years it has been documented

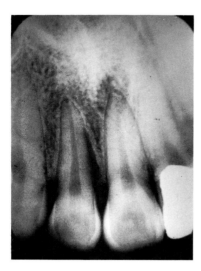

Fig. 26-2. Residual widening of the periodontal space on the mesial side of the lateral incisor. The tooth had a very deep periodontal pocket that was treated with subgingival curettage 3 years prior to this roentgenogram. Probing did not reveal any pocket at the time, and reexamination over a period of 6 years never showed a reopening of the pocket. Note the well-defined lamina dura bordering the anatomical defect in the alveolar bone, indicating that the defect is inactive pathologically.

that teeth may be maintained in a state of health and good function, without further loss of periodontal support, even when the intrabony lesions have not been filled in by new bone functionally attached to the adjacent tooth surfaces.[68] Thus, periodontal treatment of intrabony lesions may be successful even when bone did not regenerate to fill the defects (Fig. 26-2).

A gradual regeneration of bone over 2 years following the modified Widman flap procedure has been reported in patients with intrabony lesions.[73] Thus, the postsurgical presence of a residual defect that can be penetrated by a thin periodontal probe along the root surface, without bleeding and without exudate, should not be interpreted as an indication of failure or need for further pocket elimination procedures. In such treated intrabony lesions, there may be a long thin epithelial attachment between the tooth and the regenerated bone,[11] and the "fill in" of bone may occur over several years.

Bone and other implants

Bone grafting has been used for almost 100 years in attempts to stimulate healing of bony defects.[48,86] The first attempt to rebuild bone loss by periodontal disease through implants was reported by Hegedus in 1923.[36] He initially used bone from the alveolar process, but later he transplanted bone from the tibia over the alveolar process to areas that had been reduced in height by periodontal disease. He used Neumann's flap procedure (see chapter 23) and emphasized proper coverage of the graft by the flap. He also warned against stretching the flap too much during the suturing. No further reports on this procedure appeared.

Materials such as plaster of Paris,[58] heterogenous bone powder,[4,5] and other bone preparations[60] were also tried for implantation into intrabony periodontal defects during the 1930's. They supposedly had some success,[2,3] although this has not been well documented.

Bone implants, like other tissue grafts, may be classified according to the donor source; *autogenous* grafts indicate that both donor and recipient are the same individual; *isografts* refer to donors and recipients that are either identical twins or animals belonging to the same breed strain; *homogenous* grafts, or *allografts*, indicate that the donor and the recipient are different individuals within the same species; and *heterogenous* grafts, or *xenografts*, indicate that the donor and the recipient are of different species. Implantation materials of crystalline or biodegradable substances other than bone are also considered xenografts.

When bone transplantation is done between immunocompetent individuals with genetic differences, the grafted tissue will normally be rejected within about 2 weeks by an immunological mechanism that

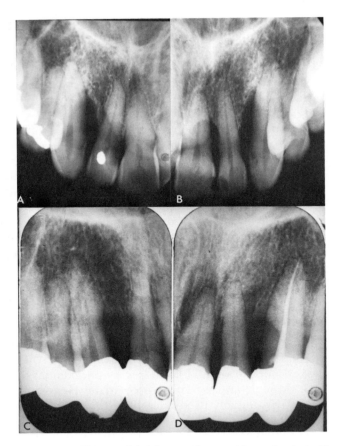

Fig. 26-3. *A,* This mesial defect on the cuspid was treated with flap surgery and autogenous osseous implant. *B,* Similar defects on the cuspid and the central incisor in the same patient were treated with modified Widman flap surgery without an implant. *C,D,* Roentgenograms 2 years after treatment. Note that the intrabony defects have been eliminated. The roentgenograms in *C* and *D* show equally good "fill in" of bone in the treated areas.

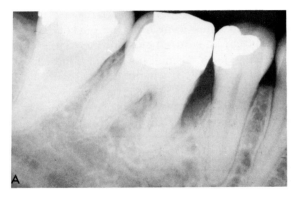

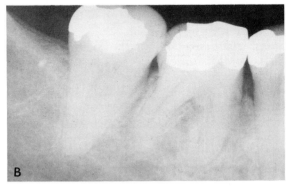

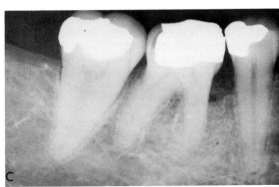

Fig. 26-4. *A,* Intrabony defects before treatment. *B,* One week after bony implant. The implanted bone fills the defect. *C,* One year later. The implanted bone has been resorbed and partially replaced by new bone. Note the well-defined alveolar crest over the treated interproximal area.

depends upon the antigenic differences between the donor and the host.[6] The principal mechanism of this immunological rejection is a cell-mediated immune reaction. Sensitized lymphocytes are found in the lymph nodes, which drain the graft site within 6 to 10 days after grafting. At the time of the first clinical signs of graft rejection at 10 to 14 days postoperatively, an increasing number of sensitized lymphocytes appear as mediators of allograft rejections and infiltrating the graft bed. Destruction of the allograft is due to vascular damage, which leads to thrombosis. However, the precise manner in which vascular injuries are produced is still a controversial subject. Although allograft rejection may be prevented or minimized by the administration of antimetabolites, adrenal corticosteroids, or antilymphocytic serum, such therapy appears much too risky for the patient's general health and therefore impractical in periodontics.

Unfavorable immunological reactions can be avoided if grafting is performed within the same in-

dividual (autografts) or between genetically identical individuals (isografts). Therefore, autografts are often used in periodontics.[13,33,34,39,53,54,72,75] Most free bony autografts are obtained from edentulous areas,[13,28,39,72] mandibular retromolar regions,[71,72] maxillary tuberosities,[39] or recent extraction sites.[34] Chips from osteoplasty or ostectomy have also been used.[53,54] Cancellous bone generally is preferred as graft material because its numerous marrow spaces make vascularization and acceptance easier and more predictable.[71,72] However, cortical bone may be used if it is applied in small chips to reduce the chance of sequestration.[53,54]

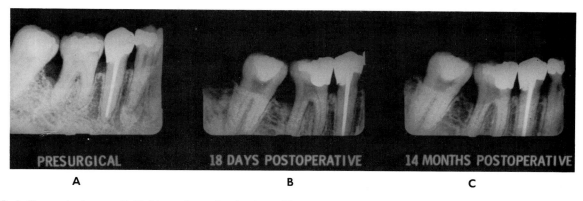

Fig. 26-5. *A,* Presurgical x-ray. *B,* Eighteen days after implant of bone in distal defect of first molar. *C,* Fourteen months later, there is evidence of partial regeneration of the lost bone, but this does not fill the entire intrabony lesion shown in the initial presurgical roentgenogram.

Some investigators prefer to remove the cortical plate and use only cancellous bone for grafts onto the intrabony periodontal lesions.[71,72] It has been claimed that the osteoid tissues from extraction sites would provide the most desirable material for grafting;[34] such osteoid tissue may be removed 4 to 8 weeks following an extraction using trephine or ronguer. Regeneration or "filling in" of bone may definitely take place following autogenous bone implants from oral donor sites, but similar healing may also occur with no implants (Fig. 26-3). Roentgenographic evidence of bone regeneration must be evaluated on a long-term basis, after at least 2 to 3 years, because the implanted bone may remain at an inert state, with very slow resorption and with or without replacement of the implanted bone. Thus, it is not possible to assess from short-term roentgenographic studies if the bone present in a bony lesion is old implanted bone or new regenerated bone (Fig. 26-4, 26-5).

Another form of autogenous implant is the *osseous coagulum,*[70] which is made up of small particles or shavings of bone mixed with blood. The shavings may be obtained during osteoplasty or following exposure of edentulous alveolar ridges. A large-sized round bur may be used to remove bone shavings or chips of bone that, mixed with blood, may be triturated in an amalgamator in a sterile capsule for 60 seconds.[15] The consistency of such a mixture will allow for efficient packing into an intrabony defect. The use of osseous coagulum is based on the assumptions that small bone particles are more readily resorbed and replaced than larger particles and that these mineralized fragments may induce osteogenesis.[70] Good results have been reported following the use of osseous coagulum,[25,26,28,70] and the short-term healing was better than that following curettage alone.[12] However, meaningful long-term comparisons with other methods under controlled conditions are not available.

Healing studies of free osseous auto grafts in humans[27,54,75] and animals[12,62] have demonstrated that bone grafts are resorbed and replaced by new bone formation. The autograft is first surrounded by a blood clot and then partially resorbed. New bone is deposited on the autograft and new cementum on the exposed dentin. An active remodeling of the graft, with new supporting bone being deposited, has been observed up to 8 months postoperatively.[75] It appears that excellent root planing is highly significant for the success of grafting.[54] If the intrabony defect is covered by a well-defined cortical plate, the plate may be perforated by a #1 round bur to establish a good blood clot and communication with the bone-forming bone marrow. Use of antibiotic coverage in order to avoid postsurgical infection has also been recommended.[53] However, the value of these latter two recommendations has never been established. It appears that minimal inflammation at the graft site is favorable to success.[62]

Another approach to bone grafting, especially for one-wall intrabony defects, is bone swaging (Fig. 26-6). This represents a contiguous or pedicle bony autograft utilizing the principle of greenstick fractures of long bones.[23] The ideal indication for bone swaging is in the case of a mesial intrabony pocket on a tipped mandibular second or third molar adjacent to an edentulous alveolar ridge,[8,23,76] but bone swaging may also be used in other, similar cases. Following complete removal of the soft tissue lining of the pocket and thorough root planing, a gingival incision may be made parallel to the slope of the bone defect 1 to 2 mm away from the defect. A thin chisel is then inserted into the incision and with blows from a mallet the intervening bone is swaged toward the root surface.[53] The swaging may also be performed after exposure of the bone by a mucoperiosteal flap. The graft should be of adequate width to prevent complete fracture, and the flap must cover the graft completely to allow for optimal healing.[76] The relative merit of this procedure compared with other methods of treatment of intrabony pockets has not been established.

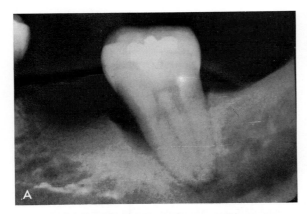

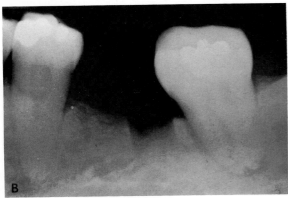

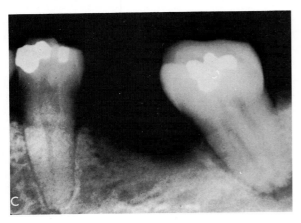

Fig. 26-6. *A,* Deep intrabony defect on mandibular third molar. *B,* Six months after attempt at bone swaging. Note mesial fragment of bone. Other smaller fragments had been resorbed. *C,* One and one half years after the bone swaging. Remains of the moved bone are still visible. There is no periodontal pocket, but there is obvious reduction in ridge height.

AUTOGENOUS BONE MARROW GRAFTS

The osteogenic potential of bone marrow has been recognized for a long time.[46] Since Schallhorn introduced the use of hematopoietic marrow for grafting into periodontics in 1967,[80] great interest in this modality of treatment has been evident.[9,16,17,18,38,39,81,83,84] It was hoped that implantation of viable hematopoietic cells would stimulate bone formation in periodontal

defects.[39,80,83,84] Hematopoietic hip marrow may be obtained by a hematologist or surgeon using a biopsy needle either through a small incision or directly through the skin over the posterior iliac crest.[16,80] The marrow may be placed in a glycerol solution, frozen,[80] and stored until the periodontal surgery is scheduled. It also may be implanted fresh, without freezing,[17] or stored for a limited time in tissue culture fluid.[9,85] One extensive report by Schallhorn and co-workers in 1970 included a follow-up of 182 autogenous iliac marrow transplants in 52 patients.[84] The graft material for this study was obtained and stored in minimal essential medium. A full- or partial-thickness flap was reflected over the periodontal defect, all soft tissue was removed from the intrabony defect, and the roots were planed. The bony walls of the defect were perforated with a bur to gain communication with the adjacent marrow. The hip marrow transplant was placed into the defect until it was over-filled. The flaps were sutured tightly in place to cover the implant, and the patient was placed on antibiotic therapy.

Reevaluation after various periods of healing revealed that crestal defects gained a mean of 2.57 mm in crestal height, two bony wall defects filled in almost completely, but furcations and one bony wall defects showed only partial regeneration of bone. The total mean increase in bone height in all types of defects was 3.33 mm. Other papers have reported similar good results.[17,18]

However, problems associated with iliac transplants have occurred. Schallhorn, in 1972, listed five potential complications: 1) postoperative infections; 2) sequestration of the graft material; 3) varying rates of healing that can complicate evaluation and subsequent treatment; 4) rapid recurrence of the defect; and 5) root resorption with ankylosis.[82] Other reports of root resorption associated with bone marrow transplants have also appeared.[9,18,20] Most cases of root resorption and ankylosis have been reported with fresh, unfrozen bone marrow, and it has been suggested that resorption can be avoided by the use of frozen marrow and careful control of postsurgical inflammation.[18] Since Rosling[73] and co-workers found 2.5-3.0 mm fill-in of bone after modified Widman flap surgery without any bone implant, the interest in bone implants has decreased.

ALLOGRAFTS AND XENOGRAFTS

Most promising are the recently reported good results from the use of freeze-dried, crushed cortical bone allografts.[51] The freeze-dried bone appeared to be nonautogenic and easily replaced by host tissues. It has been postulated that small particle size (100 to 300 μm) is essential for the success of such grafts, and the material has been called "bone blend."[26]

Despite potentially unfavorable immune reactions,

allografts and xenografts have been used rather extensively in periodontics. Various forms and preparations of bovine bone have been advocated as implant materials,[3,14,24,49,50,85] but, regardless of the numerous reports claiming success, none of these materials has any established usefulness in periodontal therapy. The same can be said of lyophilized cartilage,[37,78,89] cementum and dentin with or without gel foam,[61] and plaster of Paris, which acts as a nonirritating scaffold but does not stimulate new bone formation.[1,79] Biodegradable ceramics have also been found to act as a scaffold without interfering with healing,[10,55] as have hydroxyapatite crystals, but without any proven benefit to osteogenesis.

Homogenous bone from "bone banks" and other sources has been used experimentally in intrabony pockets,[14,42] with claimed success. However, because these studies were made without sham-operated controls, it is impossible to assess the value of the implant in the regeneration of bone. Recently, the interest in placing bone allografts into periodontal pockets has been revised as a result of reports of excellent results in applying decalcified lyophilized bone allografts into intrabony defects.[47] These materials are easily available and easily applied. It appears that the potential for connective tissue reattachment is slightly enhanced in the presence of such materials.[7] However, the clinical significance of such a slight gain in connective tissue attachment has not been established, and this procedure cannot be recommended as a routine clinical procedure.

Cross-matched frozen iliac marrow allografts have also been used, with about the same degree and number of good results as the autogenous hip marrow transplants.[38,83] However, despite freezing and cross-matching, ten of the patients developed cytotoxic antibodies to human lymphocyte antigen. Therefore, the procedure cannot be considered completely safe.

Summary of grafts

Equally or almost equally good results have been reported in the treatment of intrabony pockets with or without implants,[19,63,65,73] and, as far as future maintenance of the teeth is concerned, the filling-in of bone may not be of essential importance.[68]

Until criteria for predicting success of the various grafting procedures under various anatomic and maintenance conditions have been established, routine use of grafts in treating intrabony pockets cannot be recommended.

At present, it appears that technical skill in treatment procedures and meticulous professional maintenance care are more important determinants for success than is the type of material placed into the intrabony pocket.

TREATMENT OF FURCATION INVOLVEMENT

The extensions of periodontal pockets that may occur between the roots of multirooted teeth are called *furcation involvements*.[32] It is important to determine if the involvement has bearing on pulpal pathology,[59,87] since the furcation area may have accessory pulp canals and, if there is pulpal involvement, root canal therapy should precede the periodontal treatment.

There is no difference in basic etiology and pathology between furcation involvements and other periodontal pockets. However, the anatomical and morphological features of the furcations and their relationship to the adjacent structures pose specific problems in treatment of involved teeth.

A long projection of junctional epithelium along enamel projections toward furcations may predispose to pocket formation in this area, although the significance of this anatomical aberration in the development of furcation involvement has never been established.[45] Another common anatomical aberration in the furcation area is enamel pearls and atypical hypoplastic cementum with a very irregular morphology (Fig. 26-7). Therefore, if bacterial plaque has gained access after furcation involvement, it is often very difficult to create a root surface that is biologically acceptable to the surrounding soft tissues to the extent that attachment or close adaptation of the surrounding tissue will occur.

From the standpoint of management, it may be expedient to divide the furcation involvements into three classes: Class 1 constitutes beginning involvement, not extending more than 2 mm into the furcation; Class 2 includes involvement extending deeper than 2 mm but not passing entirely through the furcation; and Class 3 comprises the through-and-through involvement, in which a probe can be passed

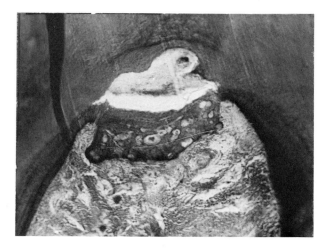

Fig. 26-7. Photomicrograph of furcation of mandibular first molar. Note enamel pearl (gray-white area) covered by irregular cementum.

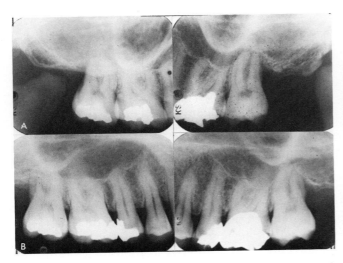

Fig. 26-8. *A,* Extensive bone loss and very deep distal pockets with furcation involvement between the distobuccal and palatal roots of both maxillary second molars. Treatment at that time was extensive subgingival curettage with assumed poor prognosis. *B,* The same teeth as in *A* 18 years later. At this time, it was not possible to probe the furcations that were involved at the time of the initial treatment.

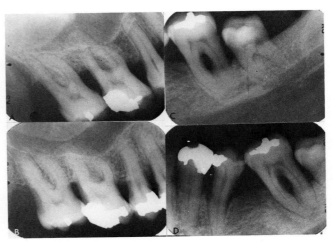

Fig. 26-9. *A,* Class II furcation involvement between mesial and distal roots and between distal and palatal root on maxillary first molar treated with modified Widman flap surgery without bone surgery. *B,* Ten years after the initial treatment. At this time, it is not possible to probe the furcations. *C,* Mandibular second molar with Class III (through and through) furcation involvement in same patient as in *A* and *B.* This was treated with surgical opening of the furcation for patient home care. *D,* Six years after the initial treatment. An abscess developed in the furcation and the tooth was extracted.

between the roots through the entire furcation.

The best treatment for the Class 1 involvement is usually a modified Widman or reverse bevel flap, which will provide access to the area of beginning involvement. The most important part of the treatment is to remove accretions and plane the root surface in such a way that all contaminated surface material is removed. If the furcation is narrow and wedge-shaped, a small groove must be created by a fine-pointed diamond stone to ensure complete removal of all contaminated surface cementum as far as the bottom of the furcation. The open part of the furcation should be reshaped by the diamond point so that a curette can be used for future cleaning of the area. Then the ground surface should be polished by steel finishing burs. The flap should be sutured into close approximation to the tooth and held in place by a firm dressing.

In general, it has been found that teeth with Class 1 furcation involvement have as good a prognosis following such treatment as teeth without furcation involvement or single rooted teeth.

The main exception is the maxillary first bicuspid, for which access for adequate treatment, even of a beginning furcation involvement, is often poor.

Early furcation involvement of the Class 1 type may also be treated with scaling and root planing only. However, if there is a definite horizontal involvement, a modified Widman or reverse bevel flap procedure is preferred. No bone surgery should be performed unless proliferative osteitis has led to a pathological lipping of the bone associated with the furcation in-

volvement. If such a protrusion is present, it should be removed with a bone chisel.

With Class 2 furcation involvement, treatment becomes increasingly difficult with increasing extent of involvement, and the prognosis will be related to the accessibility of the lesion for treatment. Deep involvement from the lingual aspect of the mandibular molars, the distal palatal aspects of the maxillary molars, and the distal aspects of the maxillary first biscuspids are all very difficult to treat successfully.

For the Class 2 involvement, the modified Widman or reverse bevel flap is again the best surgical approach for providing access for complete root planing and reshaping of the roots in the exposed furcation area. A fine-pointed diamond stone is the best instrument for this purpose. All soft tissues should be removed by curettes in the area of furcation involvement. Mandibular molars sometimes have two mesiodistal furcation ledges, one toward the buccal and another toward the lingual aspects of the furcation, with a deepening or concavity of the furcation in the middle.[22] If the furcation involvement extends into such an area, it is necessary to accentuate the furcation with a diamond stone until complete access for curettage is gained into the deepest part of the furcation involvement.

Following complete root planing, the flap should be sutured back to its original position. It is not unusual at follow-up examinations to find that the previous area of furcation involvement can no longer be probed. The prognosis is dependent on the accessibility for complete instrumentation of the involved root surface, and on good maintenance care. Some teeth with Class 2 involvement have a surprisingly good long-term prognosis, as indicated in Figure 26-8.

Some minor bone surgery may be needed to gain access for cleaning and reshaping of the exposed furcation, but do not try to reshape the bone in order to facilitate homecare by the patient (Fig. 26-9). Bone implants have been used in association with the flap procedures, but a convincing advantage has never been established under acceptable controlled conditions. A report on experimental pockets in animals claimed better results with bone implants than without,[21] but such results have not been demonstrated in humans. It appears that total removal of all irritating substances from the lesions and complete flap adaptation are more important factors for the healing than is the type of material placed into the defect. Recent publications have reported spectacular results following the use of guided periodontal membrane regeneration,[31,56] as proposed by Nyman and co-workers.[56] The results indicated complete healing of furcation involvement. However, further studies are needed before this procedure can be recommended for routine clinical practice.

Treatment of Class 3 (the through-and-through furcation involvement) is the most challenging aspect of periodontal therapy. The conventional approach has been to separate the roots by sectioning,[52] and sometimes to remove the most involved root or the most difficult one to treat endodontically. However, it has become evident from retrospective studies that the periodontal prognosis for teeth with furcation involvement after periodontal flap surgery is much better than was assumed,[74] and the prognosis following root sectioning much poorer than anticipated.[44] Thus, most molars with furcation involvement are treated with flap and diamond points, followed by burnishing with steel burs and subsequent flap coverage. Only in special situations (such as one bad and one good root periodontally, hopeless root canal anatomy for one root needing endodontic care, or accidental perforation in the furca) is root sectioning the treatment of choice.

On a long-term basis, attempts to open furcations for ease of access by the patient by so-called "tunneling"[35] and then by using a pipe cleaner or some other device have not been successful. After about 5 years, there is a tendency to develop root caries or resorption of the furcation (Fig. 26-10).

The removal of a disto- or mesiobuccal maxillary molar root with a Class 3 furcation involvement has a good prognosis, provided that there is residual bone between the two remaining roots (Fig. 26-11). The

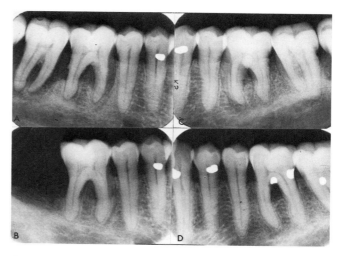

Fig. 26-10. *A,* Severe Class II furcation involvement and deep mesial and distal pockets on the mandibular first molar. The second and third molars were extracted and the first molar treated with modified Widman flap surgery. *B,* Eight years after the initial treatment, the attachment levels have improved markedly for all pockets, and the furcation cannot be probed. *C,* Furcation involvement in first mandibular molar of same patient as in *A.* Treatment consisted in opening and "tunneling" of the furcation, and instruction for the patient to use pipecleaners for plaque control in the open furcation. *D,* Eight years later, the tooth is still free of symptoms, but carious lesion in the furcation has been treated with an amalgam restoration.

endodontic therapy of the residual roots is done either prior to the sectioning or at the same time as the hemisectioning.

The separation of the roots during hemisectioning should always be done after buccal and lingual flaps have been raised, so that the sectioning can be initiated from the furcation rather than from the occlusal surface of the crowns of the teeth. During hemisectioning of mandibular molars, it is usually advisable to extract the root with the most extensive periodontal involvement and keep only one of the roots as abutment for restorative dentistry. The remaining root should be stabilized with a temporary acrylic splint (Fig. 26-12) at the time of the sectioning,[66] and the fabrication of a permanent bridge should be delayed for 2 to 3 months to allow complete healing and natural contouring of the adjacent gingival tissues. Accessibility for adequate plaque control is essential to the success of hemisectioning, as it is for other periodontal treatment procedures, and restorative procedures should aim at ease of plaque control. Removal of both buccal roots of maxillary molars in cases of Class 3 involvement of all roots has been recommended in patients needing extensive oral rehabilitation.[57] However, the combination of problems in plaque control, esthetic appearance, and distribution of occlusal forces detracts from the practicality of such procedures. Because of poor accessibility, hemisectioning of a max-

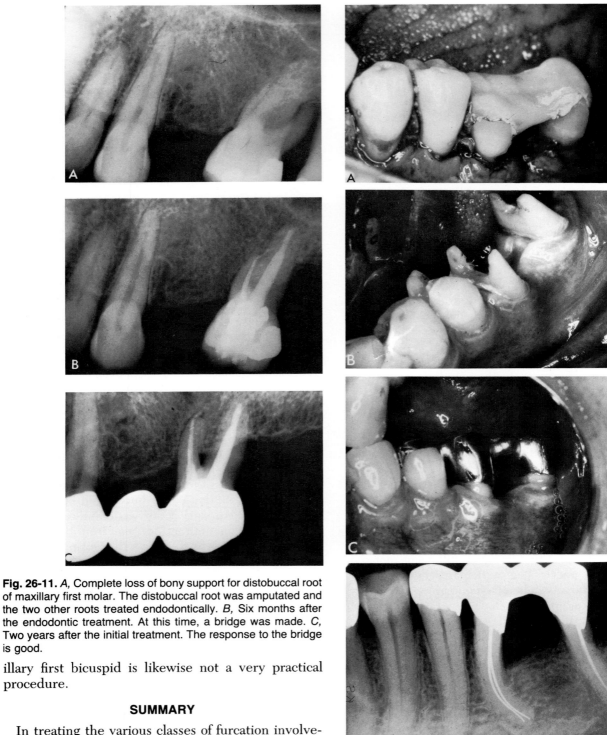

Fig. 26-11. *A,* Complete loss of bony support for distobuccal root of maxillary first molar. The distobuccal root was amputated and the two other roots treated endodontically. *B,* Six months after the endodontic treatment. At this time, a bridge was made. *C,* Two years after the initial treatment. The response to the bridge is good.

illary first bicuspid is likewise not a very practical procedure.

SUMMARY

In treating the various classes of furcation involvement:

Class 1 (2 mm or less) should be treated with modified Widman or reverse bevel flap surgery. Odontoplasty may enhance access for cleaning and maintenance care.

Class 2 involvement (more than 2 mm, but not through-and-through involvement) should be treated similarly to Class 1.

Fig. 26-12. *A,* Temporary plastic bridge cemented to hold the remaining roots in proper position following hemisectioning and removal of the distal roots. *B,* After healing took place, the temporary bridge was removed and the abutments prepared for a fixed bridge. *C,* The fixed bridge in place. Note supragingival margins for the full crowns. *D,* Roentgenograms 3 years after the insertion of the bridge. Good periodontal response.

Class 3 involvement (through and through) may be treated similarly to class 1 and class 2 involvement. In selected cases, root sectioning may also be used.

REFERENCES

1. Alderman, M.E.: Sterile plaster of paris as an implant in the infrabony environment. A preliminary study, J Periodont. 40:11, 1969.
2. Beube, F.E.: Observations on the formation of cementum, periodontal membrane and bone, 20 months postoperatively, with the use of boiled cow-bone powder, J. Dent. Res. 21:298, 1942.
3. Beube, F.E.: A study on reattachment of the supporting structures of the teeth, J. Periodont. 18:55, 1947.
4. Beube, F.E., and Silvers, H.F.: Influence of devitalized heterogenous bone powder on regeneration of alveolar and maxillary bone of dogs, J. Dent. Res. 14:15, 1934.
5. Beube, F.E., and Silvers, H.F.: Further studies on bone generation with the use of boiled heterogenous bone, J. Periodont. 7:17, 1936.
6. Billingham, R.E.: The immunobiology of tissue transplantation, Int. Dent. J. 21:478, 1971.
7. Bowers, G.M., et al.: Histologic evaluation of new attachment in humans: A preliminary report, J. Periodontol. 56:381, 1985.
8. Burnette, D.: Treatment of an isolated severe osseous crater. A case report, J. Periodont. 38:148, 1967.
9. Burnette, D.: Fate of an iliac crest graft, J. Periodont. 43:88, 1972.
10. Bump, R.L., et al.: The use of woven ceramic fabric as a periodontal allograft, J. Periodont. 46:453, 1975.
11. Caton, J., and Zander, H.A.: Osseous repair of an infrabony pocket without new attachment of connective tissues, J. Clin. Periodontol. 3:51, 1976.
12. Coverly, L., Toto, P., and Gargiulo, A.: Osseous coagulum: A histologic evaluation, J. Periodont. 46:596, 1975.
13. Cross, W.G.: Bone grafts in periodontal disease. A preliminary report, Dent. Pract. 6:98, 1955.
14. Cross, W.G.: Bone implants in periodontal disease. A further study, J. Periodont. 28:184, 1957.
15. Diem, G., Bowers, B.M., and Muffitt, W.C.: Bone blending: A technique for osseous implants, J. Periodont. 42:295, 1972.
16. Dragoo, M.R., and Irwin, R.K.: A method of producing iliac bone utilizing a trephine needle, J. Periodont. 43:82, 1972.
17. Dragoo, M.R., and Sullivan, H.C.: A clinical and histological evaluation of autogenous iliac bone grafts in humans. Part I. Wound healing 2 to 8 months, J. Periodont. 44:599, 1973.
18. Dragoo, M.R., and Sullivan, H.C.: A clinical and histological evaluation of autogenous iliac bone grafts in humans. Part II. External root resorption, J. Periodont. 44:614, 1973.
19. Ellegaard, B., and Löe, H.: New attachment of periodontal tissues after treatment of intrabony lesions, J. Periodont. 42:648, 1971.
20. Ellegaard, B., et al.: New attachment after treatment of interradicular lesions, J. Periodont. 44:209, 1973.
21. Ellegaard, B., et al.: New attachment after treatment of intrabony defects in monkeys, J. Periodont. 45:368, 1974.
22. Everett, F.G.: The intermediate bifurcation ridge: A study of the morphology of the bifurcation of the lower first molar, J. Dent. Res. 37:162, 1958.
23. Ewen, S.J.: Bone swaging, J. Periodont. 36:57, 1965.
24. Forsberg, H.: Transplantation of os purum and bone chips in the surgical treatment of periodontal disease, Acta Odont. Scand. 13:235, 1956.
25. Froum, S.J.: Comparison of different autograft materials for obtaining bone fill in human periodontal defects, J. Periodont. 45:240, 1974.
26. Froum, S.J., et al.: Osseous autografts. I. Clinical responses to bone blend or hip marrow grafts, J. Periodont. 46:515, 1975.
27. Froum, S.J., et al.: Osseous autografts. II. Histological responses to osseous coagulum-bone blend grafts, J. Periodont. 46:656, 1975.
28. Froum, S.J., et al.: Osseous autografts. III. Comparison of osseous coagulum-bone blend implants with open curettage, J. Periodont. 47:287, 1976.
29. Glickman, I.: Clinical Periodontology, 4th ed., Philadelphia, 1972, W.B. Saunders Co.
30. Goldman, H.M., and Cohen, D.W.: The infrabony pocket: Classification and treatment, J. Periodont. 29:272, 1958.
31. Gottlow, J., et al.: New attachment formation in the human periodontium by guided tissue regeneration. Case reports, J. Clin. Periodontol. 13:604, 1986.
32. Goldman, H.M., and Cohen, D.W.: Periodontal Therapy, 5th ed., St. Louis, 1973, C.V. Mosby Co.
33. Haggerty, P.C., and Maeda, J.: Autogeneous bone grafts: A revolution in the treatment of vertical bone defects, J. Periodont. 42:626, 1971.
34. Halliday, D.G.: The grafting of newly formed autogeneous bone in the treatment of osseous defects, J. Periodont. 40:511, 1969.
35. Hamp, W.E., Nyman, S., and Lindhe, J.: Periodontal treatment of multirooted teeth. Results after five years, J. Clin. Periodontol. 2:126, 1975.
36. Hegedus, Z.: The rebuilding of the alveolar process by bone transplantation, Dent. Cosmos 65:736, 1923.
37. Held, A.J., and Spingi, M.: Treatment of complex periodontitis by insertion of lyophilized cartilaginous grafts, Parodontologie 14:9, 1960.
38. Hiatt, W.H., and Schallhorn, R.G.: Human allografts of iliac cancellous bone and marrow in periodontal osseous defects. I. Rationale and methodology, J. Periodont. 42:642, 1971.
39. Hiatt, W.H., and Schallhorn, R.G.: Intraoral transplants of cancellous bone and marrow in periodontal lesions, J. Periodont. 44:194, 1973.
40. Jackson, D.B.: Gingival contour and coronal level changes following three periodontal treatment procedures. Thesis, The University of Michigan, 1973.
41. Kramer, G.M.: Grafts to repair alveolar lesions, Dental Times 9:6, 1966.
42. Kroemer, H.: Bone homografts in surgical treatment of cysts of the jaw and periodontal pockets, Odontol. Tidskr. 68:1, 1960.
43. Kroemer, H.: Implantation of bone homografts in periodontal pockets, Dent. Clin. North Am. p. 471, 1962.
44. Langer, B., et al.: An evaluation of root resections. A ten-year study, J. Periodontol. 53:719, 1982.
45. Leib, A.M.: Furcation involvements correlated with enamel projections from the cementoenamel junction, J. Periodont. 38:330, 1967.
46. Levander, G.: An experimental study of the bone marrow in bone regeneration, Acta Chir. Scand. 83:545, 1940.
47. Libin, B.M., Ward, H.L., and Fishman, L.: Decalcified lyophilized bone allograft for use in human periodontal defects, J. Periodont. 46:51, 1975.
48. McWilliams, C.: A discussion of bone transplantation and the use of a rib as a graft, Ann. Surg. 56:377m, 1912.
49. Melcher, A.H.: The use of heterogenous anorganic bone in periodontal bone grafting. A preliminary report, J. Dent. Ass. South Africa 13:80, 1958.
50. Melcher, A.H.: Use of heterogenous anorganic bone as an implant material in oral procedures, Oral Surg. 15:996, 1962.
51. Mellonig, J.T., et al.: Clinical evaluation of freeze-dried bone allografts in periodontal osseous defects, J. Periodont. 47:125, 1976.

52. Messinger, T.F., and Orban, B.J.: Elimination of periodontal pockets by root amputation, J. Periodont. 26:213, 1954.

53. Nabers, C.L., and O'Leary, T.J.: Autogeneous bone transplants in the treatment of osseous defects, J. Periodont. 36:5, 1965.

54. Nabers, C.L., Reed, O.M., and Hammer, J.E.: Gross and histologic evaluation of an autogenous bone graft 57 months postoperatively, J. Periodont. 43:702, 1972.

55. Nery, E.B., et al.: Bioceramic implants in surgically produced infrabony defects, J. Periodont. 46:328, 1975.

56. Nyman, S., et al.: New attachment following surgical treatment of human periodontal disease, J. Clin. Periodontol. 9:290, 1982.

57. Nyman, S., Lindhe, J., and Lundgren, D.: The role of occlusion for the stability of fixed bridges in patients with reduced periodontal tissue support, J. Clin. Periodontol. 2:53, 1975.

58. Nyström, B.: Plugging of bone cavities with rivanol-plaster-porridge, Acta Chir. Scand. 63:296, 1928.

59. Orban, B.J., and Johnston, H.B.: Interradicular pathology as related to accessory root canals, J. Endod. 3:21, 1948.

60. Orell, S.: The use of "os purum" and "boiled bone" in surgical bone grafting, J. Bone Joint Surg. 19:873, 1937.

61. Packer, M.W., and Schaffer, E.: Cementum-dentine and gel foam implants in surgical periodontal pockets in dogs, Oral Surg. 18:722, 1964.

62. Patterson, R.L., Collings, C.K., and Zimmerman, E.R.: Autogenous implants in the alveolar process of the dog with induced periodontitis, Periodontics 5:19, 1967.

63. Patur, B.: Osseous defects: Evaluation of diagnostic and treatment methods, J. Periodont. 45:623, 1974.

64. Prichard, J.F.: The intrabony technique as predictable procedure, J. Periodont. 28:202, 1957.

65. Prichard, J.F.: Advanced Periodontal Disease, 2nd ed., Philadelphia, 1972, W.B. Saunders Co.

66. Ramfjord, S.P.: Periodontal aspects of restorative dentistry, J. Oral Rehabil. 1:107, 1974.

67. Ramfjord, S.P., et al.: Longitudinal study of periodontal therapy, J. Periodont. 44:66, 1973.

68. Ramfjord, S.P., et al.: Results following three modalities of periodontal therapy, J. Periodont. 46:522, 1975.

69. Rivault, A.F., et al.: Autogenous bone grafts: Osseous coagulum and osseous retrograde procedures in primates, J. Periodont. 42:787, 1971.

70. Robinson, R.: Osseous coagulum for bone induction, J. Periodont. 40:503, 1969.

71. Rosenberg, M.M.: Free osseous tissue autografts as a predictable procedure, J. Periodont. 42:195, 1971.

72. Rosenberg, M.M.: Reentry of an osseous defect treated by a bone implant after a long duration, J. Periodont. 42:360, 1971.

73. Rosling, B., Nyman, S., and Lindhe, J.: The effect of systemic plaque control on bone regeneration in intrabony pockets, J. Clin. Periodontol. 3:38, 1976.

74. Ross, J.E., and Thompson, R.H.: Furcation involvement in maxillary and mandibular molars, J. Periodontol. 51:450, 1980.

75. Ross, S.E., and Cohen, D.W.: The fate of a free osseous tissue autograft. A clinical and histological case report, Periodontics 6:145, 1968.

76. Ross, S.E., Malmed, E.H., and Amsterdam, M.: The contiguous autogeneous transplant. Its rationale, indications and technique, Periodontics 4:246, 1966.

77. Saphos, S.W.: The use of periograf in periodontal defects. Histologic findings, J. Periodontol. 57:7, 1986.

78. Schaffer, E.M.: Cartilage grafts in human periodontal pockets, J. Periodont. 29:176, 1958.

79. Schaffer, C.D., and App, G.R.: The use of plaster of paris in treating infrabony periodontal defects in humans, J. Periodont. 42:685, 1971.

80. Schallhorn, R.G.: Eradication of bifurcation defects utilizing frozen autogenous hip marrow implants, Periodont. Abstr. 15:101, 1967.

81. Schallhorn, R.G.: The use of autogenous hip marrow biopsy implants for bone crater defects, J. Periodont. 39:145, 1968.

82. Schallhorn, R.G.: Postoperative problems associated with iliac transplants, J. Periodont. 43:3, 1972.

83. Schallhorn, R.G., and Hiatt, W.H.: Human allografts of iliac cancellous bone and marrow in periodontal osseous defects. II. Clinical observations, J. Periodont. 43:67, 1972.

84. Schallhorn, R.G., Hiatt, H.W., and Boyce, W.: Iliac transplants in periodontal therapy, J. Periodont. 41:566, 1970.

85. Scopp, J.W., et al.: Bovine bone (Boplant) implants for infrabony oral lesions (clinical trial in humans). Periodontics 4:169, 1966.

86. Senn, N.: On the healing of aseptic bone cavities by implantation of antiseptic decalcified bone, Am. J. Med. Sci. 98:219, 1889.

87. Simring, M.: The pulpal pocket approach: Retrograde periodontitis, J. Periodont. 35:22, 1964.

88. Sottosanti, J.S., and Bierly, J.A.: The storage of bone marrow and its relation to periodontal grafting procedure, J. Periodont. 46:162, 1975.

89. Standnicki, J., and Rassumowska, D.: Ueber die chirugische Behandlung von Parodontopathien mit Implanteten lyophilisierten heterologen Knorpelgewebes, Dtsch. Zahnarztl. Ztschr. 19:615, 1964.

27

PERIODONTAL CONSIDERATIONS IN RESTORATIVE AND OTHER ASPECTS OF DENTISTRY

In restorative dentistry, endodontics, and oral surgery, one should consider the health and maintenance of the periodontium. For the most effective periodontal therapy, the following must be considered: the health of the periodontium prior to restorative dental procedures; placement of gingival margins of restorations; preparation of the teeth; impression techniques; temporization of restorations and cementation; and polishing of restorations. The design of contours, contact areas, and pontics is also important for periodontal health. The importance of occlusion in restorative procedures was discussed in chapter 19. The significance of endodontics and pulpal disease to periodontitis must also be considered, inasmuch as periodontal disease and pulpitis complicate effective periodontal and endodontal therapy. Finally, the potential periodontal hazards associated with oral surgery procedures will be discussed here.

RESTORATIVE DENTISTRY

The goal of restorative dentistry is to restore optimal functional and esthetic features of the teeth in a way that is also conducive to the maintenance of periodontal health. Dental restorations should be performed without injury to the periodontal tissues, and the completed restoration should be nonirritating, allow for optimal plaque control, and afford comfortable, nontraumatic function.[52]

PRERESTORATIVE PERIODONTAL HEALTH

In order to minimize the risk of trauma to the gingival tissues during preparation and impression procedures, and to determine a lasting optimal relationship between the margins of the restorations and the gingiva, a physiological gingival sulcus and healthy resilient gingival tissues must be established prior to the restorative procedures. When selecting surgical procedures, never use resective techniques in the an-

terior part of the mouth. Modified Widman flap surgery allows much less recession than pocket elimination surgery.[46] However, in the great majority of cases, scaling and root planing is the only needed therapy.[48] In cases of extensive periodontal surgery, it may take 2 to 3 months or more before the new adaptive relationships between the gingival tissues and the teeth are developed with respect to the position of the free gingival margins and the interdental papillae.[54] But even in instances of severe gingival inflammation that do not require periodontal surgery, it takes a month or more after scaling and the commencement of good oral hygiene before healing and collagen maturation have established a resilient gingival fiber structure that will allow the safe opening and physiological closure of the gingival sulcus and junctional epithelium associated with impression techniques. Margins of restorations that were placed subgingivally in relation to swollen and inflamed gingival tissues or periodontal pockets have a tendency to become exposed and become an esthetic liability following healing and subsequent gingival recession. The opposite often occurs with restorations placed supragingivally a short time after extensive periodontal surgery; they may be covered by regenerating gingival tissues and act as a source of subgingival irritation in the future.

Technically, it is much easier to make precise preparations and obtain accurate impressions when the gingiva is healthy than when it is hemorrhagic and inflamed.

If the restorations will be related to the gingiva or to occlusal function, only temporary restorations needed for plaque control and protection against injury from deep caries should be placed prior to the hygienic phase.

Gingival margin of restorations

Black's concept of "extension for prevention"[8] went

unchallenged for more than 50 years. However, several recent investigators have reported that there is always an inflammatory gingival response to all types of subgingivally placed restorations,[3,27,32,34] and that subgingival placement of margins does not provide predictable protection against caries.[10,64,65]

The subgingival irritation associated with restorations may be due to (1) toxic products released from the restorative materials; (2) an increased plaque retention potential on the restorations; and (3) imperfections at the junction between the restorations and the teeth.

The most common restorative materials (amalgam, gold, porcelain, heat-cured acrylic, and composites) do not release tissue irritants if they are sterilized and implanted under aseptic conditions. Phosphate cements and silicates are slightly irritating, and acrylic restorations extended subgingivally may absorb bacterial toxins and cause irritation, although the material itself is nonirritating when fully polymerized. Gingival tissues adjacent to composite resin restorations extended subgingivally will develop gingivitis even in the presence of good oral hygiene.[33]

Clinical and histological studies have indicated a more favorable gingival response to gold than to amalgam restoration,[3] and a more severe irritation from subgingival silicate and plastic than from either of the two alloys.[67] There may be a difference in plaque-retaining potentials related to chemical differences in the materials,[71] and the bacterial composition of the plaque may also be influenced by the material. It appears, for example, that more plaque accumulates on gold than on a tooth surface under similar conditions,[53] but the gingival response remains the same if the restorations do not extend subgingivally. Restorations that were extended subgingivally showed more inflammation than those restorations terminating at the gingival margin, although the plaque scores were the same in both cases;[53] this inflammation indicates an adverse gingival effect even on these well-fitting margins. Crown margins placed at the free gingival margin will react less favorably than margins placed completely supragingivally.[40]

It is a common clinical observation that rough surfaces on teeth, restorations, and dental appliances lead to faster and more extensive plaque and calculus formation than highly polished surfaces. Roughening the subgingival aspect of a tooth has been shown to enhance subgingival plaque formation.[63]

Although no standards of acceptable surface smoothness for restorations have been established, and some materials such as composites cannot be polished or worn to a smooth finish,[22] it is generally accepted that surface smoothness facilitates both natural and artificial cleansing.

The junction between a restoration and the tooth is always a source of retention of bacteria and other irritating substances.[56] None of the commonly used restorative materials will provide a hermetic seal between the restoration and the tooth.

Mechanical imperfections, cement margins, and variations in thermal expansion between the restoration and the tooth are unavoidable sources of bacterial retention and gingival irritation of subgingival margins. The margin of a restoration should ideally be placed supragingivally on enamel. This allows for optimal finishing of the restoration. It is much more difficult to get a good finish of a margin contacting cementum, even if it is located supragingivally.

Although subgingival margins are periodontal hazards, and caries prevention can be better achieved with fluorides, diet, and plaque control than with subgingival restorations, there are some valid reasons for placing restorations subgingivally, such as (1) subgingival extension of caries, previous restorations, and tooth fractures; (2) esthetic appearance; and (3) retention and prevention of root fractures. When preparations have to be extended subgingivally because of caries or previous restorations, this extension should be limited to the minimum dictated by the conditions. It has been shown in a longitudinal study over 5 years that well-fitted supragingival margins were of no periodontal significance, and margins of restorations placed at the free gingival margin resulted in only an insignificant increase in gingivitis. By far the greatest increases in gingivitis, in pocket depth, and in loss of attachment occurred with subgingival margins.[64,65] In a cross-sectional survey,[7] it was shown that when margins had less than 0.2 mm of imperfections, the effect on the alveolar crest was insignificant compared to the effect of restorations with greater imperfections. It has also been shown that the subgingival bacterial flora will be similar in cases with well-fitting subgingival margins and in cases with no fillings, while in cases with poorly fitting margins, the bacterial flora will change to potentially pathogenic flora.[29]

These findings emphasize that preparations should be extended subgingivally only to the minimal extent needed for the specific purpose of covering tooth defects, and should be finished as well as possible, preferably under rubber dam.

The second reason for subgingival placement of margins is esthetic appearance, especially if the junction between the restoration and the tooth will be visible during normal lip function. In such instances, extend the margin only 0.5 to 1.0 mm into the gingival sulcus, and stay at least 0.5 mm away from the connective tissue attachment as measured by a thin periodontal probe. With crown preparations, place subgingivally only the part of the margin that would be visible, and place the margins on the lingual side supragingivally unless more extensive restorations are needed for the prevention of fractures or for proper occlusal function. Leaving a band of undisturbed junctional epithelium between the restoration and the connective tissue attachment is very important, because this band will prevent the unavoidable gingival inflammation related to the margin from extending to the fiber attachment of the periodontium. A common mistake is to place the margins too deep into the gingival crevice interproximally.

The third reason for subgingival extension of margins, related to retention, can usually be solved by pin techniques[15] without having to extend the margins. If the crown of a tooth has been lost and the tooth has a root canal filling, it may be necessary to place a band of supporting metal around the neck of the tooth to guard against future fracture. However, such instances are rare.

In restorative dentistry, including fixed prosthetics, for patients with advanced loss of periodontal support, the margins of the restorations should be placed at least 2 to 3 mm away from the gingival margins[42] and end in enamel wherever feasible.

Modern technical procedures in restorative dentistry, combined with advances in the prevention of caries and periodontal disease, have eliminated many of the past reasons for placing margins subgingivally. The main problem now is to educate members of the dental profession to reassess their procedures in line with the new scientific information.

Preparation and impression techniques

Ideally, the preparation of the teeth for restorations should be done under rubber dam to assure that the gingiva is protected from injury. However, this is cumbersome if "washed field" techniques are used, and may be impractical for some types of restorations. Careful use of small diamond points or burs for subgingival preparations makes it possible to complete such preparations with little or no gingival injury, provided that the gingival tissues were healthy prior to the preparation. Small injuries to the soft crevicular tissues will heal readily and without any alteration of gingival relations to the tooth. Probing or separation of the gingival tissues from the teeth[60] with scalers,[47] separating packs, or rubber dam clamps will commonly extend to the connective tissue attachment at the bottom of the junctional epithelium. However, the junctional epithelium will become attached to the tooth surface again within a week,[62] provided that the gingiva was healthy prior to the procedure and the injury was minor.

Any preparation extended beyond the bottom of this clinically determined sulcus is potentially a periodontal hazard, especially if the preparation or an accidentally slipped stone or bur touches cementum with attached fibers. Usually, new junctional epithelium will cover this injured cementum and prevent regeneration of the fiber attachment.[49] It is a good rule with all preparations to stay at least 0.5 mm coronally to the clinically determined bottom of the gingival sulcus, both to assure that permanent injury does not occur during the preparation and impression procedures and to avoid harmful irritation from the finished restoration.

Special care should be exercised when the free gingiva is thin and only a narrow zone of attached gingiva is present, because traumatic gingival recession may easily be induced in such cases by careless procedures. Careless placement of a rubber dam clamp, especially when combined with the use of local anesthetics, may also lead to necrosis of periodontal tissues, and the following regeneration may only be partial.

Routine placement of separating gingival packs in preparation for impressions will sever the attachment of the junctional epithelium to the tooth. When performed in a reasonably careful manner on healthy gingival tissues, such procedures have no prolonged harmful effect on the periodontal tissues.[2,36] However, if the gingival tissues are highly inflamed and to a great extent composed of exudate instead of being held firmly together by dense fibrous connective tissue, careless use of tissue packs, especially under anesthesia, may separate the gingival tissues from the cementum apically to the epithelial attachment, and permanent loss of attachment may result. Forceful, lengthy packing and high epinephrine content of the pack may induce ischemic necrosis and result in gingival recession. Special care must be taken when the zone of attached gingiva is narrow and when there is very thin free gingiva. It is true that tube impression will sever the epithelial attachment, but so will other impression methods, without causing any lasting harmful effect if the impression tube is not forced beyond the bottom of the junctional epithelium. It is especially important that the cemental surface not be scratched beyond the bottom of the epithelial attachment, because such injury may not heal with connective tissue attachment; thus, a very tightly fitting tube forced too far down during impression procedures is worse than a wider tube, which may inflict only soft tissue injury.

Various electrosurgical techniques have been advocated in order to facilitate impression procedures.[38] A recent study of rhesus monkeys indicates that there is a distinct hazard of loss of periodontal attachment following intracrevicular "troughing" by a thin needle electrode and high frequency electrosurgery.[69] Electrosurgery is discussed in chapters 20 and 22. Although electrosurgery may facilitate accurate impression procedures, it is not a safe technique from a periodontal standpoint, and is not needed if the gingival

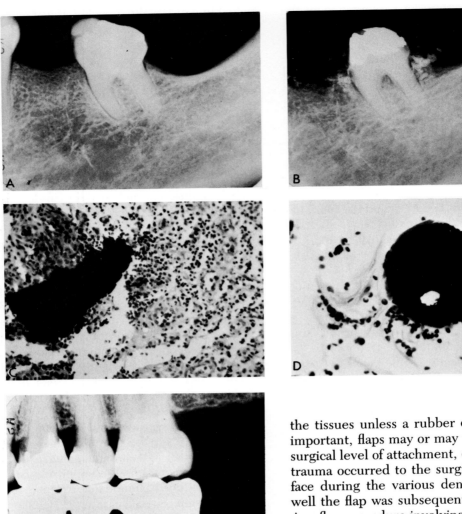

Fig. 27-1. *A,* Mandibular molar prior to crown preparation. *B,* After crown preparation with extensive soft tissue trauma and rubber base impression. Note infiltration of foreign material around the tooth and into the bone. *C,* Highly inflamed connective tissues removed from the gingiva around the tooth. Note foreign body (rubber base). *D,* Rubber base material within a distended blood vessel. *E,* Follow-up 1 year after placement of bridge. Note lowering of alveolar crest compared with *A,* before preparation.

tissues were healthy before a careful preparation was initiated. Hyperplastic gingival tissues may be safely removed with an electrosurgical needle, provided that the needle does not touch the cementum apically to the epithelial attachment.[19] A surgical dressing should then be applied, and the area should have a chance to heal before preparation for restorations is initiated.

Performing periodontal flap procedures in order to gain access for impressions should be avoided because of the hazard that impression materials will get into the tissues unless a rubber dam is used; even more important, flaps may or may not heal back to the presurgical level of attachment, depending on how much trauma occurred to the surgically exposed tooth surface during the various dental procedures and how well the flap was subsequently adapted to the tooth. Any flap procedure involving exposure of the alveolar crest is contraindicated as part of impression technique, because surgical exposure of the alveolar crest invariably leads to subsequent bone resorption.[25]

Severe periodontal reactions will occur if rubber base impression material is introduced into the gingival tissues during impression procedures.[44,45] This may occur following electrosurgical "troughing,"[44] or in other instances of inflamed traumatized tissues.[45] It appears that the rubber base material may be forced into opened vascular lumens and thus spread into the bone, as well as infiltrating soft tissues (Fig. 27-1). The periodontal reaction to this material is very severe and painful and may necessitate the removal of both bone and soft tissues around the involved tooth. Impressions taken with rubber base should be postponed until gingival wounds have healed.

Temporary Restorations

Any temporary restoration extended subgingivally is a source of gingival irritation.[16] Rough surfaces and poorly fitting margins of temporary restorations will enhance plaque accumulation and predispose the pa-

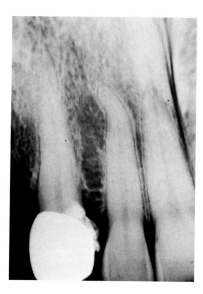

Fig. 27-2. Residual cement and beginning bone resorption 1 year after cementation of full crown on maxillary cuspid.

tient to gingival irritation even if the restoration does not come into direct contact with the gingival tissues. However, short-term irritation at the free gingival margin is not by any means as significant in the preservation of periodontal support as is irritation at the bottom of the gingival crevice, because inflammation in the latter area may lead to loss of connective tissue attachment to the cementum. Temporary restorations or cements should never be extended apically to the border of the subgingival preparation. It is often advisable to make temporary crowns slightly short and to seat them with a zinc oxide eugenol periodontal dressing, which will fill the void and be only mildly irritating at the border of the temporary restoration. Surface compression displacement of the free gingival margins and the interdental papillae may be of limited, if any, permanent significance if present for a few days. The tendency is for such displaced tissues to rebound to the normal position when allowed to do so. However, such compression may result in progressive periodontal destruction if allowed to persist over a prolonged period of time.

Temporary restorations should also maintain stable interproximal and occlusal contact relations; otherwise, the teeth may move, and it may become difficult to force such teeth back to their initial position at the time of the insertion of the permanent restorations.

Newly formed bone at the alveolar fundus of a rapidly erupting tooth is resistant to resorption, and such a tooth is not readily intruded by occlusal function to its normal position.

Permanent gingival recession following temporary restorations is most likely to occur where the gingival crevice was deeper than normal prior to the prepa-

ration for the restoration. The reason is that a rebound is not likely to go beyond the restoration of the physiological crevice depth, especially if the gingival tissues are relatively thin.

Cementation and Polishing of Restorations

It is often advisable to have the patient wear temporarily seated cast restorations for a 2-3 week trial period to assess the gingival response to the restorations and the effectiveness of the patient's home care. It is much easier to make adjustments to the design and finish of the restorations before than after they are seated permanently. This is especially true for all types of fixed prosthetic restorations. If gingival inflammation appears after the trial period, the restorations and the patient's oral hygiene habits have to be revised and a new trial period implemented. Complete removal of excess cement following cementation has to be checked carefully, since it may take years for such excess cement to be eliminated by body fluids, and in the meantime it will act as a serious source of irritation (Fig. 27-2).

Unfortunately, the polishing of subgingival amalgam surfaces is often neglected and thus makes subgingival plaque control difficult, even if dental floss is used. Ideally, the surface finish and marginal fit of restorations should be checked under rubber dam. Interproximal margins should always be tested with dental floss and finished to a point at which they do not interfere with the passing of the floss.

Periodontal Significance of Design of Restorations

The design of restorations in relation to periodontal health has not been studied extensively, and many assumptions are cited in lack of scientific evidence. The relationship between the design of pontics and periodontal health, gingival contour of restorations, and interproximal contacts will be discussed briefly here. Faulty design and its effect on food impaction, plaque formation, and effective home care procedures should receive careful consideration.

Contour

It has been stated frequently that a prominent buccolingual contour on the crowns of the teeth is of essential importance in protecting the gingiva against bruising and trauma from hard food and in preventing food from being packed into the gingival crevice.[68] There is no scientific evidence to validate this assumption, and it is becoming increasingly evident that the main cause of periodontal disease is plaque on teeth and restorations.[37] With adequate plaque control, the gingival tissues may be healthy with or without prominent contour on the teeth. However, when the gingiva contacts a flat (non-contoured) tooth surface, there is a tendency to develop a thick free gin-

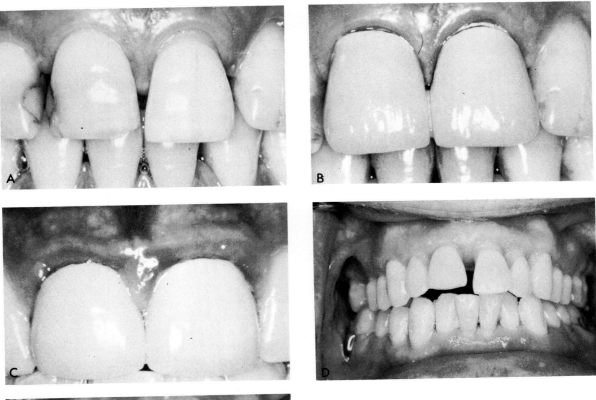

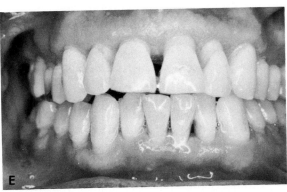

Fig. 27-3. *A,* Healthy gingiva before crown preparations. *B,* Same patient after placement of two gold-porcelain combination crowns. Thick, irritating crown margins. *C,* Overcontoured gold-porcelain combination crowns are causing severe gingivitis. *D,* Before orthodontic treatment. Distema is present between central incisors. *E,* Same patient after orthodontic treatment and with the teeth held in position by pin-ledge inlay splint on palatal side, avoiding contact with the gingiva.

gival margin, whereas a thin gingival margin can be maintained only with a normal tooth contour against the free gingiva.[39] A thin gingival margin is esthetically pleasing and may facilitate plaque control with a roll or sweep method of toothbrushing, but a thick margin is equally compatible with gingival health if the patient uses a Bass or circular scrub method for oral hygiene. There are no valid health reasons for making crowns with subgingival margins and contour to promote an anatomically normal gingival contour if subgingival placement of margins is not otherwise needed.

Overcontouring of restorations or faulty placement of contour is a much greater hazard to periodontal health than is lack of contour, since both supra- and subgingival plaque accumulation may be enhanced by overcontoured crowns.[72] A common mistake is to make bulging rounded buccal surfaces on artificial crowns,[16] especially gold porcelain combination crowns (Fig. 27-3). One reason for this faulty design is inadequate removal of labial tooth substance during preparation of vital teeth, so that the technician has to make an exaggerated contour in order to get space for both metal and porcelain. Such subgingival overcontouring interferes with the sealing "cuff" effect of the gingiva against the tooth, and the physiological self-cleansing of the gingival sulcus is impaired, with resultant bacterial retention and gingivitis. Often crown preparations are not extended to the cementoenamel junction, but the artificial crowns are designed as complete dental crowns. The result is a "double-chin" effect relative to the gingival margin, with two cervical contours and problems in plaque control (Fig. 27-4).

In order to avoid overcontouring of the crowns corresponding to the furcations, special consideration has to be given to the preparation and fabrication of crowns on teeth with partial exposure of furcations. A concave dip in the preparation and marginal aspect of the crown should be made to correspond to the ex-

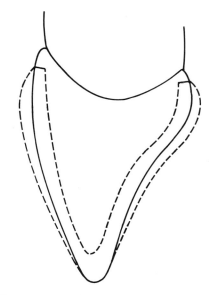

Fig. 27-4. Crown contour designed as if the preparation extended to the cementoenamel junction, thus creating an unfavorable contour.

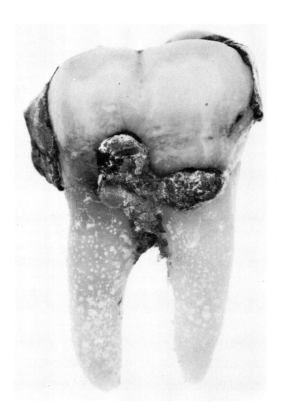

Fig. 27-5. Overextended and poorly finished amalgam restoration involving furcation of mandibular molar.

posed furcation. Far too often, restorations are poorly finished in furcation extensions, having overhanging or thick margins in this most periodontally vulnerable location (Fig. 27-5).

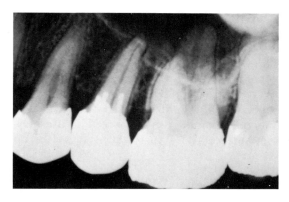

Fig. 27-6. Roentgenogram of overcontoured restorations.

Interproximal overcontouring of restorations and crowns may be even more common and more harmful than buccolingual overcontouring (Fig. 27-6). The proximal surfaces of natural teeth gingivally to the contact areas are either flat or concave,[68] but in restorative dentistry, too much emphasis is given to excessive contouring of matrix bands for amalgam restorations and carving of contour in cast restorations. In patients in whom the interproximal spaces of anterior teeth are not filled with gingival papillae, as is often seen after pocket elimination surgery, there is a common tendency to make artificial crowns too wide mesiodistally toward the gingival margin in order to close the open spaces. This produces ugly-looking teeth, and gingival irritation related to the overcontoured interproximal margins occurs. The result is a deeper-than-normal col, and hyperplastic buccal and lingual papillae between posterior teeth. These will enhance accumulation and complicate removal of plaque. A larger-than-normal interproximal space is not a periodontal handicap if the surfaces are readily accessible for hygiene procedures. Thus, it is better to lean toward under- than overcontouring of interproximal restorations, and to place contact areas and interproximal soldering connections as far occlusally as possible.

Interproximal Contacts

The periodontal significance of proper interproximal contacts in the prevention of food impaction and gingival irritation was keenly observed and described by Hirschfeld many years ago.[24] The periodontal hazard of uneven marginal ridges, plunger cusps, and so on, is discussed in chapter 10.

Open contacts without food impaction are of no periodontal significance, and they should not be closed with dental restorations or orthodontic therapy if the occlusion is stable and the teeth are intact. No experimental studies have assessed the periodontal significance of the buccolingual width of the contact areas, but the prevailing clinical impression is that the most significant aspect of interproximal contact is the ability to prevent both vertical and horizontal food impaction that does not necessarily relate to the width of the contacts. The width of contact increases considerably with age and physiological mesial drift of teeth subsequent to interproximal wear. This does not pose any periodontal problem except in cases in which concomitant occlusal wear has worn away the normal contact areas.

Pontics

Pontics should both esthetically and functionally replace lost teeth, and at the same time be nonirritating to the mucosa and allow effective plaque control. In the mandibular molar areas, where esthetics are usually not a problem, a simple solution is to use pontics that do not contact the mucosa and have a smooth rounded undersurface. These are called *sanitary* or *hygienic* pontics. Properly finished, such a pontic does not interfere with normal occlusal and phonetic function and is easy to keep clean with dental floss and "proxi-brushes." In all other areas of the dentition, the pontics, for esthetic reasons, should make light contact with the alveolar ridge mucosa. This mucosal contact should be to firmly attached gingiva without hyperplastic aberrations. If loss of bone and attached gingiva has resulted in a thin alveolar ridge without attached gingiva, free gingival grafts or pedicle grafts have to be placed prior to the construction of the bridge, in order to establish a contact area of attached gingiva for the pontic (Fig. 26-7A). Ridge defects in a pontic area should be corrected by soft- or hard-tissue submucosal grafts. For this purpose, hydroxyapatite graft material may be used.[1]

If the edentulous ridge that the pontic is going to contact is irregular in shape, with hyperplastic tissues, a gingivoplasty should be made and the wound given time to heal prior to the placement of the bridge.

With a well-structured ridge, a pontic should barely touch the labial aspect of the ridge mucosa for a distance dictated by esthetics and the space needed for interdental papillae. Ridge lapping makes plaque removal under the pontic impossible.[61] The labial contour should, as much as possible, match the neighboring teeth. The surface of the pontic facing the ridge should be polished to a high gloss and be accessible for complete plaque removal by the patient. A common mistake is to make the interproximal spaces too narrow, which results in gingival hyperplasia and poor access for hygiene (Fig. 27-7). It is also important that the interproximal soldering points be convex, well rounded, and easy to clean. In general, pontics will increase plaque retention, gingivitis levels, and pocket depth compared with surfaces not adjacent to pontics.[58]

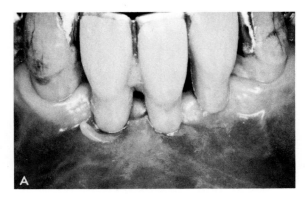

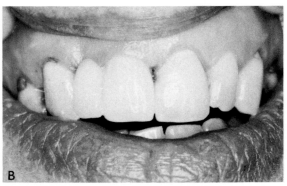

Fig. 27-7. *A,* Mucosal irritation from pontics extended over alveolar mucosa. *B,* Pontic replacing maxillary right lateral incisor and attached to central incisor. No space for papilla or for cleaning has been left.

The gingival space requirements for partial denture abutments are similar to those for fixed bridges. Emphasis should be placed on ample space for papillae and free gingiva. Even with overdentures,[9] it is important to maintain a healthy gingival sulcus. This can be achieved only if there is no infringement on the space needed for normal gingival contour. Clasps, indirect retainers, and attachments for partial dentures should have no unfavorable periodontal impact and be easy to clean. Common sources of irritation are impingement from clasps and indirect retainers, and overcontoured gingival contact areas of precision attachments.

OCCLUSION AND PERIODONTAL HEALTH

An appraisal of the patient's occlusion should precede all restorative procedures. If occlusal corrections are indicated, they should be accomplished prior to the preparations for the restorations so that they may be made to fit an optimal occlusal pattern for the patient.[50]

Such occlusal corrections may involve the use of orthodontics, biteplanes, occlusal adjustment, and a number of other restorative procedures (see chapter 19).

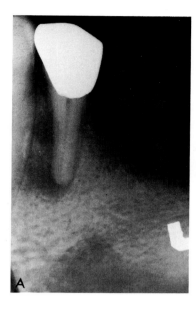

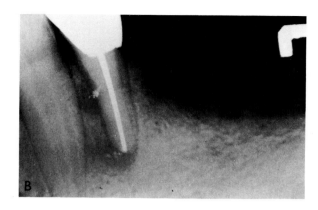

Fig. 27-8. *A,* Retrograde periodontitis with mesial pocket caused by pulpal abscess. *B,* Same tooth after root canal therapy. Note accessory canals.

ENDODONTICS AND PERIODONTAL TREATMENT

It has been shown for a long time that periodontal disease may be related to, or even cause, pulpal disease,[11,13,121] and that pulpal disease may cause periodontal lesions that behave somewhat differently than chronic destructive periodontal disease. The effect of periodontal disease on the pulp,[6] as well as the potential for healing of certain periodontal lesions following endodontic therapy,[59] have been documented extensively.

It is usually assumed that infection from a periodontal pocket may spread to the pulp through accessory canals, which occur most often in the furcation and close to the apex of teeth.[30,55] Advanced periodontitis may eventually spread to the apical foramen and cause pulp necrosis.[31] Inflammatory cells in the pulp have been observed in relation to bacteria on the root surface. When the bacterial plaque on the root surface covered the entrance of lateral canals, there was also common pulpal inflammation. However, the vitality of the pulp was usually maintained until the apical foramina were involved by bacterial plaque.[31] It has been our clinical experience, however, that pulpal infection and necrosis may occur subsequent to root planing in pockets extending close to the apex of teeth.[51] This does not happen often enough to suggest routine endodontic therapy for all teeth with pockets extending close to the apex. Unfortunately, vitality tests of the pulp will not indicate most cases of focal pulpal inflammation associated with exposed accessory pulp canals. Infection in such canals may prevent healing of periodontal pockets following therapy. In cases of reinfection of periodontal pockets following subgingival curettage or modified Widman flap procedures, endodontic therapy may be instituted in vital teeth on a trial basis, although this may not completely eliminate the inaccessible infection in the accessory canal. Old reports indicate positive bacterial cultures from the pulp of as many as 30% of teeth with vital pulp and periodontal disease,[12] and even greater frequency with increasing severity of the disease. These proportions are surprisingly high. Pulpal infection through accessory canals in the furcation of teeth with furcation periodontal involvement is rare.

Pulpal disease is a cause of periodontal disease has received much attention during the last 10 to 20 years.[23,59] Pulpal infection may release toxins and allow the spread of bacteria to the periodontium, as well as allowing the start of destructive inflammatory process in the periodontal membrane and adjacent bone. The latter manifested as an abscess (Fig. 27-8). This so-called retrograde periodontitis is not the same disease as marginal destructive periodontitis, and often is not even preceded by periodontitis. The treatment and the prognosis are also different for the two types of lesions, so a differential diagnosis is important.

Retrograde periodontitis[59] starts from a partially vital or nonvital pulp. However, in multirooted teeth, vitality tests may be misleading, because one root may have vital pulp while another root has dead pulp. Obviously, the treatment for a pulpally caused lesion must be endodontic to eliminate the source of infection. The problem is how much periodontal therapy to include with the endodontic therapy.[23] Spectacular results have been reported from endodontic therapy alone[59] and from combined endodontic and periodontal therapy.[23] The most rational approach seems to be applying endodontic therapy first and then waiting some months before assessing the need for periodontal surgery. If calculus and plaque are eliminated, the

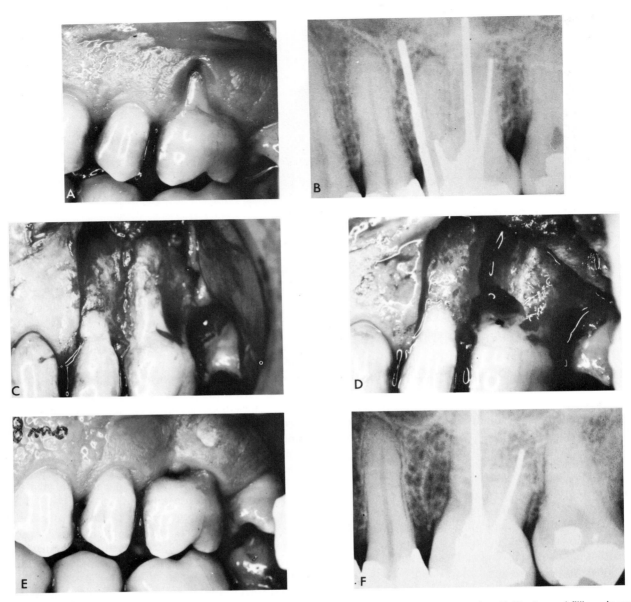

Fig. 27-9. *A,* Gingival recession and pocket to the apex on mesiobuccal root of maxillary first molar. *B,* Root canal fillings in palatal and distobuccal root, with only partial filling of mesiobuccal root due to obstructed canal. Silver point indicating the deep mesiobuccal pocket. *C,* Flap exposure of denuded mesiobuccal root. *D,* Mesiobuccal root has been amputated. *E,* Eight months postoperatively, with good healing. *F,* Roentgenographic evidence of excellent bone response to the therapy.

periodontal lesion will usually heal to the attachment level that existed prior to the pulpally caused lesion. Periodontal flap surgery at the time of the endodontic therapy is an additional insult to the already injured tissues, and root planing of surfaces involved in the abscess may remove vital remains of collagen fibers that may promote regeneration.

Periodontal pockets extending into the bifurcation of nonvital teeth may heal following root canal treatment of the teeth, provided that the pocket formation was the result of pulpal infection extended through accessory canals in the furcation.

If a molar with nonvital or partially vital pulp and

furcation involvement is the only tooth in the mouth with advanced periodontal disease, there is a good chance that the furcation involvement may be of pulpal origin. Endodontic therapy may be tried. Occasionally, intact teeth without caries or restorations may develop a periapical abscess, which may drain along the root surfaces and even involve the furcation. It must be assumed that the pulpal infection is hematogenous, and it may be associated with pulpal changes related to trauma from occlusion.[14,26] For such teeth, endodontic therapy is indicated. However, if the patient has generally advanced periodontitis or juvenile periodontitis, experimental endodontic therapy for possible healing of the lesion in the furcation is not indicated, even if the tooth or teeth happen to be devitalized.

There seems to be a time factor involved in the healing potential of pulpal as well as of marginal periodontal lesions. Lesions of short (a few weeks') duration have much better potential for healing than of chronic lesions (months or years).[41] Whether this difference is related to lack of epithelialization of the fistulous tract in the acute lesions, or to less toxin penetration of the root surface, is not known. So-called endodontic implants[5,18] with metal posts extended through the root canal and into the supporting bone in order to stabilize loose teeth are of questionable value and cannot be recommended. For deep pockets involving a single root of a multirooted tooth, the involved root may be amputated (Fig. 27-9). For a discussion of periodontal treatment of furcation involvement, root amputations, and hemisections, see chapter 26.

PERIODONTICS AND ORAL SURGERY

Mucoperiosteal flaps are used extensively for access in oral surgery. If such flaps are raised carefully and replaced without any trauma to the exposed root surfaces, they will heal back without significant permanent loss of attachment or loss of alveolar bone.[28] However, there is always some bone resorption following any kind of flap surgery,[25] and the smaller the flaps and the less the bone exposure, the better for the periodontium.

Sometimes the flaps are pulled up on the crowns of the teeth during suturing. Pseudopocket formation results, because no connective tissue attachment will develop to enamel. This can also lead to loss of attached gingiva, which would be significant when there is a narrow band of attached gingiva, as is often seen on the buccal aspect of mandibular second molars. In such cases, a slight apical positioning of a reverse bevel flap would be better than the conventional crevicular mucogingival flap procedure. The greatest periodontal hazard in oral surgery is development of distal pockets on second molars following extraction of impacted third molars (Fig. 27-10). It was found in a longitudinal study that extraction of completely and partially covered third molars resulted in a high incidence of periodontal pocket formation on the distal side of the second molars.[4] Except in young patients, apically placed, completely covered third molars should not be extracted simply because they are impacted. After completion of the roots of third molars, or in patients older than their early twenties, the potential for loss of periodontal support of 2nd molars is significantly greater from extraction of impacted third molars than from their retention. It is important that scratching of the root surface of the second molar be avoided during

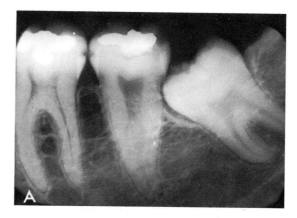

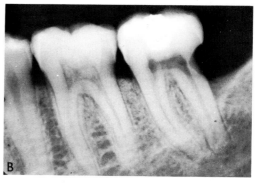

Fig. 27-10. *A,* Before removal of impacted third molar. *B,* Another case after removal of impacted molar. Note residual intrabony defect at the distal surface of the second molar.

the extraction of the third molar. All areas of injury to fiber attachment to the root cementum tend to become covered by epithelium wherever located in the mouth.[49] Such injuries should be avoided in all oral surgery procedures.[35]

Fibrotomy of the supra alveolar fibers following orthodontic treatment apparently may be done without any permanent loss of attachment,[20,43] so long as the fiber attachment to the cementum is not eliminated by trauma. However, surgical exposure of impacted teeth for orthodontic treatment should be made as conservatively as possible; otherwise, there may be permanent loss of attachment.[70]

REFERENCES

1. Allen, E.P., et al: Improved technique for localized ridge augmentation, J. Periodontol. 56:195, 1985.
2. Anneroth, G., and Göransson, P.: Exposing the gingival margin by taking impressions with elastic material—some clinical and histopathological aspects, Odont. Tidskr. 73:394, 1965.
3. App, G.R.: Effect of silicate, amalgam, and cast gold on the gingiva, J. Prosthet. Dent. 11:522, 1961.
4. Ash, M.M., Jr., Costich, E.R., and Hayward, J.R.: A study of periodontal hazards of third molars, J. Periodont. 33:209, 1962.
5. Baumhammers, A., and Baumhammers, I.: Periodontal considerations of endosseous endodontic implants, J. Periodont. 43:135, 1972.

6. Bender, J.B., and Seltzer, S.: The effect of periodontal disease on the pulp, Oral Surg. 33:458, 1972.

7. Björn, A.L., Björn, H., and Grkovic, B.: Marginal fit of restorations and its relation to periodontal bone level, Odont. Revy. 21:337, 1970.

8. Black, G.V.: Operative Dentistry. Vol. 2. Chicago: MedicoDental Publishing Co., 1908.

9. Brewer, A.A., and Morrow, R.M.: Overdentures, St. Louis, 1975, C.V. Mosby Co.

10. Budtz-Jörgensen, V.: Gingival health and secondary caries adjacent to cervical restorations, Proceedings of the Annual Meeting of the Scandinavian Association for Dental Research, Copenhagen, 1970.

11. Cahn, L.R.: The pathology of pulp found in pyorrhetic teeth, Dent. Items Int. 49:598, 1927.

12. Canby, C.P.: Incidence of pupal infection in periodontoclasia, J.A.D.A. 23:1871, 1936.

13. Colyer, F.: Bacteriological infection in pulps of pyorrhetic teeth, Br. Dent. J. 5:558, 1924.

14. Cooper, M.B., Landay, M.A., and Seltzer, S.: The effect of excessive occlusal force on the pulp. II. Heavier and longer term forces, J. Periodont. 42:353, 1971.

15. Courtade, G.L., and Timmermans, J.J.: Pins in Restorative Dentistry, St. Louis, 1971, C.V. Mosby Co.

16. Donaldson, D.: Gingival recession associated with temporary crowns, J. Periodont. 44:691, 1973.

17. Eissman, H.F., Radke, R.A., and Noble, W.A.: Physiologic design criteria for fixed dental restorations, Dent. Clin. North Am. 15:543, 1971.

18. Frank, A.L.: Improvement of crown-root ratio by endosseous endodontic implants, J.A.D.A. 74:451, 1967.

19. Glickman, J., and Imber, L.R.: Comparison of gingival resection with electrosurgery and periodontal knives. A biometric and histologic study, J. Periodont. 41:142, 1970.

20. Hansson, C., and Linder-Aronson, S.: Periodontal health following fibrotomy of the supra-alveolar fibers, Scand. J. Dent. Res. 84:11, 1976.

21. Häupl, K., and Lang, F.J.: Die Marginale Paradentitis, Berlin, 1927, H. Meusser.

22. Heath, J.R., and Wilson, H.J.: Surface roughness of restorations, Br. Dent. J. 140:131, 1976.

23. Hiatt, W.H.: Periodontal pocket elimination by combined endodontic-periodontic therapy, Periodontics 1:152, 1963.

24. Hirschfeld, I.: Food impaction, J.A.D.A. 17:1504, 1930.

25. Hoag, P.M., et al. Alveolar crest reduction following full and partial thickness flaps, J. Periodont. 43:141, 1972.

26. Ingle, J.L. Occupational bruxism and its relation to periodontal disease, J. Periodont. 23:7, 1952.

27. Karlsen, K. Gingival reaction to dental restorations, Acta Odont. Scand. 28:895, 1970.

28. Kohler, C., and Ramfjord, S.P.: Healing of gingival mucoperiosteal flaps, Oral Surg. 13:89, 1960.

29. Lang, N.P., et al. Clinical and microbiological effects of subgingival restorations with overhanging or clinically perfect margins, J. Clin. Periodontol. 10:563, 1983.

30. Langeland, K.: The histopathologic basis in endodontic treatment, Dent. Clin. N. Am., Nov. 1967, p. 491.

31. Langeland, K., Rodrigues, H., and Dowden, W.: Periodontal disease bacteria and pulpal histopathology, Oral Surg. 37:257, 1974.

32. Larato, D.C.: The effect of crown margin extension on gingival inflammation, J. S. Calif. Dent. Ass. 3:7, 476, 1969.

33. Larato, D.C.: Influence of a composite resin restoration on the gingiva, J. Prosthet. Dent. 28:402, 1972.

34. Leon, A.R.: Amalgam restoration and periodontal disease, Br. Dent. J. 140:377, 1976.

35. Levine, H.L., and Stahl, S.S.: Repair following periodontal flap surgery with retention of gingival fibers, J. Periodont. 43:99, 1972.

36. Löe H., and Silness, J.: Tissue reaction to string packs used in fixed restorations, J. Prosthet. Dent. 13:318, 1963.

37. Löe, H., Theilade, E., and Jensen, S.B.: Experimental gingivitis in man, J. Periodont. 36:177, 1965.

38. Malone, W.F., and Manning, J.L.: Electrosurgery in restorative dentistry, J. Prosthet. Dent. 20:417, 1968.

39. Morris, M.L.: Artificial crown contour and gingival health, J. Prosthet. Dent. 12:1146, 1962.

40. Muller, H.P.: The effect of artificial crown margins of the gingival margin on the periodontal condition in a group of periodontally supervised patients treated with fixed bridges, J. Clin. Periodontol. 13:97, 1986.

41. Nabers, J.M., et al.: Chronology, an important factor in the repair of osseous defects, Periodontics 22:304, 1964.

42. Nyman, S., Lindhe, J., and Lundgren, D.: The role of occlusion for the stability of fixed bridges in patients with reduced periodontal tissue support, J. Clin. Periodontol. 2:53, 1975.

43. Nielsen, I.L.: Transsection of supraalveolar fibers on orthodontically rotated teeth in monkeys, Tandlaegebladet 75:1330, 1971.

44. O'Leary, T.J., Standish, S.M., and Bloomer, R.S.: Severe periodontal destruction following impression procedures, J. Periodont. 44:43, 1973.

45. Price, C., and Whitehead, F.J.H.: Impression material as foreign bodies, Br. Dent. J. 133:9, 1972.

46. Ramfjord, S.P.: Present status of the modified Widman flap procedure, J. Periodont. 48:558, 1977.

47. Ramfjord, S.P., and Kiester, G.: The gingival sulcus and the periodontal pocket immediately following scaling of teeth, J. Periodont. 25:167, 1954.

48. Ramfjord, S.P.: Aesthetics, periodontology and restorative dentistry, Quintessence Int. 9:581, 1985.

49. Ramfjord, S.P., and Costich, E.R.: Healing after simple gingivectomy, J. Periodont. 34:401, 1963.

50. Ramfjord, S.P., and Ash, M.M., Jr.: Occlusion, 3rd ed. Philadelphia, 1983, W.B. Suanders Co.

51. Ramfjord, S.P., et al.: Longitudinal study of periodontal therapy, J. Periodont. 44:66, 1973.

52. Ramfjord, S.P.: Periodontal aspects of restorative dentistry, J. Oral Rehabil. 1:107, 1974.

53. Renggli, H.H., and Regolati, B.: Gingival inflammation and plaque accumulation by well-adapted supra- and subgingival proximal restorations, Helv. Odont. Acta 16:99, 1972.

54. Rosen, H., and Gitnick, P.J.: Integrating restorative procedures into the treatment of periodontal disease, J. Prosthet. Dent. 14:343, 1964.

55. Rubach, W.C., and Mitchell, D.F.: Periodontal disease, accessory canals and pulp pathosis, J. Periodont. 36:34, 1965.

56. Saltzberg, D.S., et al.: Scanning electron microscope study of the junction between restorations and gingival cavo-surface margins, J. Prosthet. Dent. 36:517, 1976.

57. Sicher, H.: Über Pulpaerkrankungen als Folge von Paradentose, Z. Stomatol. 34:819, 1936.

58. Silness, J.: Periodontal conditions in patients treated with dental bridges, J. Periodont. Res. 9:50, 1974.

59. Simring, M., and Goldberg, M.: The pulpal pocket approach. Retrograde periodontitis, J. Periodont. 35:22, 1964.

60. Sivertson, J.F., and Burgett, F.G.: Probing of pockets related to the attachment level, J. Periodont. 47:281, 1976.

61. Stein, R.S.: Pontic-residual ridge relationship. A research report, J. Prosthet. Dent. 16:251, 1966.

62. Taylor, A.C., and Campbell, M.M.: Reattachment of gingival epithelium to the tooth, J. Periodont. 43:281, 1972.

63. Tureskey, S., Renstrup, G., and Glickman, J.: Histologic and histochemical observations regarding early calculus formation

in children and adults, J. Periodont. 32:7, 1961.

64. Valderhaug, J.: Periodontal conditions and carious lesions following the insertion of fixed prostheses. A. 10 years follow-up study, Int. Dent. J. 30:296, 1980.

65. Valderhaug, J., and Birkeland, J.M.: Periodontal conditions in the patients five years following insertion of fixed prosthesis, J. Oral Rehabil. 3:237, 1976.

66. Waerhaug, J.: Effect of rough surface upon gingival tissue, J. Dent. Res. 35:323, 1956.

67. Waerhaug, J., and Zander, H.A.: Reaction of gingival tissue to self-curing acrylic restorations, J.A.D.A. 54:760, 1957.

68. Wheeler, R.C.: Complete crown form and the periodontium, J. Prosthet. Dent. 11:722, 1962.

69. Wilhelmsen, N.R., Ramfjord, S.P., and Blankenship, J.R.: Effects of electrosurgery on the gingival attachment in rhesus monkeys, J. Periodont. 47:160, 1976.

70. Wirth, P.J., Norderval, K., and Boe, D.E.: Comparison of two surgical methods in combined surgical-orthodontic correction of impacted maxillary canines, Acta Odont. Scand. 34:53, 1976.

71. Wise, M.D., and Dykenm, R.W.: The plaque-retaining capacity of four dental materials, J. Prosthet. Dent. 33:178, 1975.

72. Yuodelis, R.A., Weaver, J.D., and Sapheos, S.: Facial and lingual contours of artificial complete crown restorations and their effect on the periodontium, J. Prosthet. Dent. 29:61, 1973.

73. Zander, H.A.: Effect of silicate and amalgam on gingiva, J.A.D.A. 55:11, 1957.

28

Periodontal disease results from an opportunistic infection by organisms commonly present in the mouth that cannot be totally eliminated for prolonged time periods.[22,23] Immune responses cannot be boosted to the extent that these organisms can be made innocuous. Perfect periodontal health has been established and maintained by complete plaque control over a short time in select populations,[21] but it has not been possible in clinical trials to keep larger population groups free of plaque and gingivitis over long periods of time. Even so, in one study conducted over 6 years, the severity of gingivitis was reduced through rigid plaque control to very small values, and periodontal support was maintained with insignificant attachment loss; while patients who received the same initial treatment, but received less supervised plaque control, had more plaque, more severe gingivitis, and lost much more attachment over the same 6 years.[1,2]

It is obvious from all clinical trials that the closer we come to a plaque-free dentition, the less the risk for return of any periodontal disease. However, perfect plaque control is almost impossible to maintain over time,[37,38,39,40,41] and the present goal of periodontal therapy and maintenance is to "restore health and function to the periodontium and to preserve the teeth for a lifetime."[17] Health in this definition does not necessarily mean total absence of gingivitis. "To preserve the teeth" means no or minimal loss of attachment over time. In this context, periodontal treatment has been proven successful,[17] but we cannot completely eliminate gingivitis in all patients, and we cannot halt all loss of periodontal support over time with any of the treatment modalities available today. There is no definitive periodontal treatment. The main focus of both treatment and maintenance care is to preserve as much as possible the connective tissue attachment to the teeth. In that context, gingivitis may or may not be significant. Gingivitis may develop into peri-odontitis with loss of attachment, but it may also go on over a long time without measurable loss of connective tissue attachment. Because we have no way to separate "dangerous" from "innocent" gingivitis, and because severe gingivitis seems more apt to be accompanied by attachment loss than is mild gingivitis,[40] it appears logical to eliminate or reduce gingivitis whenever possible through optimal plaque control. Both length of life and quality (comfort) of the human dentition are best served by keeping the attack rate of pathogenic organisms the lowest possible. Maximal efforts in oral health care should be directed towards plaque control. However, from a practical public health standpoint, and considering limitations on time and personnel, it seems justifiable to concentrate the maintenance care efforts on individuals who have already developed periodontitis and thus demonstrated their vulnerability to plaque and gingivitis.

It has been shown that for patients treated for periodontitis, professional toothcleaning is indicated every 3 to 4 months[1,2,17] during the maintenance phase, while for patients treated for gingivitis or early periodontitis, there may be no extra benefit from professional toothcleaning more often than once a year in highly motivated populations,[8] although these populations will have some plaque and gingivitis. While professional toothcleaning every 3 months in patients treated for moderate to advanced periodontitis served predictably well for prevention of significant loss of clinical attachment, it was not adequate for prevention of gingivitis when the plaque control was less than perfect.[37,38,39,41] Maintenance care should therefore be adjusted to what is needed for maintenance of attachment levels, rather than what would be needed for complete control of gingivitis. The striking effectiveness of periodic professional tooth cleaning programs in prevention of periodontal loss and caries has been well documented in a number of Swedish studies over several years both within[1,2] and outside[42] of teaching and research institutions. Similar treatment without periodic, well-supervised maintenance care led to very poor results.[33]

When should the maintenance phase start

Maintenance care should secure for the future the results obtained by the periodontal therapy, and, if possible, encourage regeneration of lost periodontal support (soft tissue and bone). It should preserve oral and dental health and intercept any upcoming threats to the health status.

Following periodontal therapy, there is a healing response directly related to the therapy, both on a histologic and clinical level. The length of this healing period depends on the nature of the periodontal lesion, the modality of therapy, type of care during the healing, and a number of host response factors. Thus, the length of the healing phase is not a set number of days or months. The initial gross clinical results after scaling and root planing were established 4 to 6 weeks after completion of the therapeutic procedures[6] in one study, but there are collagen changes and changes in gingival form for at least 6 months after surgical treatment. The return of the pretreatment bacterial flora in the pockets also varies to a great extent,[28,32] depending not only on the treatment, but on the oral hygiene and professional care after the treatment. With reasonably good post-treatment care, the results with regard to clinical attachment levels are fairly stable from 6 months after periodontal therapy,[44] while considerable variations, depending on type of care, are evident a shorter time after the therapy. After mucogingival surgery, the results appear to stabilize 4 to 6 weeks postsurgically.[14]

Westfelt et al have suggested that the first 6 months after periodontal surgery be called the "healing phase," while longer periods of observation should be called the "maintenance phase."[44] Longitudinal results in their study are documented after followup at 6 months, but most studies give the initial results of the treatment after a followup at 12 months and then rescore every 1 year for the maintenance care reports after treatment of moderate to advanced periodontal lesions, when the patients have received professional toothcleaning with oral hygiene encouragement every 3 months.[19,42,44]

Procedures of maintenance care
A. Plaque control. Mechanical.

The most important objective of maintenance care is to secure optimal supra and subgingival plaque control, first by encouraging optimal oral hygiene by the patient, and second by professional removal of all supra and subgingival calculus and plaque. The following sequence of procedures is recommended to be used during maintenance recall visits.

1. Check for change in medical status.
2. Oral examination.
3. Apply disclosing solution.
4. Review oral hygiene with the patient.
5. Probe for bleeding and/or pus.
6. Polish with EVA contraangle and fluoridated toothpaste.
7. Polish with rubber cup and toothpaste.
8. Scale and rootplane where needed.
9. Check all interproximal areas with dental floss.
10. Dry teeth and apply acidulated or other fluoride, depending whether ceramic restorations are present.
11. If bleeding or pus is present, reschedule the patient in 2 to 3 weeks to check need for retreatment. Otherwise, schedule a recall visit in 3 months.

Because we have not been able to implement a perfect and uniform plaque control in periodontitis patients,[37,38,39,41] we rely heavily on meticulous periodic supra and subgingival professional toothcleaning and the application of fluorides. Provided that a well-controlled recall program is maintained, the patient's own plaque control is more critical for optimal healing during the healing phase immediately after the treatment,[44] than for maintenance of attachment during the maintenance phase.[37,38,39,40,41]

An animal experiment appears to indicate that with perfect oral hygiene, periodic professional tooth cleaning is not needed for successful maintenance care.[31] Other reports from studies in humans also indicate that with excellent plaque control, frequent recalls are not very important.[8]

However, it has been shown convincingly that with inadequate oral hygiene and recall every 6 months, deepening of pockets and loss of attachment commonly occurs in patients treated for periodontitis.[34]

It should also be acknowledged that in spite of well controlled recall, and without relation to plaque control, some teeth have been lost due to the progress of periodontitis during the maintenance phase. All of the lost teeth in our[37] and other longitudinal studies[35] had residual old calculus and/or inaccessable furcations. Thus, both professional and personal oral hygiene proved inadequate to stop the progress of periodontitis when residual infection was left on the root surfaces.

B. Plaque control. Chemical.

Much interest is currently focused on the use of antibiotics for the treatment and the maintenance care of periodontal patients.[7] Tetracycline,[25,28] metronidazole,[25] clindamycin,[10] and other drugs have been shown to have a beneficial effect both on the pathogenic bacterial flora in periodontal pockets and, clinically, on pocket depth and attachment levels. However, at various time intervals after the antibiotics, the bacteria and the inflammation will return. For maintenance care, the drugs have to be administered repeatedly over time, but will then lead to a large percentage of the bacteria becoming resistant to the drug as with tetracycline.[20] Other effective drugs, such as clindamycin, may have serious side effects.[10] It has not been demonstrated that maintenance care is more successful if drugs are added to good mechanical care and recall every 3 months. Antibiotics during the maintenance may have some transient good effect in areas of bacterial plaque that were missed during the initial therapy,[25] and on periodontal abscesses; but the antibiotics should be followed up by mechanical therapy.

Prolonged use of antibiotics during the maintenance phase cannot be recommended because of possible side effects and because good results can be maintained by mechanical therapy.[1,17,19,27]

A number of antiseptic mouthwashes have been shown to reduce the supragingival bacterial flora,[45] but have to be specifically introduced into the periodontal pockets to be effective against subgingival bacteria. Of all mouthrinses, chlorhexidine gluconate is currently the most effective,[12] but it is not superior to good manual oral hygiene. Antimicrobial irrigation of deep pockets to supplement mechanical treatment has not been found to be better than saline irrigation.[30] Other studies have reported some benefit from pocket irrigation with snF2,[3] chlorhexidine, and other agents.[11] However, even chlorhexidine did not augment the results of good mechanical care over a prolonged time.

Chlorhexidine is now available in the U.S.A. as a prescription drug under the name of *Peridex* at a concentration of 0.12%. It may be used for oral rinse twice a day. It should be monitored for adverse side effects. Several agents may augment plaque reduction associated with mechanical oral hygiene; but there is no evidence that any antiseptic agent will augment the results of mechanical therapy in maintenance of attachment levels. If any antibacterial agent is used, it should be combined with mechanical therapy.

There is no convincing evidence that the so-called Keyes' technique[18] has any significant advantage over conventional techniques for maintenance care.[13] The long-term monitoring of maintenance care by phase-contrast microscopy needs further study.[28]

Experimental use of non-steroidal anti-inflammatory drugs such as indomethacin to prevent bone resorption cannot be recommended at the present time.[43]

Retreatment

One very important part of maintenance care is locating and re-treating pockets with progressive periodontitis, either because the irritants were not com-

pletely removed during the initial treatment or because of repopulation by infective organisms. It has been suggested that the need for re-treatment can be assessed by bacterial counts.[18] However, the significance of bacterial assessment as a diagnostic tool for a specific pocket is very controversial,[13] and its use cannot be justified at the present state of the art.

Although it has been claimed, on the basis of short-term studies, that clinical signs of redness, bleeding on probing, and suppurcation are poor predictors of periodontal destructive activity,[15] these manifestations do specify inflammation. Furthermore, it was found in one study that with no bleeding on probing, the chances for loss of support were minimal over 2 years, while pockets that bled every time they were probed had a much higher frequency of significant loss of attachment.[22] It has also been observed that with re-treatment of sites with bleeding and/or pus during the maintenance phase, progressive periodontitis could be halted if access could be gained.[37,38] As pointed out in chapter 17, incomplete removal of calculus and plaque on the root surface may occur after scaling and rootplaning and after surgery.[5] Thus, a pocket that bleeds from gentle probing should be re-scaled during maintenance therapy. If access is poor or it bleeds again the next time the patient is seen, the pocket should be exposed surgically and planed, even if no calculus is visible. With furcation involvement, it may not be possible to secure a satisfactory end result. It is important that during recall visits, bleeding from pockets that bleed from the bottom with deep probing be distinguished from gingival bleeding associated with recurrent gingivitis. The latter will be taken care of by the routine professional tooth-cleaning.

Loss of attachment greater than 2 mm during maintenance signifies a need for re-treatment. Bone loss evident on x-rays is a late sign of attachment loss,[9] but indicates a need for further therapy. Crevicular fluid measurements are not helpful for directing the maintenance care.[36]

It has often been assumed that if a crevice could be probed beyond 3 mm after treatment, the prognosis during the maintenance care would be poor. This is not true. In a recent 5-year longitudinal study, there were as high or higher percentages of loss of greater than 2 mm in shallow than in deep crevices.[41] There is no reason to re-treat a crevice of a depth over 3 mm if there is no pus or bleeding to probing. A warning should also be made against routine root planing during recall visits if there is no sign of progressive periodontitis. Tightly adapted pocket walls without appreciable subgingival plaque and calculus should be scaled only lightly, or just polished.

A very few patients will go downhill on this recommended program and lose attachment at a much more progressive rate than the average patient.[16] Some of these patients may be helped by antibiotic therapy, but others do not benefit from antibiotics, and, in any case, antibiotics give only temporary relief.

It has been observed that if such patients are given professional toothcleaning once a month over 1/2 to 1 years, their periodontal status will gradually improve.[38] They should then be placed on recall every 2 months.

Monitoring of Oral and Dental Health

In addition to routine inspection for oral lesions; caries status, occlusion, and dental restorations and appliances should be inspected at least twice a year. Roentgenograms should be obtained only for specific reasons, such as high caries rate, and for control of periapical areas. Old restorations often need replacement. Occlusion may change with loss of teeth and/or occlusal wear. If mobile teeth are becoming increasingly mobile or feel uncomfortable during normal mastication, splinting may be indicated. Teeth with a tendency towards tipping or elongation should be observed for possible need of treatment. Special attention should be given to removable prosthetic appliances and their periodontal relationships.

Maintenance care is a very important part of dental practice beyond professional toothcleaning for plaque control.

REFERENCES

1. Axelsson, P., and Lindhe, J.: Effect of controlled oral hygiene procedures on caries and periodontal disease in adults. Results after 6 years, J. Clin. Periodontol. 8:239, 1981.
2. Axelsson, P., and Lindhe, J.: The significance of maintenance care in the treatment of periodontal disease, J. Clin. Periodontol. 8:281, 1981.
3. Boyd, R.L., et al.: Effect of self-administered daily irrigation with 0.02% SnFz on periodontal disease activity, J. Clin. Periodontol. 12:420, 1985.
4. Braatz, L., Garrett, S., Cloffey, N., and Egelberg, J.: Antimicrobial irrigation of deep pockets to supplement nonsurgical periodontal therapy. II Daily irrigation, J. Clin. Periodontol. 12:630, 1985.
5. Caffesse, R.G., Sweeney, P.L., and Smith, B.A.: Scaling and root planing with and without periodontal flap surgery, J. Clin. Periodontol. 13:205, 1986.
6. Caton, J., Praze, M., and Polson, A.: Maintenance of healed periodontal pockets after a single episode of root planing, J. Periodont. 53:420, 1982.
7. Ciancio, S.G., and Genco, R.J.: The use of antibiotics in periodontal diseases, Int. J. Periodontics Restorative Dent. 6:54, 1982.
8. Eneroth, L., and Sundberg, H.: Effekten av forebyggande tannvard utfört av specialutbildade tandsköterskor. Delegationen för Social Forskning. Projekt 75/1007, Slutrapport April 1984, Stockholm.
9. Goodson, J.M., Haffajee, A.D., and Socransky, S.S.: The relationship between attachment level loss and alveolar bone loss, J. Clin. Periodontol. 11:348, 1984.
10. Gordon, J., et al.: Efficacy of clindamycin hydrochloride in refractory periodontitis, J. Periodont. (Special Issue) 56:75, 1985.
11. Gordon, J.M., Lamster, J.B., and Seiger, M.C.: Efficacy of Listerine antiseptic in inhibiting the development of plaque and gingivitis, J. Clin. Periodontol. 12:697, 1985.
12. Greenstein, G., Berman, C., and Jaffin, R.: Chlorhexidine. An adjunct to periodontal therapy, J. Periodont. 57:370, 1986.
13. Greenwell, H., et al.: The effect of Keyes' method of oral hygiene on the subgingival microflora compared to the effect of sealing and/or surgery, J. Clin. Periodontol. 12:327, 1985.
14. Guinard, E.A., and Caffessee, R.G.: Treatment of localized gingival recessions. Part III. Comparison of results obtained with lateral sliding and coronally repositioned flaps, J. Periodont. 49:457, 1978.
15. Haffajee, A.E., Socransky, S.S., and Goodson, J.M.: Clinical parameters as predictors of destructive periodontal disease activity, J. Clin. Periodontol. 10:257, 1983.
16. Hirschfeld, L., and Wasserman, B.: A long-term survey of tooth loss in 600 treated periodontal patients, J. Periodont. 49:225, 1978.
17. Kakahashi, S., and Parakkal, P.F.: Proceedings from the state-of-the-art workshop on surgical therapy for periodontitis, J. Periodont. 53:476, 1982.
18. Keyes, P.H., Wright, W.E., and Harvard, S.A.: The use of phase-contrast microscopy and chemotherapy in the diagnosis and treatment of periodontal lesions—an initial report (II), Quintessence Int. 9:69, 1978.
19. Knowles, J.W., et al.: Results of periodontal treatment related to pocket depth and attachment level. Eight years, J. Periodont. 50:225, 1979.
20. Kornman, K.S., and Karl, E.H.: The effect of long-term low-dose tetracycline therapy on the subgingival microflora in refractory adult periodontitis, J. Periodont. 53:604, 1982.
21. Löe, H., Theilade, E., and Jensen, S.B.: Experimental gingivitis in man, J. Periodont. 36:177, 1965.
22. Lang, N.P., et al.: Bleeding on probing. A predictor for the progression of periodontal disease? J. Clin. Periodontol. 13:590, 1986.
23. Lang, N.P., Gusberti, F.A., and Siegrist, B.E.: Aetiologie der Parondontalerkraunkungen, Acta Parondontologica 14:1, 1985.
24. Lindhe, J., Hamp, S.E., and Löe, H.: Plaque induced periodontal disease in beagle dogs. A 4-year clinical, roentgenographical and histometric study, J. Periodont. Res. 10:243, 1975.
25. Lindhe, J., Liljenberg, B., and Adielsson, B.: Effect of long-term tetracycline therapy on human periodontal disease, J. Clin. Periodontol. 10:590, 1983.
26. Lindhe, J., Liljenberg, B., Adielsson, B., and Borjesson, I.: Use of metronidazole as a probe in the study of human periodontal disease, J. Clin. Periodontol. 10:100, 1983.
27. Lindhe, J., and Nyman, S.: Long-term maintenance of patients treated for advanced periodontal disease, J. Clin. Periodontol. 11:504, 1984.
28. Listgarten, M.A., et al.: Failure of a microbial assay to reliably predict disease recurrence in a treated periodontitis population receiving regularly scheduled prophylaxes, J. Clin. Periodontol. 13:768, 1986.
29. Listgarten, M.A., Lindhe, J., and Helldén, L.: Effect of tetracycline and/or scaling on human periodontal disease. Clinical, microbiological and histological observations, J. Clin. Periodontol. 5:246, 1978.
30. MacAlpine, R., et al.: Antimicrobial irrigation of deep pockets to supplement oral hygiene instructions and root debridement. I. Biweekly irrigation, J. Clin. Periodontol. 12:568, 1985.
31. Morrison, E.C., et al.: Effects of repeated scaling and root planing and/or controlled or hygiene on the periodontal at-

tachment level and pocket depth in beagle dogs. I. Clinical findings, J. Periodont. Res. 14:428, 1979.

32. Mousques, T., Listgarten, M., and Philip, R.A.: Effect of scaling and root planing on the composition of human subgingival microbial flora, J. Periodont. Res. 15:144, 1980.

33. Nyman, S., Lindhe, J., and Rosling, B.: Periodontal surgery in plaque-infected dentitions, J. Clin. Periodontol. 4:240, 1977.

34. Nyman, S., Rosling, B., and Lindhe, J.: Effect of professional tooth cleaning on healing after periodontal surgery, J. Clin. Periodontol. 2:80, 1975.

35. Pihlstrom, B.L., Ortis-Campos, C., and McHugh, R.B.: A randomized four-years study of periodontal therapy, J. Periodont. 52:227, 1981.

36. Polson, S., and Goodson, J.M.: Periodontal diagnosis—current status and future trends, J. Periodont. 56:25, 1985.

37. Ramfjord, S.P., et al.: Four modalities of periodontal treatment compared over 5 years, J. Clin. Periodontol. 14:445, 1987.

38. Ramfjord, S.P.: Maintenance care for treated periodontitis patients, J. Clin. Periodontol. 14:433, 1987.

39. Ramfjord, S.P., et al.: Oral hygiene and maintenance of periodontal support, J. Periodont. 53:26, 1982.

40. Ramfjord, S.P.: The periodontal status of boys 11 to 17 years old in Bombay, India, J. Periodont. 32:237, 1961.

41. Ramfjord, S.P.: Surgical pocket elimination: still a justifiable objective? J. Am. Dent. Assoc. 114:37, 1987.

42. Söderholm, G.: Effect of a dental care program on dental health conditions. A study of employees of a Swedish shipyard, Thesis, University of Lund, Malmö, 1979.

43. Voge, R.I.: The experimental use of anti-inflammatory drugs in the treatment of periodontal disease, J. Periodont. (Special Issue) 56:88, 1985.

44. Westfelt, E., Nyman, S., Socransky, S.S., and Lindhe, J.: Significance of frequency of professional tooth cleaning for healing following periodontal surgery, J. Clin. Periodontol. 10:148, 1983.

45. Wennström, J., and Lindhe, J.: The effect of mouthrinses on parameters characterizing human periodontal disease, J. Clin. Periodontol. 13:86, 1986.

Prognosis is a studied forecast of the outcome of treatment or lack of treatment. It is influenced by the modality of treatment and the biological and behavioral characteristics of the patient. Prognosis is a basic consideration in treatment planning because feasibility of treatment and selection of procedures should be based on what provides the most favorable outlook for the health and function of the dentition. The prognosis for treated or untreated dentitions, or for separate teeth, is also of decisive importance for the patient's acceptance or rejection of proposed treatment plans (Fig. 29-1).

A discussion of periodontal prognosis as related to treatment planning was included in chapter 14. The prognosis following specific procedures used in periodontal prevention and treatment was discussed in the chapters describing these procedures. This chapter attempts to summarize current philosophy and knowledge of the periodontal prognosis on the basis of the material that has been presented in this book.

Prognostication should be based on all available knowledge of natural history, etiology, pathology, diagnosis, and therapy of periodontal disease. Traditionally, such knowledge, in conjunction with past experience, provides the much-heralded "clinical judgment,"[4] which is a personal, and often poorly defined, philosophical basis for prognosis.[30]

Since the introduction of antibiotics in the 1940s, medicine in general has been undergoing transformation from an art, as it was earlier termed, to a mixture of science and technology. The successful use of penicillin against identifiable streptococci led to the randomized clinical trial technique, which was first used to evaluate streptomycin in the treatment of pulmonary tuberculosis in 1946.[18] Since that time, such clinical trials have dominated the scientific developments in therapeutic and preventive medicine. Focused clinical trials with statistical experimental design have been introduced into periodontics during the last few years. However, problems with ethics, randomization, double-blind technique, and suitable accurate measurement systems for assessing this chronic, slowly progressing disease may all explain the slow progress and limited acceptance of clinical trials in periodontics.

Medical and surgical practices have traditionally depended more on skilled professional opinion than on knowledge,[37] and experts usually have become authorities by virtue of their opinions rather than of their knowledge. Furthermore, statistical data on mean values with large standard deviations obviously have to be applied with reservations and with caution to individual patients. Variations in operator skills as well as in biological responses in the patient also tend to favor the classic clinical judgment approach over applied biostatistical knowledge. The basis for the clinical judgment has been empiricism and anecdotal case reports in various forms. The most obvious shortcoming of this method is lack of controls and randomization.

It is becoming increasingly evident in clinical research that nothing improves the performance of an innovative approach so much as lack of controls,[6] and that poorly controlled or uncontrolled studies, which when repeated are likely to agree, build up an illusion of strong evidence on the basis of numbers rather than validity. Selection of treatment methods and determination of prognosis for patients with periodontal disease have traditionally been based on "soft evidence" from empiricism, from case reports, from philosophical deductions, and from theories derived from studies on the nature of periodontal disease.

As evidence becomes available from targeted clinical trials for evaluation of various modalities of periodontal treatment and maintenance care, it is to be assumed that treatment planning and prognostication in the future will rest on a firmer scientific basis than today.

The following words regarding medicine are also applicable to periodontics: "Medicine in the future must be building, as a central part of its scientific base, a solid underpinning of biostatistical and epidemiological knowledge. Hunches and intuitive impressions are essential for getting the work started, but it is only through the quality of the numbers at the end that truth can be told."[36]

Different therapies may produce similar mortality or cure rates (the length of life factor), but the quality of life factor may be more favorable following one method than following another. This certainly applies to the selection of modalities of periodontal surgery. In this area, postoperative comfort and esthetic appearance may favor one method over another, even when the two methods may reduce morbidity and tooth mortality to a similar degree.

PROGNOSIS FOLLOWING PERIODONTAL THERAPY

Cross-sectional[25,26,34] and a few longitudinal[1,2,17,35] studies all indicate that the loss of attachment in patients with or without periodontitis tends to be progressive with time, even when the disease has been treated.[9] However, the loss is greater in untreated than in treated cases.[1,10,35] Because loss of attachment is irreversible in most instances, untreated controls are, for ethical reasons, not to be included in clinical trials of periodontal therapy. Clinical trials of periodontal therapy in humans have therefore been limited to comparisons over short and long terms of results following a variety of clinical procedures.[23] The results of the treatments have been related to pocket depth, gingivitis, plaque, tooth mobility, and tooth type in numerous studies.[10] The ultimate value of therapy is usually assessed on the basis of comparisons of clinical attachment levels and/or roentgenographic levels of the alveolar crest,[11] with lesser attention to the number of teeth lost during the time of observation.

In spite of the acknowledged shortcomings of clinical probing, it is the most practical method for assessment of successes or failure of periodontal therapy.[11,16,27,31,33]

The prediction in prognosis is based on past experience, expressed in numerical results, following the various modalities of treatment available. The quality of life (esthetics, lack of pain, low cost, etc.) enters into the choice of therapeutic modality, while the length of life of the teeth is the prime consideration.

Success of periodontal therapy has been defined as "To restore health and function to the periodontium and to preserve the teeth for a lifetime."[10] This can be accomplished for the overwhelming majority of patients.[12,15,21]

Current periodontal research has established a number of facts that all have to be considered in case analysis and presentation of the treatment plan and prognosis to the patient.

Status of periodontal therapy

Periodontal pockets from 4 to 12 mm deep will, on average, respond favorably to periodontal therapy. The pockets will be significantly reduced in depth initially and, with prophylaxis at least every 3 months, remain reduced over a long period of time.[12,14,20,29]

Attachment levels will usually improve following therapy in 4-to-12 mm pockets and, with prophylaxis at least every 3 months, either stay improved or remain at the pre-treatment level.[12,14,20,29,32]

The prognosis is as good for deep as for shallow pockets,[12,14,29] provided that the teeth have adequate support for function. The prognosis is not adversely affected by early furcation involvement of 2 mm or less.[8]

The ultimate long-term prognosis is poor for teeth with deep furcation involvement.[8] However, such

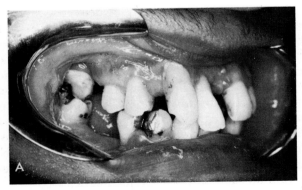 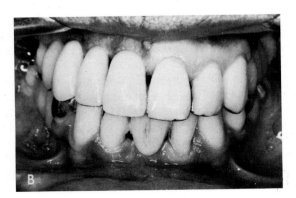

Fig. 29-1. *A,* Severe juvenile periodontitis in 19-year-old male. *B,* Seventeen-year follow-up after periodontal and reconstructive therapy. Three-quarter crowns and inlays with protected cusps used for the abutments. *Continued*

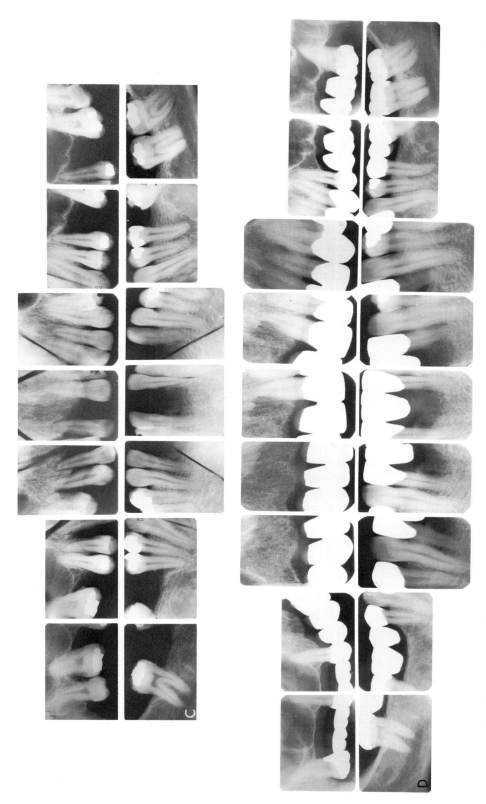

Fig. 29-1 continued. *C,* Roentgenograms before treatment. Some teeth had been lost because of periodontal disease. *D,* Seventeen-year follow-up roentgenograms. Excellent bone response. The patient has been seen for prophylaxis every 3 months.

teeth may be asymptomatic and maintained in good function for an indeterminable number of years, provided that the root surfaces in the furcation can be instrumented properly.[12]

Induced gingival recession following gingivectomy and apically positioned flaps does not have a favorable effect on the maintenance of attachment for the teeth.[12,29,33]

Surgical pocket elimination is not essential for a good prognosis of periodontal treatment.[12,23,29,33]

A gingival crevice that can be probed beyond 3 mm after periodontal therapy may be compatible with maintenance of periodontal attachment levels if there is no bleeding or exudation during probing.[12,28,29]

Although the prognosis is fairly similar following various modalities of periodontal therapy, the better postoperative attachment levels, esthetics, and comfort following conservative surgery (curettage and modified Widman Procedure) favor selection of those modalities over the more radical surgical pocket elimination procedures.[12,23,28,29,33]

The role of tooth mobility in the prognosis has not been fully determined, but it appears that teeth with increased mobility may be maintained without further loss of attachment following periodontal therapy.[14,19] Increasing mobility may have an adverse effect on the long-term prognosis.[19] Increased mobility has an adverse effect on the results after treatment of periodontal pockets.[5]

Frequency of recall for professional cleaning of the teeth may have a decisive effect on the prognosis, and apparently is much more important than the modality of initial surgical treatment.[32,33] The most desirable time intervals for recall related to the patient's oral hygiene have not been determined. In general, in patients with advanced periodontitis, good results have been reported for recall intervals of from 2 weeks[8,32,33] to 3 months,[14,28,29] and poor results for 6 to 12 month intervals.[32]

The periodontal prognosis for patients with inadequate oral hygiene may be greatly improved by frequent recall and prophylaxis, even though the personal oral hygiene practice may continue to be less than ideal[28] (Fig. 29-2).

Deviations from "physiologic" gingival contour do not influence the prognosis, provided that adequate methods for oral hygiene are instituted.[12]

With good oral hygiene, lack of attached gingiva has minimal or no effect on maintenance of attachment levels.[3] The common cause of loss of teeth after treatment is residual calculus and plaque associated with furcations.[23]

CLINICAL CONSIDERATIONS

Mathematical figures of success rates for periodontal therapy in terms of percentage of maintained treated teeth may be meaningless. Such figures are, to a great extent, dependent on inclusion or exclusion of teeth with severe lesions.

If all teeth with advanced periodontitis or furcation involvement are extracted prior to the periodontal treatment, the prognosis for the remaining teeth is usually good, with or without treatment.

The real challenge in prognostication is to forecast the results of treatment of advanced lesions under adverse conditions. Such a forecast cannot be based entirely on present scientific knowledge with assurance for individual patient success or failure, because our assessments of periodontal biological responses as well as patient behavior and operator skill are necessarily incomplete. With an increase in our knowledge of the biology of periodontal health and disease, and with an accumulation of results from controlled, targeted clinical trials, the present uncertainty and widely divergent opinions on periodontal prognosis should be reduced.

The average clinician is usually far too pessimistic regarding the prognosis for teeth with periodontal disease. In order to protect a reputation as a savior of teeth, the dentist often extracts teeth considered to be bad risks, although such teeth can often be maintained in comfortable function for many years. On the other hand, inadequate diagnosis and treatment (sloppy probing and superficial scaling) of teeth with extensive furcation involvement or with very advanced periodontitis (which may also be complicated by secondary trauma from occlusion), is an unjustifiable waste of time and money and can only serve to verify the initial impression of poor prognosis. If such teeth are to be treated, they should be given the most meticulous attention with regard to treatment and frequent maintenance recalls.

The most encouraging aspect of modern periodontics is an increasing accumulation of evidence that lost periodontal support, to some extent and under certain conditions, may be regained.[29,32,33] The prognosis for at least some types of periodontal lesions following therapy is generally considered much better today than it was a few years ago, when only pockets with three bony walls were considered good prospects for healing.[22,24] Today, reparative periodontal surgery is promising,[7] and indications are that this exciting development will continue and establish increasingly predictable bases for treatment. It also appears that the potential for healing and maintenance of health and function of teeth with very deep periodontal pockets is much better than previously assumed.[12,23,29]

REFERENCES

1. Becker, W., et al.: Untreated periodontal disease: A longitudinal study, J. Periodont. 50:234, 1979.
2. Chawla, T.N., Nanda, R.S., and Kapoor, K.K.: Dental prophylaxis procedures in control of periodontal disease in Luch-

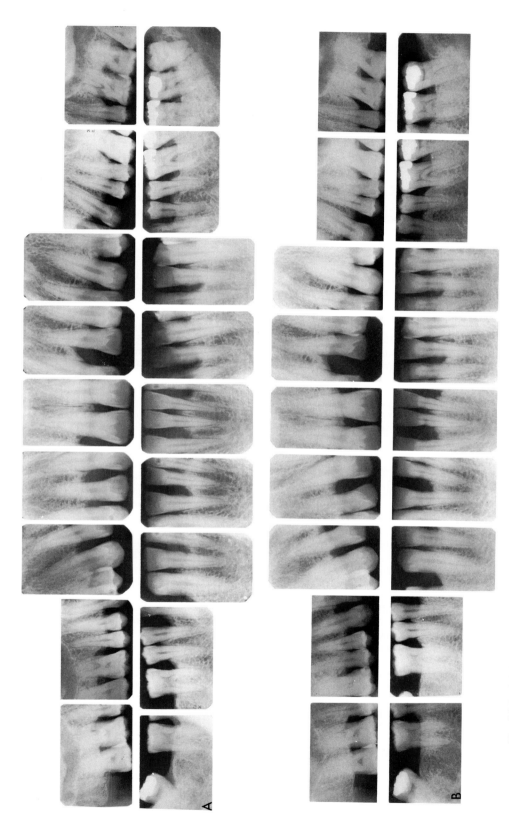

Fig. 29-2. *A,* Moderately severe periodontitis in 27-year-old male. *B,* Roentgenograms 10 years after periodontal treatment. Note well-defined alveolar crest over interproximal spaces and no progression of bone loss.

Continued

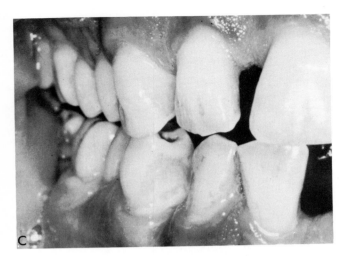

Fig. 29-2 continued. *C,* Clinical picture of the same patient showing abundant plaque at time of recall for prophylaxis. The patient was on a 3-month recall schedule. In spite of consistent poor oral hygiene and gingivitis, the roentgenograms and clinical probing indicate no loss of attachment or bone during the 10 years of observation.

now (rural) India, J. Periodont. 46:498, 1975.

3. Dorfman, H., et al.: Longitudinal evaluation of free gingival autografts, J. Clin. Periodontol. 7:316, 1980.
4. Feinstein, A.R.: Clinical Judgment, Baltimore: Williams and Wilkins, 1967.
5. Fleszar, T.J., et al.: Tooth mobility and periodontal therapy, J. Clin. Periodontol. 7:495, 1980.
6. Gilbert, J.P., McPeek, B., and Mosteller, F.: Statistics and ethics in surgery and anesthesia, Science, 198:684, 1977.
7. Gottlow, J., et al.: New attachment formation in the human periodontium by guided tissue regeneration. Case reports, J. Clin. Periodontol. 13:604, 1986.
8. Hamp, S.E., Nyman, S., and Lindhe, J.: Periodontal treatment of multirooted teeth. Results after 5 years, J. Clin. Periodontol. 2:126, 1975.
9. Hirschfeld, L., and Wasserman, B.: A long-term survey of tooth loss in 600 treated periodontal patients, J. Periodontol. 49:225, 1978.
10. Kakehashi, S., and Parakkal, P.F.: Proceedings from state-of-the-art workshop on surgical therapy for periodontitis, J. Periodontol. 53:476, 1982.
11. Kelly, G.P., et al.: Radiographs in clinical periodontal trials, J. Periodont. 46:381, 1975.
12. Knowles, J.W., et al.: Results of periodontal treatment related to pocket depth and attachment level. Eight years, J. Periodontol. 50:225, 1979.
13. Lindhe, J., and Ericsson, I.: The influence of trauma from occlusion on reduced but healthy periodontal tissues in dogs, J. Clin. Periodontol. 3:110, 1976.
14. Lindhe, J., and Nyman, S.: The effect of plaque control and surgical pocket elimination on the establishment and maintenance of periodontal health. A longitudinal study of periodontal therapy in cases of advanced periodontal disease, J. Clin. Periodontol. 2:67, 1975.

15. Lindhe, J., et al.: Long-term effects of surgical-nonsurgical treatment of periodontal disease, J. Clin. Periodontol. 11:448, 1984.
16. Listgarten, M.A.: Periodontal probing. What does it mean? J. Clin. Periodontol. 7:165, 1980.
17. Löe, H., et al.: The natural history of periodontal disease in man. The rate of periodontal destruction before 40 years of age, J. Periodontol. 40:607, 1978.
18. Mike, V., and Goode, R.A.: Old problems, new challenges, Science 198:677, 1977.
19. Nyman, S., and Lindhe, J.: Persistent tooth hypermobility following completion of periodontal treatment, J. Clin. Periodontol. 3:81, 1976.
20. Nyman, S., Rosling, B., and Lindhe, J.: Effect of professional tooth cleaning on healing after periodontal surgery, J. Clin. Periodontol. 2:80, 1975.
21. Nyman, S., and Lindhe, J.: A longitudinal study of combined periodontal and prosthetic treatment of patients with advanced periodontal disease, J. Periodont. 50:163, 1979.
22. Patur, B., and Glickman, I.: Clinical and roentgenographic evaluation of the posttreatment healing of infrabony pockets, J. Periodont. 33:164, 1962.
23. Pihlstrom, B.F., et al.: Comparison of surgical and nonsurgical treatment of periodontal disease. A review of current studies and additional results after six and one-half years, J. Clin. Periodontol. 10:574, 1984.
24. Prichard, J.: Regeneration of bone following periodontal therapy, Oral Surg. 10:247, 1957.
25. Ramfjord, S.: Survey of the periodontal status of boys 11 to 17 years old in Bombay, India, J. Periodont. 32:237, 1961.
26. Ramfjord, S.P., et al.: Epidemiological studies of periodontal diseases, Am. J. Public Health 58:1713, 1968.
27. Ramfjord, S.P.: Design of studies or clinical trials to evaluate the effectiveness of agents or procedures for the prevention or treatment of loss of the periodontium, J. Periodont. Res. 9 (Suppl. 14):78, 1974.
28. Ramfjord, S.P., et al.: Results following three modalities of periodontal therapy, J. Periodont. 46:522, 1975.
29. Ramfjord, S.P.: Present status of the modified Widman flap procedure, J. Periodont. 48:558, 1977.
30. Ramfjord, S.P.: Changing concepts in periodontics, J. Prosthet. Dent. 52:781, 1984.
31. Rosling, B., et al.: A radiographic method for assessing changes in alveolar bone height following periodontal therapy, J. Clin. Periodontol. 2:211, 1975.
32. Rosling, B., Nyman, S., and Lindhe, J.: The effect of systematic plaque control on bone regeneration in infrabony pockets, J. Clin. Periodontol. 3:38, 1976.
33. Rosling, B., et al.: The healing potential of the periodontal tissues following different techniques of periodontal surgery in plaque-free dentitions. A 2-year clinical study, J. Clin. Periodontol. 3:233, 1976.
34. Schei, D., et al.: Alveolar bone loss as related to oral hygiene and age, J. Periodont. 30:7, 1959.
35. Suomi, J.D., et al.: The effect of controlled oral hygiene procedures on the progression of periodontal disease in adults: Results after third and final year, J. Periodont. 42:152, 1971.
36. Thomas, L.: Biostatistics in medicine, Science 198:675, 1977.
37. Tukey, J.W.: Some thoughts on clinical trials, especially problems of multiplicity, Science 198:679, 1977.

INDEX